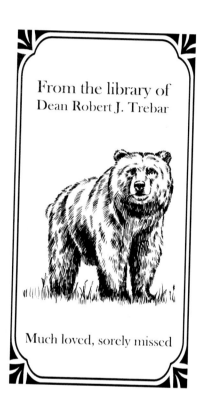

From the library of
Dean Robert J. Trebar

Much loved, sorely missed

Tension-Type and Cervicogenic Headache

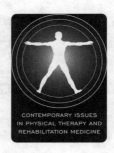

CONTEMPORARY ISSUES
IN PHYSICAL THERAPY AND
REHABILITATION MEDICINE

Jones and Bartlett's
Contemporary Issues in Physical Therapy and
Rehabilitation Medicine Series
Series Editor
Peter A. Huijbregts, PT, MSc, MHSc, DPT, OCS, MTC, FAAOMPT, FCAMT

Other books in the series:

Orthopedic Manual Therapy Diagnosis
Aad van der El
Wellness and Physical Therapy
Sharon Fair

Tension-Type and Cervicogenic Headache

Pathophysiology, Diagnosis, and Management

Edited by

César Fernández-de-las-Peñas, PT, DO, PhD
Department of Physical Therapy, Occupational Therapy,
Physical Medicine, and Rehabilitation
Esthesiology Laboratory
Universidad Rey Juan Carlos
Alcorcón, Madrid, Spain

Center for Sensory-Motor Interaction (SMI)
Department of Health Science and Technology
Aalborg University
Aalborg, Denmark

Lars Arendt-Nielsen, DMSci, PhD
Laboratory for Experimental Pain Research
Center for Sensory-Motor Interaction (SMI)
Department of Health Science and Technology
Aalborg University
Aalborg, Denmark

Robert D. Gerwin, MD
Department of Neurology
Johns Hopkins University School of Medicine
Baltimore, Maryland

President and Medical Director
Pain and Rehabilitation Medicine
Bethesda, Maryland

JONES AND BARTLETT PUBLISHERS
Sudbury, Massachusetts
BOSTON   TORONTO   LONDON   SINGAPORE

World Headquarters
Jones and Bartlett Publishers
40 Tall Pine Drive
Sudbury, MA 01776
978-443-5000
info@jbpub.com
www.jbpub.com

Jones and Bartlett Publishers
Canada
6339 Ormindale Way
Mississauga, Ontario L5V 1J2
Canada

Jones and Bartlett Publishers
International
Barb House, Barb Mews
London W6 7PA
United Kingdom

Jones and Bartlett's books and products are available through most bookstores and online booksellers. To contact Jones and Bartlett Publishers directly, call 800-832-0034, fax 978-443-8000, or visit our website, www.jbpub.com.

The authors, editor, and publisher have made every effort to provide accurate information. However, they are not responsible for errors, omissions, or for any outcomes related to the use of the contents of this book and take no responsibility for the use of the products and procedures described. Treatments and side effects described in this book may not be applicable to all people; likewise, some people may require a dose or experience a side effect that is not described herein. Drugs and medical devices are discussed that may have limited availability controlled by the Food and Drug Administration (FDA) for use only in a research study or clinical trial. Research, clinical practice, and government regulations often change the accepted standard in this field. When consideration is being given to use of any drug in the clinical setting, the health care provider or reader is responsible for determining FDA status of the drug, reading the package insert, and reviewing prescribing information for the most up-to-date recommendations on dose, precautions, and contraindications, and determining the appropriate usage for the product. This is especially important in the case of drugs that are new or seldom used.

Production Credits
Publisher: David Cella
Acquisitions Editor: Kristine Johnson
Associate Editor: Maro Gartside
Production Manager: Julie Champagne Bolduc
Production Assistant: Jessica Steele Newfell
Senior Marketing Manager: Barb Bartoszek
Manufacturing and Inventory Control Supervisor: Amy Bacus
Composition: SNP Best-set Typesetter Ltd., Hong Kong
Cover Design: Brian Moore/Kristin E. Parker
Printing and Binding: Malloy, Inc.
Cover Printing: Malloy, Inc.

Library of Congress Cataloging-in-Publication Data
Tension-type and cervicogenic headache : pathophysiology, diagnosis, and management /
[edited by César Fernández-de-las-Peñas, Lars Arendt-Nielsen, and Robert D. Gerwin.
   p. ; cm.
   Includes bibliographical references and index.
   ISBN-13: 978-0-7637-5283-5
   ISBN-10: 0-7637-5283-5
   1. Tension headache.   2. Tension headache–Physical therapy.   3. Neck pain–Physical
therapy. I. Fernández-de-las-Peñas, César. II. Arendt-Nielsen, Lars, 1958– III. Gerwin, Robert, 1938–
   [DNLM: 1. Headache–physiopathology.   2. Headache–diagnosis.   3. Headache–therapy.
4. Tension-Type Headache. WL 342 T3116 2010]
   RB128.T458 2010
   616.8'4914—dc22
                                                                                      2008043428

6048

Printed in the United States of America
13 12 11 10 09   10 9 8 7 6 5 4 3 2 1

Contents

Introduction by the Series Editor

Peter A. Huijbregts, PT, MSc, MHSc, DPT, OCS, MTC, FAAOMPT, FCAMT
Series Editor, Contemporary Issues in Physical Therapy and Rehabilitation Medicine
Victoria, British Columbia, Canada

With a lifetime prevalence of 93% in men and 99% in women, headaches are undeniably an extremely common problem (Saper et al., 1999). This book discusses two of the more common causes of headache: tension-type and cervicogenic headache. With a prevalence of over 70% reported in some populations, episodic tension-type headache (TTH) is the most common of all headache types; chronic TTH is found in 1% to 3% of the general population (World Health Organization [WHO], 2008). Approximately 78% of adults will experience TTH at least once in their lives (National Headache Foundation, 2008). Less prevalent, cervicogenic headache (CeH) has still been reported to affect 0.4% to 2.5% of the general population. However, its prevalence may be as high as 15% to 20% in those with chronic headaches (Haldeman & Dagenais, 2001). The societal impact of TTH is significant: a large, population-based U.S. study reported that 8.3% of patients with episodic TTH lost an average of 8.9 workdays and that 11.8% of patients with chronic TTH lost an average of 27.4 workdays (Schwartz et al., 1998). Of patients with TTH, 60% experience limitations in social activities and work capacity (WHO, 2000). At present, data on the societal impact of CeH are not available.

Headache is also a common reason for many patients to seek medical care. In a survey of neurologists, headache was identified as the leading cause for consultation (WHO, 2008). No data are available on the prevalence of headache as a cause for physical therapy management, but Boissonnault (1999) reported headache as a comorbidity in 22% of 2,433 patients presenting for outpatient physical and occupational therapy. However, at the same time, population-based studies show that a great many patients with headache disorders do not receive a correct diagnosis or effective management. The World Health Organization (2008) has identified a lack of knowledge among health-care providers as the principal clinical barrier to effective diagnosis and management. This text seeks to address this barrier with its in-depth discussion of both basic science and clinical aspects of the pathophysiology, diagnosis, and management of TTH and CeH.

Basic science information covered includes a discussion of the epidemiology of headache disorders, medical differential diagnosis, and the pathophysiology of TTH and CeH. Special attention is placed on the pivotal role of the trigeminocervical complex, where the convergence of cervical and trigeminal sensory pathways provides an explanation for the clinically observed bidirectional referral of painful sensations between the neck and the trigeminally innervated head and face region relevant not only to TTH and CeH but also to other headache types. Chapters on diagnosis cover history taking, posture assessment, and examination of cervical, thoracic, and temporomandibular joint and muscle function. Chapters on management include discussion of thrust and nonthrust joint and soft-tissue manipulation techniques, therapeutic and postural exercise, dry needling, botulinum toxin injections, and psychological management. Throughout the book, the emphasis is on the conservative physical therapy management of patients with these two headache disorders. Although outside of the scope of physical therapy, the chapters on infiltration and psychological management emphasize implications for physical therapy management and serve to facilitate communication and cooperation between the physical therapist and other clinicians.

This book provides a current best evidence summary on the pathophysiology, diagnosis, and management of patients with TTH and CeH, integrating the most recent clinical research data with basic science knowledge.

Chapter authors hail from various countries in Europe, North America, and Australia, and readers thereby get access to research done in various countries that was often not previously accessible. With contributors to this text being acknowledged experts in the diagnosis and management of headache hailing from the fields of physical therapy and physical medicine and with the emphasis of this text on the conservative diagnosis and management of TTH and CeH, this text is not only unique but will deservedly find a ready audience among medical and nonmedical clinicians involved in the diagnosis and management of these types of patients, including, but likely not limited to, physical therapists, osteopaths, chiropractors, general practice physicians, neurologists, physical medicine specialists, and pain specialists.

REFERENCES

Boissonnault WG. Prevalence of comorbid conditions, surgeries, and medication use in a physical therapy outpatient population: a multi-centered study. *J Orthop Sports Phys Ther* 1999;29:506–519.

Haldeman S, Dagenais S. Cervicogenic headaches: a critical review. *Spine J* 2001;1:31–46.

National Headache Foundation. 2008. Categories of headache. Available at: http://www.headaches.org/press/NHF_Press_Kits/Press_Kits_Categories_of_Headache. Accessed May 2, 2008.

Saper JR, Siberstein SD, Gordon CD, Hamel RL, Swidan S. *Handbook of Headache Management*. 2nd ed. Philadelphia: Lippincott, Williams, & Wilkins; 1999.

Schwartz BS, Stewart WF, Simon D, Lipton RB. Epidemiology of tension-type headache. *JAMA* 1998;279:381–383.

World Health Organization. *Headache Disorders and Public Health*. Geneva, Switzerland: WHO; 2000.

World Health Organization. 2008. *Headache Fact Sheet*. Available at: http://www.who.int/mediacentre/factsheets/fs277/en/index.html. Accessed May 2, 2008.

Foreword

Leon Chaitow, ND, DO
Fellow, British Naturopathic Association
Honorary Fellow, University of Westminster, London
Editor-in-Chief, *Journal of Bodywork and Movement Therapies*

Because clinicians are confronted with demands for clinical choices to be evidence-based, or evidence-informed, there is a need for clarification as to just what this means. Sackett (2000) observed that "Evidence-based practice is the integration of best research evidence, clinical expertise, and patient values," and that is precisely what this book suggests and what it has achieved in describing.

Understanding and managing headache symptoms requires sound clinical reasoning so that evidence-informed therapeutic strategies can be formulated that are both safe and effective. To achieve this requires an understanding of a number of key pieces of information, most notably background data regarding epidemiology as well as the pathophysiology of both tension-type and cervicogenic headache variants.

Fortunately, a great deal is known about the causes of, and means of differentially distinguishing between, cervicogenic and tension-type headaches as well as the potential overlap between these and other headache forms, such as cluster or migraine headaches. This information is clearly set out and discussed in this textbook, along with some red flag characteristics.

In order to offer safe patient care it is necessary for clinicians to understand and evaluate current evidence relative to a range of possible influences on different headache types (including postural, structural, muscular, myofascial, and neurologic features) in the context of basic regional and general anatomy and physiology

as well as what is now understood regarding pain mechanisms associated with spinal, muscular, fascial, trigeminocervical, dural, and orofacial structures.

Building on such essential background evidence, diagnostic protocols may then be used, involving a range of validated physical and other assessment approaches. Results that emerge from appropriate assessment are designed to offer information regarding the nature of underlying pathophysiology and dysfunction, thus pointing toward potentially beneficial intervention choices based on sound clinical reasoning. Obvious as these thoughts may be, repetition of best-practice guidelines should remind us that regrettably they are not always followed.

Are your patient's headache symptoms being referred from muscle (trigger point) sources—and, if so, which particular muscles, tendons, ligaments, and/or fascial structures are potentially involved? Or is the headache perhaps deriving from a cervical, or a thoracic, joint dysfunction? Might aspects of motor control be impaired, as a feature of your patient's cervicogenic headache? Or, might orofacial structures be involved in the etiology of the headache, and/or is there the possibility of neural (or dural) involvement? Could a number of these (or other) etiologic features be active simultaneously? Whichever of these possibilities might be operating in relation to the headache symptoms, are they being influenced by underlying maintaining factors, such as forward head posture, or other biomechanical, structural, or functional (e.g., overuse, poor ergonomics) traits?

In any given region of pain, or dysfunction, manual/physical therapists need to have appropriate palpation and assessment skills in order to differentially evaluate potentially causative features and must be able to use sound clinical reasoning to formulate treatment strategies.

Decisions as to evidence-informed treatment approaches, in any given case, should ideally consider assessment outcomes, set alongside clinical experience, together with individual features such as the individual's age, history, physical condition, associated pathology or dysfunction, and, importantly, the patient's personal preferences.

Clearly the clinician's training and skill base also refines and defines clinical choices, since in any given circumstance there are likely to be therapeutic options—for example, as to whether soft-tissue treatment, mobilization, or high-velocity manipulation could or should be employed, individually or in combination, or whether one or other variant on needling might best be utilized. Fortunately, there exist a wide range of manual therapy, exercise, and needling strategies and variations and modalities that can potentially assist in either moderating or removing headache symptoms, while also beneficially influencing whatever contributing or maintaining features may have been identified.

This book offers clear guidance toward understanding all of these options and objectives, offering as it does guidelines for physical examination and identification of underlying pathophysiologic and functional causative and maintaining features, together with manual as well as more invasive (i.e., needling, injection) treatment options.

Research evidence into the neurophysiologic effects of a number of physical medicine techniques such as soft-tissue (muscle energy, myofascial release techniques), neural (neurodynamic techniques), and manipulation (high-velocity, low-amplitude thrusts) as well as needling interventions is also described, as is pharmacologic management.

This text is the first to provide such a comprehensive compilation of the best evidence—both empirical and clinical—regarding physical therapy care of patients with tension and cervicogenic headache, and as such deserves to be read, studied, and widely used as a valuable clinical resource.

REFERENCE

Sackett DL, Strauss SE, Richardson WS, et al. *How to Practice and Teach Evidence-Based Medicine*. New York: Elsevier Science; 2000.

Acknowledgments

As editors we would first and foremost like to thank all of the coauthors of this textbook. Not only do we appreciate the time they took in their busy schedules when writing their chapters, but also we are indebted to these outstanding health-care professionals for sharing their clinical and research expertise in this area. This textbook represents numerous years of combined clinical and research experience and expertise and shows the leadership role these physical therapists, osteopaths, neurologists, and medical doctors have taken in the musculoskeletal field and, more specifically, in the area of diagnosis and management of patients with headaches.

We also want to thank Peter Huijbregts (Series Editor, Contemporary Issues in Physical Therapy and Rehabilitation Medicine) and the editorial staff at Jones and Bartlett Publishers for their support during this project. Maro Gartside, Lisa Gordon, and Julie Bolduc certainly deserve special mention for their help and enduring patience during the production of the textbook.

We would like to dedicate this textbook to our patients. It is only because of them that we all have been able to accumulate our clinical and research experience and expertise. We intended this textbook to be the first step toward a better understanding with regard to diagnosis and management of the many patients presenting to our and your clinical practice with a complaint of headache.

Finally, we very much need to acknowledge the help and—at times—the tolerance of our respective families and friends. We thank them for their continued support during all of our ongoing clinical work and research but particularly for their patience and understanding during the preparation of this book.

César Fernández-de-las-Peñas
Lars Arendt-Nielsen
Robert D. Gerwin

Contributing Authors

Fabio Antonaci, MD, PhD
Headache Centre, C. Mondino Foundation, University of Pavia, Italy

Thorsten Bartsch, MD
Department of Neurology, University of Kiel, Kiel, Germany

Lars Bendtsen, MD, PhD
Danish Headache Center, Department of Neurology, University of Copenhagen, Glostrup Hospital, Glostrup, Denmark

Josh Cleland, PT, DPT, PhD, OCS, FAAOMPT
Associate Professor, Department of Physical Therapy, Franklin Pierce College, Concord, NH; Physical Therapist, Rehabilitation Services, Concord Hospital, Concord, NH; Faculty, Regis University Manual Therapy Fellowship Program, Denver, CO, United States

Maria L. Cuadrado, MD, PhD
Departments of Neurology of Fundación Hospital Alcorcón and Universidad Rey Juan Carlos, Alcorcón, Madrid, Spain

Jan Dommerholt, PT, MPS
Myopain Seminars, LLC; Bethesda Physiocare, Inc; Bethesda, MD, United States

Bill Egan, PT, DPT, OCS, FAAOMPT
Clinical Assistant Professor, Department of Physical Therapy, College of Health Professions, Temple University, Philadelphia, PA; Physical Therapist, Sports Physical Therapy Institute, Princeton, NJ; Faculty, Regis University Manual Therapy Fellowship Program, Denver, CO, United States

Deborah Falla, PT, PhD
NHMRC Research Fellow, Centre for Sensory-Motor Interaction, Department of Health Science and Technology, Aalborg University, Denmark

Christian Fossum, DO
Associate Director, A.T. Still Research Institute, Kirksville, MO; Assistant Professor, Department of Osteopathic Manipulative Medicine, Kirksville College of Osteopathic Medicine, A.T. Still University, Kirksville, MO, United States; Faculty, European School of Osteopathy, Maidstone, United Kingdom

Gary Fryer, PhD, BSc (Osteopathy), ND
Research Associate Professor, A.T. Still Research Institute, Kirksville, MO, United States; Senior Lecturer, School of Health Science, Victoria University, Melbourne, Australia; Center for Aging, Rehabilitation and Exercise Science, Victoria University, Melbourne, Australia

Hong-You Ge, MD, PhD
Laboratory for Experimental Pain Research, Center for Sensory-Motor Interactions, Department of Health Science and Technology, Aalborg University, Denmark

Christopher Gilbert, PhD
Psychologist, Chronic Pain Management Program, Kaiser Permanente Medical Center, San Francisco, CA, United States

Paul Glynn, PT, DPT, OCS, FAAOMPT
Physical Therapy Clinical Specialist, Newton-Wellesley Hospital, Newton, MA; Owner, Glynn Physical Therapy, Sudbury, MA; Faculty, Regis University Manual Therapy Fellowship Program, Denver, CO, United States

Peter J. Goadsby, PhD
Headache Group, Institute of Neurology, National Hospital for Neurology and Neuro-surgery, Queen Square, London, United Kingdom; Department of Neurology, University of California, San Francisco, San Francisco, CA, United States

Rick Hallgren, PhDEE, PhDBME
Department of Physical Medicine and Rehabilitation, Department of Osteopathic Manipulative Medicine, College of Osteopathic Medicine, Michigan State University, East Lansing, MI, United States

Peter A. Huijbregts, PT, MSc, MHSc, DPT, OCS, MTC, FAAOMPT, FCAMT
Assistant Professor, Online Education, University of St. Augustine for Health Sciences, St. Augustine, FL, United States; Clinical Consultant, Shelbourne Physiotherapy Clinic, Victoria, British Columbia, Canada; Educational Consultant, Dynamic Physical Therapy, Cadillac, MI, United States

Tamer S. Issa, PT, BSc, DPT, OCS
Issa Physical Therapy, Inc., Rockville, MD, United States

Rigmor Jensen, MD, PhD
Danish Headache Center, Department of Neurology, University of Copenhagen, Glostrup Hospital, Glostrup, Denmark

Adriaan Louw, PT, MAppSc, CSMT
Spine Pain Specialist, President and Senior Instructor, International Spine Pain Institute, Raymore, MO; Faculty, NOI Group, United States

Siegfriede Mense, DMs, PhD
Institut für Anatomie und Zellbiologie III, Universität Heidelberg, Heidelberg, Germany

Paul Mintken, PT, DPT, OCS, FAAOMPT
Assistant Professor, Physical Therapy Program, School of Medicine, University of Colorado, Denver, CO, United States

Luis Palomeque del Cerro, PT, DO
Escuela de Osteopatía de Madrid, Spain; Department of Physical Therapy, Occupational Therapy, Physical Medicine and Rehabilitation of Universidad Rey Juan Carlos, Alcorcón, Madrid, Spain

Juan A. Pareja, MD, PhD
Departments of Neurology of Fundación Hospital Alcorcón and Universidad Rey Juan Carlos, Alcorcón, Madrid, Spain

Andrzej Pilat, PT
Director of Myofascial Induction Therapies School, Madrid, Spain

Emilio "Louie" Puentedura, PT, DPT, GDMT, CSMT, OCS, FAAOMPT
Assistant Professor, Department of Physical Therapy, University of Nevada Las Vegas, Las Vegas, NV; Faculty, International Spine Pain Institute, Raymore, MO; Faculty, NOI Group, United States

Jean Schoenen, MD, PhD
Headache Research Unit, Department of Neurology and Research Center for Neurobiology, Liège University, Liège, Belgium

David G. Simons, MD
Rehabilitation Medicine at Emory University, Atlanta, GA; Department of Physical Therapy at Georgia State University, Atlanta, GA, United States

Tina Souvlis, PT, PhD
Centre of Clinical Research Excellence in Spinal Injury, Pain and Health and Division of Physiotherapy, School of Health and Rehabilitation Sciences, The University of Queensland, Australia

Michel H. Steenks, DDS, PhD
Associate Professor, Department of Orofacial Pain and Special Dental Care, University Medical Centre Utrecht, The Netherlands

Michele Sterling, PT, PhD
Centre of Clinical Research Excellence in Spinal Injury,
Pain and Health and Division of Physiotherapy, School
of Health and Rehabilitation Sciences, The University of
Queensland; Centre of National Research on Disability
and Rehabilitation Medicine, The University of
Queensland, Australia

Bill Vicenzino, PT, PhD
Centre of Clinical Research Excellence in Spinal Injury,
Pain and Health and Division of Physiotherapy, School
of Health and Rehabilitation Sciences, The University of
Queensland, Australia

Pieter Westerhuis, PT, OMT, SVOMP
Maitland Principal Instructor (IMTA), Germany

Anton de Wijer, RPT, SCS, MT, PhD
Associate Professor, Department of Orofacial Pain and
Special Dental Care, University Medical Centre Utrecht,
The Netherlands

INTRODUCTION

Introduction

Jean Schoenen, MD, PhD

There are many books on headache in general or on migraine in particular. The added value of this one is that it focuses on two neglected, though frequent, headache types and on one pathophysiologic and therapeutic aspect of them. The editors have to be complimented on tackling two difficult and controversial headache syndromes, tension-type headache (TTH) and cervicogenic headache (CeH), and on having invited a number of internationally known experts to write on the myofascial and joint facets of these disorders as well as on their management with physical therapy.

TENSION-TYPE HEADACHE

Tension-type headache is indeed the most common headache, but it is chiefly its chronic form (CTTH), affecting 3% of the general population (Lyngberg et al., 2005), that is one of the most neglected, most disabling, and most difficult headache types. TTH is a featureless headache in which the head pain is to some degree the only symptom, and thus its differential diagnosis with other primary or secondary headache types may be difficult and misleading (Fumal & Schoenen, 2007). Despite this common denominator, TTH is a heterogeneous syndrome, as suggested by some clinical signs and by the varying response to different treatment strategies. The pathogenesis of TTH is multifactorial and

varies between forms and subjects. As readers can judge from the table of contents, this book focuses on peripheral myofascial factors (myofascial nociception), including tender and trigger points in head and neck muscles (Fernández-de-las-Peñas et al., 2007), which seem to predominate in infrequent and frequent TTH. It may therefore underestimate central mechanisms (sensitization and inadequate endogenous pain control) that are intermingled with the former and tend to become the major culprit in CTTH (Schoenen et al., 1991; Bendtsen et al., 1996). It also contains a comprehensive chapter on psychological factors in primary headache in general, including tension-type headache, which contains instructive case histories and practical tips.

If acute therapy is quite effective in TTH episodes, preventive treatment, which is indicated for frequent and CTTH, has on average poor efficacy. For most CTTH patients it is therefore recommended to combine drug therapies and nondrug therapies such as relaxation and stress management techniques or physical therapies (Schoenen, 2005). The latter, which are the mainstay here, have not frequently been evaluated in randomized, controlled trials (Lenssinck et al., 2004), but some recent, more focused programs gave encouraging results (Van Ettekoven & Lucas, 2006). It is encouraging that in this book you will read more about such novel strategies, which are, as mentioned, urgently needed to improve management of disabled TTH patients. It has been argued that clinical improvement after physical therapies may be short-lasting once the treatment is interrupted, whereas the effect of behavioral therapies such as relaxation with or without electromyographic biofeedback may last longer because the patient is more actively involved and able to continue with home-based exercises. The reader should critically analyze the information, or lack thereof, given about the post-treatment duration of clinical improvements, but also, because of the high placebo response in headache disorders, the existence or not of randomized, controlled trials for the proposed treatment programs.

CERVICOGENIC HEADACHE

The notion that headaches may originate from disorders of the cervical spine and can be relieved by treatments directed at the neck has fascinated and stimulated researchers for centuries. Contributions and reports seeking to clarify this issue have multiplied in the past 80 or 90 years. Bartschi-Rochaix (1968) reported what seems to have been the first clinical description of cervicogenic headache, but it was not until 1983 that Ottar Sjaastad and his school defined diagnostic criteria for this syndrome. The current, revised *International Classification of Headache Disorders* (ICHD-II) by the International Headache Society (IHS, 2004) includes "cervicogenic headache," but the diagnostic criteria it gives differ from those of the International Association for the Study of Pain (IASP) and also from the most recent Cervicogenic Headache International Study Group (CHISG) definition (Sjaastad et al., 1998). The former (IHS, 2004), which requires "evidence of a disorder or lesion within the cervical spine or soft tissues of the neck" but does not accept "cervical spondylosis and osteochondritis as valid causes," seems too restrictive. The latter (Sjaastad et al., 1998), which emphasizes reduced range of neck motion, mechanical provocation, ipsilateral shoulder/arm pain, and relief by local anesthetic blocks, may lack specificity. This underlines the difficulties in establishing a differential diagnosis of unilateral pain originating in the neck and partly explains the diverging data in the literature.

Prevalence estimates for cervicogenic headache range from 0.4% to 4.1% (Sjaastad & Bakketeig, 2007) in the general population to 15% to 20% of clinical cohorts of patients with chronic headaches. Cervicogenic headache affects patients with a mean age of 42.9 years; has a female preponderance in most, but not all,

studies; and tends to be devoid of migrainous symptoms such as nausea, vomiting, or throbbing pain (Sjaastad & Bakketeig, 2007).

Cervicogenic headache encompasses most likely a heterogeneous group of headaches that refer pain from structures in the cervical spine region (e.g., joints, muscles, nerves) to various regions in the head as a result of convergence of sensory input from the cervical structures within the spinal trigeminal nucleus (see Chapter 10). However, the trigeminocervical model may not explain all forms of cervicogenic pain, in particular myogenic referred head pain that derives from myofascial trigger points of the cervical and upper back musculature. This aspect is highlighted in this book, and it is therefore no surprise that CeH and TTH are treated together in various sections.

The main differential diagnosis for CeH is indeed tension-type headache and migraine, with considerable overlap in symptoms and findings among these conditions. On physical examination, it seems clear that single signs have little diagnostic value, but a pattern of physical abnormalities associating palpably painful upper cervical joints, reduced range of neck extension, and impairment of craniocervical flexion may have useful discriminant value (Jull et al., 2007). No specific pathology has been noted on imaging or diagnostic studies.

Cervicogenic headache seems unresponsive to common headache medication. Small, noncontrolled case series have reported moderate success with surgery and injections. A few randomized controlled trials

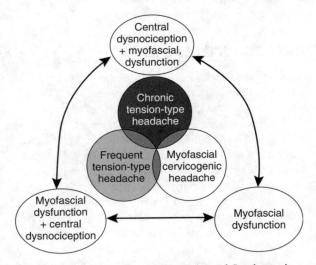

Figure 1.1 Hypothesis for Tension-Type and Cervicogenic Headache

and a number of case reports support the use of cervical manipulation, transcutaneous electrical nerve stimulation, and botulinum toxin injection. Like for TTH above, one can thus only applaud the exploration of novel physical therapies, keeping in mind that they all have to fulfill the same efficacy criteria as drug treatments—that is, to show superiority over placebo in controlled trials.

There remains considerable controversy and confusion regarding both TTH and CeH because of lack of biological markers and paucity of experimental models. However, it is anticipated that further research and aspects such as those developed in this book will help to clarify the nosography, pathophysiology, and treatment options for patients suffering from these conditions. Meanwhile, one may propose, as a working hypothesis, that at least certain forms of CeH could have in common with TTH a varying proportion of myofascial dysfunction and central sensitization (**Figure 1.1**).

REFERENCES

Bärtschi-Rochaix W. Headaches of cervical origin. In: Vinken PJ, Bruyn GW, eds. *Handbook of Clinical Neurology.* Vol. 5. *Headache and Cranial Neuralgia.* Amsterdam: North Holland Publishing; 1968:192–203.

Bendtsen L, Jensen R, Olesen J. Qualitatively altered nociception in chronic myofascial pain. *Pain* 1996;65:259–264.

Fernández-de-las-Peñas C, Cuadrado ML, Arendt-Nielsen L, Simons D, Pareja JA. Myofascial trigger points and sensitization: an updated pain model for tension-type headache. *Cephalalgia* 2007;27:383–393.

Fumal A, Schoenen J. Tension-type headache: current research and clinical management. *Lancet Neurol* 2008;7:70–83.

International Headache Society. The International Classification of Headache Disorders: 2nd edition (ICHD-II). *Cephalalgia* 2004;24(suppl 1):9–160.

Jull G, Amiri M, Bullock-Saxton J, Darnell R, Lander C. Cervical musculoskeletal impairment in frequent intermittent headache. Part 1: subjects with single headaches. *Cephalalgia* 2007;27:793–802.

Lenssinck ML, Damen L, Verhagen AP, Berger MY, Passchier J, Koes BW. The effectiveness of physiotherapy and manipulation in patients with tension-type headache: a systematic review. *Pain* 2004;112:381–388.

Lyngberg AC, Rasmussen BK, Jorgensen T, Jensen R. Incidence of primary headache: a Danish epidemiological follow-up study. *Am J Epidemiol* 2005;161:1066–1073.

Schoenen J. Tension-type headache. In: MacMahon S, Koltzenburg M, eds. *Wall & Melzack's Textbook of Pain.* 5th ed. Amsterdam: Elsevier; 2005:chap 56.

Schoenen J, Bottin D, Hardy F, Gérard P. Cephalic and extracephalic pressure pain thresholds in chronic tension-type headache. *Pain* 1991;47:145–149.

Sjaastad O, Bakketeig LS. Prevalence of cervicogenic headache: Vågå study of headache epidemiology. *Acta Neurol Scand* 2007 Nov 20 [Epub ahead of print].

Sjaastad O, Fredriksen TA, Pfaffenrath V. Cervicogenic headache: diagnostic criteria. *Headache* 1998;38:442–445.

Van Ettekoven H, Lucas C. Efficacy of physiotherapy including a craniocervical training programme for tension-type headache; a randomized clinical trial. *Cephalalgia* 2006;26:983–991.

Epidemiology of Tension-Type Headache, Migraine, and Cervicogenic Headache

Lars Bendtsen, MD, PhD, and Rigmor Jensen, MD, PhD

Headache is the most prevalent neurologic disorder (Andlin-Sobocki et al., 2005) and is experienced by almost everyone. It may represent a symptom of a serious life-threatening disease, such as a brain tumor, but in the vast majority of cases it is a benign disease, representing a primary headache such as migraine or tension-type headache (TTH) (Jensen & Rasmussen, 2004). Nevertheless, migraine and TTH may cause substantial levels of disability not only to the individual patient and his or her family but also to the entire global society because of its very high prevalence in the general population (Stovner et al., 2007). Migraine ranks as number 9 on the list of the most costly neurologic disorders in both sexes and as number 3 in women (Andlin-Sobocki et al., 2005; Olesen & Leonardi, 2003). TTH is the most common form of headache and what many people consider as their normal headache, in contrast to the more debilitating and characteristic migraine attacks. Because of its high prevalence, disability caused by TTH on the population level is larger than that for migraine. It has been shown that on the World Health Organization's ranking of the world's most disabling disorders, headache would be among the 10 most disabling disorders for the two sexes and among the 5 most disabling for women if the burden of TTH were taken into account (Stovner et al., 2007). Cervicogenic headache is a secondary headache that has been diagnosed differently by various organizations (Sjaastad et al., 1990, 1998; International Headache Society [IHS], 2004). The prevalence and impact of cervicogenic headache is therefore subject to debate (Mariano da Silva & Bordini, 2006). The objective of the present chapter is to give an overview of epidemiologic knowledge about migraine, TTH, and cervicogenic headache.

PREVALENCE OF TENSION-TYPE HEADACHE, MIGRAINE, AND CERVICOGENIC HEADACHE

Although there is a lack of biological markers for the primary headaches migraine and TTH, the clinical presentations are fairly specific, and the diagnosis is usually made on a clinical basis with relatively high precision based on the second edition of the diagnostic criteria of the *International Classification of Headache Disorders* (ICHD-II) (IHS, 2004), which now are applied on a worldwide basis.

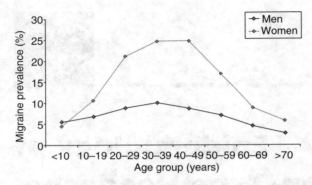

Figure 2.1 Migraine Prevalence Related to Age in Men and Women in Europe

Reproduced with permission from Stovner LJ, Zwart JA, Hagen K, Terwindt GM, Pascual J. Epidemiology of headache in Europe. *Eur J Neurol* 2006;13:333–345.

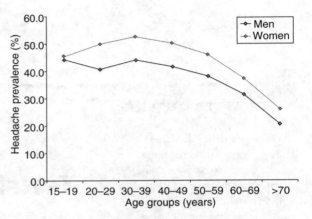

Figure 2.2 Headache Prevalence Related to Age in Men and Women in Europe

Reproduced with permission from Stovner LJ, Zwart JA, Hagen K, Terwindt GM, Pascual J. Epidemiology of headache in Europe. *Eur J Neurol* 2006;13:333–345.

Cervicogenic headache is subject to more controversies. The term *cervicogenic headache* was first introduced by Sjaastad et al. (1983, 1990), who later revised their criteria (1998). The International Association for the Study of Pain published another set of criteria in 1994 (Merskey & Bogduk, 1994), the Quebec Headache Study group published its criteria in 1995 (Meloche et al., 1993), and the International Headache Society published its latest criteria in 2004 (IHS, 2004). Thus, although the term *cervicogenic headache* is adopted by a number of organizations, its diagnostic criteria are not universally accepted (for a review, read Haldeman & Dagenais, 2001), which makes it difficult to give precise epidemiologic data.

Overall, the prevalence of current headache is 47%, current migraine is 10%, current TTH is 38%, and current chronic headache is 3% (Stovner et al., 2007). The lifetime prevalences are, as expected, somewhat higher, being 66% for headache, 14% for migraine, 46% for TTH, and 3.4% for chronic headache (Stovner et al., 2007). For migraine, the prevalence is somewhat higher among boys younger than 10 years, but after this age higher rates are seen among women in all age groups (Stovner et al., 2006) (**Figure 2.1**). The prevalence increases gradually and peaks during middle age for both women and men and declines thereafter. The decline in headache prevalence with advancing age is similar, but there is little increase from youth to adulthood, and there is a smaller difference between genders compared with migraine (Stovner et al., 2006) (**Figure 2.2**).

Looking at TTH, the prevalence seems to be much higher in Europe (80%) than in Asia and the Americas

(20% to 30%). TTH varies considerably both in frequency and duration from rare, short-lasting episodes of discomfort to frequent, long-lasting or even continuous disabling headaches. Pooling these extremes in an overall prevalence may therefore be misleading. The lifetime prevalence of TTH was as high as 86% in a population-based study in Denmark, but the majority (59%) had episodic infrequent TTH (1 day a month or less) without specific need of medical attention (Lyngberg et al., 2005a–d). Nevertheless, 24% to 37% had TTH several times a month, 10% had it weekly, and 2% to 3% of the population had chronic TTH usually lasting for the greater part of a lifetime (Rasmussen et al., 1991; Göbel et al., 1994; Lyngberg et al., 2005a–d). Data on chronic headache (headache equal to 15 days per month or more) are relatively scarce and therefore probably less reliable. In clinical practice, any report of chronic headache should always raise suspicion of a secondary headache, either due to another neurologic or systemic disease or to frequent use of acute medication—so-called medication overuse headache, which according to the ICHD-II is a secondary chronic headache with more than 3 months overuse of analgesics or migraine-specific substances (IHS, 2004). The global prevalence of chronic headache is 3.4%, the condition being most common in Central and South America (5%) and least common in Africa (1.7%) (Cheung, 2000; Wang et al., 2000; Pascual et al., 2001; Kavuk et al., 2003; Lanteri-Minet et al., 2003; Stovner et al., 2007).

Prevalence rates for cervicogenic headache have varied greatly among the various studies (for reviews, see Haldeman & Dagenais, 2001; Sjaastad & Bakketeig, 2008), because different diagnostic criteria have been used, different populations have been studied (e.g., general population or headache center patients), and different methodologies have been used (e.g., prospective cohort, retrospective analysis) (Haldeman & Dagenais, 2001; Sjaastad & Bakketeig, 2008). Moreover, several studies have not even specified the criteria used to define cervicogenic headache. In the general population, prevalence rates of cervicogenic headache have varied from 0.4% to 2.5% in previous studies (Nilsson, 1995; Sjaastad & Fredriksen, 2000). However, a recent well-conducted study reported a prevalence of 4.1% (Sjaastad & Bakketeig, 2008). The prevalence of cervicogenic headache among headache patients varies between 0.4% and 2.1% in studies that have defined the criteria used for diagnosis (Haldeman & Dagenais, 2001).

INFLUENCE OF GENDER AND AGE

In migraine, the female-to-male ratio among adults varies from 2:1 to 3:1, with a more pronounced female preponderance in migraine without aura than in migraine with aura (Rasmussen, 2001; Zwart et al., 2004). In prepubertal children, there is generally no gender difference (Bille, 1996). The female-to-male ratio of TTH is 5:4, indicating that, unlike for migraine, females are only slightly more affected than men (Andlin-Sobocki et al., 2007; Stovner et al., 2007). In both sexes the prevalence seems to peak between the age of 30 to 39 years, and it appears that the prevalence of headache in general decreases with age. The migraine prevalence increases with age until a peak is reached during the fourth decade of life and thereafter declines again, more pronounced in females than in males (Rasmussen et al., 1991; Rasmussen, 2001; Zwart et al., 2004; Lyngberg et al., 2005a–d; Stovner et al., 2007). The most common age of onset is in the second or third decade of life (Rasmussen et al., 1991; Rasmussen, 2001). The average age of onset of TTH is higher than in migraine, namely 25 to 30 years in cross-sectional epidemiologic studies (Rasmussen, 2001), and TTH as well as other chronic headaches are probably lifelong disorders, because prevalences tend to increase until the fifth decade with only a minor decline with increasing age.

In cervicogenic headache, most studies have reported the female-to-male ratio to be approximately 4:1, and the mean age of patients to be approximately 43 years (Haldeman & Dagenais, 2001). However, the most recent population study found no female preponderance and a mean age of 49 years (Sjaastad & Bakketeig, 2008).

INCIDENCE OF TENSION-TYPE HEADACHE AND MIGRAINE

The incidence of developing headache de novo has only rarely been estimated, and the results are uncertain. In a Danish epidemiologic follow-up study, the annual incidence for migraine was 8.1 per 1,000 person years (female-to-male 6:1) and 14.2 per 1,000 person years for frequent TTH (female-to-male 3:1) (Lyngberg et al., 2005a–d). Both rates decreased with age. Risk factors for developing migraine were familial disposition, no secondary education, high workload, and frequent TTH. For TTH, risk factors were poor self-rated health, inability to relax after work, and sleeping few hours per night. The incidence of migraine was higher than previously calculated from cross-sectional studies. The gender difference in TTH differed from migraine, and no association with educational level was observed (Lyngberg et al., 2005a–d). At present, there are no data on incidence of cervicogenic headache.

DISABILITY INDUCED BY TENSION-TYPE HEADACHE AND MIGRAINE

In a U.S. migraine cost study, it was calculated that migraine was the cause of 112 million bedridden days per year, corresponding to 300,000 persons staying in bed each day (24 hours) due to headaches (Hu et al., 1999). In population-based studies from Sweden, migraine patients have reported impairment between attacks as well (Dahlof & Dimenas, 1995), and 9% have stated that they do not recover completely from the attack (Linde & Dahlof, 2004). A Swedish study has shown that 27% of patients have 70% of the migraine attacks, and thereby carry most of the burden of migraine (Dahlof & Dimenas, 1995). This is also shown by application of the Migraine Disability Assessment Scale (MIDAS) (Stewart et al., 2000). In France, 22% of those with active migraine (corresponding to 1.5% of the whole population) had MIDAS grade III or IV, which indicates 11 days or more during a 3-month period with work absence or 50% or greater reduction in productivity (job or household chores) or with inability to participate in social activities (Lucas et al., 2005). In the United States

(Hamelsky et al., 2005) and in some Latin American countries, the proportion of migraine sufferers with MIDAS III or IV was more than 50%. A review of the global prevalence and burden of headaches (Stovner et al., 2007) reported that the migraine burden was relatively similar for the four continents with sufficient data (Europe, Asia, North America, and South and Central America). The study also showed that the burden of TTH was greater than that of migraine, which indirectly supports the tentative conclusion that the overall cost of TTH is greater than that of migraine (see "Costs" section).

Patients with cervicogenic headache have demonstrated substantial declines in quality of life measurements that are comparable to patients with migraine and episodic TTH (van Suijlekom et al., 2003).

COSTS OF TENSION-TYPE HEADACHE AND MIGRAINE

Most of the cost of migraine is due to the indirect cost, that is, work absence or reduced efficiency when working with headache. In the United States, the estimated total cost was $14.4 billion for 22 million migraine sufferers between ages 20 and 65 years (Hu et al., 1999). The direct costs (medication, consultations, investigations, and hospitalization) accounted for only $1 billion, whereas $13.3 billion was indirect costs. An important conclusion of the study was that the burden of migraine disproportionally falls on the patients and their employers (Hu et al., 1999). In Europe it has been estimated that of a total cost for migraine of €579 per patient, totalling €27 billion among the 41 million sufferers between ages 18 and 65 years (Andlin-Sobocki et al., 2005), close to 90% were indirect costs (Berg, 2004). Of all the purely neurologic disorders, migraine was by far the most prevalent, and although it had the lowest cost per patient, it was more costly than other neurologic disorders such as stroke, multiple sclerosis, Parkinson disease, and dementia (Andlin-Sobocki et al., 2005).

Relatively little is known about the cost of TTH. Two Danish studies have shown that the number of workdays missed in the population was three times higher for TTH than for migraine (Rasmussen et al., 1992; Lyngberg et al., 2005a–d), and a U.S. study has also found that absenteeism due to TTH is considerable (Schwartz et al., 1997). Also, it has been stated that the indirect costs of all headaches are several times higher than those of migraine alone, indicating that the costs of nonmigraine headaches (mainly TTH) are higher than

that of migraine (Berg & Stovner, 2005). Assuming that for TTH as well the indirect costs far outweigh the direct costs, one may at least assume that the cost of TTH is greater than that of migraine (Schwartz et al., 1997; Berg & Stovner, 2005; Lenaerts, 2006; Stovner et al., 2007). However, this conclusion is somewhat speculative, and good studies on the cost of TTH are urgently needed to appraise the real cost of headache. We are not aware of any such data on cervicogenic headache.

COMORBIDITY

Co-occurrence of such highly prevalent diseases as TTH and migraine with other disorders requires very careful statistical analysis before any clear conclusions about causality can be made. First of all, several headache disorders may occur within the same individual, and in clinical populations patients may have up to five different ICHD-II diagnoses (Bigal et al., 2002; Zeeberg et al., 2005). In the general population, 94% of migraineurs suffer from TTH, and 56% of those experience frequent episodic TTH (Lyngberg et al., 2005a–d). In contrast, TTH occurs with similar prevalence in those with and without migraine, leading to the assumption that migraine may trigger TTH whereas TTH may not trigger migraine (Lyngberg et al., 2005a–d). The very prevalent secondary headache and potentially preventable medication-overuse headache occur by definition most frequently in patients with primary headaches and are closely linked via a common, but yet unknown, neurobiological denominator (Katsarava & Jensen, 2007). Depending on the diagnostic criteria used for cervicogenic headache, there may be a considerable overlap between this diagnosis and migraine and TTH (Haldeman & Dagenais, 2001; Sjaastad & Bakketeig, 2008).

In general, headache disorders and especially migraine have been linked to a variety of illnesses, some very well defined, such as stroke, hypertension, diabetes, asthma, and obesity (Scher et al., 2005; Aamodt et al., 2007), and some less defined, such as fibromyalgia, various bodily pains (Hagen et al., 2002), and anxiety and depression (Zwart et al., 2003; Tietjen et al., 2007). Migraine, hypertension, and obesity are all independent risk factors for cardiovascular diseases, especially stroke, and the risk factor of stroke is 2.3 to 8.7 in younger (<45 years) women with migraine with aura and 1.8 in migraine without aura, increasing significantly when migraine with aura is associated with smoking and use of oral contraceptives (Bousser &

Welch, 2005; Kurth et al., 2006). Likewise, there is an increased risk of stroke in females with migraine with aura (OR = 2.25) but not with migraine without aura between the ages of 45 and 55, whereas this risk was not identified in older women (Kurth et al., 2006). A study reported an increased risk of cardiovascular disease in men aged 40 to 84 years with migraine (aura status not determined), with the highest OR of 1.4 for myocardial infarction (Kurth et al., 2007).

The relation between depression and migraine is reported to be bidirectional, because migraineurs have a fivefold increased risk of depression, and patients with depression have a threefold higher risk of migraine (Breslau et al., 2003). Likewise, there is a similar bidirectional relation between anxiety and migraine, all together supporting theories of a common neurobiology (McWilliams et al., 2004). However, when population-based data were adjusted for coexisting TTH, it was clear that TTH but not pure migraine was the main predictor for depression and anxiety (Lyngberg et al., 2005a–d). In future epidemiologic long-term studies, and in our work as headache doctors, it is therefore very important to identify comorbid disorders, including coexisting headache diagnoses, because both the neurobiology and the management and outcome of headache seem to be closely correlated to comorbidity.

PROGNOSIS

In a 12-year longitudinal epidemiologic study from Denmark, 549 persons participated in the follow-up study. Of 64 migraineurs at baseline, 42% had experienced remission, 38% had low-frequency migraine, and 20% had more than 14 migraine days per year (poor outcome) at follow-up. Poor outcome was associated with high migraine frequency at baseline and age of onset below 20 years (Lyngberg et al., 2005a–d), which accords with the results of a U.K. study on the prognosis of headache in general (Boardman et al., 2006). Among 146 subjects with frequent episodic TTH and 15 with chronic TTH at baseline, 45% experienced remission, 39% had unchanged frequent episodic TTH, and 16% had unchanged or newly developed chronic TTH at follow-up. Poor outcome was associated with baseline chronic TTH, coexisting migraine, not being married, and sleeping problems (Lyngberg et al., 2005a–d). Thus, the prognosis of migraine and frequent TTH was favorable.

SUMMARY

The societal and individual burden associated with headache constitutes a major public health issue, the magnitude of which has previously not been fully acknowledged. Globally, the percentage of the adult population with an active headache disorder is 47% for headache in general, 10% for migraine, 38% for tension-type headache, and 3% for chronic headache. Studies from the United States and Europe have demonstrated large societal costs of migraine, mostly indirect costs through loss of work time. Some data indicate that tension-type headache may be even more costly. On the individual level, many studies have shown that headaches result in disability, suffering, and loss of quality of life on par with other chronic disorders. Most of the headache burden is carried by a minority of the patients, and these also suffer from significant comorbidity that complicates their overall management and outcome. In the last decades general acceptance and scientific interest have amplified and important insights into epidemiology and pathophysiology have been achieved.

It is hoped that a better understanding of the epidemiology and risk factors of headache, along with better insights into the primary pathogenic mechanisms, may lead to an improved prevention strategy and an early identification of persons at risk.

REFERENCES

Aamodt AH, Stovner LJ, Midthjell K, Hagen K, Zwart JA. Headache prevalence related to diabetes mellitus: the Head-HUNT study. *Eur J Neurol* 2007;14:738–744.

Andlin-Sobocki P, Jonsson B, Wittchen HU, Olesen J. Cost of disorders of the brain in Europe. *Eur J Neurol* 2005; 12(suppl 1):1–27.

Berg J. Economic evidence in migraine and other headaches: a review. *Eur J Health Econ* 2004;5(suppl 1):S43–S54.

Berg J, Stovner LJ. Cost of migraine and other headaches in Europe. *Eur J Neurol* 2005;12(suppl 1):59–62.

Bigal ME, Sheftell FD, Rapoport AM, Lipton RB, Tepper SJ. Chronic daily headache in a tertiary care population:

correlation between the International Headache Society diagnostic criteria and proposed revisions of criteria for chronic daily headache. *Cephalalgia* 2002;22: 432–438.

Bille B. Migraine and tension-type headache in children and adolescents. *Cephalalgia* 1996;16:78.

Boardman HF, Thomas E, Millson DS, Croft PR. The natural history of headache: predictors of onset and recovery. *Cephalalgia* 2006;26:1080–1088.

Bousser MG, Welch KM. Relation between migraine and stroke. *Lancet Neurol* 2005;4:533–542.

Breslau N, Lipton RB, Stewart WF, Schultz LR, Welch KM. Co-morbidity of migraine and depression: investigating potential etiology and prognosis. *Neurology* 2003;60: 1308–1312.

Cheung RT. Prevalence of migraine, tension-type headache, and other headaches in Hong Kong. *Headache* 2000;40:473–479.

Dahlof CG, Dimenas E. Migraine patients experience poorer subjective well-being/quality of life even between attacks. *Cephalalgia* 1995;15:31–36.

Göbel H, Petersen-Braun M, Soyka D. The epidemiology of headache in Germany: a nationwide survey of a representative sample on the basis of the headache classification of the International Headache Society. *Cephalalgia* 1994;14:97–106.

Hagen K, Einarsen C, Zwart JA, Svebak S, Bovim G. The co-occurrence of headache and musculoskeletal symptoms amongst 51,050 adults in Norway. *Eur J Neurol* 2002;9:527–533.

Haldeman S, Dagenais S. Cervicogenic headaches: a critical review. *Spine J* 2001;1:31–46.

Hamelsky SW, Lipton RB, Stewart WF. An assessment of the burden of migraine using the willingness to pay model. *Cephalalgia* 2005;25:87–100.

Hu XH, Markson LE, Lipton RB, Stewart WF, Berger ML. Burden of migraine in the United States: disability and economic costs. *Arch Intern Med* 1999;159: 813–818.

International Headache Society. The International Classification of Headache Disorders: 2nd edition. *Cephalalgia* 2004;24(suppl 1):9–160.

Jensen R, Rasmussen BK. Burden of headache. *Expert Rev Pharmacoeconomics Outcomes Res* 2004;4:353–359.

Katsarava Z, Jensen R. Medication-overuse headache: where are we now? *Curr Opin Neurol* 2007;20:326–330.

Kavuk I, Yavuz A, Cetindere U, Agelink MW, Diener HC. Epidemiology of chronic daily headache. *Eur J Med Res* 2003;8:236–240.

Kurth T, Gaziano JM, Cook NR, Logroscino G, Diener HC, Buring JE. Migraine and risk of cardiovascular disease in women. *JAMA* 2006;19;296:283–291.

Kurth T, Gaziano JM, Cook NR, et al. Migraine and risk of cardiovascular disease in men. *Arch Intern Med* 2007;167:795–801.

Lanteri-Minet M, Auray JP, El Hasnaoui A, et al. Prevalence and description of chronic daily headache in the general population in France. *Pain* 2003;102:143–149.

Lenaerts ME. Burden of tension-type headache. *Curr Pain Headache Rep* 2006;10:459–462.

Linde M, Dahlof C. Attitudes and burden of disease among self-considered migraineurs: a nation-wide population-based survey in Sweden. *Cephalalgia* 2004;24:455–465.

Lucas C, Chaffaut C, Artaz MA, Lanteri-Minet M. FRAMIG 2000: medical and therapeutic management of migraine in France. *Cephalalgia* 2005;25:267–279.

Lyngberg AC, Rasmussen BK, Jorgensen T, Jensen R. Has the prevalence of migraine and tension-type headache changed over a 12-year period? A Danish population survey. *Eur J Epidemiol* 2005a;20:243–249.

Lyngberg AC, Rasmussen BK, Jorgensen T, Jensen R. Prognosis of migraine and tension-type headache: a population-based follow-up study. *Neurology* 2005b;65:580–585.

Lyngberg AC, Rasmussen BK, Jorgensen T, Jensen R. Secular changes in health care utilization and work absence for migraine and tension-type headache: a population based study. *Eur J Epidemiol* 2005c;20:1007–1014.

Lyngberg AC, Rasmussen BK, Jorgensen T, Jensen R. The association between poor well-being and migraine is related to coexisting tension-type headache. *Cephalalgia* 2005d;24: 968.

Mariano da Silva H Jr, Bordini CA. Cervicogenic headache. *Curr Pain Headache Rep* 2006;10:306–311.

McWilliams LA, Goodwin RD, Cox BJ. Depression and anxiety associated with three pain conditions: results from a nationally representative sample. *Pain* 2004;111:77–83.

Meloche JP, Bergeron Y, Bellavance A, Morand M, Huot J, Belzile G. Painful inter-vertebral dysfunction: Robert Maignes' original contribution to headache of cervical origin: The Quebec Headache Study Group. *Headache* 1993;33:328–334.

Merskey H, Bogduk N, eds. Cervicogenic headache. In: *Classification of Chronic Pain: Descriptions of Chronic Pain Syndromes and Definitions of Pain Terms*. 2nd ed. Seattle: IASP; 1994.

Nilsson N. The prevalence of cervicogenic headache in a random population sample of 20–59 year olds. *Spine* 1995;20:1884–1888.

Olesen J, Leonardi M. The burden of brain diseases in Europe. *Eur J Neurol* 2003;10:471–477.

Pascual J, Colas R, Castillo J. Epidemiology of chronic daily headache. *Curr Pain Headache Rep* 2001;5:529–536.

Rasmussen BK. Epidemiology of headache. *Cephalalgia* 2001;21:774–777.

Rasmussen BK, Jensen R, Schroll M, Olesen J. Epidemiology of headache in a general population: a prevalence study. *J Clin Epidemiol* 1991;44:1147–1157.

Rasmussen BK, Jensen R, Olesen J. Impact of headache on sickness absence and utilisation of medical services: a Danish population study. *J Epidemiol Community Health* 1992;46:443–446.

Scher AI, Bigal ME, Lipton RB. Comorbidity of migraine. *Curr Opin Neurol* 2005;18:305–310.

Schwartz BS, Stewart WF, Lipton RB. Lost workdays and decreased work effectiveness associated with headache in the workplace. *J Occup Environ Med* 1997;39:320–327.

Sjaastad O, Bakketeig LS. Prevalence of cervicogenic headache: Vaga study of headache epidemiology. *Acta Neurol Scand* 2008;117:173–180.

Sjaastad O, Fredriksen TA. Cervicogenic headache: criteria, classification and epidemiology. *Clin Exp Rheumatol* 2000;18:S3–S6.

Sjaastad O, Saunte C, Hovdahl H, Breivik H, Gronbaek E. "Cervicogenic" headache: an hypothesis. *Cephalalgia* 1983;3:249–256.

Sjaastad O, Fredriksen TA, Pfaffenrath V. Cervicogenic headache: diagnostic criteria. *Headache* 1990;30:725–726.

Sjaastad O, Fredriksen TA, Pfaffenrath V. Cervicogenic headache: diagnostic criteria—The Cervicogenic Headache International Study Group. *Headache* 1998;38:442–445.

Stewart WF, Lipton RB, Kolodner KB, Sawyer J, Lee C, Liberman JN. Validity of the Migraine Disability Assessment (MIDAS) score in comparison to a diary-based measure in a population sample of migraine sufferers. *Pain* 2000;88: 41–52.

Stovner LJ, Zwart JA, Hagen K, Terwindt GM, Pascual J. Epidemiology of headache in Europe. *Eur J Neurol* 2006;13:333–345.

Stovner L, Hagen K, Jensen R, et al. The global burden of headache: a documentation of headache prevalence and disability worldwide. *Cephalalgia* 2007;27:193–210.

Tietjen GE, Herial NA, Hardgrove J, Utley C, White L. Migraine co-morbidity constellations. *Headache* 2007;47:857–865.

van Suijlekom HA, Lame I, Stomp-van den Berg SG, Kessels AG, Weber WE. Quality of life of patients with cervicogenic headache: a comparison with control subjects and patients with migraine or tension-type headache. *Headache* 2003;43:1034–1041.

Wang SJ, Fuh JL, Lu SR, et al. Chronic daily headache in Chinese elderly: prevalence, risk factors, and biannual follow-up. *Neurology* 2000;54:314–319.

Zeeberg P, Olesen J, Jensen R. Efficacy of multidisciplinary treatment in a tertiary referral headache centre. *Cephalalgia* 2005;25:1159–1167.

Zwart JA, Dyb G, Hagen K, et al. Depression and anxiety disorders associated with headache frequency: the Nord-Trondelag Health Study. *Eur J Neurol* 2003;10:147–152.

Zwart JA, Dyb G, Holmen TL, Stovner LJ, Sand T. The prevalence of migraine and tension-type headaches among adolescents in Norway: the Nord-Trondelag Health Study (Head-HUNT-Youth), a large population-based epidemiological study. *Cephalalgia* 2004;24:373–379.

Medical Approach to Headaches

Maria L. Cuadrado, MD, PhD, and Juan A. Pareja, MD, PhD

Headache is one of the most common types of human pain, as well as one of the most common reasons for medical consultation (Rasmussen, 1995). Overall, headaches can be classified as primary and secondary or symptomatic (Bigal & Lipton, 2006a, 2006b; Olesen & Lipton, 2006; International Headache Society, 2004). In primary headaches the etiology and pathogenesis are largely unknown, the head pain itself being the problem, whereas in secondary headaches the pain is a symptom of an underlying disorder (**Table 3.1**).

Table 3.1 Classification of Headache Disorders

Primary headaches

1. Migraine
2. Tension-type headache
3. Cluster headache and other trigeminal autonomic cephalalgias
4. Other primary headaches

Secondary headaches

5. Headache attributed to head and/or neck trauma
6. Headache attributed to cranial or cervical vascular disorder
7. Headache attributed to nonvascular intracranial disorder
8. Headache attributed to a substance or its withdrawal
9. Headache attributed to infection
10. Headache attributed to disorder of homeostasis
11. Headache or facial pain attributed to disorder of cranium, neck, eyes, ears, nose, sinuses, teeth, mouth, or other facial or cranial structures
12. Headache attributed to psychiatric disorder

Cranial neuralgias, central and primary facial pain, and other headaches

13. Cranial neuralgias and central causes of facial pain
14. Other headache, cranial neuralgia, central or primary facial pain

Modified from International Headache Society, 2004.

Diagnosis of headaches is based on the recognition of a characteristic clinical pattern and relies on the diagnostic criteria that have been settled by the International Headache Society (IHS) (Olesen, 2005; IHS, 2004). This task is not always straightforward, since some patients present with atypical features or with a combination of two or more headache disorders. Essential elements are a thorough history and a general medical and neurologic examination (Olesen & Dodick, 2006; Lance & Goadsby, 2005). The assessment is often done while the patient is asymptomatic, but the clinician may occasionally have the opportunity to witness the attacks. In selected patients, supplementary laboratory testing and neuroimaging may be indicated (Evans et al., 2001).

An important first step in headache diagnosis is to identify or exclude secondary headaches (Evans & Purdy, 2006). Deciphering whether a headache is primary or secondary is crucial because secondary headaches may reflect an important, dangerous—and

Table 3.2 Red Flags That Increase the Suspicion of Secondary Headaches

Sudden-onset headache (thunderclap headache)
Worsening-pattern headache
Change in pattern of previous headaches
Fixed laterality
Triggered by cough, exertion, or postural changes
Nocturnal or early morning onset
New onset after age 50
New onset in a patient with systemic illness (cancer, AIDS)
Systemic symptoms and signs such as fever, stiff neck, or cutaneous rash
Seizures
Focal neurologic symptoms or signs other than typical visual or sensory migraine aura
Papilledema
Cognitive impairment or personality change

even potentially lethal—disorder. The features that suggest the possibility of a secondary headache are called *red flags*, and their recognition must be followed by the appropriate workup to diagnose or exclude any secondary headache that may be present (**Table 3.2**). If such headache alarms are lacking but the headache is atypical and difficult to classify among primary headaches, or does not respond to conventional therapy, the possibility of a secondary headache should be reconsidered (**Figure 3.1**).

When secondary headaches are not suspected or are adequately excluded, the physician should proceed to diagnose a primary headache (Lipton & Bigal, 2006). Because there are no biological markers or neuroimaging signs for primary headaches, their identification is entirely based on the clinical features. Accordingly, the characteristics of the head pain and any possible accompaniments must be carefully recorded. Bearing in mind the IHS diagnostic criteria, a careful analysis of the symptoms and signs usually provides an accurate clinical distinction. In the atypical cases that do not fit the IHS descriptions, the diagnosis of primary headaches can only be established after secondary headaches have been ruled out with appropriate investigations.

CASE HISTORY

General History

The family history of headache is sometimes relevant, particularly in migraine. Past medical and psychiatric

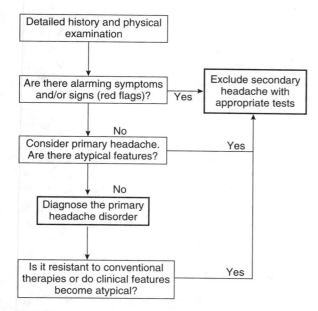

Figure 3.1 Algorithm for Headache Diagnosis
Modified from Lipton & Bigal, 2006.

diseases or previous trauma to the head, neck, or face should be recorded. Some diseases or injuries may be the origin of a secondary headache. Addiction to coffee, tobacco, alcohol, or recreational drugs must be investigated, as well as the use of medications and their effects. In headache-prone patients, particularly in those with migraine or tension-type headache, the overuse of analgesics and other symptomatic drugs for headache can cause rebound or medication-overuse headache. The social history and the exposure to physically or emotionally stressing circumstances may be important in certain patients.

Age of Onset

The age of onset may be helpful. Migraine often begins in childhood, adolescence, or early adulthood. Cluster headache usually starts around the third decade of life. Tension-type headache can begin at any age. Headaches that start after age 50 are mostly secondary (Evans & Purdy, 2006), although some primary headaches (e.g., hypnic headache) are more common in the elderly.

Location of Pain

The exact location of the pain can be a clue to the type of headache. Head pain may be unilateral or bilateral,

and may predominate in the anterior or posterior regions of the head. Migraine headache is frequently hemicranial, and usually shifts sides from attack to attack. It is also common for migraine patients to complain of occipital or nuchal pain and tenderness during a migraine attack. Most patients with trigeminal autonomic cephalalgias (i.e., cluster headache, paroxysmal hemicrania, and short-lasting, unilateral, neuralgiform headache attacks with conjunctival injection and tearing [SUNCT]) have attacks that are exclusively unilateral and invariably restricted to the same side, usually in the periorbital or temporal areas. Bilateral generalized headaches are typically tension-type headaches, but other headaches (e.g., those due to mass lesions) may take the same pattern. Cervicogenic headache is usually unilateral and is perceived mostly over the occipital region, although it may eventually extend to the oculofrontotemporal areas. The extension, borders, and shape of the painful area must be clearly specified. This is crucial for the diagnosis of neuralgias, where the pain is typically confined within the territory of a nerve. The area where the pain starts and its possible radiation or spread to other regions should also be noted. For instance, pain from the masticatory apparatus can be referred to the temple.

Duration of Attacks

The duration of the attacks can also be a critical point for diagnosis (Lipton & Bigal, 2006). Headaches may last from 1 second or less to "never-ending" days, weeks, or months. Short-lasting headaches (<4 hours) include primary stabbing headache, trigeminal neuralgia, trigeminal autonomic cephalalgias, and primary headaches induced by cough, exertion, sex, or sleep. In contrast, migraine and tension-type headache, the most common primary headache disorders, usually last longer than 4 hours, and often up to 24 hours or more. Hemicrania continua and new daily persistent headache are primary headaches of long duration. Some organic lesions give rise to recurrent attacks of short-lasting headache, but most secondary headaches have a persistent or long duration.

Intensity and Character of Pain

There is a huge variability in pain level among different headaches. The intensity of the pain should be graded either with descriptive terms (mild, moderate, or severe) or with a Visual Analogue Scale (VAS) ranging from 0 (no pain) to 10 (the worst pain imaginable) (Chapman et al., 1985). Thunderclap headache, either idiopathic or symptomatic, is probably the most severe and dramatic headache, with pain beginning abruptly and quickly reaching its maximum. Trigeminal autonomic cephalalgias and trigeminal neuralgia are also characterized by a severe, even excruciating pain. Migraine normally presents with a moderate to severe pain, whereas pain in tension-type headache ranges from "a painless discomfort" to moderate pain. Cervicogenic headache, like tension-type headache, is often a moderate, boring ache.

The character of pain is important in distinguishing between migraine and tension-type headache. A throbbing or pulsatile quality is characteristic of migraine, whereas tension-type headache sufferers usually describe a pressing pain. Some migraine patients indicate that the pain is throbbing only when they are moving about or when pain is at its worst. The quality of the pain is often described as "a needlelike pain" in primary stabbing headache, as "an electric shock" in trigeminal neuralgia, or as an atrocious pain with "the eyeball apparently being pushed out" in trigeminal autonomic cephalalgias. Explosive pain is distinctive of thunderclap headache. An instantaneous and severe head pain can also occur in those headaches specifically triggered by cough, vigorous exercise, or sexual intercourse.

Associated Phenomena

Autonomic accompaniments, such as conjunctival injection, lacrimation, nasal stuffiness, or rhinorrhea, are typical features of trigeminal autonomic cephalalgias. Migraine attacks may be accompanied by nausea, vomiting, photophobia, and phonophobia. Migraine with aura may start with focal neurologic symptoms such as visual disturbances, paresthesia, and, less frequently, aphasia. Systemic or neurologic symptoms other than those typical of migraine attacks should raise suspicion of a secondary headache. Some headaches generally lack associated features. That is the case with tension-type headache, cervicogenic headache, and most neuralgias.

Precipitating or Aggravating Factors

The recognition of precipitating or aggravating mechanisms can be helpful for both diagnosis and treatment. Several factors may trigger or exacerbate the pain. These include normal physical activity, psychological stress, menstruation, weather changes, certain foods, alcoholic beverages, missed meals, oversleeping and undersleeping (migraine); vasoactive substances such as alcohol and nitroglycerin (cluster headache); neck movements (cervicogenic headache, and occasionally paroxysmal hemicrania); jaw movements (temporomandibular disorders); sexual activity, coughing, straining, or exertion (provoked headaches, either primary or secondary); standing up (low intracranial pressure); lying down (intracranial hypertension); and sleep (hypnic headache). In SUNCT and trigeminal neuralgia, multiple mechanical stimuli over trigeminal and extratrigeminal areas may trigger the pain paroxysms.

Temporal Pattern

Several headaches have a circadian pattern. Patients are awoken from sleep by some primary headaches, particularly cluster headache and hypnic headache, and also by some secondary headaches, such as those related to intracranial tumors and intracranial hypertension. A headache of nocturnal or early morning onset should alert the physician about the possibility of a secondary headache. Conversely, the pain of tension-type headache, SUNCT, or trigeminal neuralgia appears mostly during the daytime.

The frequency of pain attacks is quite variable (Lipton & Bigal, 2006). Low- to moderate-frequency headaches of long duration include migraine and episodic tension-type headache. These disorders present with pain-free periods of variable duration between individual attacks. High-frequency primary headaches of long duration include chronic migraine, chronic tension-type headache, new daily persistent headache, and hemicrania continua. In migraine and tension-type headache patients suffering from chronic daily headache, medication overuse must be excluded. Short-lasting headaches such as cluster headache usually present with several pain attacks within the same day and in a daily fashion for variable periods of time. The symptomatic periods or "cluster periods" may last weeks to months, and are interrupted by remission periods lasting months to years. In a few patients, these short-lasting headaches become chronic and occur on a daily basis without remission. Organic headaches may be episodic, but are more often daily and continuous without pain-free intervals, and are commonly progressive.

PHYSICAL EXAMINATION

General Examination

A general physical examination and a neurologic examination should be performed in every patient complaining of headache (Olesen & Dodick, 2006; Lance & Goadsby, 2005). Vital signs should be assessed and may demonstrate fever or high blood pressure. Auscultation over the neck and the orbits may disclose bruits in case of atherosclerotic disease, arterial dissection, or arteriovenous malformation. The skull and the scalp should be examined if indicated by the history, looking for any local lesions. A large head in children may be indicative of hydrocephalus. The bones overlying inflamed sinuses may become sensitive to percussion. Palpation of the superficial temporal arteries may find enlarged, indurated, and tender arteries in aged patients suffering from temporal arteritis. The greater occipital nerve is located approximately 2 cm lateral to the occipital protuberance, just medial to the pulsation of the occipital artery. Careful palpation at this location elicits tenderness in occipital neuralgia and upper cervical syndromes, as well as in many patients with migraine. Other pericranial and facial nerves can also be palpated on their emergence or along their course: minor occipital nerve (in the groove behind the mastoid process), supraorbital nerve (supraorbital notch, in the eyebrow), infraorbital nerve (below the eye, on the cheek), and auriculotemporal nerve (immediately in front of the tragus). Craniocervical muscles should be palpated in search of local tenderness (tender points) or distant referred pain (muscle trigger points). The temporomandibular joint should be palpated while the jaw is opened and closed, seeking tenderness or crepitus. The joint is best palpated by inserting a finger in each ear and pressing forward. The cervical spine must also be tested for active and passive mobility and localized tenderness. Both meningitis and subarachnoid hemorrhage provoke nuchal rigidity (i.e., resistance of the neck to passive flexion) and other signs of meningeal irritation (the Kernig and Brudzinski signs).

Neurologic Examination

The neurologic examination must detect any abnormal sign likely to occur with headaches secondary to an underlying disease. It should always include an assessment of the cranial nerves. Inspection of the optic fundi is an essential part of the evaluation of a patient with headache. Evidence of papilledema may be indicative of an intracranial space-occupying lesion or idiopathic intracranial hypertension. Oculomotor nerve palsies may indicate compression from an intracranial lesion, an orbital lesion, or intracranial hypertension, although they may also happen in "ophthalmoplegic migraine." An ocular Horner syndrome—with ptosis and miosis on one side—may indicate a carotid dissection, although it can also be seen during and outside of attacks of cluster headache and paroxysmal hemicrania. Trigger zones on the face are characteristic of trigeminal neuralgia; if there is any facial sensory deficit, the patient may have a lesion compressing the trigeminal nerve or a pontine plaque of multiple sclerosis. The remainder of the neurologic examination should assess for any focal signs in motor power, tone, coordination, sensation, tendon stretch reflexes, and plantar responses. A complete evaluation also includes appropriate assessment of the patient's mental status and screening for psychiatric comorbidity, particularly anxiety and depression.

ANCILLARY STUDIES

Blood Tests

The erythrocyte sedimentation rate (ESR) or the C-reactive protein (CRP), or both, should be measured in all patients older than 50 presenting with a new-onset headache in order to exclude a temporal arteritis. Blood workup is also useful to detect hypercoagulability states, thyroid dysfunction, and other disorders of homeostasis that may cause or contribute to headache.

X-Ray Examinations

X-ray examination of the cranium, the sinuses, the teeth, and the cervical spine is indicated on suspicion of secondary headaches related to these structures.

Neuroimaging

Not all patients with headache require neuroimaging procedures. However, if there is any warning symptom or sign (red flags; see Table 3.2), or if the set of symptoms is atypical for a primary headache, brain imaging is indicated to exclude secondary headache etiologies. Neuroimaging can also be considered in those patients who are anxious and fear they might have a serious disease. The choice of a computed tomography (CT) scan or magnetic resonance imaging (MRI) depends on the individual patient. MRI is more sensitive than CT for lesions located in the posterior fossa, the pituitary sella, or the cavernous sinus, where CT pictures may show bone artifacts. MRI is also more sensitive for vascular malformations and venous thrombosis, and may disclose abnormal signs in meningeal carcinomatosis and in cerebrospinal fluid (CSF) hypotension. It is also a better technique for demonstrating a Chiari type I malformation or neck disorders. Conversely, CT is better for showing recent bleeding. When available, MRI is the preferred neuroimaging study for the evaluation of headaches, with the exception of patients with head trauma, acute headache to rule out subarachnoid hemorrhage, and contraindications to MRI (Evans & Purdy, 2006).

Vascular Imaging

Catheter angiography is an invasive procedure and is very rarely used. It is the gold standard for detecting intracranial aneurysms that can be the source of a subarachnoid hemorrhage, as well as carotid or vertebral dissections or cerebral vasculitis. However, most classic indications of angiography may be currently studied with noninvasive tests such as magnetic resonance angiography (MRA) and computed tomography angiography (CTA).

Cerebrospinal Fluid Examination

A lumbar puncture is mandatory when meningitis or meningoencephalitis is suspected. It is always necessary to measure the CSF pressure to diagnose intracranial hypertension or hypotension. It can also confirm the diagnosis of subarachnoid hemorrhage in the rare instances where the CT is negative.

Anesthetic Blockades

A prompt but transitory relief provided by local injections of anesthetics may support the diagnosis of neuralgias or cervicogenic headache.

Referral to Different Specialists

Many headaches can be managed by general practitioners. However, some patients must be evaluated by a neurologist or a headache specialist. Overall, neurologists should assess headaches that may be symptomatic of an underlying disorder (Table 3.2), uncommon headache disorders that may be difficult to treat (e.g., neuralgias and trigeminal autonomic cephalalgias), and

common primary headaches (migraine and tension-type headache) that have atypical features, do not respond to usual therapies, or become chronic. Sometimes the patient has to visit another specialist. An ophthalmologic examination is required if pain is confined to the orbit, if there is prolonged visual loss, or if any ocular disorder is suspected. On the other hand, an ear, nose, and throat specialist must assess the patient whenever encountering unexplained hearing loss or vertigo or if there is pain in the throat, ears, or sinuses. Dentists should be consulted if there is atypical facial pain, tooth pain, temporomandibular dysfunction, or evidence of bruxism.

SYNOPTIC DESCRIPTION OF THE MAIN HEADACHE DISORDERS

Primary Headaches

Migraine

Migraine is a common disorder that afflicts a tenth of the population (Scher et al., 1999). The pathogenesis of migraine is not completely understood, but it probably involves a genetically induced hypersensitivity of pain pathways (Rothrock, 2008; Goadsby, 2005; Silberstein, 2004). Generally speaking, it is characterized by recurrent attacks of headache and associated symptoms. However, migraine is a heterogeneous condition that results in different clinical profiles (IHS, 2004). There are two main subtypes of migraine: migraine without aura and migraine with aura.

Migraine without aura consists of headache with specific features and some associated symptoms. Typical characteristics of the headache are unilateral location, pulsating ("throbbing") quality, moderate or severe intensity, and aggravation by routine physical activity (**Table 3.3**). Yet, only two of these four pain features are required for diagnosis, and sometimes the distinction from tension-type headache is not simple. Typical accompaniments are nausea and/or vomiting, and photophobia and phonophobia. Similarly, only one of these two kinds of symptoms is required. Most patients with migraine have exclusively attacks without aura.

Migraine with aura is primarily characterized by focal neurologic symptoms that usually precede and sometimes accompany the headache. The typical aura develops gradually over 5 to 20 minutes, and lasts less than 60 minutes (Table 3.3). The most common aura symptoms are visual, including positive features (e.g., flickering lights, spots, or lines) and negative features (i.e., loss of

Table 3.3 Diagnostic Criteria for Migraine Without Aura and Migraine Headache with Typical Aura

---

Migraine without aura

A. At least five attacks fulfilling criteria B–D
B. Headache attacks lasting 4–72 hours (untreated or unsuccessfully treated)
C. At least two of the following pain characteristics:
   1. Unilateral location
   2. Pulsating quality
   3. Moderate or severe intensity
   4. Aggravation by or causing avoidance of routine physical activity (e.g., walking or climbing stairs)
D. At least one of the following:
   1. Nausea and/or vomiting
   2. Photophobia and phonophobia
E. Not attributed to another disorder

Migraine headache with typical aura

A. At least two attacks fulfilling criteria B–D
B. Aura consisting of at least one of the following but no motor weakness:
   1. Fully reversible visual symptoms including positive features (e.g., flickering lines, spots or lines) and/or negative features (i.e., loss of vision)
   2. Fully reversible sensory symptoms including positive features (i.e., pins and needles) and/or negative features (i.e., numbness)
   3. Fully reversible dysphasic speech disturbances
C. At least two of the following:
   1. Homonymous visual symptoms and/or unilateral sensory symptoms
   2. At least one aura symptom develops gradually over ≥5 min and/or different symptoms occur in succession
   3. Each symptom lasts ≥5 min and ≤60 min
D. Headache that meets criteria B–D for migraine without aura begins during the aura or follows aura within 60 min
E. Not attributed to another disorder

Modified from International Headache Society, 2004.

vision). Sensory symptoms are the second most common aura, and may include positive features (i.e., pins and needles) as well as negative features (i.e., numbness). The distribution is often cheiro-oral (face and hand), but can be hemisensory. Dysphasia is also typical, but is less frequent. More rarely the aura consists of motor weakness (familial or sporadic "hemiplegic migraine"), or symptoms and signs of brainstem dysfunction ("basilar migraine"). Finally, some patients may present otherwise typical aura without headache. The precise diagnosis of migrainous aura and its distinction from other conditions with reversible neurologic symp-

toms (e.g., transient ischemic attacks or seizures) may require appropriate investigations in some cases, especially when the aura begins after age 40 or is not typical.

Retinal migraine is a particular subtype of migraine that is characterized by monocular positive and/or negative visual phenomena preceding or accompanying migraine headache. Other causes of transient monocular blindness (e.g., ischemia) must be ruled out.

Migraine headache occurring on 15 or more days per month for more than 3 months is diagnosed as chronic migraine. Chronicity is regarded as a complication of episodic migraine. Other complications of migraine are status migrainous (debilitating attack lasting for more than 72 hours), persistent aura without infarction, migrainous infarction, and migraine-triggered seizure.

Tension-Type Headache

Tension-type headache is the most frequent primary headache, with 1-year prevalence rates higher than 30% (Schwartz et al., 1998). In contrast to migraine, the usual pain features are bilateral location, nonthrobbing quality, mild to moderate intensity, and lack of aggravation by physical activity (**Table 3.4**). Pain is frequently described as pressing or constrictive, sometimes reminiscent of a tight band around the head. Either photophobia or phonophobia may be present, but there is no significant nausea or vomiting. According to the temporal pattern, the IHS (2004) distinguishes three forms of tension-type headache: infrequent episodic (<1 attack per month), frequent episodic (1–14 attacks per month), and chronic (≥15 attacks per month). The chronic form always evolves from an episodic form. Pericranial tenderness recorded by manual palpation is a remarkable abnormal finding in some patients (Jensen et al., 1993). A conspicuous presence of active muscle trigger points has been found in various craniocervical muscles (Fernández-de-las-Peñas et al., 2007).

Trigeminal Autonomic Cephalalgias

Trigeminal autonomic cephalalgias (TACs) share the clinical features of short-lived unilateral pain and prominent autonomic dysfunction ipsilateral to the pain. This group of headache syndromes includes cluster headache, paroxysmal hemicrania, and SUNCT. The pathophysiology of TACs apparently depends on the activation of the trigeminal system, with pain felt in the area supplied by the first division (V1) of the trigeminal

Table 3.4 Diagnostic Criteria for Tension-Type Headache

Episodic tension-type headache (infrequent and frequent)[a]

A. At least 10 episodes occurring on <1 day per month (infrequent episodic) or ≥1 but <15 days per month, and fulfilling criteria B–D
B. Headache lasting from 30 min to 7 days
C. At least two of the following pain characteristics:
    1. Bilateral location
    2. Pressing or tightening (nonpulsating) quality
    3. Mild or moderate intensity
    4. Not aggravated by routine physical activity such as walking or climbing stairs
D. Both of the following:
    1. No nausea or vomiting (anorexia may occur)
    2. No more than one of photophobia and phonophobia
E. Not attributed to another disorder

Chronic tension-type headache[a]

A. Headache occurring on ≥15 days per month on average for >3 months, and fulfilling criteria B–D
B. Headache lasts hours or may be continuous
C. At least two of the following pain characteristics:
    1. Bilateral location
    2. Pressing or tightening (nonpulsating) quality
    3. Mild or moderate intensity
    4. Not aggravated by routine physical activity such as walking or climbing stairs
D. Both of the following:
    1. No more than one of photophobia, phonophobia, or mild nausea
    2. Neither moderate or severe nausea nor vomiting
E. Not attributed to another disorder

[a]Each of these forms of tension-type headache can be further classified into forms associated and not associated with pericranial tenderness.
Modified from International Headache Society, 2004.

nerve, together with a disinhibition of a trigeminofacial (parasympathetic) reflex, responsible for the oculofacial autonomic accompaniments. Although the symptoms and signs are roughly similar, TACs differ in several clinical variables, such as the duration and temporal distribution of attacks, the precipitating mechanisms, and the therapeutic response (Goadsby et al., 2007; IHS, 2004).

Cluster headache usually presents with attacks of excruciating unilateral orbital, periorbital, and/or temporal pain, associated with ipsilateral autonomic accompaniments such as conjunctival injection, lacrimation, nasal congestion, rhinorrhea, miosis, and/or ptosis (Bahra et al., 2002). Most patients are restless or agitated during the pain exacerbations. The attacks tend to appear in the evening or night, normally last 15 to 180 minutes, and occur from once every other day to eight times a day. They can be triggered by vasoactive substances such as alcohol or nitroglycerin. Age at onset is usually 20 to 40 years, and the prevalence is three to four times higher in men than in women. Attacks typically turn out in cycles ("cluster periods") lasting weeks or months, separated by remission periods lasting months or years (episodic cluster headache). However, a minority of patients have daily or near-daily headaches for more than 1 year without remission or with remissions that last less than 1 month (chronic cluster headache).

The attacks of *paroxysmal hemicrania* have similar characteristics of pain and associated features to those of cluster headache, but they are shorter (usually 2 to 30 minutes) and more frequent (>5 per day for more than half of the time). This disorder is more common in females, and responds absolutely to indomethacin. In fact, a complete effect of therapeutic doses of indomethacin is a compulsory criterion for diagnosis (Sjaastad & Dale, 1974). In a minority of patients, attacks may be precipitated upon movements of the neck or pressure over certain neck areas (Sjaastad et al., 1982). Like cluster headache, paroxysmal hemicrania has both episodic and chronic variants.

SUNCT is a rare syndrome with an impressive clinical presentation characterized by short-lasting attacks of unilateral pain that are accompanied by prominent conjunctival injection and tearing of the ipsilateral eye (Pareja & Cuadrado, 2005; Sjaastad et al., 1989). The attacks are much briefer than those seen in any other TAC (around 1 minute, range 5–250 seconds), and occur with a frequency of from 3 to 200 per day, mainly during the daytime. They are typically triggered by mechanical stimuli over trigeminal and extratrigeminal areas.

Primary Stabbing Headache

Primary stabbing headache is the shortest of all known headaches. It emerges as transient jabs of pain in localized areas of the head, mostly in the distribution of the first division of the trigeminal nerve (orbit, temple, and parietal area). The stabs occur spontaneously, in the absence of secondary causes. Pain lasts for up to a few seconds (usually 1 to 3 seconds) and recurs at irregular intervals (IHS, 2004; Pareja et al., 1996). The stabs may move from one area to another in either the same or the opposite hemicranium. Primary stabbing headache is more prevalent in people with migraine and other headaches than in control matched subjects.

Primary Cough, Exertional, and Sexual Headaches

Primary cough, exertional, and sexual headaches are elicited by a specific behavior or maneuver (IHS, 2004; Pascual et al., 1996). These headaches are strictly dependent on the provocative factor and do not exist if the precipitating mechanisms are avoided. Appropriate examinations are mandatory to rule out secondary causes, such as an Arnold-Chiari malformation type I (cough headache) or a subarachnoid hemorrhage (exertional and sexual headaches).

Hypnic Headache

Hypnic headache is a primary headache that develops only during sleep. The attacks typically last from 15 to 180 minutes, and awaken the patient at a consistent time each night. Pain is usually bilateral and lacks the autonomic accompaniments of cluster headache (IHS, 2004; Raskin, 1988). The onset normally occurs after the age of 50, and the prevalence is highest in the elderly. Intracranial disorders must be excluded before the diagnosis is established.

Primary Thunderclap Headache

Primary thunderclap headache is a violent headache of abrupt onset that reaches maximum intensity in less than 1 minute, and lasts from 1 hour to 10 days (Schwedt et al., 2006; IHS, 2004). The pain may recur within the first week, but does not recur regularly over subsequent weeks or months. It mimics the pain of a ruptured cerebral aneurysm, and the diagnosis requires that a subarachnoid hemorrhage be satisfactorily excluded. An expanding but unruptured aneurysm and other intracranial and extracranial disorders can also cause a similar picture. A reversible cerebral vasospasm has been documented in some instances of primary thunderclap headache (Dodick et al., 1999).

Hemicrania Continua

Hemicrania continua is a persistent and strictly unilateral headache, which is responsive to indomethacin. It is usually continuous, but there is also a remitting form. Baseline pain is of moderate intensity, but exacerbations of severe pain may be superimposed. During such exacerbations, ipsilateral autonomic features can occur. Even so, the autonomic signs are less prominent than those of TACs. As in the case of paroxysmal hemicrania, an absolute response to indomethacin is required for diagnosis (IHS, 2004; Pareja et al., 2001; Sjaastad & Spierings, 1984).

New Daily Persistent Headache

New daily persistent headache is unique in that headache is daily and unremitting from or almost from the moment of onset (within 3 days at most). Patients must clearly recall such an onset, and they can often tell the exact date their headache began (IHS, 2004; Rozen, 2003). The clinical features usually resemble those of chronic tension-type headache, but instead of having evolved from episodic tension-type headache, this type of headache has become persistent from the beginning. Secondary headaches such as those due to high or low CSF pressure, cerebral venous thrombosis, or infection must be excluded.

Secondary Headaches
Post-Traumatic Headache

Post-traumatic headache includes headaches that occur in close temporal relation to a known head trauma (Packard, 1999). Patients themselves often ascribe their present headache to a trauma in the past, although the causal relationship may be difficult to establish in the single patient. To properly diagnose post-traumatic headache, the headache must develop within 7 days after head trauma or after regaining consciousness following head trauma. Most of these headaches usually have the pattern of tension-type headache. If there is remission within 3 months, the headache should be classified as acute post-traumatic headache. Otherwise, it should be considered chronic (IHS, 2004). Post-traumatic headache is often associated with a combination of other symptoms such as poor concentration, memory difficulties, emotional lability, irritability, insomnia, and equilibrium disturbances. Together these symptoms constitute the so-called post-traumatic syndrome. The extent to which litigation plays a role in the persistence of post-traumatic headache is a matter under discussion (Solomon, 2005).

Whiplash Injury

Whiplash injury refers to a sudden acceleration and/or deceleration of the neck, and is usually due to a traffic accident. The postwhiplash syndrome includes symptoms and signs related to the neck (e.g., neck pain and limited range of movement) as well as a variable combination of symptoms of the post-traumatic syndrome (Bono et al., 2000). Headache is very common in this context. The same temporal rules of post-traumatic headache apply to postwhiplash headache (IHS, 2004).

Headache in Acute Stroke

Stroke can provoke headache, among other clinical manifestations (IHS, 2004; Arboix et al., 1994; Gorelick et al., 1986). In ischemic stroke or intracerebral hemorrhage, head pain may be unrecognized because of the concomitant focal signs or disorders of consciousness. Conversely, headache is the main symptom in subarachnoid hemorrhage. Most cases of subarachnoid hemorrhage result from rupture of intracranial saccular aneurysms. Aneurysms may break because of sudden increases in blood pressure during strenuous activity, sexual activity, or any kind or strain. The headache is abrupt and extremely intense. It is commonly accompanied by neck stiffness, nausea, vomiting, and depressed consciousness. Any patient presenting with headache of abrupt onset (thunderclap headache) must be evaluated for subarachnoid hemorrhage. Diagnosis is usually confirmed by CT. If neuroimaging is negative, a lumbar puncture should be performed. Headache is also the most frequent symptom of cerebral venous thrombosis.

Giant Cell Arteritis

Giant cell arteritis, or temporal arteritis, is a disorder of the elderly that causes inflammation of head arteries, mainly branches of the external carotid artery. Its most common symptom is headache, which may be variably associated with other manifestations (e.g., polymyalgia rheumatica or jaw claudication). The temporal artery is typically affected, and it may be found to be enlarged, tortuous, and tender when examining the temple. Giant cell arteritis has a great risk of blindness because of anterior ischemic optic neuropathy, but this complication can be prevented by prompt steroid treatment. Any headache starting after age 60 must suggest the possibility of giant cell arteritis and lead to appropriate investigations (Solomon & Cappa, 1987). The ESR or the CRP should be measured, since they are typically elevated.

The diagnosis is confirmed by biopsy of the temporal artery (IHS, 2004).

Arterial Dissection

Arterial dissection results from an intimae tear with subsequent blood extrusion into the wall of the artery. Carotid and vertebral dissections often occur spontaneously, but some instances may be related to trivial trauma (Dziewas et al., 2003). Types of trivial trauma reported to antedate dissections include almost all varieties of sport activities, sexual activity, violent coughing, vigorous nose-blowing, and chiropractic manipulation with forceful neck rotation. The most common presenting symptom is ipsilateral throbbing pain in the neck, the face, or the head (IHS, 2004; Silbert et al., 1995). An ipsilateral Horner syndrome is frequent in carotid dissections due to dysfunction of the pericarotid sympathetic plexus. Most patients with carotid or vertebral dissections will have transient ischemic attacks or strokes, but the headache usually precedes the onset of ischemic events. Diagnosis is based on duplex ultrasonography, MRI, MRA, and/or CTA and, in doubtful cases, conventional angiography.

Hydrocephalus and Intracranial Tumors

Hydrocephalus and intracranial tumors commonly cause headache. However, headache is seldom the only symptom (Suwanwela et al., 1994); whenever it is the initial symptom, other symptoms will eventually appear. Classic headache related to intracranial tumors and hydrocephalus with intracranial hypertension has a progressive course, reaches its maximum in the morning upon awakening, is exacerbated by Valsalva maneuvers and bending the head forward, and is accompanied by nausea and vomiting (IHS, 2004). However, only a minority of patients shows this clinical pattern, and the headache features are often indistinguishable from those of tension-type headache (Forsyth & Posner, 1992). Otherwise, the presence of seizures, neurologic deficits, and/or papilledema points to a structural intracranial disorder that can be easily demonstrated by neuroimaging techniques.

Idiopathic Intracranial Hypertension (Pseudotumor Cerebri)

Idiopathic intracranial hypertension (pseudotumor cerebri) is characterized by an increase of CSF pressure with no structural lesion. It leads to a diffuse and constant headache, which is typically increased by coughing or straining, and is usually associated with papilledema. Other potential symptoms include intracranial noises, transient visual obscurations, and diplopia. Intracranial diseases (including venous sinus thrombosis) must be ruled out with neuroimaging exams. The diagnosis is confirmed by a lumbar puncture demonstrating an elevated CSF pressure and normal CSF contents (Ball & Clarke, 2006; IHS, 2004).

Low Cerebrospinal Fluid Pressure

Low CSF pressure can also provoke a diffuse headache that characteristically worsens in the upright position and improves after lying down. It may be associated with neck stiffness, tinnitus, hypoacusia, photophobia, and nausea. The most common cause of this syndrome is a transient decrease in the pressure of CSF after a lumbar puncture. The headache develops within 5 days after the procedure, and usually disappears within 1 week (IHS, 2004; Vilming & Kloster, 1997). Less frequently the low CSF pressure is spontaneous (idiopathic) or secondary to a CSF fistula. In such instances the headache may resolve after sealing the CSF leak. Contrast MRI may show a pachymeningeal enhancement in case of low CSF pressure (Schievink, 2006; IHS, 2004). Lumbar puncture can demonstrate a low opening pressure, but it may aggravate this condition and should be avoided.

Sleep Apnea Syndrome

Sleep apnea syndrome may produce nocturnal or early morning headache in addition to daytime sleepiness and other symptoms. It is unclear whether sleep apnea headache is related to hypoxia, hypercapnia, or disturbance of sleep. The diagnosis requires the demonstration of a high apnea index in overnight polysomnography (IHS, 2004; Poceta & Dalessio, 1995).

Cervicogenic Headache

Cervicogenic headache literally means "head pain with a cervical source." The physiologic basis for this sort of pain lies in the convergence between trigeminal afferents and afferents from the upper three cervical spinal nerves (see Chapter 11). Classically, cervicogenic headache has been defined by a clinical profile including unilateral pain (intermittent or continuous) stemming from the neck and eventually spreading to the head; nonradicular ipsilateral pain in the shoulder and the arm; restricted neck mobility; precipitation of attacks by neck movements or mechanical pressure against certain areas of the ipsilateral cervical region; and near-absolute, but transitory, relief of symptoms upon anesthetic blockade of the greater occipital nerve or the C2 root (Sjaastad et al., 1986). However, the second edition of the IHS classification does not consider that a particular headache phenotype substantiates a cervical cause, and requires that a disorder or lesion of the cervical spine or soft tissues of the neck be demonstrated by clinical, laboratory, or imaging evidence (IHS, 2004). The clinical signs acceptable as evidence for a cervicogenic source of headache have not been definitely established by the IHS.

The possible sources of cervicogenic headache lie in the structures innervated by the C1 to C3 spinal nerves (Bogduk, 2001). This may result from a variety of lesions. Known examples are traumatic injuries, tumors, infections, and rheumatoid arthritis. The primary mechanisms are heterogeneous, but secondary muscle spasm may contribute to pain in all cases. Cervical disc disease and spondylosis usually affect the low cervical spine and are not generally accepted as valid causes of headache. On the other hand, when muscle trigger points in the cervical muscles are the cause of headache, it should be coded as tension-type headache if the diagnostic criteria for this condition are fulfilled.

Retropharyngeal Tendonitis

Retropharyngeal tendonitis is a rare condition of unknown etiology. It presents with unilateral or bilateral pain in the back of the neck, spreading to the back of the head or even the whole head. The pain is clearly exacerbated by retroflexion of the neck, and may be aggravated by rotation of the neck and swallowing. The transverse processes of the upper cervical vertebrae are usually tender to palpation. The diagnosis is supported by X-ray or CT demonstration of swollen prevertebral soft tissues at the level between C1 and C4 (>7 mm in adults) and full recovery within 2 weeks of treatment with nonsteroidal anti-inflammatory drugs (IHS, 2004; Fahlgren, 1986).

Focal Dystonias

Focal dystonias of the head and the neck may occasionally cause pain, and the one that is most often painful is cervical dystonia (spasmodic torticollis). Dystonia is characterized by phasic or tonic involuntary muscle contractions that lead to repetitive movements or abnormal postures. Pain arising from craniocervical dystonia is either caused by muscular hyperactivity or by secondary irritation of neural structures. If the condition persists for a long time, it may give rise to degenerative changes in the cervical spine, the mandible joint, or the dentition, which may cause additional pain. Both the dystonic movements and the pain respond to local injections of botulinum toxin (Gálvez-Jiménez et al., 2004; IHS, 2004).

Ocular Disorders

Ocular disorders may be the origin of pain in the periorbital region and other regions of the head (IHS, 2004; Daroff, 1998). Acute angle-closure glaucoma provokes severe pain in the ocular and forehead areas in conjunction with a marked increase of intraocular pressure. The attacks of acute glaucoma may last several hours and are usually accompanied by conjunctival and ciliary injection, corneal cloudiness (because of edema), mydriasis, blurred vision, and nausea and vomiting. Both refractive errors and muscle imbalance (squint) may occasionally produce asthenopia, that is, a sense of tiredness and mild headache that develops with visual effort. Inflammation of different ocular structures can cause severe ocular pain and photophobia, which are sometimes associated with ciliary (pericorneal) injection.

Acute Sinusitis

Acute sinusitis causes oppressive frontal or facial pain over the infected nasal sinus. There may also be referred pain in different head areas, depending on which sinus is affected. Fluid displacement inside the sinus often makes the pain worse when moving the head or bending forward. Percussion over the involved sinus will also elicit pain. In addition there may be purulent nasal secretions, nasal obstruction, hyposmia, and/or fever (IHS, 2004; Blumenthal, 2001). Plain radiographs, CT, or MRI of the nasal sinuses can show sinus opacifications or air-fluid levels.

Temporomandibular Disorders

Temporomandibular disorders provoke headache or facial pain in some patients. These disorders are generally di-

vided into those that are joint related (arthrogenous) and those that are muscular (myogenous). Clinically the two frequently occur together, but each type may be found in isolation (Svensson & Arendt-Nielsen, 2000). Myofascial pain is the most common form of temporomandibular disorder. It is characterized by the presence of trigger points in the masticatory muscles that reproduce classic patterns of pain referral when palpated. Joint disorders may evoke pain in the joint, the jaw, and surrounding areas, which is typically aggravated by jaw movements and mastication. The examination may reveal joint tenderness, limited or asymmetric jaw movements, joint noise upon movement, and joint locking upon opening. X-ray imaging or MRI may demonstrate joint derangements (IHS, 2004). Occlusal interferences, emotional stress, and bruxism have been implicated as possible etiologic factors for temporomandibular disorders.

Cranial Neuralgias and Primary Facial Pain

Trigeminal Neuralgia

Trigeminal neuralgia is characterized by brief paroxysms of pain, abrupt in onset and termination, that are limited to the distribution of one or more divisions of the fifth cranial nerve. It usually starts in the V2 or V3 territories, affecting the cheek or the chin. Fewer than 5% start in V1, affecting the orbit and the forehead (IHS, 2004). Eventually the pain may extend to other divisions, but it hardly ever becomes bilateral. The pain is sudden, intense, shocklike, and only lasts momentarily—usually less than 10 seconds (Pareja et al., 2005). The paroxysms are regularly precipitated by minor stimuli acting in certain trigger areas. Some maneuvers, such as talking, chewing, swallowing, or touching the face or gums, may trigger the pain. Following a painful paroxysm there is usually a refractory period during which pain cannot be triggered. Surgical explorations and MRI exams have revealed that many, possibly most, patients with trigeminal neuralgia have compression of the trigeminal root by a tortuous or aberrant vessel (Cheshire, 2007; Barker et al., 1997). These cases and the cases of unknown etiology constitute the *classic trigeminal neuralgia*. When a structural lesion other than vascular compression is demonstrated, the condition is termed *symptomatic* or *secondary trigeminal neuralgia* (IHS, 2004).

Glossopharyngeal Neuralgia

Glossopharyngeal neuralgia presents with unilateral paroxysmal pain in the distribution of the auricular and pharyngeal branches of the vagus and glossopharyngeal nerves. The pain is felt in the ear and beneath the angle of the jaw, or in the base of the tongue, tonsillar fossa, and pharynx. It is commonly precipitated by swallowing, chewing, talking, coughing, and/or yawning. Akin to trigeminal neuralgia, there are classic and symptomatic forms (IHS, 2004; Bruyn, 1983).

Occipital Neuralgia

Occipital neuralgia is a paroxysmal pain in the distribution of the greater, lesser, and/or third occipital nerves, with or without persistent aching between the paroxysms. It may be bilateral, but normally one side predominates. The attacks may be initiated by sustained awkward positioning of the head and neck, which might occur during prolonged reading or sleeping in an abnormal position. It may be related either to stretching or compression of the nerve root as it exits the spine or to compression of the nerve as it goes through the various muscles of the suboccipital region. Palpation or percussion over the course of the nerve commonly triggers or exacerbates the pain, and sometimes there is associated hypoesthesia or dysesthesia in the affected area (Hammond & Danta, 1978). Local anesthetic blockade of the nerve provides a temporary relief (IHS, 2004). Occipital neuralgia can be extremely difficult to differentiate from cervicogenic headache. Both conditions have similar pain distribution, both respond to local anesthetic injections, and both may have a common deep source in the cervical spine (Sjaastad et al., 1986). However, the cause of cervicogenic headache is always in the neck, and its pain often extends beyond the occipital area. Occipital neuralgia can also be hard to distinguish from myofascial pain.

Neck-Tongue Syndrome

Neck-tongue syndrome is a rare condition characterized by the synchronous occurrence of abrupt and brief pain in the upper part of the neck and/or occiput and numbness in the ipsilateral side of the tongue. It is typically precipitated by sudden turning of the head (IHS, 2004; Lance & Anthony, 1980). When the atlantoaxial joint is subluxated, pain is perceived in the occipital region. Numbness of the tongue arises because proprioceptive fibers from the tongue are compromised when the C2 nerve is stretched. Such proprioceptive afferences are conveyed through connections between the lingual and hypoglossal nerves and between the latter and C2 (Bogduk, 1981).

Other Neuralgias

Other neuralgias may occur when the terminal branches of the trigeminal nerve (Caminero & Pareja, 2001; Sjaastad et al., 1999; De Vries & Smelt, 1990; Bruyn, 1986a) or other craniocervical nerves (Bruyn, 1986b, 1986c) are injured or entrapped. In some cases the origin can be determined, whereas in others no cause is apparent. Pain is felt in the distribution of the affected nerve, and may be paroxysmal or constant. Normally the pain can be abolished by local anesthetic blockades.

Persistent Idiopathic Facial Pain

Persistent idiopathic facial pain (previously known as *atypical facial pain*) is a facial pain that does not have the characteristics of the cranial neuralgias described previously and is not attributed to another disorder. It is daily and almost continuous, though fluctuating in intensity. The pain is deep and poorly localized, but it may be confined at onset to a limited area on one side of the face, mostly the nasolabial fold or the chin. There is no sensory loss or other physical signs, and the ancillary examinations are consistently normal (Agostoni et al., 2005; IHS, 2004). Many patients have depressive symptoms, but these might be reactive. In fact, there is some evidence for an organic cause. The pain is remarkably similar from patient to patient, and often starts after a dental procedure or a minor facial trauma.

REFERENCES

Agostoni E, Frigerio R, Santoro P. Atypical facial pain: clinical considerations and differential diagnosis. *Neurol Sci* 2005;26(suppl 2):S71–S74.

Arboix A, Massons J, Oliveres M, Arribas MP, Titus F. Headache in acute cerebrovascular disease: a prospective clinical study in 240 patients. *Cephalalgia* 1994;14:37–40.

Bahra A, May A, Goadsby PJ. Cluster headache: a prospective clinical study in 230 patients with diagnostic implications. *Neurology* 2002;58:354–361.

Ball AK, Clarke CE. Idiopathic intracranial hypertension. *Lancet Neurol* 2006;5:433–442.

Barker FG II, Janetta PJ, Bissonette DJ, Larkins MV, Jho HD. The long-term outcome of micro-vascular decompression for trigeminal neuralgia. *N Engl J Med* 1997;334:1077–1083.

Bigal ME, Lipton RB. Headache. In: McMahon SB, Koltzenburg M, eds. *Wall and Melzack's Textbook of Pain*. 5th ed. Philadelphia: Elsevier Churchill Livingstone, 2006a: 837–850.

Bigal ME, Lipton RB. Headache classification. In: Lipton RB, Bigal ME, eds. *Migraine and Other Headache Disorders*. New York: Informa Healthcare; 2006b:1–21.

Blumenthal HJ. Headaches and sinus disease. *Headache* 2001;41:883–888.

Bogduk N. An anatomical basis for the neck-tongue syndrome. *J Neurol Neurosurg Psychiatry* 1981;44: 202–208.

Bogduk N. Cervicogenic headache: anatomic basis and patho-physiologic mechanisms. *Curr Pain Headache Rep* 2001;5:382–386.

Bono G, Antonaci F, Ghirmai S, D'Angelo F, Berger M, Nappi G. Whiplash injuries: clinical picture and diagnostic work-up. *Clin Exp Rheumatol* 2000;18(suppl 19):S23–S28.

Bruyn GW. Glossopharyngeal neuralgia. *Cephalalgia* 1983;3: 143–157.

Bruyn GW. Charlin's neuralgia. In: Rose FC, ed. *Headache: Handbook of Clinical Neurology*. Amsterdam: Elsevier; 1986a:483–486.

Bruyn GW. Nervus intermedius neuralgia. In: Rose FC, ed. *Headache: Handbook of Clinical Neurology*. Amsterdam: Elsevier; 1986b:487–494.

Bruyn GW. Superior laryngeal neuralgia. In: Rose FC, ed. *Headache: Handbook of Clinical Neurology*. Amsterdam: Elsevier; 1986c:495–500.

Caminero AB, Pareja JA. Supra-orbital neuralgia: a clinical study. *Cephalalgia* 2001;21:216–223.

Chapman CR, Casey KL, Dubner R, Foley KM, Gracely RH, Reading AE. Pain measurement: an overview. *Pain* 1985;22:1–31.

Cheshire WP Jr. Trigeminal neuralgia. *Curr Pain Headache Rep* 2007;11:69–74.

Daroff RB. Ocular causes of headache. *Headache* 1998;38:661.

De Vries N, Smelt WL. Local anaesthetic block of posttraumatic neuralgia of the infraorbital nerve. *Rhinology* 1990;28:103–106.

Dodick DW, Brown RD, Britton JW, Huston J. Nonaneurysmal thunderclap headache with diffuse, multifocal, segmental and reversible vasospasm. *Cephalalgia* 1999;19:118–123.

Dziewas R, Konrad C, Dräger B, et al. Cervical artery dissection: clinical features, risk factors, therapy and outcome in 126 patients. *J Neurol* 2003;250:1179–1184.

Evans RW, Purdy RA. Identification or exclusion of secondary headaches. In: Lipton RB, Bigal ME, eds. *Migraine and Other Headache Disorders*. New York: Informa Healthcare; 2006:131–143.

Evans RW, Rozen TD, Adelman JU. Neuroimaging and other diagnostic testing in headache. In: Silberstein SD, Lipton RB, Dalessio DJ, eds. *Wolffs' Headache and Other Head Pain*. 7th ed. New York: Oxford University Press; 2001:27–49.

Fahlgren R. Retropharyngeal tendinitis. *Cephalalgia* 1986;6:169–174.

Fernández-de-las-Peñas C, Cuadrado ML, Arendt-Nielsen L, Simons DG, Pareja JA. Myofascial trigger points and sensitization: an updated pain model for tension-type headache. *Cephalalgia* 2007;27:383–393.

Forsyth PA, Posner JB. Headaches in patients with brain tumors: a study of 111 patients. *Neurology* 1992;43: 1678–1683.

Gálvez-Jiménez N, Lampuri C, Patiño-Picirrillo R, Hargreave MJ, Hanson MR. Dystonia and headaches: clinical features and response to botulinum toxin therapy. *Adv Neurol* 2004;94:321–328.

Goadsby PJ. Migraine patho-physiology. *Headache* 2005; 45(suppl 1):S14–S24.

Goadsby PJ, Cohen AS, Matharu MS. Trigeminal autonomic cephalalgias: diagnosis and treatment. *Curr Neurol Neurosci Rep* 2007;7:117–125.

Gorelick PB, Hier DB, Caplan LR, Langenberg D. Headache in acute cerebrovascular disease. *Neurology* 1986;36: 1445–1450.

Hammond SR, Danta A. Occipital neuralgia. *Clin Exp Neurol* 1978;15:258–270.

International Headache Society. The International Classification of Headache Disorders: 2nd edition. *Cephalalgia* 2004;24(suppl 1):9–160.

Jensen R, Rasmussen BK, Pederken B, Olesen J. Muscle tenderness and pressure pain threshold in headache: a population study. *Pain* 1993;52:193–199.

Lance JW, Anthony M. Neck-tongue syndrome on sudden turning of the head. *J Neurol Neurosurg Psychiatry* 1980;43:97–101.

Lance JW, Goadsby PJ. *Mechanisms and Management of Headache*. Philadelphia: Elsevier Butterworth Heinemann; 2005.

Lipton RB, Bigal ME. Differential diagnosis of primary headaches: an algorithm-based approach. In: Lipton RB, Bigal M, eds. *Migraine and Other Headache Disorders*. New York: Informa Healthcare; 2006:145–153.

Olesen J. The International Classification of Headache Disorders, 2nd edition (ICHD-2). The 10th International Classification of Diseases, neurological adaptation (ICD 10NA) classification of headache disorders. In: Olesen J, ed. *Classification and Diagnosis of Headache Disorders*. New York: Oxford University Press; 2005:12–19.

Olesen J, Dodick DW. The history and examination of headache patients. In: Olesen J, Goadsby PJ, Ramadan NM, Tfelt-Hansen P, Welch KMA, eds. *The Headaches*. 3rd ed. Philadelphia: Lippincott Williams & Wilkins; 2006: 43–53.

Olesen J, Lipton RB. Classification of headache. In: Olesen J, Goadsby PJ, Ramadan NM, Tfelt-Hansen P, Welch KMA, eds. *The Headaches*. 3rd ed. Philadelphia: Lippincott Williams & Wilkins; 2006:9–15.

Packard RC. Epidemiology and pathogenesis of posttraumatic headache. *J Head Trauma Rehabil* 1999;14:9–21.

Pareja JA, Cuadrado ML. SUNCT syndrome: update. *Expert Opin Pharmacother* 2005;6:591–599.

Pareja JA, Ruiz J, de Isla C, Al-Sabbah H, Espejo J. Idiopathic stabbing headache (jabs and jolts syndrome). *Cephalalgia* 1996;16:93–96.

Pareja JA, Vincent M, Antonaci F, Sjaastad O. Hemicrania continua: diagnostic criteria and nosologic status. *Cephalalgia* 2001;21:874–877.

Pareja JA, Cuadrado ML, Caminero AB, Barriga FJ, Barón M, Sánchez del Río M. Duration of attacks of first division trigeminal neuralgia. *Cephalalgia* 2005;25:305–308.

Pascual J, Iglesias F, Oterino A, Vázquez-Barquero A, Berciano J. Cough, exertional, and sexual headaches: an analysis of 72 benign and symptomatic cases. *Neurology* 1996;46:1520–1524.

Poceta JS, Dalessio DJ. Identification and treatment of sleep apnea in patients with chronic headache. *Headache* 1995;35:586–589.

Raskin NH. The hypnic headache syndrome. *Headache* 1988;28:534–536.

Rasmussen BK. Epidemiology of headache. *Cephalalgia* 1995;15:45–68.

Rothrock JF. What is migraine? *Headache* 2008;48:330.

Rozen TD. New daily persistent headache. *Curr Pain Headache Rep* 2003;7:218–223.

Scher AI, Stewart WF, Lipton RB. Migraine and headache: a meta-analytic approach. In: Crombie IK, ed. *Epidemiology of Pain*. Seattle: IASP Press; 1999:159–170.

Schievink WI. Spontaneous spinal cerebrospinal fluid leaks and intracranial hypotension. *JAMA* 2006;295:2286–2296.

Schwartz BS, Stewart WF, Simon D, Lipton RB. Epidemiology of tension-type headache. *JAMA* 1998;279:381–383.

Schwedt TJ, Matharu MS, Dodick DW. Thunderclap headache. *Lancet Neurol* 2006;5:621–631.

Silberstein SD. Migraine patho-physiology and its clinical implications. *Cephalalgia* 2004;24(suppl 2):2–7.

Silbert PL, Mokri B, Schievink WI. Headache and neck pain in spontaneous internal carotid and vertebral artery dissections. *Neurology* 1995;45:1517–1522.

Sjaastad O, Dale I. Evidence for a new (?), treatable headache entity. *Headache* 1974;14:105–108.

Sjaastad O, Spierings ELH. Hemicrania continua: another headache absolutely responsive to indomethacin. *Cephalalgia* 1984;4:65–67.

Sjaastad O, Russell D, Saunte C, Horven I. Chronic paroxysmal hemicrania. VI. Precipitation of attacks: further studies on the precipitation mechanisms. *Cephalalgia* 1982;2:211–214.

Sjaastad O, Fredriksen TA, Stolt-Nielsen A. Cervicogenic headache, C2 rhizopathy, and occipital neuralgia: a connection? *Cephalalgia* 1986;6:189–195.

Sjaastad O, Saunte C, Salvesen R, Fredriksen TA, Seim A, Roe OD, Fostad K, Lobben O-P, Zhao JM. Shortlasting, unilateral, neuralgiform headache attacks with conjunctival injection, tearing, sweating, and rhinorrhea. *Cephalalgia* 1989;9:147–156.

Sjaastad O, Stolt-Nielsen A, Pareja JA, Vincent M. Supra-orbital neuralgia: the clinical manifestations and a possible therapeutic approach. *Headache* 1999;39:204–212.

Solomon S. Chronic post-traumatic neck and head pain. *Headache* 2005;45:53–67.

Solomon S, Cappa KG. The headache of temporal arteritis. *J Am Geriatr Soc* 1987;35:163–165.

Suwanwela N, Phanthumchinda K, Kaoropthum S. Headache in brain tumor: a cross-sectional study. *Headache* 1994;34:435–438.

Svensson P, Arendt-Nielsen L. Clinical and experimental aspects of temporomandibular disorders. *Curr Rev Pain* 2000;4:158–165.

Vilming ST, Kloster R. Post-lumbar puncture headache: clinical features and suggestions for diagnostic criteria. *Cephalalgia* 1997;17:778–784.

Pathophysiology of Tension-Type Headache

Nature of Muscle Pain

Siegfriede Mense, DMs, PhD

The knowledge that the mechanisms and central nervous sequelae of muscle pain are not identical to those of cutaneous pain has only recently become an established fact for the scientific community (see Mense & Simons, 2001). Some of the subjective differences between muscle and skin pain are listed in **Table 4.1**. The terms *first* and *second pain* in the skin describe the observation that after an electrical stimulus to a skin nerve, two separate pain sensations are felt, namely, an early-occurring pain that is due to activation of the relatively fast conducting thin myelinated fibers, and a late pain caused by activity in slowly conducting unmyelinated fibers. In a muscle nerve, thin myelinated pain-mediating fibers likewise exist, but their number is small, and apparently their activation does not cause subjective sensations. Muscle pain is more diffuse (less well localized) than cutaneous pain. One possible reason for this difference is the lower innervation density of muscle tissue. Quantitative comparisons between the innervation density of muscle and skin have not been undertaken so far and are difficult to make because muscle tissue is three-dimensional and skin largely two-dimensional. Another factor that determines the capacity of localizing a stimulus is the degree of convergence in the central nervous system (CNS). Convergence means that many afferent fibers originating in different body regions contact one neuron. A high spatial resolution of a neuronal network requires a combination of a high innervation density of the peripheral tissue with little convergence in the CNS.

For the differences in the subjective character between muscle and skin pain, no explanation is readily available, except that different brain regions are activated by muscle and skin pain. The frequent occurrence of referral in patients with muscle pain but not in cases of skin pain

Table 4.1 Subjective Differences Between Muscle and Skin Pain

Muscle Pain	Skin Pain
Upon electrical nerve stimulation, just second pain	Upon electrical nerve stimulation, first and second pain
Ill localizable	Well localizable
Tearing, cramping, pressing sensation	Stabbing, burning, cutting sensation
Strong tendency for pain referral	No pain referral
Strong affective component, not well tolerable	Weak affective component, better tolerable

may be due to differences in the spinal connectivity of nociceptive afferents from muscle and skin. Nociceptive input from muscle is known to be more effective for the induction of central hyperexcitability than is cutaneous input (Wall & Woolf, 1984). Lesion-induced hyperexcitability of dorsal horn neurons is one of the possible explanations for pain referral. The strong affective-emotional component of muscle pain could be explained by different limbic centers to which the nociceptive neurons project: apparently, nociceptive neurons mediating muscle pain have stronger connections with those parts of the limbic system that are responsible for the affective-emotional component of pain.

Objectively, the information from muscle nociceptors is processed differently in the CNS. For instance, muscle pain has a special relay in the mesencephalon (Keay & Bandler, 1993) and is more strongly inhibited by the descending pain-modulating pathways than is cutaneous pain (Yu & Mense, 1990; for a review on pain-modulating pathways, see Fields & Basbaum, 1999). In addition, cortical imaging data have shown that muscle pain activates areas in the human cortex that differ in location from those activated by cutaneous pain (Svensson et al., 1997). This chapter deals with peripheral and central nervous mechanisms of muscle pain and their possible relevance for symptoms in pain patients.

PERIPHERAL MECHANISMS

It has long been known that small-diameter afferent fibers have to be excited in order to elicit muscle or cutaneous pain. These fibers conduct at a velocity of below 30 m/s; histologically, they include thin myeli-

nated (group III) and nonmyelinated (group IV) fibers. The conduction velocity of group IV fibers is approximately 0.5 to 2.5 m/s, and that of group III fibers, 2.5 to 30 m/s. The nomenclature with Roman numerals (groups I–IV) was introduced by Lloyd (1943) for muscle afferent fibers. Group III fibers correspond to cutaneous Aδ, group IV to C fibers. These small-caliber or slowly conducting fibers are not composed exclusively of nociceptive fibers; they also include thermoreceptive and mechanoreceptive fibers. Therefore, C fibers or group IV fibers are not identical to nociceptive fibers (**Figure 4.1**).

Nociceptive afferent fibers are equipped with a special type of sodium channel that cannot be blocked by tetrodotoxin (TTX), the toxin of the puffer fish. These channels are TTX resistant. TTX blocks the conduction of action potentials in nerve fibers that possess TTX-sensitive sodium channels (mostly nonnociceptive large-diameter fibers); therefore, one of the first sensations after eating toxin-containing meat of the puffer fish is numbness of the tongue and mouth. The toxin does not affect conduction in nociceptive fibers. A substance that blocks selectively the TTX-resistant sodium channels of nociceptive fibers would be the ideal analgesic, because it could eliminate pain without affecting other sensations (Jarvis et al., 2007; Djouhri & Lawson, 2004, for review).

Morphologically, nociceptors are free nerve endings. Similar to the small-caliber fibers, the term *free nerve ending* must not be used as a synonym for *nociceptor*. The term *free nerve ending* indicates that in the light microscope it lacks a visible (corpuscular) receptive structure (Stacey, 1969). Free nerve endings are not really free, because most of them are unsheathed by Schwann cells. However, the sheath is incomplete, so that parts of the cell membrane of the ending are exposed. In the light microscope, the receptive ending looks like a string of beads of relatively wide diameter (so-called varicosities) connected by very thin stretches of axon. The diameter of a branch of a free nerve ending is 0.5 to 1.0 μm. The varicosities contain mitochondria and vesicles that contain neuropeptides. The exposed membrane areas are assumed to be the sites where external stimuli act. No light or electron microscopic characteristic is known by which thermoreceptive, mechanoreceptive, and nociceptive free nerve endings can be distinguished. The first comprehensive report on the morphology of free nerve endings in skeletal muscle was published by Stacey (1969). He focused on endings supplied by group III and IV fibers. The majority of the latter had a diameter of 0.35 μm, with the unmyelinated

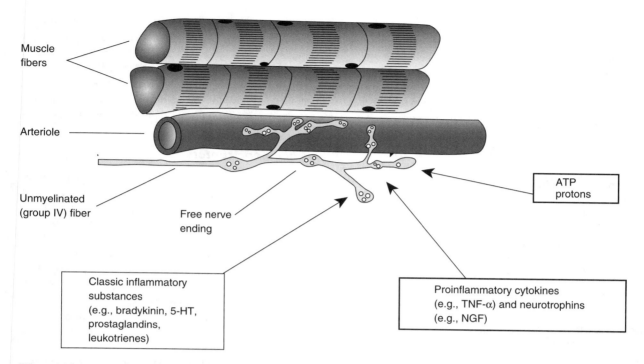

Figure 4.1 Schematic Drawing of a Nociceptive Free Nerve Ending Situated Close to an Arteriole. The vesicles inside the widening (varicosities) of the ending contain neuropeptides (in nociceptive endings, mainly substance P). The text boxes list endogenous substances that are released from muscle tissue under pathophysiologic circumstances and that sensitize or excite the nerve ending.

Source: Courtesy of S. Mense.

afferents outnumbering the myelinated ones by a factor of 2. The predominant location of free nerve endings supplied by group IV fibers was the adventitia of arterioles and venules. Surprisingly, muscle fibers themselves did not receive direct innervation by free nerve endings. Group III afferents generated not only free nerve endings but also paciniform corpuscles, whereas group IV fibers terminated exclusively in free nerve endings.

Neuropeptide Content of Muscle Nociceptors

Neuropeptides in nociceptive endings are functionally important, because when a nociceptor is excited it releases the neuropeptides into the surrounding tissue. This means that a nociceptor is not a passive sensor for tissue-threatening stimuli, but actively changes the micromilieu in its vicinity by releasing neuropeptides, many of which have a strong action on the microcirculation. Therefore, the release of neuropeptides from free nerve endings plays an important role in edema forma-

tion at the site of a lesion. Free nerve endings contain several neuropeptides in the same ending, but no combination of peptides has been found that is specific for afferent fibers from muscle. Dorsal root ganglion (DRG) cells projecting in a muscle nerve contain substance P (SP), calcitonin gene-related peptide (CGRP), and somatostatin (SOM) and thus exhibit a peptide pattern similar to that of cutaneous nerves (Molander et al., 1987; O'Brien et al., 1989).

To visualize free nerve endings, antibodies can be used. The antibodies are connected to a marker molecule and bind to the neuropeptides to form a visible reaction product at the site where the neuropeptide is situated; that is, the technique shows only endings that are immunoreactive for a given neuropeptide. In DRG cells, SP-like immunoreactivity—and to a lesser extent, also CGRP-like—appears to be present predominantly in nociceptive units (Lawson et al., 1997; Djouhri & Lawson, 2004). However, there is also evidence speaking against a relation between nociceptive function and the presence of SP (Leah et al., 1985). The presence of CGRP does not distinguish between high- and low-threshold muscle receptors with group IV afferent fibers: the neuropeptide was found in both types (Hoheisel et al., 1994b).

In a quantitative evaluation of neuropeptide-immunoreactive free nerve endings in the rat gastrocnemius-soleus (GS) muscle, most endings were found around small blood vessels (arterioles or venules) (Reinert et al., 1998). The marked sensitivity of free nerve endings to chemical stimuli, particularly to those set free during ischemia and inflammation, may be related to their location in or close to the wall of blood vessels. CGRP-immunoreactive endings were most numerous, followed by endings with immunoreactivity for SP, vasoactive intestinal polypeptide (VIP), nerve growth factor (NGF), and growth-associated protein 43 (GAP-43). Many endings exhibited immunoreactivity for more than one peptide—for example, for SP and CGRP or for SP and VIP.

Functional Properties of Muscle Nociceptors

In the skin, the following types of nociceptor are generally distinguished (data from monkeys, after Djouhri & Lawson, 2004).

- Type I A mechano-heat receptors (AMHs, supplied by Aδ and Aβ fibers. These endings respond to both innocuous mechanical and heat stimuli.
- Type II A mechano-heat nociceptors (AMHs, supplied by Aδ fibers).
- C-fiber mechano-heat nociceptors (CMHs).
- Cold nociceptors that respond specifically to painful cold.
- Polymodal nociceptors. The term *polymodal* indicates that the endings can be excited by mechanical, chemical, and thermal stimuli.

For muscle nociceptors, no generally accepted classification is available. Most studies used graded mechanical stimuli and intramuscular injection of algesic substances to obtain a coarse characterization of the endings.

High-Threshold Mechanosensitive Receptors

These receptors have a high threshold to mechanical stimulation and require noxious (tissue-threatening, subjectively painful) stimuli such as squeezing for excitation. They are supplied by group III or group IV afferent fibers. A high-threshold mechanosensitive (HTM) nociceptor

does not respond to everyday stimuli such as contractions or weak muscle stretch (Mense & Meyer, 1985; Mense, 1997). Approximately 60% of those group IV endings that responded to mechanical stimulation at all have been found to be HTM receptors (Hoheisel et al., 2005a). Among the mechanosensitive group III muscle units, the proportion of HTM endings was smaller.

Chemonociceptors

Sometimes, nerve endings are encountered that respond to algesic agents but not to mechanical stimuli. Examples are receptors that are strongly excited by ischemic contractions but not (or only weakly) by contractions alone under physiologic conditions (Kaufman et al., 1984). All receptors that showed strong reactions to ischemic contractions had group IV afferent fibers (Mense & Stahnke, 1983). Therefore, the pain of intermittent claudication may be exclusively due to activity in group IV afferent units. In the cat, the proportion of these units was approximately 10% of the group IV units (Mense & Stahnke, 1983). This type of nociceptor would be well suited to mediate the pain of tonic muscle contractions that become ischemic if they exceed a certain amount of maximum muscle force. An important point in this context is that the force must not necessarily be high for the entire muscle, but if only parts of a muscle are contracted, pain will ensue if compartments of that muscle or just small fiber bundles are overloaded. This mechanism may play a role in the pain of those patients with tension-type headache who display increased electromyographic (EMG) activity.

Polymodal Nociceptors

These units respond to high-intensity pressure stimulation and algesic substances. When free nerve endings in muscle are tested with a defined set of mechanical and chemical stimuli, they show all possible response combinations (Kniffki et al., 1978). The classic inflammatory substances, such as bradykinin (BKN), serotonin (5-hydroxytryptamine, 5-HT), and prostaglandins of the E group, have long been known to sensitize and excite muscle group IV receptors (Kumazawa & Mizumura, 1977; Mense & Meyer, 1985; Figure 4.1). Functionally, there is a marked interaction between the inflammatory agents at the receptive nerve ending: prostaglandin E2 (PGE2) and 5-HT enhance the excitatory action of BKN on slowly conducting muscle afferents (Mense, 1981). The pain elicited in human subjects by injection of a combination of BKN and 5-HT into the temporal muscle is likewise stronger than that caused by each stimulant alone (Jensen et al., 1990). These interactions are probably of clinical significance, because in damaged tissue the substances are released together.

The concentration of PGE2 and 5-HT required for enhancing the BKN action is lower than that for exciting the receptive ending. Therefore, in the beginning of a pathologic tissue alteration, when the concentrations of sensitizing endogenous agents start to increase, the receptive endings are first sensitized and then excited. Clinical observations point in the same direction: during the development of a pathologic alteration, the patient

first experiences tenderness (due to nociceptor sensitization, see below) and then spontaneous pain (due to nociceptor excitation).

Microneurographic recordings demonstrated that in human muscle receptors also exist that respond to both noxious squeezing and injection of algesic substances (e.g., capsaicin) (Marchettini et al., 1996). The chemical sensitivity of group IV endings is often restricted to only some of the algesic agents. For instance, intramuscular injection of an acidic buffer solution (pH 6) excited approximately 60% of the group IV units tested (Hoheisel et al., 2004). The only chemical stimulus that excited every unit tested was hypertonic saline (**Figure 4.2**).

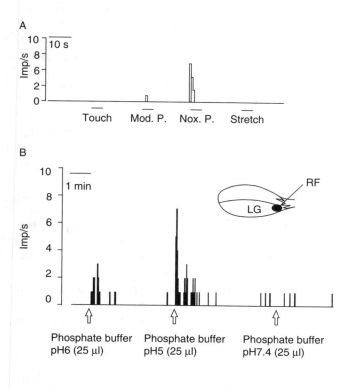
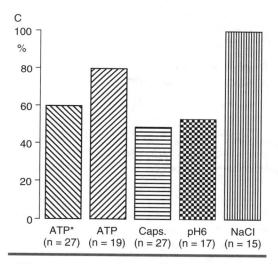

Figure 4.2 Effects of Mechanical and Chemical Stimuli on Free Nerve Endings in the Rat Gastrocnemius-Soleus (GS) Muscle.
A: Identification of a high-threshold mechanosensitive ending (a presumable nociceptor) with mechanical stimuli. The receptor did not respond to touching or stretching the muscle; stimulation with moderate pressure (Mod. P.) was likewise ineffective. The unit required noxious pressure (Nox. P., forceful squeezing) for activation. **B:** Responses of the same nociceptor as in **A** to acidic phosphate buffer solutions (pH 5 and 6). The injections were given intramuscularly into the mechanosensitive receptive field (RF) in the lateral head of the GS muscle (LG). The receptor reacted more strongly to pH 5 than to pH 6; a solution of pH 7.4 (normal tissue pH) did not elicit a response. Upward arrows mark the time of injection. **C:** Proportion of free nerve endings in the rat GS muscle responding to injections of adenosine triphosphate (ATP), capsaicin, acidic phosphate solution, and hypertonic saline into their RFs. Left bar (ATP*): ATP dissolved in tyrode. The final ATP solution had a pH of 5.5. Second bar from left (ATP): ATP dissolved in tyrode with pH adjusted to neutral (7.4). Third bar (Caps.): capsaicin. Fourth bar (pH6): phosphate solution with pH adjusted to 6.0. Fifth bar (NaCl): hypertonic saline (5%). Note that hypertonic saline activated all units tested, whereas the other agents excited only a certain fraction of them. The injection volume was 25 µl throughout. n, number of free nerve endings tested with the respective solution.

Source: Courtesy of S. Mense.

Some groups consider all muscle nociceptors to be polymodal (Kumazawa & Mizumura, 1976; Kumazawa, 1996).

Not all muscle group IV afferent units are nociceptors. In the rat and cat GS muscle, approximately 40% are low-threshold mechanosensitive (LTM) receptors (Mense & Meyer, 1985; Light & Perl, 2003; Hoheisel et al., 2005a). Many of these units can be excited by weak innocuous pressure stimuli such as slight deformation of the tissue. These endings probably mediate nonpainful pressure sensations from muscle (Graven-Nielsen et al., 2004). Other nonnociceptive types of group IV afferent units are the so-called ergoreceptors. These endings are either activated by physiologic contractions and strong stretch or by muscle metabolites; they are assumed to mediate the adjustment of respiration and circulation during physical exercise (Kalia et al., 1981; McCloskey & Mitchell, 1972).

Receptor Molecules in the Membrane of a Nociceptive Ending

In their cell membrane, muscle free nerve endings possess specific binding sites for endogenous and external stimulants that can bind to these molecules and change the response properties of the ending. The receptor molecules are either connected to ion channels or intracellular signal proteins. When the specific ligand binds to a receptor molecule connected to an ion channel, the ion channel opens and the ensuing influx of cations changes the membrane potential of the ending (in most cases in the direction of a depolarization). If the receptor molecule is connected to an intracellular signal protein, second messengers such as cyclic adenosine monophosphate (cAMP) are activated or inhibited. Both processes change the excitability of the ending. An activation of second messengers results in facilitated generation of action potentials or increased sensitivity to external stimuli (sensitization of the ending). No data are available concerning specifically the receptor molecules that are present in the membrane of muscle nociceptors. Judging from their responsiveness to pain-producing agents, the receptor molecules described in the following paragraphs are likely to be relevant for muscle pain (Mense & Meyer, 1985; Caterina & David, 1999; McCleskey & Gold, 1999; Mense, 2007).

Endogenous inflammatory substances such as BKN, 5-HT, and PGE2 are important stimulants for muscle nociceptors. Receptors for BKN are the B1 and B2 receptor molecules, for 5-HT the 5-HT3 receptor, and for prostaglandin E2 the prostanoid (EP2) receptor. In intact tissue, BKN influences the ending through the B2 receptor; when a tissue is inflamed, B1 receptors are synthesized and mediate the effects of BKN (Perkins & Kelley, 1993). This is an example of a neuroplastic change in the nociceptive ending. It shows that neuroplasticity is present in places other than the CNS and that the receptor molecules that are present in the nociceptor membrane can change depending on the state of the tissue.

Protons (H^+ ions) are among the most important chemical stimuli for muscle nociceptors, because almost all pathologic alterations of a muscle are associated with a drop in tissue pH. A pH value of around 6 is known to occur in inflamed or ischemic tissue. Besides acid-sensing ion channels (e.g., ASIC1 and 3), the vanilloid receptor (VR1 or TRPV1) (Caterina & David, 1999; Caterina & Julius, 2001) has been found to be present in DRG cells that supply receptive endings in skeletal muscle (Hoheisel et al., 2004). Capsaicin is the specific ligand of the TRPV1 receptor; it is also sensitive to H^+ ions and heat. In microneurographic recordings from muscle nerves in humans, muscle nociceptors were found that could be activated by intramuscular injections of capsaicin (Marchettini et al., 1996). The capsaicin injections were associated with strong muscle pain. Because capsaicin is assumed to be a specific stimulant for the TRPV1 receptor, these data show that this receptor molecule is present also in human muscle nociceptors. In a recent study on rats, capsaicin activated approximately 50% of muscle group IV units (Hoheisel et al., 2004; Figure 4.2). The proton-sensitive receptors are probably activated during exhaustive muscle work, ischemia, and inflammation, which all are conditions with a low tissue pH. The proton-sensitive nociceptors may be of particular importance for the induction of chronic muscle pain. Repeated intramuscular injections of acidic solutions have been reported to induce a long-lasting hyperalgesia (Sluka et al., 2001). The pain during tooth clenching and bruxism as well as tension-type headache could be mediated by proton-sensitive receptor molecules, because head muscles are overloaded and likely have a low pH.

Purinergic receptors bind adenosine triphosphate (ATP) and the products of ATP degradation. When injected in human muscle, ATP causes pain (Mörk et al., 2003). P2X3 receptors are the molecules that are responsible for ATP-induced pain (Burnstock, 2000; Cook & McCleskey, 2002). They have been reported to be present in cutaneous nociceptors, and have also been shown to exist in DRG cells supplying the rat GS muscle (Hoheisel & Mense, unpublished data). Concentrations of ATP that are normally present in muscle cells are sufficient to excite muscle nociceptors in rat GS muscle (Reinöhl et al., 2003; Figure 4.2). Because ATP is present in all body cells and is released in all disorders that damage tissue cells, ATP has been considered to be the basic pain stimulus by some.

Even neuroprotective substances such as nerve growth factor (NGF) are stimulants for muscle nociceptors. The binding site for NGF is the TrkA (tyrosine kinase A) receptor. Data from our group (Hoheisel et al., 2005a) showed that NGF excites exclusively HTM muscle receptors (presumable nociceptors). NGF is the only substance encountered so far that exclusively excites nociceptive endings in muscle. All the other established substances used in pain research to stimulate nociceptors excite also group III/IV LTM receptors that do not have a nociceptive function.

Nociceptors in the deep tissues around the temporomandibular joint are activated by glutamate (Cairns et al., 1998), the main neurotransmitter in the CNS. Apparently, glutamate receptors are present also on nociceptors of deep somatic tissues in the body periphery.

A very effective chemical pain stimulus that does not bind to specific receptor molecules is a hypertonic Na⁺ solution. A large increase in extracellular Na⁺ does not occur under (patho) physiologic conditions, but it can be easily induced in studies on muscle pain mechanisms by injecting or infusing hypertonic saline intramuscularly (Graven-Nielsen et al., 1997). In these experiments, the high Na⁺ concentration—and not the hypertonicity of the solution—appears to be the effective stimulus (Mense, 2007). Hypertonic saline may also excite muscle nociceptors indirectly by releasing glutamate (Tegeder et al., 2002; Svensson et al., 2003a).

One of the characteristic properties of a mechanonociceptor is its high mechanical stimulation threshold. The high mechanical threshold is surprising when the structure of a free nerve ending is considered, which is a fragile structure with a semifluid membrane. An ion channel has been found that is mechanosensitive and has a high mechanical threshold, the TRPV4 channel (Liedtke, 2005).

Sensitization of Nociceptors

Sensitization of nociceptors leads to an increased excitability of the nociceptive ending; it is the peripheral neurophysiologic basis of tenderness, pain during physiologic muscle contraction, and hyperalgesia. Many substances that are released from pathologically altered tissue increase the mechanical sensitivity of nociceptors. For instance, during ischemia and inflammation, BKN is cleaved from a precursor molecule in the blood plasma and sensitizes muscle nociceptors to mechanical stimuli. The sensitization is associated with a decrease in the mechanical threshold of the receptor, so that it responds to weak pressure stimuli. The sensitized muscle receptor is still connected to nociceptive central nervous neurons and, therefore, elicits subjective pain when weak mechanical stimuli act on the muscle. This sensitization of muscle nociceptors is the best established peripheral mechanism explaining local tenderness and pain during movement of a pathologically altered muscle (allodynia). Moreover, the response magnitude of a sensitized nociceptor to noxious stimuli increases (hyperalgesia). However, tenderness and hyperalgesia also have an important central nervous component (see below).

Longer-lasting pathologic alterations of muscle tissue not only sensitize nociceptors but also increase the innervation density of muscle tissue with neuropeptide-containing nerve endings. Experiments on rat GS muscle showed that an inflammation of 12 days' duration—which can be considered chronic for a rat—is associated with an increase in innervation density of neuropeptide-expressing fibers. The effect was particularly marked in endings that contained SP; the density of these SP-immunoreactive fibers increased by a factor of about 2 (Reinert et al., 1998). Since the SP-immunoreactive endings are assumed to be nociceptors, the increased innervation density is probably associated with enhanced pain sensations (hyperalgesia). The reason for this hyperalgesia could be as follows: when a given painful stimulus acts on a muscle that has an increased density of nociceptors, that stimulus will excite more nociceptors and, therefore, elicit more pain.

CENTRAL MECHANISMS

Many patients with muscle pain show signs of sensitization such as allodynia, hyperalgesia, and referred pain. Basically, two forms of sensitization have to be distinguished, namely, sensitization of muscle nociceptors in the body periphery (peripheral sensitization) and that of central nervous neurons (central sensitization). We know from many basic science and clinical studies that every long-lasting or strong input from muscle nociceptors to the spinal cord or to neurons in the trigeminal nucleus caudalis of the brainstem is likely to lead to changes in excitability of central neurons. These neuroplastic changes are the beginning of the transition from acute to chronic pain. Contrary to former beliefs, these changes do not take long to develop; in animal experiments (rats), they can be found a few minutes after applying a painful stimulus to skeletal muscle. One example is the appearance of new receptive fields in dorsal horn neurons within a few minutes after intramuscular injection of the algesic agent bradykinin (Hoheisel et al., 1993). The hyperexcitability of central neurons is the most obvious expression of central sensitization. However, it is just the first step in a chain of processes leading to chronic pain. If the pain is not treated at an early stage, it is followed by changes in connectivity, and finally structure, of dorsal horn neurons and glial cells. Input from muscle nociceptors is known to be more effective in inducing increased central excitability than is input from cutaneous nociceptors (Wall & Woolf, 1984).

Excitability Changes in the Dorsal Horn Neuron Induced by an Experimental Muscle Inflammation (Myositis)

In animal experiments (rats), changes in spinal neuronal excitability and connectivity are clearly visible a few hours after induction of a long-lasting experimental lesion. At the spinal level, three effects induced by an inflammation of the GS muscle were found: increase in background (or spontaneous) activity of dorsal horn neurons, increase in response magnitude to mechanical stimulation, and expansion of the neuron population that can be excited by input from the muscle (Hoheisel et al., 1994a). The expansion of the excited neuron population extends also to adjacent spinal segments that do not normally receive input from the GS muscle. In intact (noninflamed rats), this muscle sends its input mainly to the segments L4 and L5; if the GS is inflamed, dorsal horn neurons in the segments L3 and L6 also respond to input from that muscle. This expansion of the muscle-induced excitation to adjacent segments is also present with electrical stimulation of the muscle nerve, that is, in a condition where—in contrast to mechanical stimulation of the muscle—the sensitized nociceptors in the muscle are not involved. Therefore, the observed change must be due to central sensitization.

One possible explanation for the expansion of the myositis-induced excitation to adjacent segments is that existing—but ineffective—synaptic connections be-

tween muscle afferents and neurons in these segments became more effective (Li & Zhuo, 1998). The opening of ineffective or silent synapses leads to hyperexcitability of the neurons that now respond to an input that does not normally excite them. In patients, the hyperexcitability is likely to elicit pain during movements (allodynia) and increased pain during noxious stimulation (hyperalgesia), whereas the expansion of the muscle-induced excitation in the dorsal horn may be the reason for the spread and referral of muscle pain.

The processes underlying the opening of silent synapses are complex. One possible mechanism is that the nociceptive afferent activity releases glutamate together with SP from presynaptic boutons of muscle afferent fibers. The membrane of the postsynaptic cell is equipped with a multitude of receptor molecules, including several for glutamate, for example, N-methyl-D-aspartate (NMDA) and AMPA (α-amino-3 hydroxy-5 methyl-4-isoxazole propionic acid; the so-called non-NMDA) ion channels. These channels are permeable to cations—the NMDA channels mainly to Ca^{2+}, and the AMPA channels mainly to Na^+.

Under normal circumstances, many of the AMPA channels are ineffective or silent; that is, only a few ions pass through them per time unit. This means that presynaptic activity of low frequency or short duration is not sufficient to depolarize the postsynaptic neuron to an extent that it fires action potentials. However, during a longer-lasting nociceptive input, the amount of Na^+ ions entering the postsynaptic cell is large enough to cause a depolarization of the cell (depolarization means that the membrane potential becomes more positive and thus approaches firing threshold). The positive charges that enter the cell expel the Mg^{2+} ions that normally block the NMDA channels. Ca^{2+} ions can now enter the cell and activate intracellular enzymes such as protein kinases A and C. Kinases are enzymes that can phosphorylate the AMPA and NMDA channels; that is, they couple a phosphate residue to the channel proteins. Phosphorylated ion channels are more permeable for ions and cause larger ion currents when impulse activity arrives presynaptically and releases neurotransmitters such as glutamate. The phosphorylation and ensuing higher effectiveness of the ion channels are the first changes in response to a nociceptive input to the dorsal horn.

In the long run, the gene expression in the nucleus of the postsynaptic neuron also changes, so that a de novo synthesis of ion channel proteins can occur. The result of these neuroplastic processes is that the dorsal horn neu-

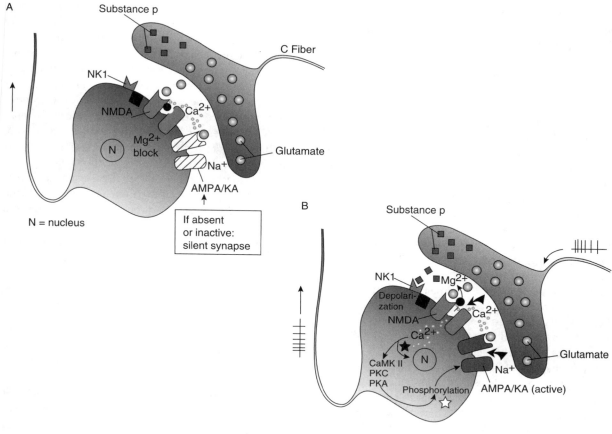

Figure 4.3 Mechanisms Involved in Central Sensitization. In the upper right of both panels, an unmyelinated fiber is shown that enters the dorsal horn and forms a presynaptic button that contains vesicles with glutamate and the neuropeptide substance P (SP). To the lower left is a postsynaptic neuron that projects with its axon to the thalamus. In the membrane of the postsynaptic cell, receptor molecules for SP (neurokinin 1, NK1) and glutamate (NMDA and AMPA/KA) are shown. The two latter ones control ion channels. The NMDA channel is normally blocked by a magnesium ion (Mg2+). **A:** Normal state before sensitization. The NMDA channel is blocked, and the AMPA/KA channel is ineffective (i.e., only a few Na+ ions can pass through it). When glutamate is released presynaptically, the postsynaptic cell does not fire action potentials, because the amount of Na+ that passes through the AMPA/KA channel is too small to excite the cell (silent synapse). **B:** Sensitized state. Because of a long-lasting or high-frequency presynaptic activity, enough Na+ ions have entered the postsynaptic cell through the AMPA/KA channel so that the cell is depolarized. The depolarization removes the Mg2+ block from the NMDA channel, and Ca2+ ions enter the cell. The Ca2+ ions activate intracellular kinases (CaMK II, PKC, PKA) that phosphorylate the NMDA and AMPA/KA channels. The channels become highly permeable to ions, and therefore the postsynaptic cell is hyperexcitable. A long-term sensitizing process is a change in gene expression leading to a de novo synthesis of NMDA and AMPA/KA channels. A sensitized dorsal horn neuron is equipped with a higher than normal density of well-permeable NMDA and AMPA/KA channels in its membrane.

Source: Courtesy of S. Mense.

rons have a larger number of highly effective ion channels in their membrane. These structural changes lead to a long-lasting hyperexcitability of the neuron to noxious and innocuous stimuli. A further factor involved in the sensitizing process is the action of SP on postsynaptic G protein-coupled neurokinin 1 (NK1) receptors (Liu & Sandkühler, 1998; Millan, 1999; Usunoff et al., 2006) (**Figure 4.3**). For the patient, all these neuroplastic alterations mean that nonpainful stimuli are felt as painful (allodynia) and that painful stimuli elicit more pain (hyperalgesia). The whole chain of events leads to a functional reorganization of the CNS.

Neurotransmitters and Neuropeptides Involved in Myositis-Induced Central Sensitization

The above-described activation of NMDA and NK1 receptors appears to contribute also to the myositis-induced central sensitization. Evidence for this assumption stems from rat experiments, in which intrathecal administration of antagonists to NK1 and NMDA receptors prevented the expansion of the spinal excitation to the segment L3 in animals with a myositis of the GS muscle (Hoheisel et al., 1997). Interestingly, a block of the AMPA receptors had no significant influence on the expansion. This result is in accordance with the general view that AMPA channels are more important for the spinal transmission under normal circumstances, whereas NMDA channels are responsible for central sensitization under pathologic conditions. With regard to the importance of AMPA channels for central sensitization, a difference between muscle- and joint-induced hyperalgesia may exist, because the latter has been reported to be reduced by administration of an AMPA receptor antagonist (Sluka et al., 1994).

When the central nervous sensitization has become chronic, it is largely independent of further input from the damaged muscle. In their model of acid-induced muscle hyperalgesia, Sluka et al. (2001) have shown that an interruption of the muscle input by local anesthesia or dorsal rhizotomy 24 hours after induction of the sensitization did not abolish the hyperalgesia. This finding clearly shows the importance of an early and effective therapy of patients with muscle pain. If therapy is delayed or ineffective, the transition to a chronic pain state is likely to occur.

Allodynia and hyperalgesia are generally expressions of increased sensitivity to stimulation. In electrophysiologic experiments on animals, the correlate of spontaneous pain is assumed to be the resting or spontaneous activity of central nociceptive neurons—that is, impulse activity in the absence of intentional stimulation. Normally, nociceptive neurons do not exhibit resting activity, but in the presence of a longer-lasting peripheral lesion they do. The increase in resting activity does not appear to be due to activation of NMDA channels but rather to a change in the release of nitric oxide (NO) (Hoheisel et al., 2000). A spinal block of the NO-synthesizing enzyme (nitric oxide synthase [NOS]) with L-NAME led to a significant increase in background activity only in nociceptive neurons. This finding was interpreted as indicating that NO is released tonically in the dorsal horn and inhibits the background discharge of the neurons. In contrast to the increased background activity induced by L-NAME, the mechanical responsiveness of the neurons was decreased by L-NAME intrathecally. Apparently, under normal circumstances enough NO is released in the spinal cord or brainstem to prevent the occurrence of resting activity in nociceptive neurons. However, in the presence of nociceptive input from a peripheral lesion, the release of NO is reduced, and this leads to resting activity in dorsal horn neurons and to spontaneous pain or dysesthesia in patients. Simultaneously, the reduced NO release should prevent hyperalgesia, because an experimental reduction of the NO level led to a decreased mechanical responsiveness (see above). However, apparently the allodynia- and hyperalgesia-promoting influence of an activation of NMDA channels and NK1 receptors is stronger than the action of NO in this respect.

The role of NO in nociception and pain is controversial in the literature; some groups regard it as a pronociceptive (pain-promoting) and some as an antinociceptive (pain-inhibiting) agent. Recently, our group was able to present data that may resolve at least some of the discrepancies in the literature. The data show that NO and cGMP (cyclic guanosine monophospate, a second messenger that needs NO for synthesis) have different actions at the spinal and supraspinal level. When administered selectively at the supraspinal level, NO and cGMP were found to be pronociceptive in animal experiments (they increased the activity of nociceptive neurons), and when applied spinally, antinociceptive (Hoheisel et al., 2005b). If blockers of the NO synthesis such as L-NAME are administered systemically, apparently the supraspinal antinociceptive action prevails. This may explain why NOS-blocking drugs can be used to alleviate hyperalgesia.

Other explanations of the seeming discrepancy in the published literature are that NO has different actions on neurons in different locations of the spinal gray matter (Pehl & Schmidt, 1997), that it sensitizes nociceptive neurons to external stimuli (Lin et al., 1999) but inhibits background activity (our results), or that low doses of NO reduce, and high doses increase, allodynia and hyperalgesia in animal experiments (Sousa & Prado, 2001).

The Role of Glial Cells in Central Sensitization

It has long been known that in the CNS the number of glial cells (astrocytes, oligodendrocytes, and microglia) is approximately 10 times greater than that of neurons. Only recently, however, has the involvement of glial cells in pain mechanisms been appreciated. The oligodendrocytes do not appear to be of importance for nociception and central sensitization, but microglia (immunocompetent brain macrophages) and astrocytes have been shown to be activated by peripheral pathologic changes, including inflammation (Dong & Benveniste, 2001; Watkins & Maier, 2002). The phrase "activation of glial cells" describes mainly changes in the metabolism of the cells and in addition morphologic changes that concern the length and arborization of the dendritic processes of these cells. Activated glia release cytokines such as proinflammatory interleukins, tumor necrosis factor alpha (TNF-α), NO, prostaglandins, ATP, and brain-derived neurotrophic factor (BDNF) in the CNS. These substances can sensitize sensory neurons; that is, they increase central neuronal excitability. Altogether these changes are called neuroinflammation; they are considered to be a central part of central sensitization (Hunt & Mantyh, 2001; Marchand et al., 2005).

After a chronic inflammation (12 days' duration) of the rat GS muscle, astrocytes in the dorsal horn exhibited a rounder shape in the morphologic evaluation; apparently, they had retracted some of their processes. In addition they showed an increase in the content of the characteristic intermediary filament, the glial fibrillary acidic protein (GFAP), and synthesized more fibroblast growth factor 2 (FGF2) as signs of an activation (Tenschert et al., 2004). Activated astrocytes are known to be capable of releasing proinflammatory cytokines such as interleukin 6 and TNF-α and therefore may contribute to the myositis-induced sensitization of nociceptive dorsal horn neurons (Dong & Benveniste, 2001; Kostrzewa & Segura-Aguilar, 2003). More recent data from our group showed that microglial cells are also activated by a chronic experimental myositis; they likewise exhibited a rounder shape with fewer arborizations. Blocking the microglia for the entire duration of the myositis with minocycline normalized the reduced exploratory activity of awake myositis rats almost completely (D. Lambertz, U. Hoheisel, and S. Mense, unpublished data) (**Figure 4.4**).

Central Sensitization Induced by Nerve Growth Factor

Nerve growth factor is not only a neurotrophic substance in the nervous system but is also synthesized in muscle and represents a major sensitizing substance for nociceptors in pathologically altered tissue (Pezet & McMahon, 2006). The action of NGF as a stimulant for muscle nociceptors has been studied with intramuscular injections in humans. The growth factor had peculiar properties in that it did not evoke any sensation upon injection but induced a sensitization of the injected muscle that lasted for more than a week. The sensitization was associated with muscle allodynia and hyperalgesia (Svensson et al., 2003b). At the time of the study, it was unknown whether the sensitization was due to peripheral or central processes, or whether both contributed to the effect.

Although the intramuscular injection of NGF did not evoke immediate pain, recent rat experiments of our group showed that NGF injected into the GS muscle excited a large proportion of group IV muscle afferents. All activated receptors had a high mechanical stimulation threshold and were assumed to be nociceptors (Hoheisel et al., 2005a). Despite the strong excitation of muscle nociceptors, rats did not show any pain-related behavior during NGF injection into the GS muscle. One possible explanation for the lack of pain is that the NGF-induced input excited just a few spinal neurons at a low frequency or evoked mainly subthreshold synaptic potentials in dorsal horn neurons. This hypothesis was tested in our group by recording intracellularly the reactions of dorsal horn neurons to NGF injections into the GS. Intracellular recordings were required because only with this technique can subthreshold synaptic potentials be seen. The results supported the working hypothesis, as NGF elicited mainly subthreshold synaptic potentials in dorsal horn neurons. Only a few neurons fired action potentials at a low frequency (Graven-Nielsen et al., 2006; Hoheisel et al., 2007). In superficial dorsal horn neurons, low-frequency stimulation of afferent C fibers also has been reported to induce long-term potentiation (Ikeda et al., 2006). In these cells, Ca^{2+} is mobilized from intracellular stores during low-level presynaptic activation, which then could lead to a sensitization (see above).

These NGF effects at the spinal level may explain why human subjects and our experimental animals did not have subjective sensations when the growth factor was injected: the spinal activity level was too low to excite higher nociceptive centers, and therefore the excitation was "stuck" in the dorsal horn. However, the long-lasting allodynia and hyperalgesia following intramuscular NGF injection raised the question of whether low-frequency activation or even subthreshold potentials in dorsal

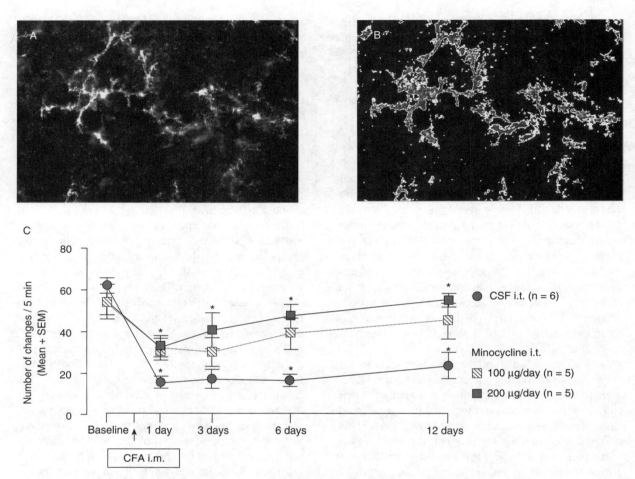

Figure 4.4 Microglia and Myositis-Induced Reduction in Exploratory Behavior. A: Visualization of rat microglial cells in the spinal dorsal horn with fluorescent antibodies to a surface molecule of the microglia cell membrane. The white network is formed by the processes of the microglial cells. **B:** Evaluation of panel **A** with image analyzing software that outlines the boundaries of the immunostained cells. After 12 days of a chronic myositis, the length of the microglia boundaries was decreased, indicating that the microglia had retracted their processes as a sign of activation. **C:** Results from behavioral experiments on rats after induction of a chronic myositis in the gastrocnemius-soleus (GS) muscle with intramuscular injections of complete Freund's adjuvant (CFA). The results were obtained in a test of spontaneous locomotion, in which the animals explored a large cage, the bottom of which was divided into squares. On the ordinate, the number of changes between the squares is shown. Before the test, the rats had been implanted with a subcutaneous osmotic pump that contained either artificial cerebrospinal fluid (CSF, vehicle), or minocycline (a blocker of microglia) at two concentrations. The pump delivered the fluids intrathecally (i.t.) through a catheter. After CFA, the exploratory movements were significantly reduced for the entire period of the experiments (filled circles). Minocycline (hatched and filled squares) led to a slow normalization of the exploratory activity. The data show that the reduction in exploratory locomotion was largely due to a myositis-induced activation of the microglia.

Source: Courtesy of S. Mense.

horn neurons are sufficient to sensitize the cells. In the literature there are many studies on the sensitization of CNS neurons, and in these studies generally high-frequency electrical stimulation (around 100 Hz) was used to induce long-term potentiation, a long-lasting increase in neuronal excitability after a single bout of stimuli. Low-frequency stimulation, on the other hand,

was reported to induce mainly long-term depression or depotentiation, a long-lasting decrease in excitability (Froc & Racine, 2005; Ikeda et al., 2006). Recently, the sensitizing action of low-frequency stimulation has attracted more interest. In rat slices of the hippocampus in vitro, low-frequency stimulation at 1 Hz was found to induce a novel form of long-term potentiation characterized by slow onset and independence from activation of NMDA receptors (Lante et al., 2006).

In intracellular recordings of dorsal horn neurons, the first signs of sensitization were seen already a few minutes after NGF injection into the GS muscle. Neurons that had reacted to electrical stimulation of the GS muscle nerve with subthreshold potentials before NGF injection fired action potentials after NGF. Because electrical stimulation was used, the possibly sensitized muscle nociceptors were not involved: the observed effect must have been due to an increase of the excitability of the recorded dorsal horn neurons—that is, to central sensitization. In studies on NGF-induced sensitization in rat and mouse, an early allodynia/hyperalgesia has likewise been reported (Malik-Hall et al., 2005; Hathway & Fitzgerald, 2006).

In clinical muscle pain research, hypertonic saline (5%) is a well-established pain stimulus. It causes immediate pain of moderate intensity when injected intramuscularly (Capra and Ro, 2004; Schmidt-Hansen et al., 2006). For rat group IV receptors from muscle, NaCl 5% is likewise a strong stimulus, but it differs from NGF in that it excites not only nociceptors but also low-threshold mechanosensitive free nerve endings that presumably do not have a nociceptive function (Hoheisel et al., 2004). Thus, the spectrum of afferent fibers excited by NGF and hypertonic saline is different. In our group, we have tested the sensitizing action of both NGF and 5% saline on dorsal horn neurons. In contrast to NGF, the same amount of hypertonic saline injected into the GS excited many dorsal horn neurons at a high frequency.

One day after NGF injection into the GS, the proportion of dorsal horn neurons responding with action potentials to electrical stimulation of the GS muscle nerve had increased significantly. In contrast, in rats that had been treated with an injection of NaCl 5% 1 day prior to testing, the dorsal horn neurons just showed an insignificant increase in the electrically induced responses (Hoheisel et al., 2007). This smaller sensitizing effect of hypertonic saline was surprising, because it elicited much stronger responses in dorsal horn neurons. The strong sensitizing action of NGF—which must be due mainly to subthreshold potentials, because only a few neurons fired action potentials—may indicate that conscious sensations are not required for a sensitizing effect of peripheral stimulation.

As pointed out earlier, the action of NGF on muscle free nerve endings is unique in that it excites exclusively nociceptive units (Hoheisel et al., 2005a). Nociceptive

afferent fibers from muscle and other tissues have been shown to possess tetrodotoxin-resistant Na$^+$ channels (Akopian et al., 1999; Steffens et al., 2003). Fibers equipped with these channels appear to carry information to the spinal cord that is particularly effective in sensitizing sensory neurons. In contrast, intramuscular NaCl 5% excited both nociceptive and nonnociceptive group IV units (Hoheisel et al., 2004). Therefore, the overall input to the spinal cord evoked by NaCl 5% is different from that elicited by NGF and includes also nonnociceptive fibers.

One possible explanation for the greater sensitizing action of NGF on central neurons in comparison with hypertonic saline is that the simultaneous input in nonnociceptive group IV units elicited by hypertonic saline has an inhibitory action on the sensitizing effects of the nociceptive NGF-induced input.

In behavioral experiments in which mechanical stimulation of the GS muscle was used to study allodynic and hyperalgesic effects of NGF in comparison with NaCl 5%, the sensitizing action of NGF was likewise much stronger. In these experiments, the NGF-induced sensitization involved the activation of NMDA ion channels, because the simultaneous injection of NGF and ketamine—a noncompetitive antagonist of the NMDA receptor—into the GS prevented the NGF-induced allodynia and hyperalgesia to mechanical stimulation. Because the muscle was mechanically stimulated in these experiments, peripheral sensitization may have been involved. However, recent recordings from single GS group IV fibers showed that the peripheral sensitization after intramuscular NGF took 5 days to fully develop. Therefore, the main sensitizing effects of NGF observed in the behavioral experiments must have been central.

The sensitizing action of low-frequency input to the CNS—such as induced by NGF—may be of particular importance for the development of chronic muscle pain, because painful conditions of muscle tissue are typically associated with low-frequency (and not high-frequency) activation of nociceptors. For instance, in inflamed muscle, free nerve endings with group IV afferent fibers—most of which are nociceptors—were shown to have an average discharge frequency of less than 1 Hz (Diehl et al., 1993). The sensitizing action of subthreshold or low-frequency spinal activity offers an intriguing explanation for some chronic muscle pain syndromes such as work-related musculoskeletal disorders (Novak, 2004; Sbriccoli et al., 2004) that are not well understood at present. It is conceivable that persons who perform tonic contractions with the same muscle or muscle compartments at low force repeatedly (e.g., musicians) develop microtraumas in the overused muscle. The microtraumas may elicit subthreshold potentials or low-frequency discharges at the spinal level. Apparently, these potentials do not evoke subjective sensations in the beginning but sensitize central neurons. If the work is continued, the central sensitization may develop into a chronic muscle pain syndrome. The danger of developing a work-related muscle disorder is particularly great if the work has to be performed under time pressure and psychic stress (Clays et al., 2007). This may be because under these circumstances the muscles or parts of a muscle are contracted involuntarily in an uncoordinated way.

THE TRANSITION FROM ACUTE TO CHRONIC MUSCLE PAIN

The above-discussed neuroplastic changes in the CNS are an important step in the transition from acute to chronic pain because they can persist under unfavorable circumstances. Another step in the direction of chronic pain is lesion-induced metabolic changes in sensory spinal neurons. An example of such metabolic changes is data from cells that synthesize NO. These cells can be visualized histologically using histochemical or immunohistochemical techniques.

In spinal cord sections from animals with an acute myositis (10 hours' duration), the number of cells with NOS immunoreactivity (cells that could be visualized with antibodies to the enzyme that synthesizes NO) was significant increased. However, after a chronic myositis (12 days' duration), the cell number was decreased. Apparently, the afferent input from a chronically inflamed muscle reduces the NOS activity in dorsal horn cells. The NO-synthesizing neurons behave like a sensor for peripheral lesions and signal a chronic painful lesion by a decrease in NOS activity. Because a lack of NO in the spinal cord has been shown to increase the resting activity in nociceptive dorsal horn neurons (see above and Hoheisel et al., 2000), the reduction in the number of NO-synthesizing neurons may be responsible for the spontaneous muscle pain or dysesthesia in patients.

The last step in the transition from acute to chronic muscle pain is morphologic changes in the circuitry of the spinal dorsal horn or brainstem. These changes consist of sprouting of the spinal terminals of afferent fibers and of de novo formation and broadening of synaptic contacts (Sperry & Goshgarian, 1993). Through these structural alterations, the initially functional changes become permanent, and the function of the spinal cord is persistently altered.

Other data indicate that hyperexcitability of neurons and chronic pain can also be induced through the mechanism of excitotoxicity (Yezierski et al., 1998). Excitotoxicity means that a strong nociceptive input releases large amounts of SP and glutamate simultaneously. This leads to simultaneous opening of all calcium-permeable ion channels. The postsynaptic cells are swamped with Ca^{2+}, which activates all enzymes that are present in the cytoplasm. Among these enzymes are some that are dangerous for the cell because they activate the genetic mechanism for the programmed cell death (apoptosis). This can lead to disintegration of the cell. An important aspect of this mechanism is that inhibitory interneurons are particularly sensitive to excitotoxicity. Normally, these interneurons depress tonically the activity of nociceptive central neurons. Therefore, after excitotoxic death of the interneurons, this region of the spinal cord is devoid of tonic inhibition, and the nociceptive neurons in that area are chronically disinhibited and hyperactive. This mechanism may be of importance for patients who develop fibromyalgia pain after a whiplash injury. Actually, more than 20% of these patients were reported to develop fibromyalgia (Buskila et al., 1997).

MECHANISMS OF REFERRAL OF MUSCLE PAIN

Referral of pain means that the patient feels pain not only at the site of the lesion but also at a distance from the lesion. Sometimes, only the referred pain is present. Referral of pain is typical of muscle pain and does not occur in cutaneous pain. The mechanisms underlying pain referral are still unsolved. The expansion of the excitation in the spinal cord observed in rats with an inflammatory lesion of a skeletal muscle may be one of these mechanisms (Hoheisel et al., 1994a). The processes evoked in the spinal cord by the peripheral muscle lesion may be as follows: When a muscle is damaged, the patient will first perceive local pain at the site of the lesion. If the nociceptive input from the muscle has a long duration or includes mainly afferent fibers with TTX-resistant sodium channels, central sensitization in the dorsal horn neurons is induced that opens silent synapses in adjacent segments and leads to an expansion of the muscle-induced excitation in the spinal cord or brainstem. As soon as the expansion reaches sensory neurons that supply peripheral areas other than the damaged muscle, the patient will feel pain in that area outside the initial pain site. It is important to note that in the area of pain referral no nociceptor is active, and the tissue is normal. The referral is simply due to the fact that the excitation induced by the original pain source spreads in the central nervous system and excites neurons that supply the body region in which the referred pain is felt. In this way a trigger point in the temporalis muscle can induce pain in the teeth of the maxilla when the trigger-point-induced central excitation spreads to sensory neurons that supply the teeth (Simons et al., 1999). For further explanation of muscle referred pain, see Chapter 5 of the current textbook.

CONCLUSIONS

The data obtained in studies on nociceptive nerve endings in muscle show that the sensitization of the endings following a muscle lesion is not an unspecific process, but is due to the binding of sensitizing agents (e.g., bradykinin, serotonin, E prostaglandins) to specific receptor molecules in the membrane of the muscle nociceptor. Of particular significance to headache patients with chronically increased EMG activity of their head muscles are the proton-sensitive receptor molecules (TRPV1 and ASICs) that are activated when the tissue pH is low. Tonic muscle contractions cause ischemia that is associated with a drop in pH. The pain in patients who present with clenching, bruxism, or tonic contraction of the temporal muscle may be partly due to the activation of the TRPV1 and ASIC receptors.

The transition from acute to chronic muscle pain is considered to consist of a series of processes that all start with the muscle lesion but have a different time course. Functional changes in the spinal or medullary dorsal horn are fastest; metabolic changes are slower. The slowest processes are morphologic alterations in neurons and glial cells. The lesion-induced structural reorganization of the CNS fixes the initially functional changes. It is generally assumed that all longer-lasting muscle lesions lead to such central nervous alterations. The fact that not all patients with muscle lesions become chronic pain patients can be explained by the complexity of the mechanisms involved (not all mechanisms are operative in all patients). Moreover, mechanisms that counteract the transition from acute to chronic pain also exist and vary in strength from patient to patient. One example is the descending antinociceptive system that originates in the brainstem and tonically inhibits the dorsal horn neurons at the origin of the spinothalamic tract. The main conclusion to be drawn from the presented data is to abolish the muscle pain as early and effectively as possible to prevent the central nervous reorganization.

REFERENCES

Akopian AN, Souslova V, England S, et al. The tetrodotoxin-resistant sodium channel SNS has a specialized function in pain pathways. *Nature Neurosci* 1999;2:541–548.

Burnstock G. P2X receptors in sensory neurones. *Br J Anaesth* 2000;84:476–488.

Buskila D, Neumann L, Vaisberg G. Increased rates of fibromyalgia following cervical spinal injury: a controlled study of 161 cases of traumatic injury. *Arthritis Rheum* 1997;40:446–452.

Cairns BE, Sessle BJ, Hu JW. Evidence that excitatory amino acid receptors within the temporomandibular joint region are involved in the reflex activation of the jaw muscles. *J Neurosci* 1998;18:8056–8064.

Capra NF, Ro JY. Human and animal experimental models of acute and chronic muscle pain: intramuscular algesic injection. *Pain* 2004;110:3–7.

Caterina MJ, David J. Sense and specificity: a molecular identity for nociceptors. *Curr Opin Neurobiol* 1999;9:525–530.

Caterina MJ, Julius D. The vanilloid receptor: a molecular gateway to the pain pathway. *Ann Rev Neurosci* 2001;24:487–517.

Clays E, De Bacquer D, Leynen F, et al. The impact of psychosocial factors on low back pain: longitudinal results from the Belstress study. *Spine* 2007;32:262–268.

Cook SP, McCleskey EW. Cell damage excites nociceptors through release of cytosolic ATP. *Pain* 2002;95:41–47.

Diehl B, Hoheisel U, Mense S. The influence of mechanical stimuli and of acetylsalicylic acid on the discharges of slowly conducting afferent units from normal and inflamed muscle in the rat. *Exp Brain Res* 1993;92:431–440.

Djouhri L, Lawson SN. Aβ-fiber nociceptive primary afferent neurons: a review of incidence and properties in relation to other afferent A-fiber neurons in mammals. *Brain Res Rev* 2004;46:131–145.

Dong Y, Benveniste EN. Immune functions of astrocytes. *Glia* 2001;36:180–190.

Fields HL, Basbaum AI. Central nervous system mechanisms of pain modulation. In: Wall PD, Melzack R, eds. *Textbook of Pain*. New York: Churchill Livingstone; 1999:309–329.

Froc DJ, Racine RJ. Interactions between LTP- and LTD-inducing stimulation in the sensorimotor cortex of the awake freely moving rat. *J Neurophysiol* 2005;93:548–556.

Graven-Nielsen T, Arendt-Nielsen L, Svensson P, Jensen T. Experimental muscle pain: a quantitative study of local and referred pain in humans following injection of hypertonic saline. *J Musculoskel Pain* 1997;5:49–69.

Graven-Nielsen T, Mense S, Arendt-Nielsen L. Painful and non-painful pressure sensations from human skeletal muscle. *Exp Brain Res* 2004;59:273–283.

Graven-Nielsen T, Curatolo M, Mense S. Central sensitization, referred pain, and deep tissue hyperalgesia in musculoskeletal pain. In: Flor H, Kalso E, Dostrovsky JO, eds. *Proceedings of the 11th World Congress on Pain*. Seattle: IASP Press; 2006:217–230.

Hathway GJ, Fitzgerald M. Time course and dose-dependence of nerve growth factor-induced secondary hyperalgesia in the mouse. *J Pain* 2006;7:57–61.

Hoheisel U, Mense S, Simons DG, Yu XM. Appearance of new receptive fields in rat dorsal horn neurons following noxious stimulation of skeletal muscle: a model for referral of muscle pain? *Neurosci Lett* 1993;153:9–12.

Hoheisel U, Koch K, Mense S. Functional reorganisation in the rat dorsal horn during an experimental myositis. *Pain* 1994a;59:111–118.

Hoheisel U, Mense S, Scherotzke R. Calcitonin gene-related peptide-immuno-reactivity in functionally identified primary afferent neurones in the rat. *Anat Embryol* 1994b;189:41–49.

Hoheisel U, Sander B, Mense S. Myositis-induced functional reorganisation of the rat dorsal horn: effects of spinal super-fusion with antagonists to neurokinin and glutamate receptors. *Pain* 1997;69:219–230.

Hoheisel U, Unger T, Mense S. A block of the nitric oxide synthesis leads to increased background activity predominantly in nociceptive dorsal horn neurons in the rat. *Pain* 2000;88:249–257.

Hoheisel U, Reinöhl J, Unger T, Mense S. Acidic pH and capsaicin activate mechano-sensitive group IV muscle receptors in the rat. *Pain* 2004;110:149–157.

Hoheisel U, Unger T, Mense S. Excitatory and modulatory effects of inflammatory cytokines and neurotrophins on mechano-sensitive group IV muscle afferents in the rat. *Pain* 2005a;114:168–176.

Hoheisel U, Unger T, Mense S. The possible role of the NO-cGMP pathway in nociception: different spinal and supra-spinal action of enzyme blockers on rat dorsal horn neurones. *Pain* 2005b;117:358–367.

Hoheisel U, Unger T, Mense S. Sensitization of rat dorsal horn neurones by NGF-induced sub-threshold potentials and low-frequency activation. A study employing intracellular recordings in vivo. *Brain Res* 2007;1169:34–43.

Hunt SP, Mantyh PW. The molecular dynamics of pain control. *Nature Rev Neurosci* 2001;2:83–91.

Ikeda H, Stark J, Fischer H, et al. Synaptic amplifier of inflammatory pain in the spinal dorsal horn. *Science* 2006;312:1659–1662.

Jarvis MF, Honore P, Shieh CC, et al. A-803467, a potent and selective Nav1.8 sodium channel blocker, attenuates neuropathic and inflammatory pain in the rat. *Proc Natl Acad Sci USA* 2007;15:8520–8525.

Jensen K, Tuxen C, Pedersen-Bjergaard U, Jansen I, Edvinsson L, Olesen J. Pain and tenderness in human temporal muscle induced by bradykinin and 5-hydroxytryptamine. *Peptides* 1990;11:1127–1132.

Kalia M, Mei SS, Kao FF. Central projections from ergoreceptors (C-fibers) in muscle involved in cardiopulmonary responses to static exercise. *Circ Res* 1981;48:148–162.

Kaufman MP, Rybicki KJ, Waldrop TG. Effect of ischemia on responses of group III and IV afferents to contraction. *J Appl Physiol* 1984;57:644–650.

Keay KA, Bandler R. Deep and superficial noxious stimulation increases Fos-like immunoreactivity in different regions of the midbrain periaqueductal grey of the rat. *Neurosci Lett* 1993;154:23–26.

Kniffki K, Mense S, Schmidt RF. Responses of group IV afferent units from skeletal muscle to stretch, contraction and chemical stimulation. *Exp Brain Res* 1978;31:511–522.

Kostrzewa RM, Segura-Aguilar J. Novel mechanisms and approaches in the study of neurodegeneration and neuroprotection. A review. *Neurotox Res* 2003;5:375–383.

Kumazawa T. The polymodal receptor: bio-warning and defense system. In: Kumazawa T, Kruger L, Mizumura K, eds. *Progress in Brain Research*. Vol. 113. Amsterdam: Elsevier Science; 1996:3–18.

Kumazawa T, Mizumura K. The polymodal C-fiber receptor in the muscle of the dog. *Brain Res* 1976;101:589–593.

Kumazawa T, Mizumura K. Thin-fiber receptors responding to mechanical, chemical and thermal stimulation in the skeletal muscle of the dog. *J Physiol* 1977;273:179–194.

Lante F, Cavalier M, Cohen-Solal C, Guiramand J, Vignes M. Developmental switch from LTD to LTP in low frequency-induced plasticity. *Hippocampus* 2006;16:981–989.

Lawson SN, Crepps BA, Perl ER. Relationship of substance P to afferent characteristics of dorsal root ganglion neurons in guinea-pig. *J Physiol* 1997;505:177–191.

Leah JD, Cameron AA, Snow PJ. Neuropeptides in physiologically identified mammalian sensory neurones. *Neurosci Lett* 1985;56:257–263.

Li P, Zhuo M. Silent glutamatergic synapses and nociception in mammalian spinal cord. *Nature* 1998;393:695–698.

Liedtke WB. TRPV4 plays an evolutionary conserved role in the transduction of osmotic and mechanical stimuli in live animals. *J Physiol* 2005;567:53–58.

Light AR, Perl ER. Unmyelinated afferent fibers are not only for pain anymore. *J Comp Neurol* 2003;461:137–139.

Lin Q, Wu J, Peng YB, Cui M, Willis WD. Nitric oxide-mediated spinal disinhibition contributes to the sensitization of primate spinothalamic tract neurons. *J Neurophysiol* 1999;81:1086–1094.

Liu XG, Sandkühler J. Activation of spinal N-methyl-D-aspartate or neurokinin receptors induces long-term potentiation of spinal C-fibre-evoked potentials. *Neuroscience* 1998;86:1209–1216.

Lloyd DPC. Neuron patterns controlling transmission of ipsilateral hind limb reflexes in cat. *J Neurophysiol* 1943;6:293–315.

Malik-Hall M, Dina OA, Levine JD. Primary afferent nociceptor mechanisms mediating NGF-induced mechanical hyperalgesia. *Eur J Neurosci* 2005;21: 3387–3394.

Marchand F, Perretti M, McMahon SB. Role of the immune system in chronic pain. *Nature Rev Neurosci* 2005;6: 521–532.

Marchettini P, Simone DA, Caputi G, Ochoa JL. Pain from excitation of identified muscle nociceptors in humans. *Brain Res* 1996;40:109–116.

McCleskey EW, Gold MS. Ion channels of nociception. *Ann Rev Physiol* 1999;61:835–856.

McCloskey DI, Mitchell JH. Reflex cardiovascular and respiratory responses originating in exercising muscle. *J Physiol* 1972;224:173–186.

Mense S. Sensitization of group IV muscle receptors to bradykinin by 5-hydroxytryptamine and prostaglandin E_2. *Brain Res* 1981;225:95–105.

Mense S. Pathophysiologic basis of muscle pain syndromes. *Phys Med Rehab Clin North Am* 1997;8:23–53.

Mense S. Muscle nociceptors and their neurochemistry. In: Schmidt RF, Willis WD, eds. *Encyclopedic Reference of Pain.* Berlin: Springer; 2007:1203–1207.

Mense S, Meyer H. Different types of slowly conducting afferent units in cat skeletal muscle and tendon. *J Physiol* 1985;363:403–417.

Mense S, Simons DG. *Muscle Pain: Understanding Its Nature, Diagnosis and Treatment.* Baltimore: Lippincott, Williams & Wilkins; 2001.

Mense S, Stahnke M. Responses in muscle afferent fibres of slow conduction velocity to contractions and ischaemia in the cat. *J Physiol* 1983;342:383–397.

Millan MJ. The induction of pain: an integrative review. *Prog Neurobiol* 1999;57:1–164.

Molander C, Ygge I, Dalsgaard CJ. Substance P-, somatostatin-, and calcitonin gene-related peptide-like immunoreactivity and fluoride resistant acid phosphatase-activity in relation to retrogradely labeled cutaneous, muscular and visceral primary sensory neurons in the rat. *Neurosci Lett* 1987;74:37–42.

Mörk H, Ashina M, Bendtsen L, Olesen J, Jensen R. Experimental muscle pain and tenderness following infusion of endogenous substances in humans. *Eur J Pain* 2003;7:145–153.

Novak CB. Upper extremity work-related musculoskeletal disorders: a treatment perspective. *J Orthop Sports Phys Ther* 2004;34:628–637.

O'Brien C, Woolf CJ, Fitzgerald M, Lindsay RM, Molander C. Differences in the chemical expression of rat primary afferent neurons which innervate skin, muscle or joint. *Neuroscience* 1989;32:493–502.

Pehl U, Schmidt HA. Electrophysiological responses of neurons in the rat spinal cord to nitric oxide. *Neuroscience* 1997;77:563–573.

Perkins MN, Kelly D. Induction of bradykinin-B1 receptors in vivo in a model of ultra-violet irradiation-induced thermal hyperalgesia in the rat. *Br J Pharmacol* 1993;110: 1441–1444.

Pezet S, McMahon SB. Neurotrophins: mediators and modulators of pain. *Annu Rev Neurosci* 2006;29:507–538.

Reinert A, Kaske A, Mense S. Inflammation-induced increase in the density of neuropeptide-immunoreactive nerve endings in rat skeletal muscle. *Exp Brain Res* 1998;121: 174–180.

Reinöhl J, Hoheisel U, Unger T, Mense S. Adenosine triphosphate as a stimulant for nociceptive and non-nociceptive muscle group IV receptors in the rat. *Neurosci Lett* 2003;338:25–28.

Sbriccoli P, Solomonow M, Zhour BH, Baratta RV, Lu Y, Zhu MP, Burger EL. Static load repetition is a risk factor in the development of lumbar cumulative musculoskeletal disorder. *Spine* 2004;29:2643–2653.

Schmidt-Hansen PT, Svensson P, Jensen TS, Graven-Nielsen T, Bach FW. Patterns of experimentally induced pain in pericranial muscles. *Cephalalgia* 2006;26:568–577.

Simons DG, Travell JG, Simons LS. *Travell and Simons' Myofascial Pain and Dysfunction: The Trigger Point Manual.* Vol. 1. *Upper Half of Body.* 2nd ed. Baltimore: Williams and Wilkins; 1999.

Sluka KA, Jordan HH, Westlund KN. Reduction in joint swelling and hyperalgesia following post-treatment with a non-NMDA glutamate receptor antagonist. *Pain* 1994;59: 95–100.

Sluka KA, Kalra A, Moore SA. Unilateral intramuscular injections of acidic saline produce a bilateral long-lasting hyperalgesia. *Muscle Nerve* 2001;24:37–46.

Sousa AM, Prado WA. The dual effect of a nitric oxide donor in nociception. *Brain Res* 2001;897:9–19.

Sperry MA, Goshgarian HG. Ultrastructural changes in the rat phrenic nucleus developing within 2 h after cervical spinal cord hemisection. *Exp Neurol* 1993;120:233–244.

Stacey MJ. Free nerve endings in skeletal muscle of the cat. *J Anat* 1969;105:231–254.

Steffens H, Eek B, Trudrung P, Mense S. Tetrodotoxin block of A-fibre afferents from skin and muscle: a tool to study pure C-fibre effects in the spinal cord. *Pflügers Arch Eur J Physiol* 2003;445:607–613.

Svensson P, Minoshima S, Beydoun A, Morrow TJ. Cerebral processing of acute skin and muscle pain in humans. *J Neurophysiol* 1997;78:450–460.

Svensson P, Cairns BE, Wang K, et al. Glutamate-evoked pain and mechanical allodynia in the human masseter muscle. *Pain* 2003a;101:221–227.

Svensson P, Cairns BE, Wang K, Arendt-Nielsen L. Injection of nerve growth factor into human masseter muscle evokes long-lasting mechanical allodynia and hyperalgesia. *Pain* 2003b;104:241–247.

Tegeder L, Zimmermann J, Meller ST, Geisslinger G. Release of algesic substances in human experimental muscle pain. *Inflamm Res* 2002;51:393–402.

Tenschert S, Reinert A, Hoheisel U, Mense S. Effects of a chronic myositis on structural and functional features of spinal astrocytes in the rat. *Neurosci Lett* 2004;361: 196–199.

Usunoff KG, Popratiloff A, Schmitt O, Wree A. Functional anatomy of pain. *Adv Anat Embryol Cell Biol* 2006;184: 1–115.

Wall PD, Woolf CJ. Muscle but not cutaneous C-afferent input produces prolonged increases in the excitability of the flexion reflex in the rat. *J Physiol* 1984;356: 443–458.

Watkins LR, Maier SF. Glia: a novel drug discovery target for clinical pain. *Nat Rev Drug Discov* 2002;2:973–985.

Yezierski RP, Liu S, Ruenes GL, Kajander KJ, Brewer KL. Excitotoxic spinal cord injury: behavioral and morphological characteristics of a central pain model. *Pain* 1998;75: 141–155.

Yu XM, Mense S. Response properties and descending control of rat dorsal horn neurons with deep receptive fields. *Neuroscience* 1990;39:823–831.

Pathophysiology of Referred Muscle Pain

Lars Arendt-Nielsen, DMSci, PhD, and Hong-You Ge, MD, PhD

REFERRED MUSCLE PAIN

Referred pain has been known and described for more than a century and has been used extensively as a diagnostic tool in the clinic. Originally the term *referred tenderness and pain* was used. Pain from deep structures such as muscle, joints, ligaments, tendons, and viscera is typically described as deep, diffuse, and difficult to locate precisely, in contrast to superficial types of pain, such as skin and mucosal pain (Bonica, 1990; Lewis, 1938; Mense, 1994). Pain located at the source of pain is termed *local pain* or *primary pain*, whereas pain felt in a different region away from the source of pain is termed *referred pain* (Bonica, 1990). Sometimes referred muscle pain dominates the clinical pain symptoms; the perceived localization of deep pain might be different from the original source of pain.

Pain drawings can be valuable tools for illustrating the localization and extent of muscle pain areas (Escalante et al., 1996; Margolis et al., 1988; Fernández-de-las-Peñas et al., 2007), although the perceived size of body areas is variable and can be influenced by pain-induced changes in central somatosensory maps (Gandevia & Phegan, 1999). Pain drawings have so far not been used on a regular basis in clinical research conducted on myofascial pain syndrome. A few studies have applied systematic pain maps to patients with myofascial pain in the trigeminal region (Gray, 1986; Hagberg, 1991; Turp et al., 1998). Use of pain drawings in both clinical diagnosis and research settings could provide a more detailed description of referred pain patterns in patients with local myofascial pain and generalized fibromyalgia syndrome, and help to find the main myofascial trigger points (MTrPs) that are responsible for patients' pain complaints.

CLINICAL SIGNIFICANCE OF REFERRED MUSCLE PAIN

It is a common clinical experience that referred muscle pain could be the main complaint in patients with chronic tension-type headache (CTTH), in which pain in the craniofacial area could be referred from active TrPs in the neck and shoulder muscles (Simons et al., 1999; Fernández-de-las-Peñas et al., 2007). For example, headache pain could be referred from active TrPs in the upper trapezius muscle, sternocleidomastoid, the levator scapulae, and supraspinatus muscle. Another typical example is pain deep in the shoulder joint, posterior deltoid region, and upper arm, which could be referred from active TrPs in the ipsilateral infraspinatus muscle (Simons et al., 1999; Ge et al., 2006). In these two circumstances, patients feel referred pain as their pain complaints; they do not feel pain at the local area where active TrPs harbor.

Under these circumstances, screening the active TrPs responsible for the patient's main complaint is a challenging process. Good clinical skills in muscle palpation are needed to reliably identify TrPs from which the pain emanates. The common manifestations of this syndrome can be identified and treated with limited training, but the more complex and esoteric presentations require detailed knowledge of functional anatomy and factors that perpetuate the condition. A further challenge to this process is the fact that in some chronic musculoskeletal pain patients, a patient's pain complaints or referred pain pattern could be a summation of referred pains from several muscles and that active TrPs in the upper body regions can refer pain to more distal regions, such as the lower body parts (**Figure 5.1**). Therefore, a further insight into the neuropathophysiology of referred muscle pain would enhance the correct diagnosis and treatment of muscle TrPs and provide a theoretical basis for the development of therapeutic modalities.

Clinical Characteristics of Referred Muscle Pain

1. Referred muscle pain is evoked by direct stimulation of a TrP within a taut muscle band.

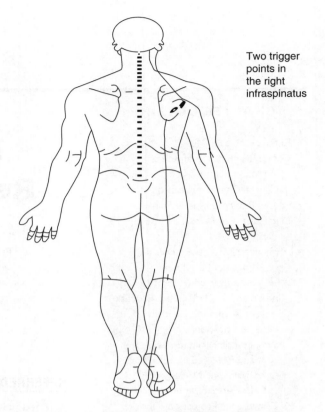

Two trigger points in the right infraspinatus

Figure 5.1 Body Chart Showing the Referred Pain Pattern from Two Trigger Points in the Right Infraspinatus Muscle

2. The duration of referred muscle pain could last for as short as a few seconds or as long as a few hours or days, presenting as spontaneous pain.
3. The quality of referred muscle pain has the characteristics of muscle pain rather than neuropathic pain and can be felt in the deep tissue or superficially in the skin.
4. Referred muscle pain may have rostral or caudal propagation depending on the location of the TrP.
5. The referred pain intensity and referred pain area are positively correlated with the degree of TrP activity.
6. Referred muscle pain is usually accompanied by other symptoms, such as numbness, coldness, stiffness, weakness of the body parts, and general motor dysfunction (stiffness and restricted range of motion).
7. Inactivation of active TrPs would effectively relieve referred muscle pain.

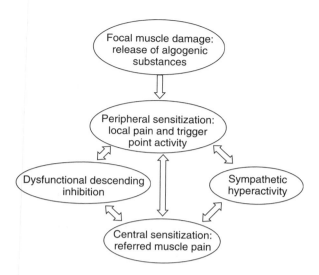

Figure 5.2 Mechanisms of Referred Muscle Pain

MECHANISMS OF REFERRED MUSCLE PAIN

Referred muscle pain is a process of central sensitization that is mediated by a peripheral activity and sensitization and can be facilitated by sympathetic activity and dysfunctional descending inhibition (**Figure 5.2**).

Myofascial Trigger Point Is a Focus of Peripheral Sensitization (Allodynia)

Local muscle pain is known to be associated with the activation of muscle nociceptors by a variety of endogenous substances, including neuropeptides, arachidonic acid derivatives, and inflammatory mediators, among others. Many kinds of algogenic substances have been used intramuscularly to induce local and referred pain. The most commonly used method is intramuscular infusion of hypertonic saline (6%). Kellgren and Lewis introduced the method in 1938 (Kellgren, 1938; Lewis, 1938), and intramuscular infusion of hypertonic saline subsequently has been used extensively (for review, Arendt-Nielsen et al., 2000; Arendt-Nielsen & Svensson, 2001; Graven-Nielsen, 2006). A variety of parameters have been shown to correlate with the infusion of hypertonic saline (e.g., saline concentration, infusion rate and pressure, and amount of saline infused) (Graven-Nielsen et al., 1997a, 1997b; Vecchiet et al., 1993). Infusion of hypertonic saline has several advantages. It is easy and safe to use, and it induces local and referred muscle pain in most individuals (40% to 85%), depend-

ing on the actual muscle of injection (Graven-Nielsen et al., 1997a, 1997b, 1997c; Vecchiet et al., 1993).

In recent years, more potent algogenic substances have been tested as muscle pain models. Bradykinin, serotonin, capsaicin (Witting et al., 2000), and substance P (Jensen et al., 1990; Babenko et al., 1999a, 1999b), glutamate (Svensson et al., 2003a), nerve growth factor (Svensson et al., 2003b), and acidic saline (Sluka et al., 2001) have been used separately or in combination to induce muscle pain. Injection of these substances into the muscle induced local and referred pain. The induced referred pain patterns have largely confirmed the referred pain patterns described in the *Trigger Point Manual* (Simons et al., 1999). In particular, repetitive intramuscular injections of glutamate (Svensson et al., 2003a; Ge et al., 2005), nerve growth factor (Svensson et al., 2003b), and acidic saline (Sluka et al., 2001) induced long-lasting primary hyperalgesia at the injection site. Hyperalgesia or decreased pain threshold within a muscle area is one of the clinical manifestations of TrPs.

It is interesting to note that more recent microdialysis studies show that concentrations of protons, bradykinin, calcitonin gene-related peptide, substance P, tumor necrosis factor alpha, interleukin-1β, serotonin, norepinephrine, and pH were found to be significantly higher in the active TrP than either the latent TrP or control nontrigger points. Furthermore, the concentrations of these substances are significantly lower after the induction of local twitch response (Shah et al., 2005). The intramuscular concentration of glutamate is also found to be higher in patients with trapezius myalgia compared with normal control subjects (Rosendal et al., 2004). These microdialysis studies further confirm that the human experimental models largely mimic the sensory manifestations of a TrP. All the above evidence suggests that there exists nociceptor hypersensivity at a TrP. Increased nociceptor sensitivity causes the local muscle tissue to respond to normally innocuous stimulation and perceive it as painful, presenting as muscle hyperalgesia or allodynia.

Referred Muscle Pain Is a Process of Reversible Central Sensitization

When the muscle is in the state of hyperalgesia or allodynia, the sensitized muscle nociceptors are more easily activated and may respond to normally innocuous and weak stimuli such as light pressure and muscle movement. The continued presence of hyperalgesia (involving temporal summation) and the presence of multiple trigger points (involving spatial summation) can sensitize the spinal cord and supraspinal structures by continued nociceptive afferent barrage to the central nervous system. The sensitized central nervous system (central sensitization) may modulate the manifestation of referred muscle pain. Ketamine (NMDA antagonist) infusion in patients with fibromyalgia has been shown to reduce the referred pain area (Graven-Nielsen et al., 2000).

Animal studies have found a development of new receptive fields via noxious muscle stimuli (Cook et al., 1987; Hoheisel et al., 1993). Recordings from a dorsal horn neuron with a receptive field located in the biceps femoral muscle indicated new receptive fields in the tibialis anterior muscle and in the paw after intramuscular injection of bradykinin into the tibialis anterior muscle. In the context of referred pain, revealing new receptive fields could be the mechanism behind referred pain because of central sensitization or hyperexcitability (Mense, 1994). The formation of new receptive fields has been suggested to be behind the phenomenon of secondary hyperalgesia in deep tissue. Similar findings are shown in humans after intradermal injection of capsaicin, in which a rapid development of central hyperexcitability (seen as secondary cutaneous hyperalgesia) is found (Witting et al., 2000). The time needed for revealing (in the range of seconds) may account for the time delay between local pain and the development of referred pain and for the increased number of individuals developing referred pain during repeated hypertonic saline infusions or tonic infusion (Graven-Nielsen et al., 1997b).

Several studies have found that the area of the referred pain correlated with the intensity and duration of the muscle pain (Graven-Nielsen et al., 1997b; Laursen et al., 1997; Inman & Saunders, 1944; Stohler & Lund, 1995). All the evidence suggests that referred muscle pain or central sensitization is maintained by peripheral sensitization or by active myofascial trigger points (MTrPs) in the muscle. It is necessary to point out that central sensitization is a reversible process in patients with local myofascial pain syndrome, although animal studies suggest that central sensitization is an irreversible process (Sluka et al., 2001). From the clinical point of view, the inactivation of active TrPs can effectively abolish the existence of referred muscle pain; thus, local myofascial pain syndrome is simply a curable disease. Evidence has shown that dry-needle-evoked inactivation of a primary (key) TrP inhibits the activity in

satellite TrPs situated in its zone of pain referral (Hsieh et al., 2007). Trigger point injection into neck muscles produces rapid relief of palpable scalp or facial tenderness (mechanical hyperalgesia and allodynia pain) and alleviates associated symptoms of nausea, photophobia, and phonophobia in patients with migrainous headache (Gary et al., 2003).

This evidence suggests that the central sensitization in local myofascial pain syndrome is a reversible process. Probably the degree of central sensitization in local myofascial pain syndrome is not as high as that in fibromyalgia or neuropathic pain syndromes, or the descending inhibitory control mechanisms are dysfunctional temporarily in local myofascial pain syndromes. A dysfunction of the descending inhibitory control system might have effects similar to those of a central sensitization state. In healthy subjects, generalized hypoalgesia to pressure is found during strong experimentally induced muscle pain. In contrast, fibromyalgia patients do not show such modulation, indicating a dysfunction of the descending inhibitory control system (Kosek & Hansson, 1997). The mechanism of descending inhibition is intact in short- and long-term osteoarthritis arthritis patients compared with control subjects (Kosek & Ordeberg, 2000). Before surgery (e.g., hip replacement), osteoarthritis patients lacked the generalized hypoalgesic effect to pressure during a strong experimental pain, in contrast to the normalized descending inhibition seen after hip surgery (Kosek & Ordeberg, 2000). This might indicate that the descending system is maximally involved in the condition with continuous pain (before surgery) and that after surgery the dynamic of the system is reestablished and effectively modulates the sensitivity to pressure. Thus, a dysfunction of the descending inhibitory control system might be involved in chronic muscle pain conditions.

Sympathetic Facilitation of Local and Referred Muscle Pain

Scientific evidence (Ge et al., 2006) suggests that TrP sensitivity is maintained by sympathetic outflow activity. The sympathetic nervous system has, under normal conditions, only minimal influence on sensory endings and on somatosensation (Janig et al., 1996; Bruce et al., 2002). However, under pathologic conditions a sympathetic-sensory and sympathetic-motor interaction can be established; thus, the increased sympathetic efferent discharge can facilitate mechanical hyperalgesia and allodynia and increase spontaneous electrical activity at TrPs.

The sympathetic contribution to deep tissue pain has long been recognized. Using deep tissue injury models, several studies do indicate the contribution of sympathetic activation to the symptoms of arthritis (Levine et al., 1986a) and muscle pain in animals (Gillette et al., 1994) and in human arthritis (Levine et al., 1986b; Gentili et al., 1996). Clinical studies suggest the involvement of sympathetic activity in tender points and TrPs (Bengtsson & Bengtsson, 1988; Martinez-Lavin, 2004). Evidence in rabbits (Chen et al., 1998) and in humans (McNulty et al., 1994; Hubbard, 1996; Chung et al., 2004) has shown sympathetic contribution to the modulation of spontaneous electrical activity at TrPs. Increased sympathetic efferent discharge increased both the frequency and the amplitude of spontaneous electrical activity of muscle TrPs, whereas sympathetic blocker decreased the frequency and amplitude of spontaneous electrical activity. Increased sympathetic efferent discharge has also been shown to increase TrP sensory sensitivity (Ge et al., 2006), and sympathetic blocker decreased the trigger point sensory sensitivity (Bengtsson & Bengtsson, 1988; Martinez-Lavin, 2004). These results correspond to the microdialysis study showing higher concentration of norepinephrine at active MTrPs (Shah et al., 2005).

Of particular interest is that increased referred pain intensity has been getting by sympathetic hyperactivity at muscle TrPs (Ge et al., 2006). This suggests sympathetic contribution to the mechanisms responsible for the generation of referred pain. Because pain perception and referred pain are a central sensitization process mediated by a peripheral sensitization (for a review see Arendt-Nielsen et al., 2000), the mechanism of sympathetic facilitation of referred pain may therefore involve specific peripheral, spinal, and supraspinal sensory and sympathetic structures. A study shows that sympathetic efferent discharge recruits neural structures throughout the rostrocaudal extent of the brain (Macefield et al., 2006). How the sensory and sympathetic systems interact in the central nervous system is unknown.

The above evidence laid the foundation to conclude that trigger point sensitivity is maintained by sympathetic hyperactivity. Currently, the mechanisms behind the sympathetic-sensory and sympathetic-motor coupling at TrPs are still unknown. Several mechanisms may be involved in this coupling process. One of the putative mechanisms is that increased sympathetic activity at TrPs enhances the sympathetic release of norepi-

nephrine and ATP, among others. These sympathetic transmitters have been shown to interact with nociceptors (Burnstock, 2002; Cook & McCleskey, 2002; Roatta et al., 2003), probably mediating the decreased pressure pain threshold at trigger point. Evidence has shown that both extracellular and endogenous ATP and other nucleotides have an important role in pain signaling at both the periphery and in the central nervous system and that they might be activated in chronic pathologic pain states, particularly in neuropathic and inflammatory pain (Inoue, 2007). Evidence also suggests that ATP and its receptors (P2X) on primary afferent neurons are involved in mechanical hyperalgesia in a rat model of muscle pain (Shinoda et al., 2008). Purinergic receptors may be of particular importance in muscle pain given that large amounts of ATP are released during muscle damage and that muscle nociceptive afferents can be activated by ATP (Reinohl et al., 2003). Furthermore, ATP provides a rapid (within seconds) nociceptive signal transmission (Cook & McCleskey, 2002); therefore, ATP is more likely one of the candidates involved in pressure-induced pain and referred pain at TrPs.

Another possible mechanism is that of an increased level of muscle sympathetic (vasoconstrictor) nerve activity (Macefield & Wallin, 1995). Increased vasoconstrictor activity may reduce the blood flow in the resting limb (Macefield & Wallin, 1995) and lead to delayed clearance of inflammatory substances and change the local chemical milieu at TrPs.

NEUROPHYSIOLOGIC MODELS FOR REFERRED PAIN

The exact neuropathways mediating referred muscle pain are still not clear. Several neuroanatomic and neurophysiologic theories regarding the appearance of referred pain have been suggested, and basically they state that nociceptive dorsal horn or brainstem neurons receive convergent inputs from various tissues. Consequently, higher centers cannot identify correctly the actual input source. Most recently the models have included newer theories in which sensitization of dorsal horn and brainstem neurons plays a central role.

Inman and Saunders (1944) systematically investigated the distribution of referred pain in relation to the activated muscle groups. Based on their observations, it was suggested that referred pain followed more frequently the distribution of sclerotomes (muscle, fascia, and bone) than the classic dermatomes. The neuropathways responsible for the mediation of referred pain are still unclear.

Convergent-Projection Theory

Ruch (1961) proposed that afferent fibers from different tissues converge onto common spinal neurons. The core of this suggestion is that the nociceptive activity from the spinal cord is misinterpreted as originating from other structures. This could explain the segmental nature of referred muscle pain and the increased referred pain intensity recorded when local muscle pain was intensified. It does not adequately explain, however, the apparent delay in the development of referred pain following onset of local pain (Graven-Nielsen et al., 1997a, 1997b). Referred pain has not been demonstrated to be a stereotyped bidirectional phenomenon (e.g., muscle pain in the anterior tibial muscle produces pain in the ventral part of the ankle, but the opposite condition has not been demonstrated). However, jaw muscle pain can be referred to the teeth, and tooth pain can be referred to the jaw muscles. Finally, the threshold for eliciting local and referred muscle pain is different (Laursen et al., 1998).

Convergence-Facilitation Theory

MacKenzie (1893) believed that viscera were totally insensitive and that nonnociceptive afferent input to the spinal cord created an irritable focus in the spinal cord. This focus would make other somatic inputs appear in an abnormal fashion and in some cases even be perceived as referred pain. The theory was not recognized, mainly because it did not accept true visceral pain. In recent years, however, MacKenzie's simple idea of an irritable focus has reclaimed awareness under another term—central sensitization. The somatosensory sensitivity changes reported in referred pain areas could in part be explained by similar mechanisms in the dorsal horn and brainstem neurons, and the delay in appearance of referred pain demonstrated in various studies (Graven-Nielsen et al., 1997a, 1997b) could also be explained because the creation of central sensitization may take time.

Axon-Reflex Theory

Bifurcation of afferents from two different tissues has been suggested as an explanation of referred pain (Sinclair et al., 1948). Although bifurcation of nociceptive afferents from different tissues (muscle and skin, and intervertebral discs and skin) exists, it is generally agreed that these types of neurons are rare (McMahon, 1994). Moreover, this theory cannot explain the time delay in the appearance of referred pain, the different thresholds required for eliciting local and referred muscle pain, and the somatosensory sensitivity changes associated with referred pain.

Thalamic-Convergence Theory

Theobald (1949) suggested that referred pain appeared as a summation of input from the injured area and the referred pain area within neurons in the brain, and not in the spinal cord. A study of referred pain in monkeys applying computer simulations has demonstrated several pathways, which converge on different subcortical and cortical neurons (Apkarian et al., 1995). Numerous experimental and clinical studies (e.g., Laursen et al., 1998) have documented pain reduction following anesthetization of a referred pain area. This finding suggests that peripheral processes contribute to referred pain, although central processes are assumed to be the most predominant.

Central Hyperexcitability Theory

The above theories do not account for all the characteristics of referred pain previously described in this chapter. Mense (1994) suggested an interesting theory, especially from a referred muscle pain point of view, which is known as the central hyperexcitability theory.

Recordings from dorsal horn neurons in animals have revealed that within minutes after noxious stimuli was applied to a receptive field in a muscle, new receptive fields at a distance from the original receptive field emerged (Hoheisel et al., 1993). That is, following nociceptive input, dorsal horn neurons that were previously responsive to only one area within a muscle began to respond to nociception from areas that previously had not provoked a response. The appearance of new receptive fields could indicate that latent convergent afferents on the dorsal horn neuron might be opened by noxious stimuli arising from muscle tissue (Mense, 1994), and that this facilitation of latent convergence connections could appear as referred pain. Recent observations from the same group have demonstrated that substance P released from the terminal ends of primary afferents plays a role in the connectivity in the dorsal horn. Furthermore, an expansion of the receptive fields proximal to the normal receptive field was found in a study in which experimental myositis was induced, and afterward application of antagonists to three different neurokinin receptors was effective in preventing the induced hyperexcitability (Sessle et al., 1986).

The central hyperexcitability theory is consistent with several of the characteristics of referred muscle pain (dependency on stimulus and a delay in appearance of referred pain compared with local pain). Nevertheless, if the emergence of new receptive fields is construed as the neurophysiologic basis for referred pain, the fact that such fields are sometimes *proximal* to a site of nociceptive input conflicts with the majority of studies on experimentally induced referred pain in healthy subjects (Arendt-Nielsen et al., 2000). These studies demonstrate the development of referred pain distal to a site of induced pain, but not proximal to it. Clinical studies looking at the spread of experimentally induced referred pain in patients suffering from whiplash syndrome, fibromyalgia, and tension-type headache have demonstrated proximal as well as distal referral of pain (Graven-Nielsen et al., 2000; Johansen et al., 1999; Fernández-de-las-Peñas et al., 2007). We have seen proximal spread of referred muscle pain in a few healthy volunteers following intramuscular injection of capsaicin. A possible explanation of the divergence between findings in healthy humans and those in people with clinically significant pain is that the preexisting pain in the latter might have induced a state of hyperexcitability in the spinal cord, resulting in proximal and distal referral compared with the predominant distal referral in healthy subjects.

The hyperexcitability theory is based on animal studies in which receptive fields appeared within minutes. This does not fit exactly with the development of referred pain in humans, which occurs within seconds. We think, however, that the idea of latent connections between dorsal horn neurons is convincing.

SUMMARY AND PERSPECTIVE

Referred muscle pain probably reflects a combination of peripheral and central sensitization facilitated by sympathetic hyperactivity and dysfunctional descending inhibitory mechanisms. It is still not clear which muscle afferents are involved in the mediation of referred muscle pain. As far as central processing is concerned, research conducted in relation to the central hypersensitivity theory supports the role of altered functioning in the dorsal horn as a contributor to referred pain. It is also likely that supraspinal mechanisms contribute to referred pain, although they have not been extensively studied. The molecular mechanisms of sympathetic facilitation of MTrP activity are still unknown. It is expected that a further elucidation of referred pain mechanisms would provide new approaches for the treatment of myofascial pain syndromes.

REFERENCES

Apkarian AV, Brüggemann J, Shi T, Airapetiam LR. A thalamic model for true and referred visceral pain. In: Gebhart GF, ed. *Visceral Pain: Progress in Pain Research and Management.* Seattle: IASP Press; 1995:217–259.

Arendt-Nielsen L, Svensson P. Referred muscle pain: basic and clinical findings. *Clin J Pain* 2001;17:11–19.

Arendt-Nielsen L, Laursen RJ, Drewes AM. Referred pain as an indicator for neural plasticity. *Prog Brain Res* 2000;129: 343–356.

Babenko V, Graven-Nielsen T, Svensson P, Drewes AM, Jensen TS, Arendt-Nielsen L. Experimental human muscle pain and muscular hyperalgesia induced by combinations of serotonin and bradykinin. *Pain* 1999a;82:1–8.

Babenko V, Graven-Nielsen T, Svensson P, Drewes AM, Jensen TS, Arendt-Nielsen L. Experimental human muscle pain induced by intra-muscular injections of bradykinin, serotonin, and substance P. *Eur J Pain* 1999b;3:93–102.

Bengtsson A, Bengtsson M. Regional sympathetic blockade in primary fibromyalgia. *Pain* 1988;33:161–167.

Bonica JJ. General considerations of acute pain. In: Bonica JJ, ed. *The Management of Pain.* 2nd ed. Philadelphia: Lea & Febiger; 1990:159–179.

Bruce S, Tack C, Patel J, Pacak K, Goldstein DS. Local sympathetic function in human skeletal muscle and adipose tissue assessed by microdialysis. *Clin Auton Res* 2002;12: 13–19.

Burnstock G. Structural and chemical organization of the autonomic neuro-effector system. In: Bolis CL, Licinio J, Govoni S, eds. *Handbook of the Autonomic Nervous System in Health and Disease.* New York: Marcel Dekker; 2002: 1–53.

Chen JT, Chen SM, Kuan TS, Chung KC, Hong CZ. Phentolamine effect on the spontaneous electrical activity of active loci in a myofascial trigger spot of rabbit skeletal muscle. *Arch Phys Med Rehabil* 1998;79:790–794.

Chung JW, Ohrbach R, McCall WD Jr. Effect of increased sympathetic activity on electrical activity from myofascial painful areas. *Am J Phys Med Rehabil* 2004;83:842–850.

Cook SP, McCleskey EW. Cell damage excites nociceptors through release of cytosolic ATP. *Pain* 2002;95:41–47.

Cook AJ, Woolf CJ, Wall PD, McMahon SB. Dynamic receptive field plasticity in rat spinal cord dorsal horn following C-primary afferent input. *Nature* 1987;325:151–153.

Escalante A, Lichtenstein MJ, Lawrence VA, Roberson M, Hazuda HP. Where does it hurt? Stability of recordings of pain location using the McGill Pain Map. *J Rheumatol* 1996;23:1788–1793.

Fernández-de-las-Peñas C, Ge HY, Arendt-Nielsen L, Cuadrado ML, Pareja JA. Referred pain from trapezius muscle trigger points shares similar characteristics with chronic tension type headache. *Eur J Pain* 2007;11:475–482.

Gandevia SC, Phegan CM. Perceptual distortions of the human body image produced by local anaesthesia, pain and cutaneous stimulation. *J Physiol* 1999;15:609–616.

Gary A, Mellick DO, Larry B, Mellick MD. Regional head and face pain relief following lower cervical intramuscular anesthetic injection. *Headache* 2003;43:1109–1111.

Ge HY, Madeleine P, Arendt-Nielsen L. Gender differences in pain modulation evoked by repeated injections of glutamate into the human trapezius muscle. *Pain* 2005;113:134–140.

Ge HY, Fernández-de-las-Peñas C, Arendt-Nielsen L. Sympathetic facilitation of hyperalgesia evoked from myofascial tender and trigger points in patients with unilateral shoulder pain. *Clin Neurophysiol* 2006;117: 1545–1550.

Gentili M, Juhel A, Bonnet F. Peripheral analgesic effect of intra-articular clonidine. *Pain* 1996;64:593–596.

Gillette RG, Kramis RC, Roberts WJ. Sympathetic activation of cat spinal neurons responsive to noxious stimulation of deep tissues in the low back. *Pain* 1994;56:31–42.

Graven-Nielsen T. Fundamentals of muscle pain, referred pain, and deep tissue hyperalgesia. *Scand J Rheumatol* 2006; 122(suppl):1–43.

Graven-Nielsen T, Arendt-Nielsen L, Svensson P, Jensen TS. Quantification of local and referred muscle pain in humans after sequential intra-muscular injections of hypertonic saline. *Pain* 1997a;69:111–117.

Graven-Nielsen T, McArdle A, Phoenix J, Arendt-Nielsen L, Jensen TS, Jackson MJ, Edwards RH. In vivo model of muscle pain: quantification of intramuscular chemical, electrical, and pressure changes associated with saline-induced muscle pain in humans. *Pain* 1997b;69: 137–143.

Graven-Nielsen T, Arendt-Nielsen L, Svensson P, Jensen TS. Stimulus response functions in areas with experimentally induced referred muscle pain: a psychophysical study. *Brain Res* 1997c;744:121–128.

Graven-Nielsen T, Aspegren-Kendall S, Henriksson KG, Bengtsson M, Sorensen J, Johnson A, Gerdle B, Arendt-Nielsen L. Ketamine attenuates experimental referred muscle pain and temporal summation in fibromyalgia patients. *Pain* 2000;85:483–491.

Gray RJ. How reliable is your patient? A comparison of subjective complaints and clinical findings in a group of temporomandibular joint patients. *J Dent* 1986;14:223–225.

Hagberg C. General musculoskeletal complaints in a group of patients with cranio-mandibular disorders (CMD). A case control study. *Swed Dent J* 1991;15:179–185.

Hoheisel U, Mense S, Simons DG, Yu XM. Appearance of new receptive fields in rat dorsal horn neurons following noxious stimulation of skeletal muscle: a model for referral of muscle pain? *Neurosci Lett* 1993;153:9–12.

Hsieh YL, Kao MJ, Kuan TS, Chen SM, Chen JT, Hong CZ. Dry needling to a key myofascial trigger point may reduce the irritability of satellite MTrPs. *Am J Phys Med Rehabil* 2007; 86:397–403.

Hubbard DR Jr. Chronic and recurrent muscle pain: pathophysiology and treatment, and review of pharmacological studies. *J Musculoskeletal Pain* 1996;4: 123–143.

Inman VT, Saunders JBCM. Referred pain from skeletal structures. *J Nerv Ment Dis* 1944;99:660–667.

Inoue K. P2 receptors and chronic pain. *Purinergic Signalling* 2007;3:135–144.

Janig W, Levine JD, Michaelis M. Interactions of sympathetic and primary afferent neurons following nerve injury and tissue trauma. *Prog Brain Res* 1996;113:161–184.

Jensen K, Tuxen C, Pedersen-Bjergaard U, Jansen I, Edvinsson L, Olesen J. Pain and tenderness in human temporal muscle induced by bradykinin and 5-hydroxytryptamine. *Peptides* 1990;11:1127–1132.

Johansen MK, Graven-Nielsen T, Olesen AS, Arendt-Nielsen L. Generalised muscular hyperalgesia in chronic whiplash syndrome. *Pain* 1999;83:229–234.

Kellgren JH. Observation on referred pain arising from muscle. *Clin Sci* 1938;3:175–190.

Kosek E, Hansson P. Modulatory influence on somatosensory perception from vibration and heterotopic noxious conditioning stimulation (HNCS) in fibromyalgia patients and healthy subjects. *Pain* 1997;70:41–51.

Kosek E, Ordeberg G. Lack of pressure pain modulation by heterotopic noxious conditioning stimulation in patients with painful osteoarthritis before, but not following, surgical pain relief. *Pain* 2000;88:69–78.

Laursen RJ, Graven-Nielsen T, Jensen TS, Arendt-Nielsen L. Quantification of local and referred pain in humans induced by intramuscular electrical stimulation. *Eur J Pain* 1997;1:105–113.

Laursen RJ, Graven-Nielsen T, Jensen TS, Arendt-Nielsen L. Referred pain is dependent on sensory input from the periphery: a psychophysical study. *Eur J Pain* 1998;1: 261–269.

Levine JD, Dardick SJ, Roizen MF, Helms C, Basbaum AI. Contribution of sensory afferents and sympathetic efferents to joint injury in experimental arthritis. *J Neurosci* 1986a;6:3423–3429.

Levine JD, Fye K, Heller P, Basbaum AI, Whiting-O'Keefe Q. Clinical response to regional intravenous guanethidine in patients with rheumatoid arthritis. *J Rheumatol* 1986b;13: 1040–1043.

Lewis T. Suggestions relating to the study of somatic pain. *BMJ* 1938;1:321–325.

Macefield VG, Wallin BG. Modulation of muscle sympathetic activity during spontaneous and artificial ventilation and apnoea in humans. *J Auton Nerv Syst* 1995;53: 137–147.

Macefield VG, Gandevia SC, Henderson LA. Neural sites involved in the sustained increase in muscle sympathetic nerve activity induced by inspiratory capacity apnea: a fMRI study. *J Appl Physiol* 2006;100:266–273.

MacKenzie J. Some points bearing on the association of sensory disorders and visceral disease. *Brain* 1893;16:321–353.

Margolis RB, Chibnall JT, Tait RC. Test-retest reliability of the pain drawing instrument. *Pain* 1988;33:49–51.

Martinez-Lavin M. Fibromyalgia as a sympathetically maintained pain syndrome. *Curr Pain Headache Rep* 2004;8:385–389.

McMahon SB. Mechanisms of cutaneous, deep and visceral pain. In: Wall PD, Melzack R, eds. *Textbook of Pain*. Edinburgh: Churchill Livingstone; 1994:129–151.

McNulty WH, Gevirtz RN, Hubbard DR, Berkoff GM. Needle electromyographic evaluation of trigger point response to a psychological stressor. *Psychophysiology* 1994;31:313–316.

Mense S. Referral of muscle pain. *Am Pain Society J* 1994;3:1–9.

Reinohl J, Hoheisel U, Unger T, Mense S. Adenosine triphosphate as a stimulant for nociceptive and non-nociceptive muscle group IV receptors in the rat. *Neurosci Lett* 2003;338:25–28.

Roatta S, Kalezic N, Passatore M. Sympathetic nervous system: sensory modulation and involvement in chronic pain. In: Johansson H, Windhorst U, Djupsjobacka M, Passatore M, eds. *Chronic Work-Related Myalgia, Neuromuscular Mechanisms Behind Work-Related Chronic Muscle Pain Syndrome*. Gävle, Sweden: Gävle University Press; 2003:265–267.

Rosendal L, Larsson B, Kristiansen J, Peolsson M, Sogaard K, Kjaer M, Sorensen J, Gerdle B. Increase in muscle nociceptive substances and anaerobic metabolism in patients with trapezius myalgia: microdialysis in rest and during exercise. *Pain* 2004;112:324–334.

Ruch TC. Pathophysiology of pain. In: Ruch TC, Patton HD, Woodbury JW, Towe AL, eds. *Neurophysiology*. Philadelphia: W.B. Saunders; 1961:350–368.

Sessle BJ, Hu JW, Amano N, Zhong G. Convergence of cutaneous, tooth pulp, visceral, neck and muscle afferents onto nociceptive and non-nociceptive neurones in trigeminal subnucleus caudalis (medullary dorsal horn) and its implication for referred pain. *Pain* 1986;27:219–235.

Shah JP, Phillips TM, Danoff JV, Gerber LH. An in-vivo microanalytical technique for measuring the local biochemical milieu of human skeletal muscle. *J Appl Physiol* 2005;99:1977–1984.

Shinoda M, Ozaki N, Sugiura Y. Involvement of ATP and its receptors on nociception in rat model of masseter muscle pain. *Pain* 2008;134:148–157.

Sinclair DC, Weddell G, Feindel WH. Referred pain and associated phenomena. *Brain* 1948;71:184–211.

Simons DG, Travell JG, Simons LS. *Myofascial Pain and Dysfunction: The Trigger Point Manual*. Vol. 1. Philadelphia: Lippincott William & Wilkins; 1999:278–307.

Sluka KA, Kalra A, Moore SA. Unilateral intramuscular injections of acidic saline produce a bilateral, long-lasting hyperalgesia. *Muscle Nerve* 2001;24:37–46.

Stohler CS, Lund JP. Psychophysical and orofacial motor response to muscle pain: validation and utility of an experimental model. In: Morimoto T, Matsuya T, Takada K, eds. *Brain and Oral Functions*. Amsterdam: Elsevier Science; 1995:227–237.

Svensson P, Cairns BE, Wang K, Arendt-Nielsen L. Glutamate-evoked pain and mechanical allodynia in the human masseter muscle. *Pain* 2003a;101:221–227.

Svensson P, Cairns BE, Wang K, Arendt-Nielsen L. Injection of nerve growth factor into human masseter muscle evokes long-lasting mechanical allodynia and hyperalgesia. *Pain* 2003b;104:241–247.

Theobald GW. The role of the cerebral cortex in the apperception of pain. *Lancet* 1949;257:41–47.

Turp JC, Kowalski CJ, O'Leary N, Stohler CS. Pain maps from facial pain patients indicate a broad pain geography. *J Dent Res* 1998;77:1465–1472.

Vecchiet L, Dragani L, De Bigontina P. Experimental referred pain and hyperalgesia from muscles in humans. In: Vecchiet L, Albe-Fessard D, Lindblom U, eds. *New Trends in Referred Pain and Hyperalgesia*. Amsterdam: Elsevier Science; 1993:239–249.

Witting N, Svensson P, Gottrup H, Arendt-Nielsen L, Jensen TS. Intramuscular and intra-dermal injection of capsaicin: a comparison of local and referred pain. *Pain* 2000;84:407–412.

Muscle Trigger Points in Tension-Type Headache

César Fernández-de-las-Peñas, PT, DO, PhD, David G. Simons, MD,
Robert D. Gerwin, MD, Maria L. Cuadrado, MD, PhD,
and Juan A. Pareja, MD, PhD

The second edition of the *Classification of Headache Disorders* of the International Headache Society (IHS) has maintained the former clinical criteria for the diagnosis of tension-type headache (IHS, 1988; IHS, 2004). According to the IHS (2004), tension-type headache is characterized by attacks lasting from 30 minutes to 7 days, with at least two of the following features: bilateral location, pressing and tightening pain, mild or moderate intensity, and lack of aggravation during routine physical activity. In addition, patients should not report photophobia, phonophobia, vomiting, or evident nausea during headache, although one of these features is sometimes permitted.

The second edition of the IHS classification has withdrawn electromyography (EMG) or pressure algometry from the diagnostic features for subdivision, because only tenderness with manual palpation has proved to be useful to distinguish different subtypes (IHS, 2004). Pericranial tenderness is usually recorded by the Total Tenderness Score (Langemark & Olesen, 1987), which has previously been proved to be reliable (Bendtsen et al., 1995). Briefly, the procedure is as follows: Eight pairs of muscles and tendon insertions (masseter, temporal, frontal, sternocleidomastoid, trapezius, and suboccipital muscles, as well as coronoid and mastoid processes) are palpated. Palpation is usually done with small rotational movements of the assessors' second and third fingers for 4 to 5 seconds. Tenderness is scored on a 4-point (0–3) scale at each location (local tenderness score), and values from both left and right sides are summed to a total tenderness score (maximum possible score = 48 points) (Langemark & Olesen, 1987). According to the tenderness score, patients are classified as associated (total tenderness score greater than 8 points) or not associated (total tenderness score less than 8 points) with pericranial tenderness.

In addition, depending on the frequency of the attacks (IHS, 2004), patients are classified as having:

- *Infrequent episodic tension-type headache:* At least 10 episodes occurring less than 1 day per month on average (less than 12 days per year)
- *Frequent episodic tension-type headache:* At least 10 episodes occurring more than 1 but less than 15 days per month for at least 3 months (more than 12 but less than 180 days per year)
- *Chronic tension-type headache:* Headaches occurring more than 15 days per month for at least 3 months (more than 180 days per year)

Although some patients may present with two types of headaches simultaneously (tension-type headache with migraine features, cervicogenic headache with tension-type headache characteristics, etc.), it seems that the pain quality and features of these headache disorders are distinctly different. Differences in pain features and quality of headache attacks may implicate different structures as being responsible for nociceptive irritation of the trigeminal nucleus caudalis (Nillson, 2000).

For instance, *cervicogenic headache* is characterized by unilateral nonlancinating pain, which is increased by head movement, maintained neck postures, or external pressure over the upper cervical joints (Sjaastad et al., 1998). Therefore, joint dysfunctions in the upper cervical spine (C0 to C2) can be implicated in the etiology of this headache (Jull & Niere, 2004).

Previous studies have found that patients with tension-type headache described their head pain as pressing, tightening, or soreness (Rasmussen et al., 1991, 1992). Dull and tight heaviness are also pain quality features of tension-type headache attacks (Chun, 1985). These pain features are similar to those provoked by muscle referred pain elicited by injection of hypertonic saline (Graven-Nielsen et al., 1997) and also resemble the descriptions of referred pain elicited by muscle trigger points (Simons et al., 1999). Therefore, it seems that tension-type headache is a headache in which neck and shoulder muscles may play a relevant role in the genesis of the pain (Davidoff, 1998; Jensen et al., 1998).

Some authors have claimed that pain from pericranial head, neck, and/or shoulder muscles is referred to the head and is experienced as headache (Simons et al., 1999; Gerwin, 2005). In their comprehensive text, Simons et al. (1999) described the referred pain patterns from muscle trigger point (TrPs) in head and neck muscles that have the potential to refer pain to the head: suboccipital, upper trapezius, temporalis, splenius capitis and cervicis, sternocleidomastoid muscles, and so on.

NEUROPHYSIOLOGIC BASIS OF MYOFASCIAL TRIGGER POINTS

Basis of Muscle Referred Pain to the Head: Convergence of Neurons in the Trigeminal Nucleus Caudalis

Small-diameter group III and IV fibers from neck and shoulder muscles terminate mainly on neurons located in the superficial and intermediate dorsal horn (laminae I and V) of the spinal cord (Nyberg & Blomqvist, 1984; Abrahams & Swett, 1986; Giamberardino, 1999). Myofascial afferents from several different areas converge onto the same second-order nociceptive relay neurons in the spinal cord and the trigeminal nucleus caudalis. Both animal (Bartsch & Goadsby, 2002, 2003) and human (Piovesan et al., 2003; Ge et al., 2004a) studies have clearly shown the convergence of cervical and trigeminal afferents in the trigeminal nerve nucleus caudalis, thus providing an anatomic basis for the referred pain to the head elicited by neck and shoulder muscles. These studies have confirmed that individual nociceptive second-order neurons in the trigeminal nucleus caudalis receive inputs both from the supratentorial dura and from the cervical musculature and other cervical structures (Bartsch & Goadsby, 2002, 2003). Further, another study demonstrated that noxious inputs from cervical muscles induced central sensitization of orofacial sensory-motor processing (Makowska et al., 2005). Because nociceptive somatic afferents from muscles of the upper cervical roots, particularly C1 to C3, and the trigeminal nerve, particularly V1 (ophthalmic) and V3 (mandible) nerves, converge on the same relay neurons, it may be assumed that the message to supraspinal structures can be misinterpreted and localized as pain in other structures distant from the site of painful stimulus (muscle referred pain).

In addition, dorsal horn neurons that receive afferents from muscle tissues frequently receive input from other structures (Schaible et al., 1987; Hoheisel & Mense, 1990). This extensive convergent input to dorsal horn neurons may account for the often diffuse and poorly localized nature of deep pain in humans, particularly when pain is intense. Further, animal studies have demonstrated spinal-level spread of the pain message from one dorsal horn cell to another that is initiated by strong inputs from muscle nociceptors (Hoheisel et al., 1993; Mense, 1994) and can be interpreted as a likely contributing cause of muscle referred pain (Simons, 1994). Further theories that may explain muscle referred pain are found in Chapter 5 of the present textbook.

Experimental Pain Models with Hypertonic Saline Injections

Different experimental pain models have been used to elicit referred pain from pericranial muscles (e.g., hypertonic saline, glutamate, capsaicin). Hypertonic saline injections induce firing in a large proportion of Aδ and C fibers and cause deep, aching, referred pain in humans, similar to clinical muscle pain (Graven-Nielsen et al., 1997). Some authors have clinically described the referred pain patterns from several head and neck muscles that have the potential to refer pain to the head (Simons et al., 1999). Several pain models using hypertonic saline injections have confirmed upper trapezius and temporalis muscle clinical pain patterns as described by Simons et al. (1999) in both healthy and patient populations:

1. The referred pain elicited by infusion of hypertonic saline into the upper trapezius muscle spreads ipsilaterally to the posterior-lateral region of the neck and to the temporal region in both healthy subjects (Ge et al., 2003, 2005) and headache patients (Mörk et al., 2003).
2. The infusion of hypertonic saline into the temporalis muscle elicits referred pain to both the trigeminal territory (anterior part of the muscle) and the cervical innervated dermatome (posterior part of the muscle) (Schmidt-Hansen et al., 2006) (**Figure 6.1**).

Dynamic Balance Between Descending Facilitation and Inhibition

Anatomic convergence and dynamic changes between descending inhibition and facilitation pathways

may also contribute to TrP referred pain (Ge, 2004). Experimental studies have found mechanical hypoalgesia in the referred pain area after unilateral or bilateral injection of hypertonic saline in the upper trapezius muscle in healthy subjects (Ge et al., 2003, 2006a). These findings suggest the activation of descending inhibitory pathways as a physiologic response after peripheral nociceptive inputs (Ge et al., 2003, 2006a). If the peripheral nociceptive input decreases or ceases, the referred pain will gradually disappear, and mechanical hypoalgesia or no changes in mechanical pain sensitivity will be found in referred pain areas (Ge, 2004; Ge et al., 2003, 2006a). On the other hand, if the nociceptive input does not decrease or cease, both peripheral and central sensitization could appear; descending inhibition would decrease and can also be dysfunctional (Ge et al., 2004b). Therefore, it is proposed that in chronic pain conditions such as chronic tension-type headache, with central sensitization probably provoked by temporal summation of nociceptive barrage (Bendtsen, 2000), mechanical hyperalgesia would be registered in referred pain areas (Ge, 2004). It has been found that in patients with chronic tension-type headache there is a decrease in the gray matter substance, particularly in the periaqueductal gray matter (Schmidt-Wilcke et al., 2005), supporting the existence of dysfunctional descending inhibitory pathways in this primary headache (Pielstickera et al., 2005).

CLINICAL PRESENTATION AND DIAGNOSTIC CRITERIA OF MUSCLE TRIGGER POINTS

Simons et al. (1999) identified a muscle trigger point as a hyperirritable spot within a taut band of a skeletal muscle that is painful on compression, stretch, overload, or contraction in the shortened position and responds with a referred pain pattern that is often distant from the spot. From a clinical viewpoint, active TrPs cause pain symptoms, and their local and referred pain evoke a usual or familiar pain for the subject (Gerwin et al., 1997). In patients, the referred pain elicited by an active TrP reproduces at least part of their clinical pain pattern.

In patients suffering from headache, active TrPs are those TrPs in which the referred pain pattern evokes sensations that the patients usually perceive during their spontaneous headache attacks, or those TrPs that reproduce the patient's headache upon examination.

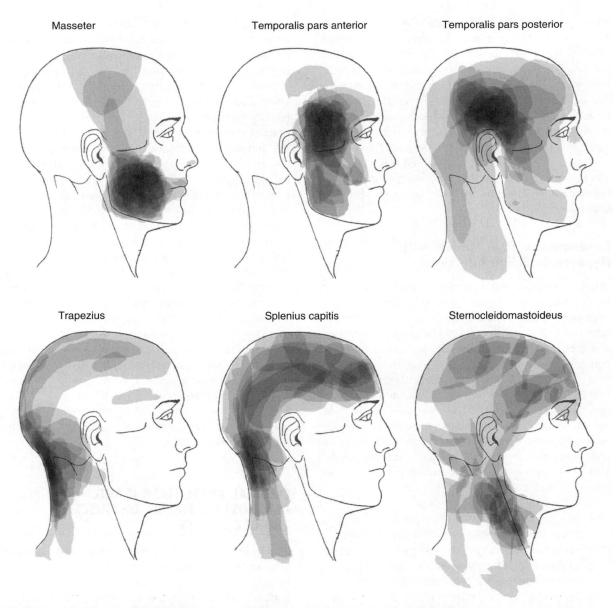

Figure 6.1 Referred Pain Elicited by the Injection of Hypertonic Saline into the Temporalis, Masseter, Upper Trapezius, Splenius Capitis, and Sternocleidomastoid Muscles

Adapted with permission from Schmidt-Hansen PT. (PhD thesis). A controlled study on muscle pain sensitivity in tension-type headache patients: experimentally induces pain in peri-cranial muscles.

Latent TrPs also evoke referred pain with mechanical stimulation, muscle contraction, or stretching, but this elicited pain is not a familiar or usual pain for the patient. Both active and latent muscle TrPs can provoke motor dysfunctions (e.g., muscle weakness) due to inhibition, increased motor irritability (spasm), muscle imbalance, or altered motor recruitment (Lucas et al., 2004) in either the affected muscle or in functionally related muscles (Simons et al., 1999). In addition, the sympathetic facilitation of mechanical sensitization and facilitation of the local and referred pain reactions in TrPs have been demonstrated, thus confirming sympathetic responses elicited by muscle TrPs (Ge et al., 2006b).

Muscle TrPs are initially identified by a history of musculoskeletal or any enigmatic pain complaint that requires examination by manual palpation. The diagnosis of a TrP for research purposes requires the identification of several features during physical examination: (a) presence of a palpable taut band in a skeletal muscle when accessible to palpation, (b) presence of a tender spot within the taut band, (c) palpable or visible local twitch response on snapping palpation (or needling) of the TrP, and (d) presence of referred pain elicited by stimulation or palpation of the sensitive spot (Simons et al., 1999). Diagnosis of TrPs requires adequate manual ability, training, and clinical practice to develop a high degree of reliability in the examination (Sciotti et al., 2001; Gerwin et al., 1997). Moreover, some muscles and examinations are consistently more reliably examined than others. The local twitch response is the least reliable because it requires so much skill.

Most important for practical clinical purposes, Simons et al. (1999) and Gerwin et al. (1997) recommend as the *minimum* acceptable criteria for active TrP diagnosis the combination of the presence of a tender spot in a palpable taut band within a skeletal muscle and the patient's recognition of the referred pain elicited by pressure applied to the tender spot as a familiar or usual symptom. These criteria have obtained a good interexaminer reliability (kappa) ranging from 0.84 to 0.88 (Gerwin et al., 1997). Latent TrPs are diagnosed in a similar way, but the difference is that the subject does not recognize the elicited referred pain as a familiar or usual symptom (Simons et al., 1999; Gerwin et al., 1997). Additional helpful clinical guides to which muscle or muscles need examination are painfully restricted stretch range of motion, muscle weakness, pain on contraction in the shortened position, and muscle tenderness to palpation. Chapter 16 provides more data about examination skills related to the exploration of muscle TrPs.

Some authors described clinically the referred pain patterns from several head and neck muscles that have the potential to refer pain to the head (Simons et al., 1999; Wright, 2000). Although referred pain patterns have much value for clinicians, these pain patterns can be different between subjects. Some subjects have more extensive patterns than others, and the extensiveness of the pattern is strongly dependent on the degree of activation of the muscle trigger point and how much test

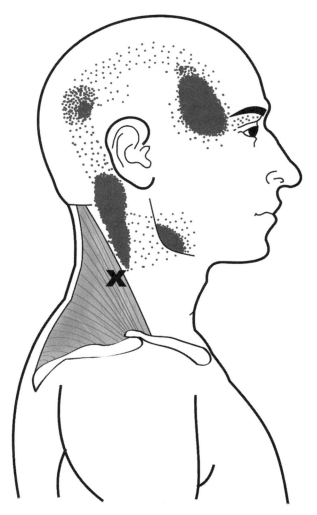

Figure 6.2 Referred Pain from Upper Trapezius Muscle Trigger Points

Modifed from Simons DG, Travell J, Simons L. *Travell and Simons' Myofascial Pain and Dysfunction: The Trigger Point Manual.* Vol. 1. 2nd ed. Baltimore: Williams & Wilkins; 1999.

pressure is applied to it (Dejung et al., 2003; Wright, 2000; Hong et al., 1996). Some of the referred pain patterns that are likely to contribute to the development of headache are the following:

- Referred pain elicited by upper trapezius muscle TrPs spreads ipsilaterally from the posterior-lateral region of the neck, behind the ear, and to the temporal region (**Figure 6.2**).
- TrPs located on the sternocleidomastoid muscle refer pain to the occiput, the frontotemporal

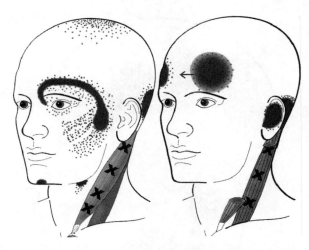

Figure 6.3 Referred Pain from Sternocleidomastoid Muscle Trigger Point

Modifed from Simons DG, Travell J, Simons L. *Travell and Simons' Myofascial Pain and Dysfunction: The Trigger Point Manual.* Vol. 1. 2nd ed. Baltimore: Williams & Wilkins; 1999.

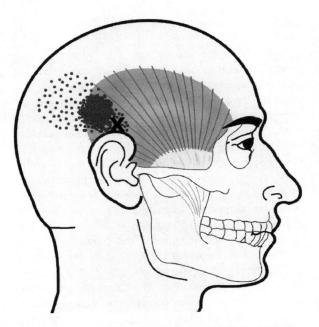

Figure 6.4 Referred Pain from Temporalis Muscle Trigger Point

Modifed from Simons DG, Travell J, Simons L. *Travell and Simons' Myofascial Pain and Dysfunction: The Trigger Point Manual.* Vol. 1. 2nd ed. Baltimore: Williams & Wilkins; 1999.

area, the retroauricular area, the forehead, and to the cheek (**Figure 6.3**).

- Referred pain from temporalis muscle TrPs is located in the temporoparietal region and perceived inside the head (**Figure 6.4**).
- Referred pain from suboccipital muscle TrPs spreads to the side of the head over the occipital, temporal, and frontal bones and is usually perceived as bilateral head pain (**Figure 6.5**).

Readers are referred to Simons et al. (1999) for more comprehensive details of a greater number of referred pain patterns.

ETIOLOGY OF MUSCLE TRIGGER POINTS

The presence of active TrPs may result from a variety of factors, for example, repetitive muscle overuse, acute or chronic (sustained) overload, psychological stress, or other active (key) TrPs. Under normal conditions, pain from TrPs is mediated by thin myelinated (Aδ) and un-myelinated (C) fibers (Newham et al., 1994). Various noxious and innocuous events, such as mechanical stimuli or chemical mediators, may excite and sensitize these Aδ or C fibers and thereby play a role in the origin of muscle TrPs and pain characteristics (Mense, 1993; Mense et al., 2001).

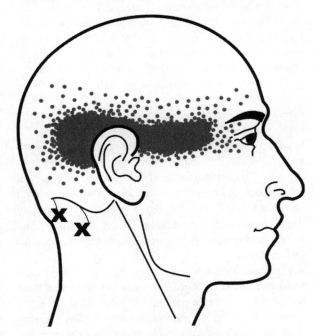

Figure 6.5 Referred Pain from Suboccipital Muscle Trigger Points

Modifed from Simons DG, Travell J, Simons L. *Travell and Simons' Myofascial Pain and Dysfunction: The Trigger Point Manual.* Vol. 1. 2nd ed. Baltimore: Williams & Wilkins; 1999.

Gerwin et al. (2004) have suggested that the pathogenesis of TrPs could result from injured or overloaded muscle fibers. For instance, direct muscle trauma may create a vicious cycle of events wherein damage to the sarcoplasmic reticulum or the cell membrane may lead to an increase of the calcium concentration, a subsequent activation of actin and myosin, a relative shortage of adenosine triphosphate (ATP), and an impaired calcium pump. The calcium pump is responsible for returning intracellular Ca^{2+} to the sarcoplasmic reticulum against a concentration gradient, which requires a functional energy supply. Based on the likelihood of these events, Simons and Travell proposed the so-called *energy crisis hypothesis*, introduced in 1981 and enhanced by subsequent research that led to integrated hypotheses (Simons et al., 1999). Chen et al. (2000) proposed that low-level muscle exertions can lead to sensitization and development of TrPs. Later, Treaster et al. (2006) demonstrated that sustained low-level muscle contractions during continuous typing for as little as 30 minutes commonly resulted in the formation of muscle TrPs. Therefore, these overloaded muscle fibers could lead to endogenous (involuntary) shortening, loss of oxygen supply, loss of nutrient supply, and increased metabolic demand on local tissues (Simons, 2004).

Nevertheless, at this time, there is no solid evidence that eccentric and submaximal concentric exercises are absolute precursors to the development of TrPs. In support of this hypothesized causal relationship, Itoh et al. (2004) found that eccentric exercise can lead to the formation of taut and tender ropy bands in exercised intrinsic hand muscle, and they hypothesized that eccentric exercise may indeed be a useful model for the development of muscle TrPs. However, further studies are now required because this was not a reliable method for postural muscles in one experimental trial.

The most credible etiologic suggestion for TrP pathogenesis is the integrated hypothesis, which proposes that abnormal depolarization of the postjunctional membrane of motor endplates enhanced by sustained muscular contraction gives rise to a localized hypoxic "ATP energy crisis" associated with sensory and autonomic reflex arcs that are sustained by central sensitization (McPartland & Simons, 2006). Qerama et al. (2004) found higher levels of pain when noxious stimuli were applied to a motor endplate region as compared with silent muscle sites. In addition, pain evoked from motor endplate regions was described as throbbing,

sharp, or aching (Qerama et al., 2004)—that is, similar features to those that have been described in TrP referred pain areas (Simons et al., 1999). Further, endplate noise and endplate spikes (EMG signals from dysfunctional motor endplate regions) have been identified and significantly associated with muscle TrPs (Simons, 2001; Couppé et al., 2001). Findings from these studies support the theory that TrPs are strongly associated with dysfunctional motor endplates (Simons et al., 2002).

Biopsy studies of TrPs indicate that the one consistent finding is evidence of seriously increased tension of some muscle fibers and that there are a number of sources for this regional sarcomere shortening. It has been previously assumed that contraction of head, neck, or shoulder muscles could play a relevant role in the development of tension-type headache. Nevertheless, numerous surface EMG studies have reported normal or, more often, only a slightly increased muscle activity in tension-type headache (Schoenen et al., 1991; Hatch et al., 1991, 1992; Goebel et al., 1992; Jensen et al., 1994; Sandrini et al., 1994; Clark et al., 1995; Jensen, 1996). A pioneer study analyzing EMG activity of the upper trapezius muscle with needle electrodes found an increase in endplate noise revealed by accurately placed needle electromyography in TrPs as compared with an adjacent nontender point (Hubbard & Berkoff, 1993). Furthermore, spontaneous EMG activity (endplate noise) in the TrP was significantly higher in patients with chronic tension-type headache compared with healthy controls (Hubbard & Berkoff, 1993). Because the endplate region of a muscle fiber is only 0.1 millimeter, at the most, in diameter, the increased EMG activity (motor endplate noise and spikes) could only be detected with needle electrodes precisely placed within the TrP. A histopathologic cause of taut bands in human TrPs has been convincingly demonstrated because the palpable band of myogelosis and of TrPs are two different names for the same thing, and clinically the symptoms of myogelosis are completely compatible with the diagnosis of muscle TrPs (Lange, 1931); on this basis, the extensive pathology described by Fassbender (1975) also applies to TrPs. Many findings confirm the presence of excessive discrete regions of hypercontracted sarcomeres and muscle fiber tension and identify several causes of sarcomere shortening and tension.

Finally, although there is evidence to support the integrated hypothesis as an etiologic origin of TrPs, the hypothesis has progressively fewer weak links that still need to be addressed in future studies in order to definitively confirm this etiologic hypothesis as the genesis of TrPs.

MUSCLE TRIGGER POINTS IN TENSION-TYPE HEADACHE

Trigger Points in Chronic Tension-Type Headache

Mercer et al. (1993) found, in a noncontrolled and non-blinded study, both active and latent TrPs in neck and shoulder muscles in subjects presenting with tension-type headache. TrPs were located in the splenius capitis, splenius cervicis, semispinalis cervicis, semispinalis capitis, levator scapulae, upper trapezius, or suboccipital muscles. In a later study from the same group, Marcus et al. (1999) found, again in a nonblinded study, that tension-type headache subjects had a greater number of either active or latent TrPs than healthy subjects. However, these authors did not specify which muscles were affected by the presence of TrPs.

More recent blinded and controlled studies have investigated the presence of either active or latent muscle TrPs in chronic tension-type headache. Two studies have described the referred pain elicited from two extraocular muscles, namely, the superior oblique (Fernández-de-las-Peñas et al., 2005) and lateral rectus (Fernández-de-las-Peñas et al., 2008), in patients with chronic tension-type headache. The referred pain elicited by the superior oblique muscle was perceived as internal, deep pain located at the retro-orbital region. This referred pain can extend to the supraorbital region, and sometimes to the homolateral forehead, whereas the referred pain elicited by the lateral rectus muscle was only located at the supraorbital region or the homolateral forehead, but not at the retro-orbital region (**Figure 6.6**).

Suboccipital muscle TrPs were found in 20 of 20 patients with chronic tension-type headache (100%), of which 13 (65%) elicited a referred pain that reproduced a familiar or usual pain similar to that perceived during their headache attacks (i.e., active TrPs) (Fernández-de-las-Peñas et al., 2006a), whereas the remaining 7 patients (35%) showed latent TrPs, that is, those which elicited a referred pain not recognized as familiar for the patient. In contrast, only 6 (30%) of the healthy subjects reported referred pain with manual exploration of the suboccipital muscles, all of them latent TrPs since no control subject recognized the elicited referred pain as a usual pain. Differences in

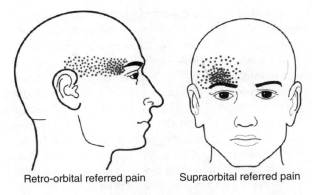

Retro-orbital referred pain   Supraorbital referred pain

Figure 6.6 Referred Pain from the Superior Oblique (both figures) and from the Lateral Rectus Muscle (right figure)

Modified from Fernández-de-las-Peñas et al. Referred pain from the trochlear region in tension-type headache: a myofascial trigger point from the superior oblique muscle. *Headache* 2005;45:731–737.

the presence of suboccipital TrPs between both groups were significant for active TrPs (P <0.001) but not for latent TrPs (P >0.05) (Fernández-de-las-Peñas et al., 2006a).

In another study with 25 patients with chronic tension-type headache, TrPs in the temporalis muscle were found in 20 of 25 (80%) on the right and 15 of 25 (60%) on the left side; TrPs in the upper trapezius muscle were found in 19 of 25 (76%) on the right and 14 of 25 (56%) on the left side; and TrPs in the sternocleidomastoid muscle were found in 16 of 25 (64%) on the right side and 12 of 25 (48%) on the left (Fernández-de-las-Peñas et al., 2006b). Within the control group, the most prevalent TrPs were located in the right upper trapezius in 12 of 25 (48%), and in the right sternocleidomastoid in 8 of 25 (32%). Differences in the distribution of active, but not latent, TrPs between groups were significant (P <0.01) for all muscles (**Table 6.1**).

Couppé et al. (2007) found that 85% of 20 patients with chronic tension-type headache had active TrPs in the upper trapezius muscle (P <0.001). In addition, they also reported that patients showed greater levels of both local and referred pain intensity than healthy controls (Couppé et al., 2007).

Nevertheless, just the presence of active TrPs in chronic tension-type headache does not establish the clinical relevance of referred pain in this disorder because the effect of treatment was not tested in these studies. Fernández-de-las-Peñas et al. (2006a) found that those patients with active TrPs in the suboccipital muscles showed significantly greater headache

Table 6.1 Distribution of Subjects with Myofascial Trigger Points (Active or Latent) in the Upper Trapezius, Sternocleidomastoid, and Temporalis Muscles in Chronic Tension-Type Headache Patients and Healthy Controls

	Upper Trapezius Muscle		Sternocleidomastoid Muscle		Temporalis Muscle	
	Left Side	Right Side	Left Side	Right Side	Left Side	Right Side
	Subjects with chronic tension-type headache					
Active TrPs (*n*)	6	9	5	6	8	9
Latent TrPs (*n*)	8	10	11	6	7	11
	Control healthy subjects					
Active TrPs (*n*)	0	0	0	0	0	0
Latent TrPs (*n*)	5	12	4	8	4	2
P value[a]	0.001	0.003	0.001	0.003	0.002	0.001

TrP, muscle trigger point; *n*, number of subjects.

[a]*P* values express differences between active TrPs. Differences between latent TrPs were not significant.

Reprinted from Fernández-de-las-Peñas et al., 2006b.

Table 6.2 Headache Intensity, Frequency and Duration Depending on Trigger Point Activity on Each Muscle Within Chronic Tension-Type Headache Patients

		Headache Intensity (VAS)	Headache Frequency (days/week)	Headache Duration (hours/day)
Right upper trapezius (*n* = 25)	Active TrPs (*n* = 9)	**5.6 (1.7)**[a]	5.1 (1.1)	**8.9 (4.2)**[a]
	Latent TrPs (*n* = 10)	**4.5 (1.6)**	4.6 (1.2)	**6.7 (5.4)**
Left upper trapezius (*n* = 25)	Active TrPs (*n* = 6)	5.6 (1.6)	5.5 (1.9)	9.2 (4.6)
	Latent TrPs (*n* = 8)	5.4 (1.2)	4.8 (1.8)	9.8 (5.1)
Right sternocleidomastoid (*n* = 25)	Active TrPs (*n* = 6)	6.1 (1.9)	5.2 (1.8)	9.6 (5.1)
	Latent TrPs (*n* = 6)	5.5 (2)	5.3 (2.3)	9.4 (5.7)
Left sternocleidomastoid (*n* = 25)	Active TrPs (*n* = 5)	**6.4 (2.5)**[a]	5.6 (1.8)	**10.8 (5.1)**[a]
	Latent TrPs (*n* = 11)	**4.5 (1.2)**	4.9 (2.4)	**7.5 (4.8)**
Right temporalis (*n* = 25)	Active TrPs (*n* = 9)	5.5 (1.8)	5.2 (2.1)	**11.6 (1.9)**[a]
	Latent TrPs (*n* = 11)	5.2 (1.9)	5.4 (1.8)	**7.2 (2.9)**
Left temporalis (*n* = 25)	Active TrPs (*n* = 8)	**5.7 (1.4)**[a]	5.1 (1.7)	9.4 (4.7)
	Latent TrPs (*n* = 7)	**4.3 (1.6)**	4.4 (2.3)	8.4 (5.5)
Suboccipital muscles (*n* = 20)	Active TrPs (*n* = 13)	**6 (3.15–9)**[a]	**6 (4–7)**[a]	8.7 (3–12)
	Latent TrPs (*n* = 7)	**4.6 (2.2–7)**	**4.9 (4–6)**	9.8 (4–13)

Values are expressed as mean (standard deviation) for all muscles, except for the suboccipital muscles, in which they are mean (min-max).

VAS, Visual Analogue Scale (0–10); TrPs, muscle trigger points.

[a]Statistically significant as compared with the latent TrP subgroup (unpaired Student *t* test, *P* <0.05).

Reprinted from Fernández-de-las-Peñas et al., 2006a, 2006b.

intensity and headache frequency, but not longer headache duration, than those patients with latent muscle TrPs (**Table 6.2**). Further, those patients with active TrPs in the right upper trapezius, left sternocleidomas-toid, or left temporalis had significantly greater headache intensity and longer headache duration, but not greater headache frequency, than those patients with latent TrPs in the same muscle (Fernández-de-las-

Table 6.3 Headache Intensity, Frequency, and Duration Depending on Myofascial Trigger Point Activity and Spatial Summation of Trigger Points Within a Chronic Tension-Type Headache Group

		Headache Intensity (VAS)	Headache Frequency (days/week)	Headache Duration (hours/day)
Right upper trapezius	Active TrPs ($n = 8$)	5.8 (1.8)[a]	5.4 (1.2)[a]	9.3 (4.4)[a]
	Latent TrPs ($n = 9$)	4.5 (1.7)	4.5 (0.6)	6.9 (5.7)
Left upper trapezius	Active TrPs ($n = 4$)	5.5 (1.3)[a]	5 (0.9)	9.8 (2.5)[a]
	Latent TrPs ($n = 7$)	4.7 (0.5)	5 (0.8)	8.3 (2.7)
Unilateral or bilateral TrPs	Bilateral TrPs ($n = 8$)	5.5 (1.9)[b]	5.3 (1)	9.9 (2.7)[b]
	Unilateral TrPs ($n = 12$)	4.6 (1.7)	4.7 (1)	7.4 (4.3)

Values are expressed as mean (standard deviation).
VAS, Visual Analogue Scale (0–10); TrPs, muscle trigger points.
[a]Statistically significant as compared with the latent TrP subgroup (unpaired Student t test, $P < 0.05$).
[b]Statistically significant differences between bilateral and unilateral TrPs (unpaired Student t test, $P < 0.05$).
Reprinted from Fernández-de-las-Peñas et al., 2007a.

Peñas et al., 2006b) (Table 6.2). These results have been confirmed in posterior studies conducted with greater sample sizes for both upper trapezius (Fernández-de-las-Peñas et al., 2007a) and temporalis muscles (Fernández-de-las-Peñas et al., 2007b). The fact that patients with chronic tension-type headache with active TrPs had greater headache clinical parameters than those patients with latent TrPs could be considered as temporal integration of neuron signals from muscle TrPs. Given that temporal summation of pain is centrally mediated (Price et al., 1994; Arendt-Nielsen et al., 1995; Vierck et al., 1997), this would suggest a temporal integration of nociceptive signals from TrPs (Shah et al., 2005) by central nociceptive neurons, contributing to central sensitization in chronic tension-type headache (Bendtsen & Schoenen, 2006; Bendtsen, 2000). In addition, it has been found that muscle pain sensitivity and temporal summation are higher in neck or shoulder muscles (e.g., upper trapezius muscle), as compared with other muscles (e.g., anterior tibialis muscle) (Ashina et al., 2003), which supports the relevance of neck or shoulder muscles in tension-type headache, particularly the upper trapezius muscle.

Finally, another interesting finding from these studies was that patients with chronic tension-type headache showed significantly greater number of TrPs (sum of both active and latent TrPs) than healthy controls ($P < 0.001$). The mean number of TrPs for each chronic tension-type headache subject was 3.9 (SD: 1.2), of which 1.9 (SD: 1.2) were active TrPs, and 1.9 (SD: 0.8) were la-

tent TrPs. Conversely, the mean number of TrPs for each healthy subject was 1.4 (SD: 0.8), all of them being latent TrPs (Fernández-de-las-Peñas et al., 2006b). Fernández-de-las-Peñas et al. (2007a) reported that patients with TrPs in both upper trapezius muscles had greater headache intensity and longer headache duration as compared with those patients with unilateral TrP (**Table 6.3**). These results suggest that higher levels of headache pain may come from spatial summation of TrP-related pain. In addition, chronic tension-type headache patients with bilateral TrPs had lower pressure pain thresholds than those patients diagnosed with unilateral muscle TrP (**Table 6.4**), which indicates that multiple muscle TrPs spatially increase mechanical pain sensitivity peripherally and centrally, because the pressure pain threshold was not measured directly on the TrP, but on a fixed point in the upper trapezius muscle (Fernández-de-las-Peñas et al., 2007a).

Trigger Points in Episodic Tension-Type Headache

It has also been demonstrated that patients with episodic tension-type headache showed active TrPs in the suboccipital, upper trapezius, sternocleidomastoid, and temporalis muscles.

Suboccipital muscle TrPs were found in 10 of 10 patients with episodic tension-type headache (100%), of which 6 (60%) reproduced a familiar or usual pain similar to that

Table 6.4 Pressure Pain Thresholds of the Upper Trapezius Muscle Depending on Trigger Point Activity in Both Chronic Tension-Type Headache Patients and Healthy Subjects

	Trigger Point	PPT Right Upper Trapezius Muscle	PPT Left Upper Trapezius Muscle
	Chronic tension-type headache		
Right upper trapezius	Active TrPs (*n* = 8)	1.3 (0.3)	1.4 (0.3)
	Latent TrPs (*n* = 9)	1.5 (0.4)	1.4 (0.4)
Left upper trapezius	Active TrPs (*n* = 4)	1.4 (0.5)	1.5 (0.5)
	Latent TrPs (*n* = 7)	1.2 (0.2)	1.3 (0.3)
Unilateral and bilateral TrPs	Bilateral TrPs (*n* = 8)	**1.1 (0.2)[a]**	**1.2 (0.2)[a]**
	Unilateral TrPs (*n* = 12)	**1.7 (0.4)**	**1.7 (0.4)**
	Control subjects		
Right upper trapezius	No TrP (*n* = 9)	2.5 (0.4)	2.5 (0.4)
	Latent TrPs (*n* = 11)	2.6 (0.5)	2.4 (0.5)
Left upper trapezius	No TrP (*n* = 15)	2.6 (0.4)	2.5 (0.4)
	Latent TrPs (*n* = 5)	2.6 (0.5)	2.5 (0.5)
Unilateral, bilateral, or no TrPs (ANOVA)	Bilateral TrPs (*n* = 2)	2.6 (0.7)	2.5 (0.6)
	Unilateral TrPs (*n* = 12)	2.6 (0.5)	2.5 (0.5)
	No TrP (*n* = 6)	2.5 (0.4)	2.5 (0.4)

Values are expressed as mean (standard deviation).
PPT, pressure pain threshold (kg/cm^2) of the upper trapezius muscle; TrPs, muscle trigger points.
[a]Statistically significant differences in PPT between bilateral and unilateral TrPs in chronic tension-type headache (unpaired Student *t* test, *P* <0.01).
Reprinted from Fernández-de-las-Peñas et al., 2007a.

perceived during their headache attacks (i.e., active TrPs), whereas the remaining 4 patients (40%) showed latent TrPs (Fernández-de-las-Peñas et al., 2006c). In contrast, only 2 healthy subjects (20%) showed referred pain with manual exploration of the suboccipital muscles, all of them latent TrPs. Differences in the presence of suboccipital muscle TrPs between both groups were significant for active TrPs (*P* <0.001) but not for latent TrPs (*P* >0.05). In another study with 15 patients with episodic tension-type headache, TrPs in the upper trapezius (*n* = 11, 75% right side; *n* = 8, 54% left side), in the temporalis (*n* = 11, 74% in either right or left sides), and in the sternocleidomastoid (*n* = 9, 60% right side; *n* = 5, 35% left side) were found (Fernández-de-las-Peñas et al., 2007c). Within the control group, the most prevalent TrPs were located in the right (*n* = 7; 47%) and left (*n* = 4; 27%) upper trapezius muscles. Differences in the distribution of active, but not latent, muscle TrPs were significant for

the right upper trapezius (*P* = 0.04), left sternocleidomastoid (*P* = 0.03), and both temporalis (*P* <0.001) muscles (**Table 6.5**).

It is interesting to note that active TrPs were present in a similar percentage in both patients with chronic or episodic tension-type headache (Fernández-de-las-Peñas et al., 2006d). **Table 6.6** summarizes the percentages of either active or latent TrPs in both episodic and chronic tension-type headache. The fact that active muscle TrPs were also present in episodic tension-type headache does not support the hypothesis that active TrPs are a consequence of central sensitization (Fernández-de-las-Peñas et al., 2006d). Because there is no evidence of central sensitization in episodic tension-type headache (Bendtsen & Schoenen, 2006; Bendtsen, 2000), one would expect fewer active and more latent muscle TrPs in episodic than in chronic tension-type headache.

Table 6.5 Distribution of Subjects with Myofascial Trigger Points (Active or Latent) in Both Episodic Tension-Type Headache and Control Groups

	Upper Trapezius Muscle		*Sternocleidomastoid Muscle*		*Temporalis Muscle*	
	Right Side	Left Side	Right Side	Left Side	Right Side	Left Side
Subjects with episodic tension-type headache						
Active TrPs (*n*)	5	2	3	2	6	7
Latent TrPs (*n*)	6	6	2	7	5	4
Control healthy subjects						
Active TrPs (*n*)	0	0	0	0	0	0
Latent TrPs (*n*)	7	4	3	2	1	3
P value[a]	0.04	NS	NS	0.02	0.001	0.004

TrP, muscle trigger point; *n*, number of subjects; NS, not significant.
[a]*P* values express differences between active TrPs. Differences between latent TrPs were not significant.
Reprinted from Fernández-de-las-Peñas et al., 2007c.

Table 6.6 Percentage of Subjects with Myofascial Trigger Points (Active or Latent) in Chronic and Episodic Tension-Type Headache Patients

	Suboccipital Muscles	*Upper Trapezius Muscle*		*Sternocleidomastoid Muscle*		*Temporalis Muscle*	
		Left Side	Right Side	Left Side	Right Side	Left Side	Right Side
Subjects with chronic tension-type headache							
Active TrPs	65%	24%	36%	20%	24%	32%	36%
Latent TrPs	35%	32%	40%	44%	24%	28%	44%
Subjects with episodic tension-type headache							
Active TrPs	60%	33%	14%	20%	14%	40%	46%
Latent TrPs	40%	40%	40%	14%	46%	33%	27%

TrP, muscle trigger point; *n*, number of subjects.
Suboccipital muscle TrPs in chronic tension-type headache (CTTH) are based on a sample of 20, whereas in episodic tension-type headache (ETTH) they are based on a sample of 10 patients.
Upper trapezius, sternocleidomastoid, and temporalis muscle TrPs in CTTH are based on a sample of 25, whereas in ETTH they are based on a sample of 15 patients.
Reprinted from Fernández-de-las-Peñas et al., 2006d.

Finally, these studies showed that headache intensity, frequency, or duration was not significantly different between episodic tension-type headache patients with active TrPs in suboccipital, upper trapezius, sternocleidomastoid, or temporalis muscles and those patients with latent TrPs (**Table 6.7**), which demonstrates that TrP activity was not related to headache parameters in episodic tension-type headache.

Table 6.7 Headache Intensity, Frequency, and Duration Depending on the Type of Trigger Point on Each Muscle Within an Episodic Tension-Type Headache Group

		Headache Intensity (VAS)	Headache Frequency (days/week)	Headache Duration (hours/day)
Right upper trapezius	Active TrPs (n = 5)	5.1 (1.4)	2.7 (0.4)	6.3 (0.7)
(n = 15)	Latent TrPs (n = 6)	4.2 (1.7)	2.7 (0.7)	4.7 (3.2)
Left upper trapezius	Active TrPs (n = 2)	5.1 (0.2)	3 (0.5)	6.4 (0.6)
(n = 15)	Latent TrPs (n = 6)	4.6 (1.8)	2.5 (0.7)	8.6 (2.1)
Right sternocleidomastoid	Active TrPs (n = 3)	5.2 (2)	2.8 (0.8)	6.8 (1.7)
(n = 15)	Latent TrPs (n = 2)	4.3 (0.3)	2.3 (1)	3.5 (3.5)
Left sternocleidomastoid	Active TrPs (n = 2)	3.9 (0.9)	2.5 (0.5)	5.7 (0.4)
(n = 15)	Latent TrPs (n = 7)	4.5 (1.3)	2.5 (0.7)	6.1 (3.8)
Right temporalis	Active TrPs (n = 6)	5 (1.4)	2.7 (0.5)	5.5 (3.1)
(n = 15)	Latent TrPs (n = 5)	4.5 (2)	3.1 (0.6)	7.3 (4.1)
Left temporalis	Active TrPs (n = 7)	4 (1.5)	2.8 (0.6)	7.3 (4)
(n = 15)	Latent TrPs (n = 4)	5.6 (1.9)	2.7 (0.7)	7 (1.4)
Suboccipital muscles	Active TrPs (n = 6)	4.8 (1.4)	2.9 (0.5)	4.2 (3.4)
(n = 10)	Latent TrPs (n = 4)	3.6 (1.4)	3 (0.5)	6.3 (0.4)

Values are expressed as mean (standard deviation) for all muscles.
VAS, Visual Analogue Scale (0–10); TrPs, muscle trigger points.
No comparison showed statistical significance (unpaired Student t test, P >0.05).
Reprinted from Fernández-de-las-Peñas et al., 2006c, 2007c.

SUMMARY

Trigger points in the superior oblique, upper trapezius, temporalis, suboccipital, and sternocleidomastoid muscles are clinically relevant for episodic and chronic tension-type headache. Nevertheless, future studies are required to investigate whether TrPs in other muscles (e.g., splenius capitis or cervicis, levator scapulae, masseter) are also prevalent in tension-type headache.

REFERENCES

Abrahams VC, Swett JE. The pattern of spinal and medullary projections from a cutaneous nerve and a muscle nerve of the forelimb of the cat: a study using transganglionic transport of HRP. *J Comp Neurol* 1986;246:70–84.

Arendt-Nielsen L, Petersen-Felix S, Fischer M, Bak P, Bjerring P, Zbinden AM. The effect of N methyl-aspartate antagonist (ketamine) on single and repeated nociceptive stimuli: a placebo-controlled experimental human study. *Anesth Analg* 1995;81:63–68.

Ashina S, Jensen R, Bendtsen L. Pain sensitivity in pericranial and extra-cranial regions. *Cephalalgia* 2003;23:456–462.

Bartsch T, Goadsby P. Stimulation of the greater occipital nerve induces increased central excitability of dural afferent input. *Brain* 2002;125:1496–1509.

Bartsch T, Goadsby P. Increased responses in trigemino-cervical nociceptive neurons to cervical input after stimulation of the dura mater. *Brain* 2003;126:1801–1813.

Bendtsen L. Central sensitization in tension-type headache: possible patho-physiological mechanisms. *Cephalalgia* 2000;29:486–508.

Bendtsen L, Schoenen J. Synthesis of tension type headache mechanisms. In: Olesen J, Goasdby P, Ramdan NM, Tfelt-Hansen P, Welch KMA. *The Headaches*. 3rd ed. Philadelphia: Lippincott Williams & Wilkins; 2006.

Bendtsen L, Jensen R, Jensen NK, Olesen J. Pressure-controlled palpation: a new technique which increases the reliability of manual palpation. *Cephalalgia* 1995;15:205–210.

Chen SM, Chen JT, Kuan TS, Hong J, Hong CZ. Decrease in pressure pain thresholds of latent myofascial trigger points in the middle finger extensors immediately after continuous piano practice. *J Musculoskeletal Pain* 2000;8(3):83–92.

Chun WX. An approach to the nature of tension type headache. *Headache* 1985;25:188–189.

Clark GT, Sakai S, Merrill R, Flack VF, McCreary C. Cross-correlation between stress, pain, physical activity, and temporalis muscle EMG in tension-type headache. *Cephalalgia* 1995;15:511–518.

Couppé C, Midttun A, Hilden J, Jorgensen U, Oxholm P, Fuglsang-Frederiksen A. Spontaneous needle electromyographic activity in myofascial trigger points in the infraspinatus muscle: a blinded assessment. *J Musculoskeletal Pain* 2001;9(3):7–16.

Couppé C, Torelli P, Fuglsang-Frederiksen A, Andersen KV, Jensen R. Myofascial trigger points are very prevalent in patients with chronic tension-type headache: a double-blinded controlled study. *Clin J Pain* 2007;23:23–27.

Davidoff RA. Trigger points and myofascial pain: toward understanding how they affect headaches. *Cephalalgia* 1998;18:436–448.

Dejung B, Gröbli C, Colla F, Weissman R. *Trigger Point Therapy*. Bern: Verlag Hans Huber; 2003.

Fassbender HG. Non-articular rheumatism. In: *Pathology of Rheumatic Diseases*. New York: Springer-Verlag; 1975:303–314.

Fernández-de-las-Peñas C, Cuadrado ML, Gerwin RD, Pareja JA. Referred pain from the trochlear region in tension-type headache: a myofascial trigger point from the superior oblique muscle. *Headache* 2005;45:731–737.

Fernández-de-las-Peñas C, Alonso-Blanco C, Cuadrado ML, Gerwin RD, Pareja JA. Trigger points in the suboccipital muscles and forward head posture in tension type headache. *Headache* 2006a;46:454–460.

Fernández-de-las-Peñas C, Alonso-Blanco C, Cuadrado ML, Gerwin R, Pareja JA. Myofascial trigger points and their relationship with headache clinical parameters in chronic tension type headache. *Headache* 2006b;46:1264–1272.

Fernández-de-las-Peñas C, Alonso-Blanco C, Cuadrado ML, Pareja JA. Myofascial trigger points in the suboccipital muscles in episodic tension type headache. *Man Ther* 2006c;11:225–230.

Fernández-de-las-Peñas C, Arendt-Nielsen L, Simons DG. Contributions of myofascial trigger points to chronic tension type headache. *J Manual Manipulative Ther* 2006d;14:222–231.

Fernández-de-las-Peñas C, Ge H, Arendt-Nielsen L, Cuadrado ML, Pareja JA. Referred pain from trapezius muscle trigger point shares similar characteristics with chronic tension type headache. *Eur J Pain* 2007a;11:475–482.

Fernández-de-las-Peñas C, Ge H, Arendt-Nielsen L, Cuadrado ML, Pareja JA. The local and referred pain from myofascial trigger points in the temporalis muscle contributes to pain profile in chronic tension-type headache. *Clin J Pain* 2007b;23:786–792.

Fernández-de-las-Peñas C, Cuadrado ML, Pareja JA. Myofascial trigger points, neck mobility and forward head posture in episodic tension type headache. *Headache* 2007c;47:662–672.

Fernández-de-las-Peñas C, Cuadrado ML, Gerwin RD, Pareja JA. Referred pain from the lateral rectus muscle in subjects with chronic tension type headache. *Pain Med* 2008 (in press).

Ge HY. Experimental neck shoulder pain: gender differences in pain modulation [PhD thesis]. Aalborg University, Denmark, 2004.

Ge HY, Madeleine P, Wang K, Arendt-Nielsen L. Hypoalgesia to pressure pain in referred pain areas triggered by spatial summation of experimental muscle pain from unilateral or bilateral trapezius muscles. *Eur J Pain* 2003;7:531–537.

Ge HY, Wang K, Madeleine P, Svensson P, Sessle BJ, Arendt-Nielsen L. Simultaneous modulation of the exteroceptive suppression periods in the trapezius and temporalis muscles by experimental muscle pain. *Clin Neurophysiol* 2004a;115:1399–1408.

Ge HY, Madeleine P, Arendt-Nielsen L. Sex differences in temporal characteristics of descending inhibitory control: an evaluation using repeated bilateral experimental induction of muscle pain. *Pain* 2004b;110:72–78.

Ge HY, Arendt-Nielsen L, Farina D, Madeleine P. Gender-specific differences in electromyographic changes and perceived pain induced by experimental muscle pain during sustained contractions of the upper trapezius muscle. *Muscle Nerve* 2005;32:726–733.

Ge HY, Madeleine P, Cairns BE, Arendt-Nielsen L. Hypoalgesia in the referred pain areas after bilateral injections of hypertonic saline into the trapezius muscles of men and women: a potential experimental model of gender-specific differences. *Clin J Pain* 2006a;22:37–44.

Ge HY, Fernández-de-las-Peñas C, Arendt-Nielsen L. Sympathetic facilitation of hyperalgesia evoked from myofascial tender and trigger points in patients with unilateral shoulder pain. *Clin Neurophysiol* 2006b;117:1545–1550.

Gerwin R. Headache. In: Ferguson L, Gerwin R, eds. *Clinical Mastery in the Treatment of Myofascial Pain*. Philadelphia: Lippincott Williams & Wilkins; 2005:1–24.

Gerwin RD, Shannon S, Hong CZ, Hubbard D, Gevirtz R. Inter-rater reliability in myofascial trigger point examination. *Pain* 1997;69:65–73.

Gerwin RD, Dommerholt D, Shah JP. An expansion of Simons' integrated hypothesis of trigger point formation. *Curr Pain Headache Rep* 2004;8:468–475.

Giamberardino MA. Visceral hyperalgesia. In: *Proceedings of the 9th World Congress on Pain*. Seattle: IASP Press; 1999.

Goebel H, Weigle L, Kropp P, Soyka D. Pain sensitivity and pain reactivity of pericranial muscles in migraine and tension-type headache. *Cephalalgia* 1992;12:142–151.

Graven-Nielsen T, Arendt-Nielsen L, Svensson P, Jensen T. Experimental muscle pain: a quantitative study of local and referred pain in humans following injection of hypertonic saline. *J Musculoskeletal Pain* 1997;5:49–69.

Hatch JP, Prihoda TJ, Moore PJ, Cyr-Provost M, Borcherding S, Boutros NN, Seleshi E. A naturalistic study of the relationships among electromyographic activity, psychological stress, and pain in ambulatory tension-type headache patients and headache-free controls. *Psychosom Med* 1991;53:576–584.

Hatch JP, Moore PJ, Provost M, Boutros NN, Seleshi E, Borcherding S. The use of electromyography and muscle palpation in the diagnosis of tension-type headache with and without pericranial muscle involvement. *Pain* 1992;49:175–178.

Hoheisel U, Mense S. Response behaviour of cat dorsal horn neurones receiving input from skeletal muscle and other deep somatic tissues. *J Physiol (Lond)* 1990;426:265–280.

Hoheisel U, Mense S, Simons DG, Yu XM. Appearance of new receptive fields in rat dorsal horn neurons following noxious stimulation of skeletal muscle: a model for referral of muscle pain? *Neurosci Lett* 1993;153:9–12.

Hong CZ, Chen YN, Twehous D, Hing DH. Pressure threshold for referred pain by compression on trigger point and adjacent areas. *J Musculoskeletal Pain* 1996;4(3):61–79.

Hubbard DR, Berkoff GM. Myofascial trigger points show spontaneous needle EMG activity. *Spine* 1993;18:1803–1807.

International Headache Society. Classification and Diagnostic Criteria for Headache Disorders, Cranial Neuralgias and Facial Pain: 1st edition. *Cephalalgia* 1988;8(suppl 7):29–34.

International Headache Society. The International Classification of Headache Disorders: 2nd edition. *Cephalalgia* 2004;24(suppl 1):8–152.

Itoh K, Okada K, Kawakita K. A proposed experimental model of myofascial trigger points in human muscle after slow eccentric exercise. *Acupunct Med* 2004;22:2–13.

Jensen R. Mechanisms of spontaneous tension-type headaches: an analysis of tenderness, pain thresholds and EMG. *Pain* 1996;64:251–256.

Jensen R, Fuglsang Frederiksen A, Olesen J. Quantitative surface EMG of pericranial muscles in headache. A population study. *Electroencephalogr Clin Neurophysiol* 1994;93:335–344.

Jensen R, Bendtsen L, Olesen J. Muscular factors are of importance in tension type headache. *Headache* 1998;38:10–17.

Jull GA, Niere R. The cervical spine and headache. In: *Grieve's Modern Manual Therapy of the Vertebral Column*. Edinburgh: Churchill Livingstone; 2004:291–311.

Lange M. *Die Muskelhärten (Myogelosen)*. Munich: JF Lehmanns; 1931.

Langemark M, Olesen J. Pericranial tenderness in tension headache. A blind controlled study. *Cephalalgia* 1987;7:249–255.

Lucas KR, Polus BI, Rich PA. Latent myofascial trigger points: their effects on muscle activation and movement efficiency. *J Bodywork Mov Ther* 2004;8:160–166.

Makowska A, Panfil C, Ellrich J. Long-term potentiation of orofacial sensorimotor processing by noxious input from the semispinal neck muscle in mice. *Cephalalgia* 2005;25:109–116.

Marcus DA, Scharff L, Mercer S, Turk DC. Musculoskeletal abnormalities in chronic headache: a controlled comparison of headache diagnostic groups. *Headache* 1999;39:21–27.

McPartland JM, Simons DG. Myofascial trigger points: translating molecular theory into manual therapy. *J Man Manipulative Ther* 2006;14:232–239.

Mense S. Peripheral mechanisms of muscle nociception and local muscle pain. *J Musculoskeletal Pain* 1993;1:133–170.

Mense S. Referral of muscle pain: new aspects. *Am Pain Soc J* 1994;3:1–9.

Mense S, Simons DG, Russell IJ. *Muscle Pain: Understanding Its Nature, Diagnosis and Treatment*. Philadelphia: Lippincott, Williams & Wilkins; 2001.

Mercer S, Marcus DA, Nash J. Cervical musculoskeletal disorders in migraine and tension type headache. Presented at the 68th Annual Meeting of the American Physical Therapy Association; Cincinnati, OH; 1993.

Mörk H, Ashina M, Bendtsen L, Olesen J, Jensen R. Induction of prolonged tenderness in patients with tension-type headache by means of a new experimental model of myofascial pain. *Eur J Neurol* 2003;10:249–256.

Newham DJ, Edwards RHT, Mills KR. Skeletal muscle pain. In: Wall PD, Melzack R, eds. *Textbook of Pain*. 3rd ed. Edinburgh: Churchill Livingstone; 1994:423–440.

Nillson N. Evidence that tension-type headache and cervicogenic headache are distinct disorders. *J Manipulative Physiol Ther* 2000;23:288–289.

Nyberg G, Blomqvist A. The central projection of muscle afferent fibers to the lower medulla and upper spinal cord: an anatomical study in the cat with the transganglionic transport method. *J Comp Neurol* 1984;230:99–108.

Pielstickera A, Haagc G, Zaudigh M, Lautenbachera S. Impairment of pain inhibition in chronic tension-type headache. *Pain* 2005;118:215–223.

Piovesan EJ, Kowacs PA, Oshinsky ML. Convergence of cervical and trigeminal sensory afferents. *Curr Pain Headache Rep* 2003;7:377–383.

Price DD, Mao J, Frenk H, Mayer DJ. The N-methyl-aspartate receptor antagonist dextromethorphan selectively reduces temporal summation of second pain in man. *Pain* 1994;59:165–174.

Qerama E, Fuglsang-Frederiksen A, Kasch H, Bach FW, Jensen TS. Evoked pain in motor endplate region of the brachial biceps muscle: an experimental study. *Muscle Nerve* 2004;29:393–400.

Rasmussen BK, Jensen R, Schroll M, Olesen J. Epidemiology of headache in a general population: a prevalence study. *J Clin Epidemiol* 1991;44:1147–1157.

Rasmussen BK, Jensen R, Schroll M, Olesen J. Interrelation between migraine and tension type headache in the general population. *Arch Neurol* 1992;49:914–918.

Sandrini G, Antonaci F, Pucci E, Bono G, Nappi G. Comparative study with EMG, pressure algometry and manual palpation in tension-type headache and migraine. *Cephalalgia* 1994;14:451–457.

Schaible HG, Schmidt RF, Willis WD. Convergent inputs from articular, cutaneous and muscle receptors onto ascending tract cells in the cat spinal cord. *Exp Brain Res* 1987;66:479–488.

Schmidt-Hansen PT, Svensson P, Jensen TS, Graven-Nielsen T, Bach FW. Patterns of experimentally induced pain in pericranial muscles. *Cephalalgia* 2006;26:568–577.

Schmidt-Wilcke T, Leinisch E, Straube A, Kampfe N, Draganski B, Diener HC, Bogdahn U, May A. Gray matter decrease in patients with chronic tension type headache. *Neurology* 2005;65:1483–1486.

Schoenen J, Gerard P, De Pasqua V, Sianard Gainko J. Multiple clinical and para-clinical analyses of chronic tension type headache associated or un-associated with disorder of pericranial muscles. *Cephalalgia* 1991;11:135–139.

Sciotti VM, Mittak VL, DiMarco L, Ford LM, Plezbert J, Santipadri E, Wigglesworth J, Ball K. Clinical precision of myofascial trigger point location in the trapezius muscle. *Pain* 2001;93:259–266.

Shah JP, Phillips TM, Danoff JV, Gerber LH. An in vitro microanalytical technique for measuring the local biochemical milieu of human skeletal muscle. *J Appl Physiol* 2005;99:1977–1984.

Simons DG. Neuro-physiological basis of pain caused by trigger points. *Am Pain Soc J* 1994;3:17–19.

Simons DG. Do endplate noise and spikes arise from normal motor endplates? *Am J Phys Med Rehabil* 2001;80:134–140.

Simons DG. Review of enigmatic MTrPs as a common cause of enigmatic musculoskeletal pain and dysfunction. *J Electromyogr Kinesiol* 2004;14:95–107.

Simons DG, Travell J, Simons LS. *Myofascial Pain and Dysfunction: The Trigger Point Manual.* Vol. 1. 2nd ed. Baltimore: Williams & Wilkins; 1999.

Simons D, Hong CZ, Simons L. Endplate potentials are common to midfiber myofascial trigger points. *Am J Phys Med Rehabil* 2002;81:212–222.

Sjaastad O, Fredriksen TA, Pfaffenrath V. Cervicogenic headache: diagnostic criteria. *Headache* 1998;38:442–445.

Treaster D, Marras W, Burr D, Sheedy J, Hart D. Myofascial trigger point development from visual and postural stressors during computer work. *J Electromyogr Kinesiol* 2006;16:115–124.

Vierck CJ Jr, Cannon RL, Fry G, Maixner W, Whitsel BL. Characteristics of temporal summation of second pain sensations elicited by brief contact of glabrous skin by a preheated thermode. *J Neurophysiol* 1997;78:992–1002.

Wright EF. Referred cranio-facial pain patterns in patients with temporo-mandibular disorder. *J Am Dent Assoc* 2000;131:1307–1315.

Suboccipital Muscle Contribution to Tension-Type Headache

Richard C. Hallgren, PhDEE, PhDBME, and
César Fernández-de-las-Peñas, PT, DO, PhD

Chronic pain syndromes are costly to both the individual and to society. Even apart from the personal implications of spending 20 to 40 years in disabling pain, the financial burden of chronic pain is estimated to cost the United States over 60 billion dollars annually, with most of this expense attributed to a small group of patients who are considered to be disabled. Chronic pain syndromes are often difficult to treat because a clear cause for the pain is often absent. Although there has been a significant effort by physicians and clinical scientists to define morphologic and physiologic abnormalities that result in head, neck, and back pain and to characterize the etiology of pathology, it has resulted in only modest success.

Because there is not always a clear understanding of the organic cause of painful syndromes, it is difficult for a physician to know how best to resolve the problem and eliminate the pain. Cherkin et al. (1995) found little consensus among physicians about which treatments are effective for low back pain, and poor correlation between treatments that physicians *believed* were effective and those that had been *shown* to be effective by well-designed studies. Surgical interventions for chronic benign pain syndromes are generally quite ineffective in providing long-term relief (Wetzel, 1992). It has been estimated that at least 10% of all medical-surgical patients have no objective evidence of disease (Deyo et al., 1990a), helping to explain at least part of this lack of success. Further, some randomized clinical trials suggested that traction (Deyo et al., 1990b), transcutaneous electrical nerve stimulation (Guieu

& Serratrice, 1992), and facet joint (Buckelew et al., 1994) or trigger point injections (Garvey et al., 1989) may also be ineffective in treating chronic low back pain. Purely educational interventions have also been shown to have no impact on symptoms, function, disability, or health-care use (Cherkin et al., 1995). It would be easy to conclude that apart from a clear definition of morphologic and physiologic pathology, the best that can be hoped for the individual who has chronic head and neck pain is spontaneous resolution of the problem.

FUNCTIONAL AND ANATOMIC CHARACTERISTICS OF THE CERVICAL SPINE

Upper Cervical Vertebrae

Vertebrae of the upper cervical spine have unique morphologic characteristics:

- No intervertebral discs separate the occiput from C1, and C1 from C2.
- C1 does not have a typical vertebral body, but instead has paired lateral masses interconnected by anterior and posterior arches (Doherty & Heggeness, 1994).

These lateral masses have superior and inferior facets that form articulations between the adjacent structures. The anterior arch of the axis vertebra is thickened centrally, forming a structure called the odontoid process (Hollinshead, 1967; Panjabi et al., 1988) that permits rotation of the skull and the atlas as a unit. These first two joints at the top of the spinal column are highly specialized to provide flexion-extension and side-bending motions at the junction of the atlas and the occiput, and head rotation at the junction of the atlas and axis.

Upper Cervical Muscles

The muscles of the upper cervical spine that are involved with flexion and extension are referred to as the capital flexors and the capital extensors (Burt, 1995). The capital extensors, collectively known as suboccipital muscles (Staubesand, 1986), consist of the rectus capitis posterior major (RCPmaj), the rectus capitis posterior minor (RCPmin), the oblique capitis inferior (OCinf), and the oblique capitis superior (OCsup).

Although suboccipital muscles can be functionally classified as extensor muscles, their small size, relative to larger muscles that act in parallel with them, minimizes their contribution to motion (Nitz & Peck, 1986; Nolan & Sherk, 1988). A parallel muscle combination—that is, short muscles acting across joints in parallel with much larger muscles—occurs often in humans. The smaller muscles of parallel muscle combinations have an average of 3.76 times as many spindles per gram of tissue as do their large counterparts. The greatest absolute value of spindle density occurs in the smaller muscles of parallel muscle combinations in the cervical spine (Peck et al., 1984). It has been suggested that the function of these small muscles is to provide proprioceptive feedback to the central nervous system related to the position and motion of the head (Cooper & Danial, 1963; Abrahams, 1977). Examination of the properties of fibers entering the upper cervical cord revealed that the majority did not have its origin in the large dorsal neck muscles under study, but rather originated from the smaller muscles. These fibers, which had spindlelike firing patterns, showed remarkably large changes in their firing response rate to even the smallest movement of vertebral joints (Abrahams, 1981).

Upper Cervical Nerves

The C1 dorsal ramus, arising from the C1 spinal nerve as it crosses the superior aspect of the posterior arch of the atlas, branches to innervate the suboccipital muscles (Gray, 1977). The C1 dorsal ramus passes dorsolaterally through the suboccipital plexus of veins, describing an upward arch to enter the suboccipital triangle, where it divides to form a branch for the RCPmin muscles. Most commonly the suboccipital muscles are innervated in their dorsal surfaces; however, the branch to the RCPmin muscles may innervate its muscle ventrally or by penetrating the RCPmaj muscle (Bogduk, 1982). Anatomic variations in these nerve/muscle relations, both intra- and interindividually, are commonly reported. In an autopsy study performed on 20 cases, the greater occipital nerve was found to penetrate the trapezius muscle in 45% of the cases, the semispinalis capitis muscle was penetrated in 90% of the cases, and the inferior oblique muscle was penetrated in 7.5% of the cases (Bovim et al., 1991).

Although C1 does not have a dermatome, there are other peripheral nerves that do not have dermatomal sensation that often cause pain when damaged, for ex-

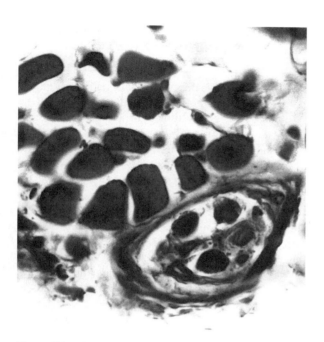

Figure 7.1 Spindle Organs in the Rectus Capitis Posterior Minor Muscle

Reprinted with permission from Hallgren RC, Greenman PE, Rechtien JJ. Atrophy of suboccipital muscles in patients with chronic pain: a pilot study. *Journal of the American Osteopathic Association* 1994;12:1032–1038, © 1994.

ample, the anterior interosseous, posterior interosseous suprascapulary, and long thoracic nerves (Polletti, 1991). C1 does have a rudimentary dorsal root ganglion (DRG) (Kerr, 1961; Gray, 1977). Although the literature does not specifically report on spindle organs in the RCPmin muscles, there is no reason to believe that they would be different from other skeletal muscles. Nevertheless, to eliminate any doubt of their existence, we dissected the RCPmin and RCPmaj muscles from embalmed cadavers. The embalmed tissue was post-fixed in 10% neutral formalin and processed according to standard paraffin procedures (Armed Forces Institute of Pathology, 1960). Sections were cut on a rotary microtome at microns and stained with hematoxylin and eosin (H&E) and Gomori trichrome (Armed Forces, 1960). We confirmed that spindle organs do exist in the RCPmin muscles (**Figure 7.1**) and that their density is similar to the density of spindles found in the RCPmaj muscles.

Bogduk (1982) demonstrated the existence of communicating branches between C1 and C2, making it conceptually possible that proprioceptive activity from structures such as muscle spindles in the RCPmin muscles is relayed to the central nervous system at the level of C1 or of C2, through the C1 communicating branch that meets the superior communicating branch of the C2 dorsal ramus (Bogduk, 1982; Haig & Parks, 1994). Intraoperative electrical stimulation of C1 dorsal rootlets in conscious patients has been shown to elicit retro-orbital and frontal pain (Kerr, 1961). These provide evidence for the existence of proprioceptive and nociceptive pathways from C1 to the spinal cord (Ehni & Benner, 1984).

Afferent fibers from the upper cervical muscles terminate within the dorsal gray matter of the spinal cord. This region, often referred to as the trigeminocervical nucleus caudalis, encompasses the pars caudalis of the spinal nucleus and also contains afferents from the first division of the trigeminal nerve (Kelly, 1985). Histologically, the pars caudalis consists of layers of cells that are identical to laminae I to V of the spinal dorsal horn. With respect to nociception, the physiologic properties of the neurons in the pars caudalis are virtually identical to those of nociceptive neurons of the dorsal horn. The trigeminocervical nucleus is important because activity within this region can be interpreted as pain referral to the frontal and orbital regions of the head regardless of the point of origin of the activity. Only structures innervated by C1 through C3 have been shown to be capable of causing headache. These include muscles, joints, and ligaments of the upper three cervical segments, as well as the dura mater of the spinal cord, posterior cranial fossa, and the vertebral artery (Bogduk, 1992).

ROLE OF ELECTROMYOGRAPHY IN DETERMINING THE ETIOLOGY OF MUSCLE ATROPHY

The presence of abnormal spontaneous electrical activity (fibrillation potentials and positive sharp waves) when a muscle is relaxed and an electromyographic (EMG) needle electrode is not being moved is an indication of abnormal nerve or muscle membrane stability (Dumitru, 1996) that most commonly accompanies lower motor neuron trauma that results in denervation of skeletal muscle (Nitz & Peck, 1986). As a rule, abnormal spontaneous activity will not be recorded in skeletal muscle weakened by disuse atrophy. Consequently, abnormal spontaneous activity, if reproducible in at least two muscle sites, suggests the existence of an abnormality that is associated with denervated muscle and certain primary muscle diseases (Kohara et al., 1993). Previous articles (Rantanen et al., 1993; Sihvonen et al., 1993) described atrophic changes in the multifidus muscle occurring after lumbar laminectomy in a group of patients who experienced significant postoperative low back pain. Denervation atrophy, resulting from lesions to the dorsal ramus nerve as a result of mechanical trauma during surgery, was confirmed from EMG data collected from the lumbar multifidus. EMG data have also been used to obtain precise determination of the anatomic root level of radiculopathy by assessment of spontaneous activity precipitated by insertion of a needle electrode into lumbar paraspinal muscles (Haig et al., 1993). Muscle wasting, as a consequence of disuse (Milne et al., 1988), results in decreased muscle volume of up to 50% of normal within 1 or 2 months (Halar & Bell, 1988) but does not result in a decrease in the number of muscle fibers. Consequently, with exercise and time, the fibers will again increase in size, and strength will be regained. In contrast, denervation of skeletal muscle results in an irreversible loss of muscle fibers, and is characterized by infiltration with fatty tissue (Bertoniri & Igarashi, 1985).

We have previously presented a technique to insert a needle and inject dye into the RCPmin muscles of cadavers that was modified from Haig et al. (1991). This technique was refined and modified for use in living subjects. A line is drawn between the inion and spinous process of the C2 vertebra. This distance is bisected, and a 50-mm monopolar needle electrode is inserted approximately 1 cm lateral to the midline at the bisected line. The electrode is angled so that the point of the needle is directed cephalad. The electrode is inserted until it encounters a bony stop (occiput). Insertional activity is observed during these insertions. Care should be taken to observe insertional activity 1 to 2 cm from the occiput, increasing the probability of sampling the RCPmin muscle. The needle electrode is withdrawn to the subcutaneous tissue, and the angle of the needle is changed approximately 20° and a new vector explored. Again, the needle electrode is inserted until the occiput is found. When the angle between the needle electrode and the skin of the neck reaches 90°, the insertions are stopped. At each insertion near the occiput bone, the needle is moved, withdrawn, and moved slightly medially-laterally to explore other "quadrants of the muscle." The electromyographer attempts 20 separate insertions with observed insertional activities performed in each RCPmin muscle.

ROLE OF MAGNETIC RESONANCE IMAGING IN DETERMINING THE EXTENT OF MUSCLE ATROPHY

Biologic tissues have intrinsic characteristics that permit reliable identification of the tissue type from magnetic resonance imaging (MRI) data. In T1-weighted images, grayscale intensity is inversely related to the value of T1, meaning that tissues having short values for T1 (fat and blood) produce bright images, whereas tissues having long values for T1 (edema and tumors) produce dark images. In T2-weighted images, grayscale intensity is directly related to T2 values, meaning that tissues having short values for T2 (tendons, cartilage, and muscle) produce dark images, whereas structures having long values for T2 (urine, edema, and fat) produce bright images (Horowitz, 1989). By manipulating imaging parameters, the image intensity of skeletal muscle (T1 = 900 msec, T2 = 30 msec) can be changed relative to fatty tissues (T1 = 250 msec, T2 = 80 msec). It is this ability to control image contrast that makes MRI a qualified noninvasive procedure for studying musculoskeletal trauma and dysfunction (Fleckenstein et al., 1989a, 1989b; Coderre et al., 1993).

CHANGES IN SUBOCCIPITAL MUSCLE MORPHOMETRY IN CHRONIC PAIN CONDITIONS

Several studies have demonstrated changes in muscle morphometry in several chronic pain conditions, for example, neck pain (Hallgren et al., 1994), whiplash (Elliott et al., 2008), or chronic tension-type headache (Fernández-de-las-Peñas et al., 2007). The first study was conducted in 1994 as follows: Control subjects were recruited from faculty, students, and staff of Michigan State University. No attempt was made to match a chronic pain subject with a specific control. A physician, using standardized methods, performed a structural examination of the cervical spine of all subjects who did not violate the exclusion criteria. The examination consisted of measurement of range of motion of the upper (C0-C1, C1-C2, and C2-C3) and lower (C2-C7) cervical complex, and determination of the presence or absence of a lesion. Evaluation was made on the basis of texture abnormalities of the skin, subcutaneous tissues, or muscles and of altered motion characteristics, particularly hypomobility and asymmetry of form and function, of the cervical spine. In order to con-

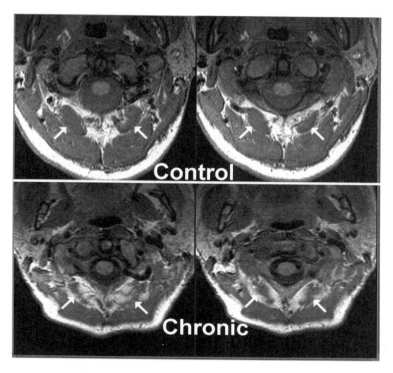

Figure 7.2 Magnetic Resonance Image from One Healthy Subject (top) and One Chronic Pain Patient (bottom)

Reprinted with permission from Hallgren RC, Greenman PE, Rechtien JJ. Atrophy of suboccipital muscles in patients with chronic pain: a pilot study. *Journal of the American Osteopathic Association* 1994;12:1032–1038. © 1994.

tinue with the project, a subject needed to fall into one of the two following categories:

- *Control group:* Free of significant motion restrictions and having no history of recurring neck and head pain
- *Chronic pain group:* Being treated for chronic pain and having significant restriction of motion thought to be provoked by abnormal neuromuscular conditions

For all subjects, axial images consisting of 4-mm-thick contiguous slices of data were collected inferior and superior to the posterior arch of the atlas using a 1.5-tesla superconducting magnet (Signa; General Electric Medical Systems, Milwaukee, WI) with TR equal to 2,000 msec, TE equal to 25 msec, a 12-cm field of view, a 128 × 256 matrix, NEX equal to 2, and a total scan time approximately equal to 8.5 minutes. The RCPmaj and the RCPmin muscles of five control subjects (three men, two women; age, 37.6 years) and six chronic pain patients (six women; age,

42.1 years) were the muscles that were of primary interest.

Figure 7.2 shows data from one subject who was considered to be representative of the control group and from one subject of the chronic pain group. There was significant difference between the appearances of the RCPmaj muscles in the two persons. For control subjects, the boundaries of muscles are well defined and the muscles are of uniform intensity. Muscles from the chronic pain group had an appearance that was characteristic of skeletal muscle that has died and been replaced with fatty tissue. Comparison of muscles in PD-weighted images with muscles in T2-weighted images (TR = 2,000 msec, TE = 80 msec) confirmed that the infiltrating tissue was a fatty type.

The average intensity of a 200 sample of pixel values taken from within the spinal cord of each subject, from eight consecutive slice levels, was used to calculate an individual normalization factor that permitted the comparison of muscle intensity values between subjects. Spinal cord data from both control and chronic pain

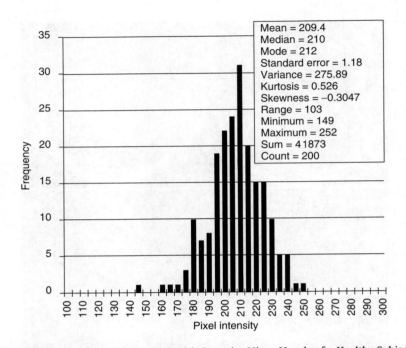

Mean = 209.4
Median = 210
Mode = 212
Standard error = 1.18
Variance = 275.89
Kurtosis = 0.526
Skewness = −0.3047
Range = 103
Minimum = 149
Maximum = 252
Sum = 41873
Count = 200

Figure 7.3 Histogram of 200 Samples from the Rectus Capitis Posterior Minor Muscle of a Healthy Subject

Reprinted with permission from Hallgren RC, Greenman PE, Rechtien JJ. Atrophy of suboccipital muscles in patients with chronic pain: a pilot study. *Journal of the American Osteopathic Association* 1994;12:1032–1038, © 1994.

subjects was, for all practical purposes, Gaussian. Samples taken from the RCPmin muscles of control subjects (**Figure 7.3**) had the same Gaussian distribution as the samples from the spinal cord. However, the histogram of pixel intensity samples taken from the RCPmin mucles of chronic pain subjects (**Figure 7.4**) was found to be skewed toward higher intensity values as a result of an increased percentage of high intensity pixels (i.e., fatty tissue). These findings were supported in a study conducted by the same group (McPartland et al., 1997).

More recent studies have been conducted with the following guideline: An axial scan of the cervical spine was planned from sagittal scout images. Axial MR slice data, aligned parallel to the C2-3 intervertebral disc, were collected from the base of the occiput down through the upper portion of the C5-C7 vertebral body so that cross-sectional area (CSA) measurements could be performed. Because CSA measurements of cervical extensor muscles above and below the C2-3 level could include a slight measurement error in both patients and controls, relative CSA (rCSA) were reported. The rCSAs of the neck extensor muscles were calculated from the region of interest that was created on the axial images at certain cervical levels. Axial scans at C1 and C2 levels were used to measure the rCSA for the RCPmin and the RCPmaj muscles on both sides, respectively. The rCSA measures for the superficial extensor muscles (i.e., semispinalis capitis and splenius capitis) were obtained at two segments (C3 and C4) on the axial slices crossing the most cephalad portion of each corresponding vertebral body (Elliott et al., 2006, 2007, 2008; Fernández-de-las-Peñas et al., 2007).

Elliott et al. (2007) have published preliminary data of normal morphometry of the cervical extensor muscles in a cohort of healthy females within a defined age range (18–45 years). These authors found significant side-to-side differences in the relative cross-sectional area for the RCPmin (P <0.001), RCPmaj (P <0.001), multifidus (P = 0.002), the semispinalis cervicis (P = 0.001), and capitis (P <0.001) muscles. There were vertebral-level differences in muscle morphometry, with a greater cross-sectional area in lower cervical levels, of the semispinalis cervicis/capitis, multifidus, splenius capitis, and upper trapezius (P <0.001) (Elliott et al., 2007).

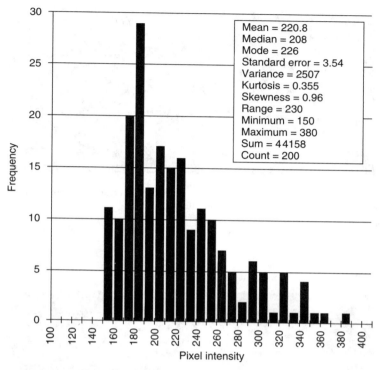

Mean = 220.8
Median = 208
Mode = 226
Standard error = 3.54
Variance = 2507
Kurtosis = 0.355
Skewness = 0.96
Range = 230
Minimum = 150
Maximum = 380
Sum = 44158
Count = 200

Figure 7.4 **Histogram of Pixel Intensity from the Rectus Capitis Posterior Minor Muscle of a Chronic Pain Patient**
Reprinted with permission from Hallgren RC, Greenman PE, Rechtien JJ. Atrophy of suboccipital muscles in patients with chronic pain: a pilot study. *Journal of the American Osteopathic Association* 1994;12:1032–1038, © 1994.

These authors analyzed fatty infiltration (Elliott et al., 2006) and cross-sectional area (Elliott et al., 2008) of the cervical extensors in patients with whiplash-associated disorders (WAD). WAD patients had significantly larger amounts of fatty infiltrate for all of the cervical extensor muscles compared with healthy control subjects (P <0.0001). In addition, the amount of fatty infiltrate varied by both cervical level and muscle, with the RCPmin, RCPmaj, and multifidus at C3 level having the largest amount of fatty infiltrate (P <0.0001). Further, intramuscular fat was independent of age, self-reported pain or disability, compensation status, body mass index, and duration of symptoms (Elliott et al., 2006). These authors suggested that the higher levels of fatty infiltrate in the RCPmin, RCPmaj, and multifidus muscles (C3 level) in the WAD group could lead to the contention that there was a greater injury with consequent change in the muscles at these segments (Elliott et al., 2006). Further, fatty infiltration in the muscles could be associated with several mechanisms, for example, generalized disuse, chronic denervation, motor-neuron

lesions, metabolic disorders, or other muscle impairments (Elliott et al., 2006). In addition, WAD patients had significantly larger rCSA at all spinal levels for the cervical multifidus muscle (P <0.0001) (Elliott et al., 2008). It is possible that the consistent pattern of larger rCSA in multifidus at all levels and the variable pattern of rCSA values in the intermediate and superficial muscles in patients with WAD may reflect morphometric changes due to fatty infiltrate in the muscles. Higher fat content may alter and expand the muscle-fascial borders, thereby creating larger rCSA values with MRI measures, which suggests that measures of rCSA of the cervical extensor musculature have to be interpreted with caution, at least in persons with persistent WAD (Elliott et al., 2008). On the contrary, Elliott et al. (2008) did not find differences in rCSA for RCPmin and RCPmaj muscles between WAD patients and healthy controls.

Fernández-de-las-Peñas et al. (2007) have demonstrated that patients with chronic tension-type headache showed reduced rCSA for both RCPmin

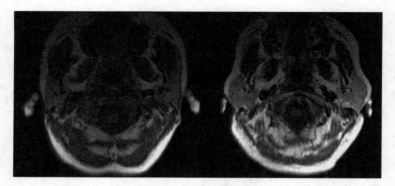

Figure 7.5 Comparison of the Cross-Sectional Area of the Rectus Capitis Posterior Minor Muscle Between a Patient with Chronic Tension-Type Headache (right) and a Healthy Subject (left)

Reprinted with permission from Fernández-de-las-Peñas C, Bueno A, Ferrando J, Elliott JM, Cuadrado ML, Pareja JA. Magnetic resonance imaging of the morphometry of cervical extensor muscles in chronic tension type headache. *Cephalalgia* 2007;27:355–362.

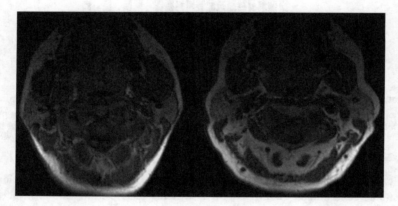

Figure 7.6 Comparison of the Cross-Sectional Area of the Rectus Capitis Posterior Major Muscle Between a Patient with Chronic Tension-Type Headache (right) and a Healthy Subject (left)

Reprinted with permission from Fernández-de-las-Peñas C, Bueno A, Ferrando J, Elliott JM, Cuadrado ML, Pareja JA. Magnetic resonance imaging of the morphometry of cervical extensor muscles in chronic tension type headache. *Cephalalgia* 2007;27:355–362.

(**Figure 7.5**) and RCPmaj (**Figure 7.6**) muscles compared with controls ($P <0.01$). On the other hand, rCSA for semispinalis capitis and splenius capitis at C3 and C4 levels in patients did not differ significantly from those in controls ($P >0.3$). **Table 7.1** summarizes the differences in rCSA between patients with chronic tension-type headache and healthy controls for each muscle (Fernández-de-las-Peñas et al., 2007). Further, there were significant negative correlations between headache intensity, duration, or frequency and rCSA for both RCPmin and RCPmaj muscles: the greater the headache intensity, duration, or frequency, the smaller

the rCSA in these two muscles (Fernández-de-las-Peñas et al., 2007).

NEUROPHYSIOLOGIC CONSEQUENCES OF MUSCLE ATROPHY

Muscle atrophy of the suboccipital muscles may play a relevant role in some chronic conditions, such as WAD or chronic tension-type headache. Peck et al. (1984) found that the suboccipital musculature showed greater concentration of muscle spindles (36 spindles per gram for RCPmin; 30.5 spindles per gram for RCPmaj) in com-

Table 7.1 Differences in Cross-Sectional Areas Between Chronic Tension-Type Headache Patients and Healthy Controls

	CTTH	Controls	*P* Value
RCPmin right side	78.2 (30.7)	122.6 (39.8)	0.002[a]
RCPmin left side	78.1 (22.6)	122.3 (35.1)	0.001[a]
RCPmaj right side	103.7 (22.2)	127.7 (29.5)	0.01[a]
RCPmaj left side	102.1 (18.4)	126.9 (30.8)	0.01[a]
Semispinalis capitis C3 right side	254.6 (52.3)	262.1 (53)	NS
Semispinalis capitis C3 left side	249.7 (57.1)	239.3 (41.7)	NS
Semispinalis capitis C4 right side	186.1 (45.8)	188.8 (36.3)	NS
Semispinalis capitis C4 left side	196.8 (43.8)	182.3 (31.1)	NS
Splenius capitis C3 right side	188.8 (39.3)	205.7 (51.8)[b]	NS
Splenius capitis C3 left side	189.4 (37.9)	191.7 (44.3)	NS
Splenius capitis C4 right side	146.3 (27.4)	153.8 (27.2)	NS
Splenius capitis C4 left side	154.2 (24.9)	153.6 (30.8)	NS

Values are expressed as mean (standard deviation).

CTTH, chronic tension-type headache; RCPmin, rectus capitis posterior minor; RCPmaj, rectus capitis posterior major; NS, nonsignificant.

[a]Significant differences between CTTH and controls (unpaired Student *t* test).

[b]Significant difference as compared with the left side (paired Student *t* test).

Reprinted with permission from Fernández-de-las-Peñas C et al. Magnetic resonance imaging of the morphometry of cervical extensor muscles in chronic tension type headache. *Cephalalgia* 2007;27:355–362.

parison with other cervical extensor muscles (e.g., 7.6 spindles per gram in the splenius capitis muscle). Such high densities of muscle spindles in both RCPmin and RCPmaj muscles suggest that these muscles act as proprioceptive monitors of the upper cervical spine. Further, we know that proprioceptive signals stemming from the muscles conveyed by large-diameter Aβ fibers may serve as a gate that blocks nociceptive (C-fiber) transmission into the spinal cord and higher centers of the central nervous system (Wall, 2005). Muscle atrophy could account for a reduction of proprioceptive output from these muscles, and may facilitate the transmission of impulses from wide dynamic range nociceptors (Wall, 2005). In that way, muscle atrophy may result in functional reorganization and central sensitization of neural structures in the dorsal root ganglion and the ventral horn (McMahon & Wall, 1984; Ilynsky et al., 1987; Beaman et al., 1993).

Second, muscle atrophy may produce functional weakness, resulting in spinal instability with the accompanying condition of chronic pain (Hayashi et al., 1992). Replacement of RCPmin muscle with fatty tissue, or a decrease in CSA, may result in spinal instability that puts abnormal demands upon synovial joints, structures that are known to be capable of producing head and

neck pain (Barnsley et al., 1995). This hypothesis is related to another possible explanation in which muscle atrophy could result from reflex inhibition associated with the development of chronic muscle pain (Hides et al., 1996; Hodges & Moseley, 2003). For example, nociceptive signals generated in suboccipital muscles may elicit referred pain (Shah et al., 2005; Fernández-de-las-Peñas et al., 2006). This referred pain may result in a guarding response by the patient that may reduce muscle function and further contribute to disuse atrophy, which might in turn perpetuate the pain cycle.

Third, muscle atrophy of the suboccipital muscles may result in decreased afferent activity from them, as a consequence of the physical loss of receptor organs or the loss of a viable afferent pathway. A decrease in afferent activity being transmitted to the central nervous system may result in dizziness or balance problems or both (Oosterveld et al., 1991; Revel et al., 1991). Head orientation in three-dimensional space makes use of visual, vestibular, and cervical proprioceptive cues (Revel et al., 1991). From a group of 262 patients suffering from the later effects of WAD, approximately 85% complained of some kind of vertigo (Oosterveld et al., 1991). Consequently, if nonspecific cervical pathology is paired with an alteration in kinesthetic sensibility that is evidenced by complaints of dizziness and disturbances of balance and equilibrium, it is possible that a proprioceptive deficit is involved, either by lesion or functional impairment of muscular or articular receptors, and could be a significant factor in the maintenance of chronic pain (Wall, 1991).

Finally, it is possible that proprioceptive muscles, such as the RCPmin and RCPmaj, may be more sensitive to muscle atrophy than other superficial muscles, such as the semispinalis capitis or splenius capitis.

ANATOMIC PARTICULARITIES OF THE SUBOCCIPITAL REGION

Hack et al. (1995) reported the existence of a connective tissue bridge between the RCPmin muscle and the dorsal spinal dura at the C0-C1 junction, providing anatomic evidence to link the two tissues. This connective tissue bridge runs perpendicular from the C0-C1 junction to the posterior atlanto-occipital membrane, which is intimately connected to the spinal dura. Rutten et al. (1997) have confirmed the existence of this connective tissue bridge and subsequently observed separate strands between the dura and the posterior wall of the vertebral canal. This muscle attachment to the cervical spine dura was later confirmed by Humphreys et al. (2003) and Zumpano et al. (2006). Further, Hack and Hallgren (2004) have reported a case of a single patient who experienced relief of chronic headache after surgical separation of this connective tissue bridge. Therefore, atrophic changes in RCPmin muscle may result in buckling of the spinal dura during movement of the head and neck that may result in pain (Alix & Bates, 1999). It is known that the dura mater is densely innervated by small-diameter A- and C-fiber afferents that are supplied by the ophthalmic division of the trigeminal nerve and the upper cervical roots (Yamada et al., 2001). Hack et al. (1995) speculated that this connective tissue bridge transmits forces from the cervical spine joint complex to the pain-sensitive dura. Therefore, when the head and neck are extended, the spinal dura folds inwardly toward the spinal cord in subjects with atrophic RCPmin muscles. We can suggest that the observed connection between the RCPmin muscle and the dura may assist in resisting dural infolding, and that this mechanism may be compromised when atrophy occurs.

In addition, Mitchell et al. (1998) observed continuity between the posterior spinal dura and the ligamentum nuchal in the dissection of 10 cadavers. A midline section of the ligamentum nuchal was observed traveling anterior toward the posterior spinal dura connection (Mitchell et al., 1998). These authors suggested that the dura–ligamentum nuchal connection aids in the spinal dura resistance to inward folding, particularly during cervical spine extension (Mitchell et al., 1998). Therefore, both studies agreed with the suggestion that the dura–ligamentum nuchal connection may contribute to the prevention of dural enfolding during upper cervical spine movements (Hack et al., 1997).

CLINICAL RELEVANCE OF SUBOCCIPITAL MUSCLES IN TENSION-TYPE HEADACHE AND CERVICOGENIC HEADACHE

All the data presented in this chapter should be taken into account by clinicians when they treat patients with either tension-type or cervicogenic headache.

In patients with tension-type headache, we would like to formulate the following hypothesis: suboccipital muscles might send nociceptive inputs to the central nervous system not only in a direct way through the trigeminal nerve nucleus caudalis, but also in an indirect way by irritating or facilitating the afferent input from dural nociceptors. Therefore, clinicians should treat suboccipital muscles in all patients with tension-type headache (Fernández-de-las-Peñas et al., 2006), not only with passive techniques (stretching, manipulative therapy, compression) but also with therapeutic exercises to restore the normal function of these muscles (Chapter 29).

In patients with cervicogenic headache, the connective tissue bridge, acting as a dynamic connection, may transmit abnormal levels of tension from suboccipital muscles to the pain-sensitive dural membrane (Alix & Bates, 1999). According to the "nuchal-dural-adhesion theory" (Driscoll & Beatty, 1997), traction on the dura, because of activation of the suboccipital muscles, stimulates nociceptive dural fibers, with resultant pain (Schaller & Baumann, 2003). Therefore, in patients with cervicogenic headache the mechanism would be as follows: The increased tension within suboccipital muscles may produce abnormal traction on the cranial dura, stimulating dural nociceptive fibers, with resultant head pain, even in the absence of pathology (Hack & Hallgren, 2004). Based on this proposed mechanism, clinicians should treat those structures responsible for mechanical traction over the cranial dura mater (e.g., upper cervical joint) with spinal manipulation, or suboccipital muscles with soft-tissue approaches. Therapeutic exercises are again recommended to restore the normal function of this region and the synergy between deep cervical flexors and neck extensors (Chapter 29).

CONCLUSIONS

There is clearly evidence showing the relevance of the suboccipital muscles in both tension-type and cervico-genic headache, particularly the rectus capitis posterior minor muscle, although by different mechanisms. Nevertheless, clinicians should include both active and passive approaches to restore normal functionality of these muscles in both headache disorders.

REFERENCES

Abrahams VC. The physiology of neck muscles: their role in head movement and maintenance of posture. *Can J Physiol Pharmacol* 1977;55:332–338.

Abrahams VC. Sensory and motor specialization in some muscles of the neck. *Trends Neurosci* 1981;4:24–27.

Alix ME, Bates D. A proposed etiology of cervicogenic headache: the neurophysiologic basis and anatomic relationship between the dura mater and the rectus posterior capitis minor muscle. *J Manipulative Physiol Ther* 1999;22:534–539.

Armed Forces Institute of Pathology. *Manual of Histology and Special Staining Techniques.* 2nd ed. New York: McGraw-Hill; 1960.

Barnsley L, Lord SM, Wallis B, Bogduk N. The prevalence of chronic cervical zygapophyseal joint pain after whiplash. *Spine* 1995;20:20–26.

Beaman DN, Graziano GP, Glover RA, Wojtys EM, Chang V. Substance P innervations of lumbar spine facet joints. *Spine* 1993;18:1044–1049.

Bertorini TE, Igarashi M. Post poliomyelitis muscle pseudohypertrophy. *Muscle Nerve* 1985;8:644–649.

Bogduk N. The cervical anatomy of the cervical dorsal rami. *Spine* 1982;7:319–330.

Bogduk N. The anatomical basis for cervicogenic headache. *J Manipulative Physiol Ther* 1992;15:67–70.

Bovim G, Bonamica L, Fredriksen TA, et al. Topographic variations in the peripheral course of the greater occipital nerve: autopsy study with clinical correlations. *Spine* 1991;16:475–478.

Buckelew SP, Parker JC, Keefe FJ, et al. Self-efficacy and pain behavior among subjects with fibromyalgia. *Pain* 1994;59:377–384.

Burt CW. *Injury-Related Visits to Hospital Emergency Departments. United States: 1992.* Hyattsville, MD: National Center for Health Statistics; 1995. Advance Data from Vital and Health Statistics, No. 261.

Cherkin DC, Deyo RA, Wheeler K, Ciol MA. Physician views about treating low back pain: the results of a national survey. *Spine* 1995;20:1–10.

Coderre TJ, Katz J, Vaccarino AL, Melzack R. Contribution of central neuro-plasticity to pathological pain: review of clinical and experimental evidence. *Pain* 1993;52:259–285.

Cooper S, Danial PM. Muscle spindles in man: their morphology in the lumbricals and the deep muscles of the neck. *Brain* 1963;86:563–594.

Deyo RA, Loeser JD, Bigos SJ. Diagnosis and treatment: herniated lumbar intervertebral disk. *Ann Intern Med* 1990a;112:598–603.

Deyo RA, Walsh NE, Martin DC, Schoenfeld LS, Somayaji RA. A controlled trial of transcutaneous electrical nerve stimulation (TENS) and exercise for chronic low back pain. *New Engl J Med* 1990b;322:1627–1634.

Doherty BJ, Heggeness MH. The quantitative anatomy of the atlas. *Spine* 1994;19:2497–2500.

Driscoll CL, Beatty CW. Pain after acoustic neuroma surgery. *Otolaryngol Clin North Am* 1997;30:893–903.

Dumitru D. Single muscle fiber discharges. Insertional activity, end-plate potentials, positive sharp waves, and fibrillation potentials: a unifying proposal. *Muscle Nerve* 1996;19:221–226.

Ehni G, Benner B. Occipital neuralgia and the C1-2 arthrosis syndrome. *J Neurosurgery* 1984;61:961–965.

Elliott JM, Jull GA, Darnell R, Galloway G, Gibbon WW. Fatty infiltration in the cervical extensor muscles in persistent whiplash-associated disorders: a magnetic resonance imaging analysis. *Spine* 2006;31:E847–E855.

Elliott JM, Jull GA, Noteboom JT, Durbridge GL, Gibbon WW. MRI study of the cross-sectional area of the cervical extensor musculature in an asymptomatic cohort. *Clin Anat* 2007;20:35–40.

Elliott J, Jull GA, Noteboom JT, Galloway G. MRI study of the cross-sectional area for the cervical extensor musculature in patients with persistent whiplash associated disorders (WAD). *Man Ther* 2008 (in press).

Fernández-de-las-Peñas C, Alonso-Blanco C, Cuadrado ML, Gerwin RD, Pareja JA. Myofascial trigger points in the suboccipital muscles and forward head posture in chronic tension type headache. *Headache* 2006;46:454–460.

Fernández-de-las-Peñas C, Bueno A, Ferrando J, Elliott JM, Cuadrado ML, Pareja JA. Magnetic resonance imaging of the morphometry of cervical extensor muscles in chronic tension type headache. *Cephalalgia* 2007;27:355–362.

Fleckenstein JL, Bertocci LA, Nunnally R, Parkey RW, Peshock RM. Exercise-enhanced MRI of variations in forearm muscle anatomy and use: importance in MR spectroscopy. *AJR* 1989a;153:693–698.

Fleckenstein JL, Weatheral PT, Parkey RW, Payne JA, Peshock RM. Sports-related muscle injuries: evaluation with MRI. *Radiology* 1989b;172:793–798.

Garvey TA, Marks MF, Wiesel SW. A prospective randomized double blind evaluation of trigger point injection therapy for low back pain. *Spine* 1989;14:962–964.

Gray H. *Anatomy, Descriptive and Surgical*. Pick T, Howden R, eds. New York: Gramercy Books; 1977.

Guieu R, Serratrice G. Identifying the afferents involved in movement-induced pain alleviation in man. *Brain* 1992;115:1073–1079.

Hack GD, Hallgren RC. Chronic headache relief after section of suboccipital muscle dural connections: a case report. *Headache* 2004;44:84–89.

Hack GD, Koritzer RT, Robinson WL, Hallgren RC, Greenman PE. Anatomic relation between the rectus capitis posterior minor muscle and the dura mater. *Spine* 1995;20: 2484–2486.

Hack GD, Koritzer RT, Robinson WL, Hallgren RC, Greenman PE. The ligamentum craniale durae matris spinalis ligament may contribute to the prevention of dural enfolding [response]. *Spine* 1997;22:925–926.

Haig AJ, Parks TJ. Para-spinal muscles: anatomy and electro-diagnostic testing in the cervical and lumbar regions. *Phys Med Rehabil Clin North Am* 1994;5:447–463.

Haig JA, Moffroid M, Henry S, Haugh L, Pope M. A technique for needle localization in paraspinal muscles with cadaveric confirmation. *Muscle Nerve* 1991;14:521–526.

Haig AJ, Talley C, Grobler LJ, LeBreck DB. Para-spinal mapping: quantified needle electromyography in lumbar radiculopathy. *Muscle Nerve* 1993;16:477–484.

Halar E, Bell K. Contracture and other deleterious effects of immobility. In: DeLisa JA, ed. *Rehabilitation Medicine: Principles and Practice*. Philadelphia: JB Lippincott Company; 1988.

Hallgren RC, Greenman PE, Rechtien JJ. Atrophy of suboccipital muscles in patients with chronic pain: a pilot study. *J Am Osteopath Assoc* 1994;12:1032–1038.

Hayashi N, Tamaki T, Yamada H. Experimental study of denervated muscle atrophy following severance of posterior rami of the lumbar spinal nerves. *Spine* 1992;17: 1001–1010.

Hides JA, Richardson CA, Jull G. Multifidus muscle recovery is not automatic following resolution of acute first episode low back pain. *Spine* 1996;21:2763–2769.

Hodges PW, Moseley GL. Pain and motor control of the lumbopelvic region: effect and possible mechanisms. *J Electromyogr Kinesiol* 2003;13:361–370.

Hollinshead WH. *Textbook of Anatomy*. New York: Harper & Row; 1967:chap 14.

Horowitz AL. *MRI Physics for Physicians*. New York: Springer Verlag; 1989.

Humphreys BK, Kenin S, Hubbard BB, Cramer GD. Investigation of connective tissue attachments to the cervical spinal dura mater. *Clin Anat* 2003;16:152–159.

Ilyinsky OB, Kozlova M, Kondrikova ES, et al. Effects of opioid peptides and naloxone on nervous tissue. *Neuroscience* 1987;22:719–735.

Kelly JP. Trigeminal system. In: Kandel E, Schwartz J, eds. *Principles of Neuroscience*. New York: Elsevier; 1985.

Kerr FWL. A mechanism to account for frontal headache in cases of posterior fossa tumors. *J Neurosurgery* 1961;18:605–609.

Kohara N, Kaji R, Kimura J. Comparison of recording characteristics of monopolar and concentric needle electrodes. *Electroencephalogr Clin Neurophysiol* 1993;89:242–246.

McMahon SB, Wall PD. Receptive fields of rat lamina I projection cells move to incorporate a nearby region of injury. *Pain* 1984;19:235–247.

McPartland JM, Brodeur RR, Hallgren RC. Chronic neck pain, standing balance, and suboccipital muscle atrophy: a pilot study. *J Manipulative Physiol Ther* 1997;20:24–29.

Milne RJ, Aniss AM, Kay N, Gandevia S. Reduction in perceived intensity of cutaneous stimuli during movement: a quantitative study. *Exp Brain Res* 1988;70: 569–576.

Mitchell BS, Humphreys BK, O'Sullivan E. Attachments of the ligamentum nuchae to cervical posterior spinal dura and the lateral part of the occipital bone. *J Manipulative Physiol Ther* 1998;21:145–148.

Nitz AJ, Peck D. Comparison of muscle spindle concentrations in large and small human muscles acting in parallel combinations. *Am Surgeon* 1986;52:273–277.

Nolan JP, Sherk H. Biomechanical evaluation of the extensor musculature of the cervical spine. *Spine* 1988;13: 9–11.

Oosterveld WJ, Kortschot HW, Kingma GG, de Jong AA, Saatci MR. Electro-nystagmographic findings following cervical whiplash injuries. *Acta Otolaryngol* 1991;111:201–205.

Panjabi M, Dvorak J, Duranceau J, et al. Three-dimensional movements of the upper cervical spine. *Spine* 1988;13: 726–730.

Peck D, Buxton DF, Nitz A. A comparison of spindle concentrations in large and small muscles acting in parallel combinations. *J Morphology* 1984;180:243–252.

Poletti CE. C2 and C3 pain dermatomes in man. *Cephalalgia* 1991;11:155–159.

Rantanen J, Hurme M, Falck B, et al. The lumbar multifidus muscle five years after surgery for a lumbar inter-vertebral disc herniation. *Spine* 1993;18:568–574.

Revel M, Andre-Deshays C, Minguet M. Cervico-cephalic kinesthetic sensibility in patients with cervical pain. *Arch Phys Med Rehabil* 1991;72:288–291.

Rutten HP, Szpak K, van Mameren H, Ten Holter J, de Jong JC. Anatomic relation between the rectus capitis posterior minor muscle and the dura mater [comment]. *Spine* 1997;22:924–925.

Schaller B, Baumann A. Headache after removal of vestibular schwannoma via the retro-sigmoid approach: a long-term follow-up study. *Otolaryngol Head Neck Surg* 2003;128: 387–395.

Shah JP, Phillips TM, Danoff JV, Gerber LH. An in vitro microanalytical technique for measuring the local biochemical milieu of human skeletal muscle. *J Appl Physiol* 2005;99:1977–1984.

Sihvonen T, Herno A, Paljarv L, et al. Local denervation atrophy of paraspinal muscles in postoperative failed back syndrome. *Spine* 1993;18:575–581.

Staubesand J, ed. *Atlas of Human Anatomy*. Munich: Urban & Schwarzenberg; 1986.

Wall PD. Neuropathic pain and injured nerve: central mechanisms. *Br Med Bull* 1991;47:631–643.

Wall PD. The dorsal horn. In: Wall PD, Melzack R, eds. *Textbook of Pain*. 2nd ed. Edinburgh: Churchill Livingstone; 2005:102–111.

Wetzel FT. Chronic benign cervical pain syndromes. *Spine* 1992;17(suppl 10):S367–S374.

Yamada H, Honda T, Yaginuma H, Kikuchi S, Sugiura Y. Comparison of sensory and sympathetic innervation of the dura mater and posterior longitudinal ligament in the cervical spine alter removal of the stellate ganglion. *J Comp Neurol* 2001;434:86–100.

Zumpano MP, Hartwell S, Jagos CS. Soft tissue connection between rectus capitis posterior minor and the posterior atlanto-occipital membrane: a cadaveric study. *Clin Anat* 2006;19:522–527.

Forward Head Posture in Headaches

César Fernández-de-las-Peñas, PT, DO, PhD,
Maria L. Cuadrado, MD, PhD, and Juan A. Pareja, MD, PhD

Proper posture is believed to be the key for musculoskeletal balance that involves a minimal amount of stress and strain on the body. Although proper posture is desired, many people do not exhibit good posture. According to Kendall et al. (1952), ideal head posture is achieved when the external auditory meatus is aligned with the vertical postural line. The vertical postural line, as seen in a side view of the patient, passes slightly in front of the ankle joint and the center of the knee joint, slightly behind the center of the hip joint, and through the shoulder joint and the external auditory meatus. However, other authors disagree with this statement (Woodhull et al., 1985). Cervical posture abnormalities have been traditionally linked to headache disorders. One of the most common cervical posture abnormalities in the clinical setting (66%) is a forward head posture, which implies that the head is anterior to a line passing through the center of gravity of the body (Griegel-Morris et al., 1992).

Forward head posture has been found in patients with neck pain (Haughie et al., 1995), temporomandibular disorders (Evcik & Aksoy, 2004), postconcussional headache (Treleaven et al., 1994), tension-type headache (Marcus et al., 1999; Fernández-de-las-Peñas et al., 2006a), and migraine (Fernández-de-las-Peñas et al., 2006b). Treleaven et al. (1994) found a lesser craniovertebral angle, that is, a greater forward head posture, but not a statistically significant one, in postconcussional headache patients (mean: 46.7° ± 2.8°) compared with control healthy subjects (mean: 50.7° ± 7.9°). Marcus et al. (1999) demonstrated that patients with tension-type headache showed a greater number of musculoskeletal abnormalities, including forward head posture, but the evaluation was based on visual inspection. Fernández-de-las-Peñas et al. (2006a) found that patients with chronic tension-type headache showed a lesser craniovertebral angle (mean: 45.3° ± 7.6°) compared with healthy subjects (mean: 54.1° ± 6.3°). In addition, those patients with a smaller craniovertebral angle (i.e., greater forward head posture) reported a higher headache frequency than those patients with greater craniocervical angle (i.e., less forward head posture) (Fernández-de-las-Peñas et al., 2006a). On the contrary, Griegel-Morris et al. (1992) did not find an association between the severity of cervical postural abnormalities and the severity and frequency of pain in patients presenting with neck pain. Nevertheless, these authors suggested that patients with more severe postural cervical abnormalities were more likely to experience pain than those patients with less severe abnormalities (Griegel-Morris et al., 1992). Causality, however, could not be demonstrated in these studies, and the possibility that head posture can be the result, rather than the cause, of headache or neck pain should be further investigated.

Forward head posture has been also found in cervicogenic headache by some authors (Watson & Trott, 1993) but not by others (Zito et al., 2006). Watson and Trott (1993) reported that patients with cervicogenic headache have a lesser craniovertebral angle (greater forward head posture) than healthy subjects (mean: 44.5° ± 5.5° vs. 49.1° ± 2.9°; *P* <0.001). On the contrary, Zito et al. (2006) did not report significant differences between the craniovertebral angle of patients with cervicogenic headache (mean: 51.1° ± 5.8°), migraine (mean: 53.3° ± 3.9°), and healthy controls (mean: 50.3° ± 4.6°). Differences between these studies may be related to the age of the subjects, because it is known that forward head posture is age related (Dalton & Coutts, 1994).

Finally, Fernández-de-las-Peñas et al. (2006b) also demonstrated that the craniovertebral angle was smaller (*P* <0.001) in patients with unilateral migraine (mean: 42.2° ± 6.4°) as compared with healthy controls (mean: 52.6° ± 7.2°). Therefore, forward head posture appears to be a feature common to several headache syndromes. However, head posture may be a consequence (i.e., an antalgic posture trying to reduce pain) rather than an etiologic factor for headache. Whether forward head posture contributes to the origin or is one of the perpetuating factors of headaches must be verified by future research.

CLINICAL ASSESSMENT OF FORWARD HEAD POSTURE

The evaluation of head posture of a patient is generally discussed in both clinical and research environments. Although clinical inspection is under criticism, clinicians usually explore the posture of their patients. Furthermore, although some patients may not be able to describe specific movements that bring on their symptoms, they will often describe certain sustained positions, such as sitting behind the computer (which implies a forward head position), as the aggravating factors of their headache symptoms.

One of the most commonly used methods for assessing forward head posture is a picture of the lateral view of the patient (Watson & Trott, 1993; Greenfield et al., 1995; Raine & Twomey, 1997; Fernández-de-las-Peñas et al., 2006a, 2006b; Zito et al., 2006). The base of the camera is set at the height of the patient's shoulder. The

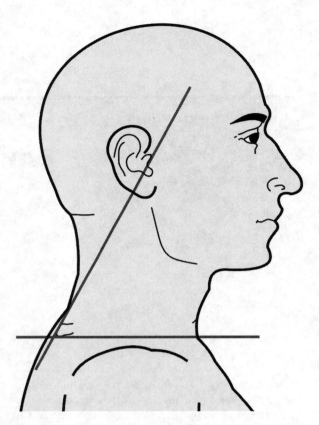

Figure 8.1 Assessment of the Forward Head Posture with the Craniovertebral Angle

tragus of the ear is marked, and a plastic pointer is taped to the skin overlying the spinous process of the C7 vertebra. Once the picture is obtained, it is used to measure the *craniovertebral angle*—the angle between the horizontal line passing through C7 and a line extending from the tragus of the ear to C7 (**Figure 8.1**). A smaller craniovertebral angle indicates a greater forward head posture. Forward head posture should be examined in both a relaxed sitting and standing position. For instance, for assessing head posture while sitting, patients can be asked to sit comfortably on a high-backed chair with both feet flat on the floor, hips and knees positioned at 90° angles, and buttocks positioned against the back of the chair. Patients are requested to rest their hands on their laps and to keep their shoulders against the back of the chair.

Griegel-Morris et al. (1992) found an intraexaminer (kappa = 0.825) and interexaminer (kappa = 0.611) reliability for postural visual assessment in clinical setting. Garret et al. (1993) evaluated the reliability of the assessment of forward head posture with a cervical range of motion goniometer in patients with orthopaedic disorders. These authors found both a high intraexaminer (ICC = 0.93) and interexaminer (ICC = 0.83) reliability (Garret et al., 1993). Raine and Twomey (1997) reported that the reliability of the assessment of forward head posture with a lateral picture of the patients was also high (ICC = 0.88).

CLINICAL SIGNIFICANCE OF FORWARD HEAD POSTURE

Postural deviations associated with a forward head posture include extension at the atlanto-occipital (C0 to C2) joints, accompanied by a flexion of the lower cervical spine (C4 to C7), and a possible reversal or "flattening" of the midcervical lordosis. This head position results in joint dysfunction that leads to abnormal afferent information affecting the tonic neck reflex and encouraging the gradual adoption of a forward head position (Darnell, 1983). The extension motion of the upper cervical joints can induce a compression of the craniocervical structures. Because of this compression, the greater and lesser occipital nerves may become involved, hence contributing to the perpetuation of headaches, particularly cervicogenic headache or migraine.

The insidious nature of repetitive minor trauma in the form of abusive postural positions and abnormal movement patterns (e.g., habitual flexed postures of the neck) may affect changes in the length-tension relationships of the cervical muscles (Darnell, 1983). A forward head position creates a musculoskeletal imbalance with shortening of the posterior cervical muscles, tightness of the anterior chest muscles, and lengthening and weakness of the anterior neck flexors and masticatory muscles. Simons et al. (1999) stated that postural abnormalities in the cervical spine might be responsible for the activation of muscle trigger points in the neck muscles. Forward head posture can result in shortening of the posterior cervical muscles that extend the neck (suboccipital, semispinalis, splenii, and upper trapezius muscles) and active trigger points. Fernández-de-las-Peñas et al. (2006c) reported that those chronic tension-type headache patients with active trigger points (those points whose elicited referred pain reproduces headache features) in the suboccipital muscles tended to have a greater forward head posture than those patients with latent trigger points (those points whose referred pain did not reproduce headache symptoms), although differences were not statistically significant. In a study, Fernández-de-las-Peñas et al. (2006d) found

that chronic tension-type headache patients with active trigger points in the sternocleidomastoid muscle (mean: 41.6° ± 7.7°) showed a smaller craniovertebral angle than those patients with latent trigger points (mean: 48.5° ± 5.8°) in the same muscle (*P* <0.01). Therefore, the shortening of some craniocervical muscles caused by a forward head position might be responsible for the activation of trigger points (Simons et al., 1999; Gerwin, 2005). However, it is equally plausible that forward head posture might be a consequence of headache, that is, an antalgic posture to try to reduce pain.

Another problem associated with forward head posture arises from the scalene muscles. The dorsal scapula nerve penetrates the scalene muscles, and it can therefore be vulnerable to the increased tension in these muscles produced by this head position. Fernández-de-las-Peñas et al. (2007) have reported an abnormal referred pain to the head elicited by trigger points located in the scalene muscles in patients with chronic tension-type headache. Therefore, shortening of the scalene muscles induced by a forward head position can perpetuate trigger points in these muscles.

In addition, a forward head posture usually involves an increased midthoracic spine kyphosis, protraction (abduction) of the scapulae with downward rotation (the inferior angle of the scapula moves medially while the glenoid fossa moves anteriorly and inferiorly), and internal rotation of the humerus bone. Therefore, in many patients, a forward head posture is not an isolated postural problem (Braun & Anundson, 1989). A rounded position of the shoulders frequently accompanies the forward head posture. This postural characteristic is traditionally detected by an anterior position of the bicipital tendon groove relative to the plumb line (Kadir et al., 1981). As the patient becomes more round shouldered, the scapula moves in a lateral and anterior direction in relation to the thorax. The change in scapula position alters the position of the humerus, and the bicipital tendon groove moves more anteriorly and medially (Braun & Anundson, 1989). Therefore, clinicians should include visual inspection of the position of the shoulder girdle, and not only the head, when they evaluate a patient with headache. Black et al. (1996) demonstrated that different sitting postures resulted in changes in cervical spine posture. Therefore, lumbar and pelvic position should also be considered when head and neck posture is evaluated.

Walmsley et al. (1996) and Ordway et al. (1999) showed that forward head posture could affect neck mobility. Limited cervical range of motion is considered to be a major feature of cervicogenic headache (Sjaastad et al., 1998), but it is not included among the clinical signs that lead to the diagnosis of tension-type headache or migraine (International Headache Society, 2004). Kidd and Nelson (1993) found that patients with tension-type and migraine headache showed more abnormalities of cervical mobility during examination compared with healthy subjects. On the contrary, Zwart (1997) did not find significant differences in neck mobility between patients with migraine, tension-type headache, or healthy subjects. Further, Fernández-de-las-Peñas et al. (2006a) found a correlation between forward head posture and neck mobility in patients with chronic tension-type headache: patients with a greater forward head posture showed lesser cervical range of motion. Haughie et al. (1995) also reported a relationship between forward head posture and neck mobility

in extension in patients with neck pain. It is expected that forward head posture may lead to excessive compression on the facet joints and posterior surfaces of the vertebral bodies, thus affecting the biomechanics of the head and the neck.

CONCLUSIONS

Posture abnormalities have been traditionally linked to headache disorders. A forward head posture has been found in postconcussional, tension-type, migraine, and cervicogenic headaches. It seems that forward head posture is a feature common to several headache syndromes. However, head posture may also be a consequence (i.e., an antalgic posture trying to reduce pain) rather than an etiologic factor for headache.

REFERENCES

Black KM, McClure P, Polansky M. The influence of different sitting positions on cervical and lumbar posture. *Spine* 1996;21:65–70.

Braun BL, Anundson LR. Quantitative assessment of head and shoulder posture. *Arch Phys Med Rehabil* 1989;70:322–329.

Dalton M, Coutts A. The effect of age on cervical posture in a normal population. In: Boyling JD, Palastanga N, Jull G, Lee D, eds. *Grieves Modern Manual Therapy. The Vertebral Column*. 2nd ed. London: Churchill Livingstone; 1994:361–370.

Darnell MW. A proposed chronology of events for forward head posture. *Phys Ther* 1983;1:50–54.

Evcik D, Aksoy O. Relationship between head posture and temporomandibular dysfunction syndrome. *J Musculoskeletal Pain* 2004;12(2):19–24.

Fernández-de-las-Peñas C, Alonso-Blanco C, Cuadrado ML, Pareja JA. Forward head posture and neck mobility in chronic tension type headache: a blinded, controlled study. *Cephalalgia* 2006a;26:314–319.

Fernández-de-las-Peñas C, Cuadrado ML, Pareja JA. Myofascial trigger points, neck mobility and forward head posture in unilateral migraine. *Cephalalgia* 2006b;26:1061–1070.

Fernández-de-las-Peñas C, Alonso-Blanco C, Cuadrado ML, Gerwin R, Pareja JA. Trigger points in the suboccipital muscles and forward head posture in tension type headache. *Headache* 2006c;46:454–460.

Fernández-de-las-Peñas C, Alonso-Blanco C, Cuadrado ML, Gerwin R, Pareja JA. Myofascial trigger points and their relationship to headache clinical parameters in chronic tension type headache. *Headache* 2006d;46:1264–1272.

Fernández-de-las-Peñas C, De la Llave Rincón AI, Miangolarra JC. Uncommon referred pain from scalene muscle trigger points in chronic tension type headache [abstract]. *J Musculoskeletal Pain* 2007;15(suppl 13):21.

Garret TR, Youdas JW, Madson TJ. Reliability of measuring forward head posture in a clinical setting. *J Orthopedic Sports Phys Ther* 1993;17:155–160.

Gerwin R. Headache. In: Ferguson L, Gerwin R, eds. *Clinical Mastery in the Treatment of Myofascial Pain*. Philadelphia: Lippincott Williams & Wilkins; 2005:1–24.

Greenfield B, Catlin PA, Coates PW, Green E, McDonald JJ, North C. Posture in patients with overuse injuries and healthy individuals. *J Orthop Sports Phys Ther* 1995;21:287–295.

Griegel-Morris P, Larson K, Mueller-Klaus K, Oatis CA. Incidence of common postural abnormalities in the cervical, shoulder, and thoracic regions and their associations with pain in two age groups of healthy subjects. *Phys Ther* 1992;72:425–430.

Haughie LJ, Fiebert IM, Roach KE. Relationship of forward head posture and cervical backward bending to neck pain. *J Manual Manipulative Ther* 1995;3:91–97.

International Headache Society. The International Classification of Headache Disorders: 2nd edition. *Cephalalgia* 2004;24(suppl 1):9–160.

Kadir N, Grayson MF, Goldberg AAJ, Swain MC. New neck goniometer. *Rheum Rehabil* 1981;20:219–226.

Kendall HO, Kendall FP, Boynton DA. *Posture and Pain*. Baltimore: Williams & Wilkins; 1952.

Kidd RF, Nelson R. Musculoskeletal dysfunction of the neck in migraine and tension headache. *Headache* 1993;33:566–569.

Marcus DA, Scharff L, Mercer S, Turk DC. Musculoskeletal abnormalities in chronic headache: a controlled comparison of headache diagnostic groups. *Headache* 1999;39:21–27.

Ordway NR, Seymour RJ, Donelson RG, et al. Cervical flexion, extension, protrusion, retraction: a radiographic segmental analysis. *Spine* 1999;24:240–247.

Raine S, Twomey LT. Head and shoulder posture variations in 160 asymptomatic women and men. *Arch Phys Med Rehabil* 1997;78:1215–1223.

Simons DG, Travell JG, Simons LS. *Myofascial Pain and Dysfunction: The Trigger Point Manual.* Vol. 1. Philadelphia: Lippincott William & Wilkins; 1999:278–307.

Sjaastad O, Fredriksen TA, Pfaffenrath V. Cervicogenic headache: diagnostic criteria. *Headache* 1998;38:442–445.

Treleaven J, Jull G, Atkinson L. Cervical musculoskeletal dysfunction in post-concussional headache. *Cephalalgia* 1994;14:273–279.

Walmsley RP, Kimber P, Culham E. The effect of initial head position on active cervical axial rotation range of motion in two age populations. *Spine* 1996;21:2435–2442.

Watson DH, Trott PH. Cervical headache: an investigation of natural head posture and upper cervical flexor muscle performance. *Cephalalgia* 1993;13:272–284.

Woodhull A, Maltrud K, Mello BL. Alignment of the human body in standing. *Eur Apply Physiol* 1985;54:109–115.

Zito G, Jull G, Stoty I. Clinical tests of musculoskeletal dysfunction in the diagnosis of cervicogenic headache. *Man Ther* 2006;11:118–129

Zwart JA. Neck mobility in different headache disorders. *Headache* 1997;37:6–11.

Sensitization in Tension-Type Headache: A Pain Model

César Fernández-de-las-Peñas, PT, DO, PhD,
Lars Arendt-Nielsen, DMSci, PhD, David G. Simons, MD,
Maria L. Cuadrado, MD, PhD, and Juan A. Pareja, MD, PhD

Despite some advances, the pathogenesis of tension-type headache is not clearly understood. It has been demonstrated that the most prominent clinical finding in both adults and children suffering from tension-type headache is an increased tenderness to palpation of pericranial tissues (Langemark & Olesen, 1987; Jensen et al., 1993; Jensen & Olesen, 1996; Lipchik et al., 1997; Metsahonkala et al., 2006). A second characteristic of chronic, but not episodic, tension-type headache is lower pressure pain threshold levels as compared with healthy subjects (Schoenen et al., 1991; Bendtsen et al., 1996a; Ashina et al., 2005). Bove and Nilsson (1999) demonstrated that pressure pain thresholds did not differ based on the presence or absence of headache in episodic tension-type headache, suggesting that pressure pain sensitivity is constant in this headache disorder. Nevertheless, the second edition of the International Headache Society's classification has withdrawn electromyography (EMG) and pressure algometry from the diagnostic features for subdivision of tension-type headache, because only tenderness on manual palpation is useful to distinguish different subtypes (IHS, 2004).

It is postulated that increased tenderness and pressure pain sensitivity in chronic tension-type headache may be due to an increased sensitivity (hyperexcitability) in the central nervous system or in the periphery. Nevertheless, the demonstration of a relation between increased tenderness and central sensitization does not reveal the cause-effect relationship between these factors. Bendtsen (2000) postulated a pain model in which the main problem in chronic tension-type headache is the central sensitization due to prolonged nociceptive inputs, provoked by the liberation of algogenic substances at the periphery, from pericranial myofascial tender tissues. His proposed model explains the sensitization at the level of the spinal dorsal horn and/or trigeminal nucleus, the slightly increased supraspinal hypersensitivity, the slightly increased muscle pain activity, the increased muscle hardness, the chronic pain, and the absence of objective signs of peripheral pathology in patients with chronic tension-type headache. However, the model does not account for the mechanisms that initiate the central sensitization, that is, the structures responsible for the nociceptive input from the periphery (Bendtsen, 2000).

PERIPHERAL AND CENTRAL SENSITIZATION IN TENSION-TYPE HEADACHE

Sensitization of Peripheral Muscle Nociceptors

Spinal dorsal horn neurons receiving inputs from muscle tissues can be classified as high-threshold mechanosensitive (HTM) neurons, which require noxious intensities of stimulation for activation, or as low-threshold mechanosensitive (LTM) neurons, which are activated by innocuous stimuli (Mense, 1993). It has been demonstrated that HTM dorsal horn neurons have a positively accelerating stimulus-response function, whereas LTM neurons have a linear stimulus-response function (Yu & Mense, 1990). This finding suggests that the linear stimulus-response function in human muscles may be caused by activity in LTM afferents, although at first this seems unlikely. Further, several studies have demonstrated that a prolonged noxious input from the periphery is capable of sensitizing spinal dorsal horn neurons, concluding that LTM afferents can mediate pain (Woolf, 1983; Mense, 1993; McMahon et al., 1993; Hoheisel et al., 1997).

It is known that chemical mediators may sensitize the nociceptive nerve endings. Particularly effective stimulants for skeletal muscle nociceptors are endogenous substances such as bradykinin or serotonin (Mense, 1993). Several studies have found that sensitization of nociceptive nerve endings was greater with the combination of both substances rather than with each sub-

stance alone (Babenko et al., 1999; Mörk et al., 2003a). Therefore, muscle pain would be produced by noxious stimuli that lead to increased synthesis and release of endogenous algogenic substances such as serotonin, bradykinin, histamine, or prostaglandins. Such stimuli may cause the antidromic release of neuropeptides (i.e., calcitonin gene-related peptide, substance P, or neurokinin A) from the nerve endings of C fibers (O'Brien et al., 1989; Mense et al., 2001). The liberation of these algogenic substances would lower tissue pH and then activate the arachidonic acid cascade, which produces a number of unsaturated lipid products. Sensitization of nociceptors would cause spontaneous neuronal discharge, a lowered threshold to stimuli that normally provoke pain, and an increased firing to stimuli that are not ordinarily perceived as painful. Other inflammatory chemicals believed to be involved include bradykinin from plasma, serotonin from platelets, and glutamate, which are known to affect the membranes of polymodal nociceptors to produce sensitization (Schmidt, 1993).

Previous studies have confirmed the presence of sensitization of peripheral muscle nociceptors in both chronic (Bendtsen, 2000) and episodic tension-type headache (Mörk et al., 2003b; Christensen et al., 2005). It seems that the most prominent clinical finding in tension-type headache is an increased tenderness to palpation of pericranial tissues (Langemark & Olesen, 1987; Jensen et al., 1993; Jensen & Olesen, 1996; Lipchik et al., 1997; Metsahonkala et al., 2006). This increased tenderness seems to be uniformly increased throughout the pericranial region, and both the muscles and tendon insertions have been found to be excessively tender (Langemark & Olesen, 1987; Jensen et al., 1993). Fernández-de-las-Peñas et al. (2007a) reported no side-to-side differences in increased pain sensitivity in patients with chronic tension-type headache. In addition, increased tenderness in both cephalic and neck regions showed a positive relationship: the greater the cephalic tenderness, the greater the neck tenderness (Fernández-de-las-Peñas et al., 2007a).

Whether increased tenderness is a primary or a secondary phenomenon to tension-type headache is under debate. Two cross-sectional studies have reported contradictory results. Jensen et al. (1993), in a headache population study, found that the degree of tenderness was correlated with the frequency and intensity of headache. In this study, the authors classified headache intensity as mild, moderate, or severe, whereas headache frequency was assessed by means of the number of days with headache during the previous year.

On the other hand, Lipchik et al. (1996) reported that tenderness was not correlated with headache frequency or intensity.

Two studies demonstrated that increased pain sensitivity is a consequence rather than a causative factor for the development of tension-type headache. Fernández-de-las-Peñas et al. (2007a), in a cross-sectional blinded case-control study, found that the increased tenderness was not related to headache intensity, frequency, or duration in patients with chronic tension-type headache. In this study, the authors used a headache diary for 4 weeks to assess headache clinical parameters. They suggested that it is possible that headache perception recorded by chronic tension-type headache patients themselves in a headache diary provided detailed data (Fernández-de-las-Peñas et al., 2007a). A 12-year follow-up longitudinal study has demonstrated that subjects who later will develop frequent episodic or chronic tension-type headache had a normal tenderness and pain threshold at baseline, that is, before the beginning of the symptoms (Buchgreitz et al., 2008). These findings demonstrate, for the first time in a longitudinal study, that increased pain sensitivity is a consequence, not a risk factor, of tension-type headache (Buchgreitz et al., 2008).

Sensitization of Second-Order Neurons in the Dorsal Horn or Trigeminal Nucleus Caudalis

It seems that central sensitization can be generated by prolonged nociceptive inputs from the periphery (Mendell & Wall, 1965). This mechanism is particularly important in patients with chronic myofascial pain, since inputs from muscle nociceptors are more effective in inducing prolonged changes in the behavior of dorsal horn neurons than inputs from cutaneous nociceptors (Wall & Woolf, 1984). During central sensitization, the dorsal horn neurons would become hyperexcitable in response to noxious stimulation of deep tissues (Hu et al., 1992; Hoheisel et al., 1993). Noxious stimuli to a specific receptive field in a muscle will generate new muscle receptive fields at a distance from the original within minutes, and referred pain located outside the lesion would be provoked by sensitization spreading to adjacent spinal segments (Mense, 1994). Significant increased excitability of the dorsal horn neurons would alter the pain perception. In this sensitized state, previously ineffective low-threshold Aβ-fiber inputs to nociceptive dorsal horn neurons may become effective (Woolf & Thompson, 1991; Hoheisel et al., 1993). The activation of these silent peripheral nociceptors might result in qualitatively changed stimulus-response function, explaining the abnormal stimulus-response function seen in patients with chronic muscle pain (Bendtsen et al., 1996b). It has been reported that the displacement of the stimulus-response function was closely associated with frequency of the attacks in chronic tension-type headache (Buchgreitz et al., 2006).

In the sensitized state, pain could be generated by low-threshold Aβ fibers, which clinically would manifest as allodynia. It has been suggested that the major cause of increased pain sensitivity in chronic pain is an abnormal response to inputs from low-threshold Aβ fibers (Woolf & Doubell, 1994). In addition, the response to activation of high-threshold afferents would be exaggerated, which clinically would manifest as hyperalgesia, that is, lower pressure pain threshold. Pressure pain threshold (i.e., the lowest pressure stimulus that is perceived as painful) in cephalic and extracephalic regions has been found to be normal in episodic tension-type headache, but lower (hyperalgesic response) in chronic tension-type headache as compared with healthy controls (Schoenen et al., 1991; Bovim, 1992; Jensen et al., 1993; Bendtsen et al., 1996a; Ashina et al., 2003a). Further, Fernández-de-las-Peñas et al. (2007a) found a positive relationship between pressure pain sensitivity in the head and in the neck, and Bendtsen et al. (1996a) reported that pressure pain thresholds between the finger and head were also positively correlated. Nevertheless, lower pressure pain thresholds were not related to headache intensity, frequency, or duration (Fernández-de-las-Peñas et al., 2007a). A second study, in which patients were asked to fill out a headache diary for 4 weeks, also reported that pressure pain threshold levels in the upper trapezius, suboccipital, and frontalis muscles were not correlated with headache frequency or duration in adolescents presenting with chronic tension-type headache (Tüzün et al., 2005). On the contrary, an older study reported a negative correlation between headache severity and pressure pain threshold levels in the temporal region; however, there was no reference to a diary in this study (Langerman et al., 1989), which could account for the discrepancy.

The pressure pain tolerance threshold (i.e., the maximal pressure stimulus that is tolerated) has only been compared between chronic tension-type headache subjects and healthy controls (Bendtsen et al., 1996a), although this pain tolerance threshold is generally considered a better and more reproducible correlate to clinical pain than the pain detection threshold (Petersen et al., 1992) that is usually studied. In this study, pressure pain tolerance thresholds in the finger were significantly lower in chronic tension-type headache patients than in healthy controls (Bendtsen et al., 1996a).

These findings, lowered pressure pain detection and tolerance thresholds, show the presence of both allodynia (i.e., pain elicited by stimuli that are normally not perceived as painful) and hyperalgesia (i.e., increased sensitivity to painful stimuli) in patients with chronic tension-type headache (Bendtsen, 2000). Finally, pressure pain detection and tolerance thresholds at both cephalic and extracephalic sites were negatively correlated with increased tenderness in patients with chronic, but not episodic, tension-type headache (Langemark et al., 1989; Bendtsen et al., 1996a; Jensen et al., 1998).

Finally, in the sensitized state, the afferent Aβ fibers (that normally inhibit Aδ and C fibers by presynaptic mechanisms in the dorsal horn) will on the contrary stimulate the nociceptive second-order (trigeminal) neurons. Therefore, the effect of Aδ- and C-fiber stimulation of the nociceptive dorsal horn (trigeminal) neurons will be promoted and the receptive fields of the dorsal horn neurons will be expanded (Coderre et al., 1993). The nociceptive input to supraspinal structures will be considerably increased, and if more spatial input exists, may result in increased excitability of these supraspinal neurons (Lamour et al., 1983) and decreased inhibition or increased facilitation of nociceptive transmission in the spinal dorsal horn or the trigeminal nucleus caudalis (Wall & Devor, 1981). The supraspinal neurons' sensitization will clinically manifest as generalized pain hypersensitivity.

Generalized pressure pain hyperalgesia has been demonstrated in chronic tension-type headache (Ashina et al., 2006). These authors found that pain ratings to both single and repetitive suprathreshold stimulation were higher in patients than in control subjects in both skin and muscle in all examined cephalic and extracephalic regions ($P < 0.04$). These findings are similar to those reported for other chronic musculoskeletal conditions, such as osteoarthritis (Bajaj et al., 2001) or fibromyalgia (Arendt-Nielsen & Graven-Nielsen, 2003).

Some studies have confirmed that individual nociceptive second-order neurons in the trigeminal nucleus caudalis receive inputs both from the supratentorial dura, the cervical musculature, and other cervical structures (Bartsch & Goadsby, 2002, 2003). It has also been demonstrated that irritation of the suboccipital muscles

evokes reflex muscle activity of the surrounding cervical muscles (Hu et al., 1993) and that activation of dural nociceptors evokes an increase of EMG activity in the suboccipital muscles (Hu et al., 1995). Further, stimulation of trigeminal afferents with a C-fiber irritant results in sensitization of cervical afferents (Bartsch & Goadsby, 2003). These findings support the hypothesis that sensitization of the trigeminal nucleus caudalis neurons occurs in a similar way to sensitization of second-order neurons in the dorsal horn. Readers are referred to Chapter 10 of this textbook for more information on the neurophysiology of the trigeminal nucleus caudalis.

PAIN MODELS FOR TENSION-TYPE HEADACHE

Integration of Nociceptive Inputs

Olesen (1991) proposed that perceived headache may be the sum of nociceptive inputs from cranial and extracranial tissues converging on the neurons of the trigeminal nucleus caudalis. In this "integration model," this author proposed how vascular, supraspinal, or myofascial inputs may be relevant for migraine or tension-type headache. Olesen (1991) proposed that in migraine with aura, vascular and supraspinal inputs would be more relevant than myofascial afferents for the genesis of head pain features (**Figure 9.1**); in migraine without aura, myofascial and supraspinal inputs would be more relevant than vascular afferents (**Figure 9.2**); and in tension-type headache, myofascial inputs would be the key (**Figure 9.3**).

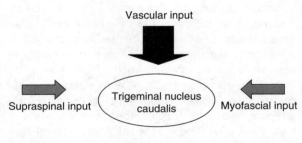

Figure 9.1 Predicted Relevance of Supraspinal, Vascular, or Myofascial Inputs in Patients with Migraine with Aura.
Vascular inputs are more relevant than supraspinal myofascial afferent inputs.

Source: Modified from Olesen, 1991.

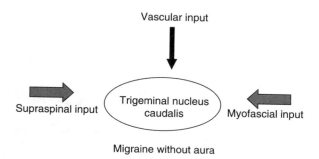

Figure 9.2 Predicted Relevance of Supraspinal, Vascular, or Myofascial Inputs in Patients with Migraine Without Aura. Myofascial and supraspinal inputs are more relevant than vascular afferents.

Source: Modified from Olesen, 1991.

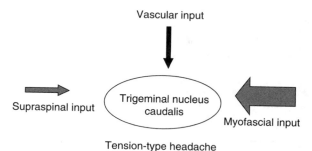

Figure 9.3 Predicted Relevance of Supraspinal, Vascular, or Myofascial Inputs in Patients with Tension-Type Headache. Myofascial inputs, which are trigger points, are more relevant than both supraspinal and vascular afferents.

Source: Modified from Olesen, 1991.

Central Mechanisms in Chronic Tension-Type Headache

Currently, it is postulated that the increased tenderness and decreased pressure pain threshold levels seen in chronic tension-type headache are due to a hyperexcitability of the central nervous system (Bendtsen, 2000), to a sensitization of peripheral endings (Svensson et al., 2003), or to both peripheral and central sensitized states.

Bendtsen (2000) established a model in which the main problem in chronic tension-type headache is the sensitization of central pathways due to prolonged nociceptive inputs, provoked by the liberation of algogenic substances at the periphery, from pericranial tender tissues. In such a way, the presence of prolonged peripheral inputs can be a mechanism of major importance for the conversion of episodic into chronic tension-type headache (Bendtsen, 2000; Bendtsen & Schoenen, 2006).

This model was based in clinical and basic pain sciences. It is known that in healthy subjects, the normal pain processing is finely regulated by multiple pathways, so that the degree of perceived pain is appropriate for each situation. The nociceptive system allows the detection of harmful events and enables the individual to react appropriately to these, for example, to avoid unphysiologic working positions that cause painful muscles and headache. The painful stimulus from the periphery is usually eliminated by actions from the individual and, if necessary, by local reparative mechanisms in the muscle tissues. Therefore, the properties of the nociceptive system will normally not be altered after a short-lasting painful episode (Bendtsen, 2000) (**Figure 9.4**).

Under other unknown conditions, the painful stimulus from muscle tissues may be more prolonged or more intense than normal, probably induced by the release of various chemical mediators in the periphery. In most subjects this condition will be self-limiting due to central pain modulatory mechanisms (descending inhibitory pathways) and local reparative processes, and will be experienced as headache episodes for a limited period of time. However, in predisposed individuals the prolonged nociceptive input originated in muscle tissues may lead to sensitization of nociceptive second-order neurons at the level of the spinal dorsal and the trigeminal nucleus caudalis. Nevertheless, the pathophysiologic basis for this susceptibility to sensitization of central pathways is not completely understood (Bendtsen, 2000) (**Figure 9.5**).

The proposed model explains the sensitization at the level of the spinal dorsal horn or trigeminal nucleus, the slightly increased supraspinal hypersensitivity, the increased muscle activity, the increased muscle hardness, and the absence of objective signs of peripheral pathology in patients with chronic tension-type headache. Nevertheless, this model does not account for the mechanisms that initiate the central sensitization, that is, the structures responsible for the liberation of algogenic substances in the periphery (Bendtsen, 2000; Bendtsen & Schoenen, 2006).

Structures Responsible for Initiating the Liberation of Chemical Mediators in the Periphery

Therefore, the question arising would be: Which structures and mechanisms are responsible for initiating the

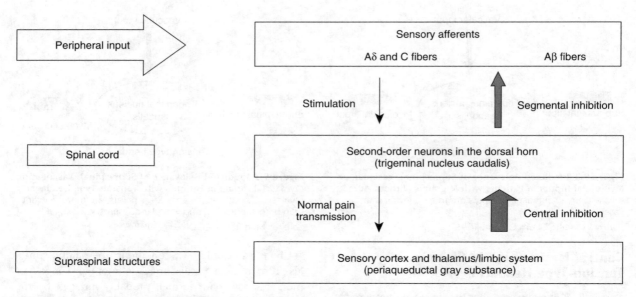

Figure 9.4 Normal Pain Processing, in Which Peripheral or Central Inhibition or Both Will Block Pain Transmission
Source: Modified from Bendtsen, 2000.

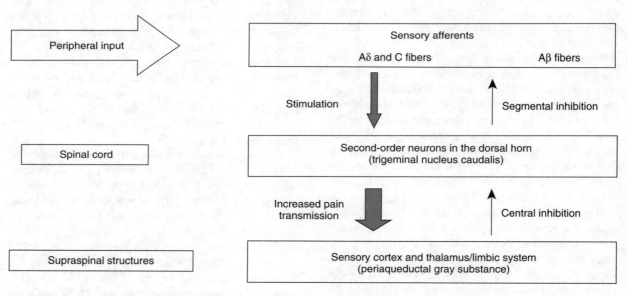

Figure 9.5 Aberrant Pain Processing, in Which Peripheral or Central Inhibition or Both Cannot Block Pain Transmission
Source: Modified from Bendtsen, 2000.

liberation of algogenic substances in the peripheral tissues? Bendtsen (2000) suggested that tender tissues should be the structure. Tender points are hypersensitive spots that, when mechanically stimulated, induce local, but not referred, pain (Simons et al.,

1999). Ashina et al. (2003b) found no significant differences in change in interstitial concentration of adenosine 5′-triphosphate (ATP), glutamate, bradykinin, prostaglandin E2, glucose, pyruvate, and urea from baseline to exercise and postexercise periods between nonspecific tender points of chronic tension-type headache patients and healthy controls. These authors concluded that tender points in chronic tension-type headache are not responsible for liberation of algogenic substances in the periphery (Ashina et al., 2003b).

In two pioneering studies, Shah et al. (2005, 2008) found significantly higher levels of algogenic substances (i.e., bradykinin, calcitonin gene-related peptide, substance P, tumor necrosis factor-α, interleukin-1β, serotonin, and norepinephrine) and lower pH levels in active muscle trigger points (TrPs) (those TrPs whose referred pain is responsible for patients' symptoms) but not in latent TrPs or non-TrPs. These substances are well-known stimulants for various muscle nociceptors and bind to specific receptor molecules of the nerve endings, including the so-called purinergic and vanilloid receptors (McCleskey & Gold, 1999; Mense, 2003). This study confirms that active muscle TrPs are the structure responsible for peripheral nociceptive inputs, and that they can contribute to both peripheral and central sensitization in tension-type headache.

Trigger Points and Sensitization in Tension-Type Headache

If one analyzed data from previous studies (Ashina et al., 2003b; Shah et al., 2005, 2008; Fernández-de-las-Peñas et al., 2006a, 2006b, 2007a, 2007b, 2007c; Couppé et al., 2007), an updated pain model for tension-type headache could be formulated. Bendtsen (2000) suggested that prolonged barrage from peripheral nociceptive inputs could be responsible for the development of central sensitization in patients with chronic tension-type headache. It seems that prolonged pain from active muscle TrPs can be explained by nociceptor activation of several algogenic substances (Shah et al., 2005). Herren-Gerber et al. (2004) demonstrated that central hypersensitivity could be most likely dependent on local nociceptive peripheral input. Because central sensitization is driven by prolonged nociceptive inputs from the periphery (Mendell & Wall, 1965), the proposed pain model could involve both peripheral sensitization of muscle nociceptors by active TrPs and sensitization of central pathways (Fernández-de-las-Peñas et al., 2007d). This model would suggest that active TrPs located in head and neck muscles innervated by C1 through C3 (e.g., upper trapezius, suboccipital, sternocleidomastoid muscles) or by the trigeminal nerve (e.g., temporalis, masseter, or extraocular muscles) would be responsible for peripheral nociceptive input,

and may produce a continuous afferent barrage into the trigeminal nerve nucleus caudalis. Connections between afferents innervating deep structures and second-order neurons could be altered by these peripheral inputs. Convergent synaptic connections on dorsal horn neurons that are not usually functional could be activated if intense nociceptive input reaches the dorsal horn. Changes in size and shape of peripheral receptive fields, and the formation of new receptive fields, would occur if the muscle TrP nociceptive barrage were prolonged. This would result in temporal and spatial integration of neuron signals, and might be one of the reasons for central sensitization in chronic tension-type headache.

In such a way, headache pain perception in tension-type headache can at least partly be explained by referred pain from TrPs in the posterior cervical, head, and shoulder muscles, mediated through the spinal cord and the brainstem trigeminal nucleus caudalis, rather than only tenderness of the muscles themselves. In this model, one could consider muscle TrPs as primary hyperalgesic zones in which referred pain areas to the head exhibit increased tenderness and decreased pressure pain thresholds (secondary hyperalgesic zones). Nevertheless, there is not sufficient evidence to claim a major role for either peripheral or central sensitization, and probably both mechanisms are involved in head pain perception in tension-type headache. **Figure 9.6** diagrams the proposed updated pain model for tension-type headache (Fernández-de-las-Peñas et al., 2007d).

One clinical phenomenon that is observed by many clinicians and that has been reported in one research paper (Hong & Simons, 1993) is the fact that the degree of chronicity is strongly correlated with the number of treatments required to inactivate TrPs. With increased duration of symptoms, there is increased central sensitization, and one of the few available clinical treatments to normalize this central sensitization is to do repeated treatment as often as necessary to maintain the patient nearly pain free. One should eliminate those muscle TrPs as a source of chronic pain that is contributing to the sensitization. In the authors' clinical practice, with recent onset of pain, one or two treatments generally suffice. With greater chronicity, the period of pain relief following a treatment is not shortened as much as it would be in acute cases, and consequently it takes more treatments to normalize this state of central sensitization and eliminate the return of spontaneous central pain (Fernández-de-las-Peñas et al., 2006c).

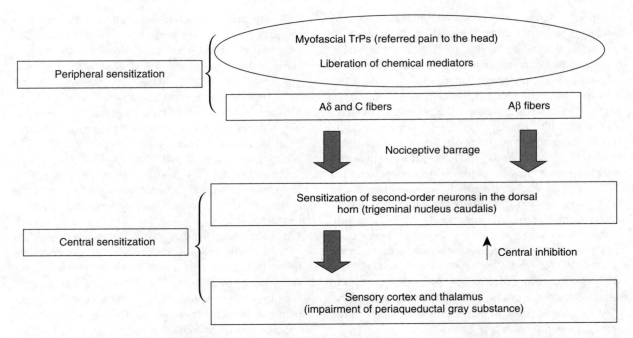

Figure 9.6 Model for Tension-Type Headache Based on Peripheral Sensitization Elicited by Muscle Trigger Points
Source: Modified from Fernández-de-las-Peñas et al., 2007d.

Finally, a muscle TrP role in headache does not negate the importance of some perpetuating factors (Simons et al., 1999), such as malalignment of upper cervical vertebrae (Bogduk, 2001), forward head posture (Fernández-de-las-Peñas et al., 2006d), muscle atrophy (Fernández-de-las-Peñas et al., 2007e), altered muscle pattern recruitment (Fernández-de-las-Peñas et al., 2007f), or psychological (e.g., anxiety or depression)

(Zwart et al., 2003) factors in exacerbating and sustaining this process. These same factors are known to aggravate and promote muscle TrP activity (Simons et al., 1999). Therefore, prolonged and perpetuated pain from active muscle TrPs, which induce the release of several algogenic substances (Shah et al., 2005, 2008), can refer pain to the head and explain chronic tension-type headache (Fernández-de-las-Peñas et al., 2007d).

REFERENCES

Arendt-Nielsen L, Graven-Nielsen T. Central sensitization in fibromyalgia and other musculoskeletal disorders. *Curr Pain Headache Rep* 2003;7:355–361.

Ashina S, Jensen R, Bendtsen L. Pain sensitivity in pericranial and extra-cranial regions. *Cephalalgia* 2003a;23:456–462.

Ashina M, Stallknecht B, Bendtsen L, Pedersen JF, Schifter S, Galbo H, Olesen J. Tender points are not sites of ongoing inflammation: in vivo evidence in patients with chronic tension-type headache. *Cephalalgia* 2003b;23:109–116.

Ashina S, Babenko L, Jensen R, Ashina M, Magerl W, Bendtsen L. Increased muscular and cutaneous pain sensitivity in cephalic region in patients with chronic tension-type headache. *Eur J Neurol* 2005;12:543–549.

Ashina S, Bendtsen L, Ashina M, Magerl W, Jensen R. Generalized hyperalgesia in patients with chronic tension-type headache. *Cephalalgia* 2006;26:940–948.

Babenko V, Graven-Nielsen T, Svenson P, Drewes MA, Jensen TS, Arendt-Nielsen L. Experimental human muscle pain and muscular hyperalgesia induced by combinations of serotonin and bradykinin. *Pain* 1999;82:1–8.

Bajaj P, Graven-Nielsen T, Arendt-Nielsen L. Osteoarthritis and its association with muscle hyperalgesia: an experimental controlled study. *Pain* 2001;93:107–114.

Bartsch T, Goadsby P. Stimulation of the greater occipital nerve induces increased central excitability of dural afferent input. *Brain* 2002;125:1496–1509.

Bartsch T, Goadsby P. Increased responses in trigemino-cervical nociceptive neurons to cervical input after stimulation of the dura mater. *Brain* 2003;126:1801–1813.

Bendtsen L. Central sensitization in tension-type headache: possible patho-physiological mechanisms. *Cephalalgia* 2000;29:486–508.

Bendtsen L, Schoenen J. Synthesis of tension type headache mechanisms. In: Olesen J, Goasdby P, Ramdan NM, Tfelt-Hansen P, Welch KMA, eds. *The Headaches*. 3rd ed. Philadelphia: Lippincott Williams & Wilkins; 2006.

Bendtsen L, Jensen R, Olesen J. Decreased pain detection and tolerance thresholds in chronic tension type headache. *Arch Neurol* 1996a;53:373-376.

Bendtsen L, Jensen R, Olesen J. Qualitative altered nociception in chronic myofascial pain. *Pain* 1996b;65:259-264.

Bogduk N. Cervicogenic headache: anatomic basis and patho-physiologic mechanisms. *Curr Pain Headache Rep* 2001;5:382-386.

Bove GM, Nilsson N. Pressure pain threshold and pain tolerance in episodic tension type headache do not depend on the presence of headache. *Cephalalgia* 1999;19:174-178.

Bovim G. Cervicogenic headache, migraine and tension-type headache: pressure pain threshold measurements. *Pain* 1992;51:169-173.

Buchgreitz L, Lyngberg AC, Bendtsen L, Jensen R. Frequency of headache is related to sensitization: a population study. *Pain* 2006;123:19-27.

Buchgreitz L, Lyngberg AC, Bendtsen L, Jensen R. Increased pain sensitivity is not a risk factor but a consequence of frequent headache: a population-based follow-up study. *Pain* 2008;137:623-630.

Christensen MB, Bendtsen L, Ashina M, Jensen R. Experimental induction of muscle tenderness and headache in tension-type headache patients. *Cephalalgia* 2005;25:1061-1067.

Coderre TJ, Katz J, Vaccarino AL, Melzack R. Contribution of central neuroplasticity to pathological pain: review of clinical and experimental evidence. *Pain* 1993;52:259-285.

Couppé C, Torelli P, Fuglsang-Frederiksen A, Andersen KV, Jensen R. Myofascial trigger points are very prevalent in patients with chronic tension-type headache: a double-blinded controlled study. *Clin J Pain* 2007;23:23-27.

Fernández-de-las-Peñas C, Alonso-Blanco C, Cuadrado ML, Gerwin RD, Pareja JA. Trigger points in the suboccipital muscles and forward head posture in tension type headache. *Headache* 2006a;46:454-460.

Fernández-de-las-Peñas C, Alonso-Blanco C, Cuadrado ML, Gerwin R, Pareja JA. Myofascial trigger points and their relationship with headache clinical parameters in chronic tension type headache. *Headache* 2006b;46:1264-1272.

Fernández-de-las-Peñas C, Arendt-Nielsen L, Simons DG. Contributions of myofascial trigger points to chronic tension type headache. *J Man Manipulative Ther* 2006c;14:222-231.

Fernández-de-las-Peñas C, Alonso-Blanco C, Cuadrado ML, Pareja JA. Forward head posture and neck mobility in chronic tension type headache: a blinded, controlled study. *Cephalalgia* 2006d;26:314-319.

Fernández-de-las-Peñas C, Cuadrado ML, Ge HY, Arendt-Nielsen L, Pareja JA. Increased pericranial tenderness, decreased pressure pain threshold, and headache clinical parameters in chronic tension type headache patients. *Clin J Pain* 2007a;23:346-352.

Fernández-de-las-Peñas C, Ge H, Arendt-Nielsen L, Cuadrado ML, Pareja JA. Referred pain from trapezius muscle trigger point shares similar characteristics with chronic tension type headache. *Eur J Pain* 2007b;11:475-482.

Fernández-de-las-Peñas C, Ge H, Arendt-Nielsen L, Cuadrado ML, Pareja JA. The local and referred pain from myofascial trigger points in the temporalis muscle contributes to pain profile in chronic tension-type headache. *Clin J Pain* 2007c;23:786-792.

Fernández-de-las-Peñas C, Cuadrado ML, Arendt-Nielsen L, Simons DG, Pareja JA. Myofascial trigger points and sensitization: an updated pain model for tension type headache. *Cephalalgia* 2007d;27:383-393.

Fernández-de-las-Peñas C, Bueno A, Ferrando J, Elliott JM, Cuadrado ML, Pareja JA. Magnetic resonance imaging of the morphometry of cervical extensor muscles in chronic tension type headache. *Cephalalgia* 2007e;27:355-362.

Fernández-de-las-Peñas C, Pérez-de-Heredia M, Molero-Sánchez A, Miangolarra-Page JC. Performance of the cranio-cervical flexion test, forward head posture, and headache clinical parameters in patients with chronic tension type headache: a pilot study. *J Orthop Sports Phys Ther* 2007f;37:33-39.

Herren-Gerber R, Weiss S, Arendt-Nielsen L, et al. Modulation of central hyper-sensitivity by nociceptive input in chronic pain after whiplash injury. *Pain Med* 2004;5:366-376.

Hoheisel U, Mense S, Simons DG, Yu XM. Appearance of new receptive fields in rat dorsal horn neurons following noxious stimulation of skeletal muscle: a model for referral of muscle pain? *Neurosci Lett* 1993;153:9-12.

Hoheisel U, Sander B, Mense S. Myositis-induced functional reorganisation of the rat dorsal horn: effects of spinal superfusion with antagonists to neurokinin and glutamate receptors. *Pain* 1997;69:219-230.

Hong CZ, Simons DG. Response to treatment for pectoralis minor myofascial pain syndrome after whiplash. *J Musculoskeletal Pain* 1993;1(1):89-131.

Hu JW, Sessle BJ, Raboisson P, Dallel R, Woda A. Stimulation of craniofacial muscle afferents induces prolonged facilitatory effects in trigeminal nociceptive brain-stem neurons. *Pain* 1992;48:53-60.

Hu JW, Yu XM, Vernon H, Sessle BJ. Excitatory effects in neck and jaw muscle activity of inflammatory irritant applied to cervical paraspinal tissues. *Pain* 1993;55:243-250.

Hu JW, Vernon H, Tatourian I. Changes in neck electromyography associated with meningeal noxious stimulation. *J Manipulative Physiol Ther* 1995;18:577-581.

International Headache Society. The International Classification of Headache Disorders: 2nd edition. *Cephalalgia* 2004;24(suppl 1):8-152.

Jensen R, Olesen J. Initiating mechanism of experimentally induced tension-type headache. *Cephalalgia* 1996;16:175-182.

Jensen R, Rasmussen BK, Pederken B, Olesen J. Muscle tenderness and pressure pain threshold in headache: a study population. *Pain* 1993;52:193-199.

Jensen R, Bendtsen L, Olesen J. Muscular factors are of importance in tension type headache. *Headache* 1998;38:10-17.

Lamour Y, Guilbaud G, Willer JC. Altered properties and laminar distribution of neuronal responses to peripheral stimulation in the SmI cortex of the arthritic rat. *Brain Res* 1983;22:183–187.

Langemark M, Olesen J. Pericranial tenderness in tension headache. A blind controlled study. *Cephalalgia* 1987;7:249–255.

Langemark M, Jensen K, Jensen TS, Olesen J. Pressure pain thresholds and thermal nociceptive thresholds in chronic tension-type headache. *Pain* 1989;38:203–210.

Lipchik GL, Holroyd KA, France CR, Kvaalm SA, Segal D, Cordingley GE, et al. Central and peripheral mechanism in chronic tension type headache. *Pain* 1996;64:467–475.

Lipchik GL, Holroyd KA, Talbot F, Greer M. Pericranial muscle tenderness and exteroceptive suppression of temporalis muscle activity: a blind study of chronic tension-type headache. *Headache* 1997;37:368–376.

McCleskey E, Gold M. Ion channels of nociception. *Annu Rev Physiol* 1999;61:835–856.

McMahon SB, Lewin GR, Wall PD. Central hyper-excitability triggered by noxious inputs. *Curr Opin Neurobiol* 1993;3:602–610.

Mendell LM, Wall PD. Responses of single dorsal cord cells to peripheral cutaneous unmyelinated fibres. *Nature* 1965;206:97–99.

Mense S. Nociception from skeletal muscle in relation to clinical muscle pain. *Pain* 1993;54:241–289.

Mense S. Referral of muscle pain: new aspects. *Am Pain Soc J* 1994;3:1–9.

Mense S. The pathogenesis of muscle pain. *Curr Pain Headache Rep* 2003;7:419–425.

Mense S, Simons DG, Russell IJ. *Muscle Pain: Understanding Its Nature, Diagnosis and Treatment.* Philadelphia: Lippincott, Williams & Wilkins; 2001.

Metsahonkala L, Anttila P, Laimi K, Aromaa M, Helenius H, Mikkelsson M, et al. Extra-cephalic tenderness and pressure pain threshold in children with headache. *Eur J Pain* 2006;10:581–585.

Mörk H, Ashina M, Bendtsen L, Olesen J, Jensen R. Experimental muscle pain and tenderness following infusion of endogenous substances in humans. *Eur J Pain* 2003a;7:145–153.

Mörk H, Ashina M, Bendtsen L, Olesen J, Jensen R. Induction of prolonged tenderness in patients with tension-type headache by means of a new experimental model of myofascial pain. *Eur J Neurol* 2003b;10:249–256.

O'Brien C, Woolf CJ, Fitzgerald M, Lindsay RM, Molander C. Differences in the chemical expression of rat primary afferent neurons which innervate skin, muscle or joint. *Neuroscience* 1989;32:493–502.

Olesen J. Clinical and patho-physiological observations in migraine and tension-type headache explained by integration of vascular, supra-spinal and myofascial inputs. *Pain* 1991;46:125–132.

Petersen KL, Brennum J, Olesen J. Evaluation of peri-cranial myofascial nociception by pressure algometry: reproducibility and factors of variation. *Cephalalgia* 1992;12:33–37.

Schmidt RF. Sensitization of peripheral nociceptors in muscle. In: Olesen J, Schoenen J, eds. *Tension-Type Headache: Classification, Mechanisms, and Treatment.* New York: Raven Press; 1993:47–59.

Schoenen J, Bottin D, Hardy F, Gerard P. Cephalic and extra-cephalic pressure pain thresholds in chronic tension type headache. *Pain* 1991;47:145–149.

Shah JP, Phillips TM, Danoff JV, Gerber LH. An in vitro microanalytical technique for measuring the local biochemical milieu of human skeletal muscle. *J Appl Physiol* 2005;99:1977–1984.

Shah JP, Danoff JV, Desai MJ, et al. Bio-chemicals associated with pain and inflammation are elevated in sites near to and remote from active myofascial trigger points. *Arch Phys Med Rehabil* 2008;89:16–23.

Simons DG, Travell J, Simons LS. *Myofascial Pain and Dysfunction: The Trigger Point Manual.* Vol. 1. 2nd ed. Baltimore: Williams & Wilkins; 1999.

Svensson P, Cairns BE, Wang K, Hu JW, Graven-Nielsen T, Arendt-Nielsen L, Sessle BJ. Glutamate-evoked pain and mechanical allodynia in the human masseter muscle. *Pain* 2003;101:221–227.

Tüzün EH, Karaduman A, Levent E. Pressure pain thresholds in adolescent patients with chronic tension type headache. *Pain Clinic* 2005;17:127–131.

Wall PD, Devor M. The effect of peripheral nerve injury on dorsal root potentials and on transmission of afferent signals into the spinal cord. *Brain Res* 1981;23:95–111.

Wall PD, Woolf CJ. Muscle but not cutaneous C-afferent input produces prolonged increases in the excitability of the flexion reflex in the rat. *J Physiol* 1984;356:443–458.

Woolf CJ. Evidence for a central component of post-injury pain hypersensitivity. *Nature* 1983;15:686–688.

Woolf CJ, Doubell TP. The pathophysiology of chronic pain increased sensitivity to low threshold A beta-fibre inputs. *Curr Opin Neurobiol* 1994;4:525–534.

Woolf CJ, Thompson SW. The induction and maintenance of central sensitization is dependent on N-methyl-D-aspartic acid receptor activation: implications for the treatment of post-injury pain hypersensitivity states. *Pain* 1991;44:293–299.

Yu XM, Mense S. Response properties and descending control of rat dorsal horn neurons with deep receptive fields. *Neuroscience* 1990;39:823–831.

Zwart JA, Dyb G, Hagen K, Odegard KJ, Dahl AA, Bovim G, et al. Depression and anxiety disorders associated with headache frequency: the Nord-Trondelag Health Study. *Eur J Neurol* 2003;10:147–152.

Pathophysiology of Cervicogenic Headache

The Anatomy and Physiology of the Trigeminocervical Complex

Peter J. Goadsby, PhD, MD, and Thorsten Bartsch, MD

Integral to understanding any of the primary headaches is an appreciation of the anatomy and physiology of the trigeminocervical complex. Patients with primary headache often report pain that involves the front of the head, in the cutaneous distribution of the first (ophthalmic) division of the trigeminal nerve (International Headache Society, 2004). At the same time, at different times, or even at different stages of the same attack, they will report pain with occipital distribution or, indeed, involving the neck (Lance & Goadsby, 2005). Furthermore, other clinical features, such as hypersensitivity of the skin of the face or scalp, neck muscle tenderness, and hyperalgesia, are often reported widely in the head (Selby & Lance, 1960; Bogduk, 1997). The relatively poor localization of pain in primary headaches produces significant diagnostic problems and certainly affects the understanding of these disorders. The current chapter sets out what is currently known of the anatomy and physiology of these pivotal structures. We have covered some aspects of these issues previously (Bartsch & Goadsby, 2005) and here provide an updated view.

CLINICAL OBSERVATIONS

Early neurosurgical studies in patients showed that stimulation of trigeminally innervated intracranial structures, such as the supratentorial dura mater and large cranial vessels, evoked painful sensations regardless of the stimuli applied and implied that the afferent input from dural structures is the neural substrate of head pain (McNaughton, 1938; Ray & Wolff, 1940; Penfield & McNaughton, 1940; Feindel et al., 1960). Hence, afferent input, or at least perceived input, from dural structures is likely to be the neural substrate of pain in primary headache syndromes (Goadsby & Oshinsky, 2007). It has been shown that spread and referral of pain can be induced by stimulation of structures in the neck that are innervated by the upper cervical roots. Posterior fossa tumor (Kerr, 1961), stimulation of infratentorial dura mater (Wolff, 1948), direct stimulation of cervical roots (Kerr, 1961; Hunter & Mayfield, 1949), vertebral artery dissection (Cremer et al., 1995; Hutchinson et al., 2000), and stimulation of subcutaneous tissue innervated by the greater occipital nerve (Feinstein et al., 1954; Piovesan et al., 2001) may be perceived as frontal head pain. Similarly, direct stimulation of the supratentorial dura mater leads to pain that is mostly referred to the ophthalmic division of the trigeminal nerve (Wolff, 1948) but may also be referred to dermatomes supplied by the upper cervical roots (Wirth & van Buren, 1971). Busch et al. (2006) examined the R2 components of the nociceptive blink reflex responses (Kaube et al., 2000) in 15 healthy subjects before and after unilateral nerve blockade of the greater occipital nerve with local anesthetic. R2 response areas (area under the curve, or AUC) decreased, and the R2 latencies increased significantly after the nerve blockade only on the side of injection. AUC and latencies on the noninjection side remained stable. These data provide objective evidence for a functional influence of trigeminal nociceptive inputs from occipital inputs.

A mechanism that could explain these clinical and experimental findings is the convergence of trigeminal and cervical afferents onto neurons in the trigeminocervical complex of the brainstem (**Figure 10.1**). Convergence taken together with sensitization of central trigeminal neurons provides a physiologic basis for the clinical phenomenon of spread and referred pain, whereby pain originating from an affected tissue is perceived as originating from a distant receptive field (Mackenzie, 1909; Ruch, 1965). Although local mechanisms at the trigeminocervical level are undoubtedly important, it is crucial to recall functional imaging evidence of altered thalamic processing in chronic migraine patients clinically well controlled by occipital nerve stimulation (Matharu et al., 2004). It seems likely that the effects we describe in the trigeminocervical complex will have more and more complex correlates in other parts of the brain that will need to be explored to understand this physiology completely.

EVIDENCE FROM THE LABORATORY

The nociceptive input from the dura mater to the first synapse in the brainstem is transmitted via small-diameter A- and C-fiber afferents in the ophthalmic division of the trigeminal nerve via the trigeminal ganglion to nociceptive second-order neurons in the superficial and deep layers of the medullary dorsal horn of the trigeminocervical complex (Burstein et al., 1998; Schepelmann et al., 1999; Bartsch & Goadsby, 2002; Levy & Strassman, 2002). The trigeminocervical complex extends from the trigeminal nucleus caudalis to the segments of C2-C3 in the rat (Strassman et al., 1994), cat (Kaube et al., 1993a), and monkey (Goadsby & Hoskin, 1997). Trigeminovascular nociceptive inputs project bilaterally in the brainstem from unilateral structures, such as middle meningeal artery dura mater (Hoskin et al., 1999). These dural-sensitive trigeminal neurons show a high degree of convergent input from other afferent sources because they typically show also facial and corneal receptive fields (Burstein et al., 1998; Schepelmann et al., 1999), although interestingly they are less susceptible to wind-up than trigeminocervical neurons with peripheral inputs (Bolton et al., 2005).

Cervical Inputs

With regard to the innervation of the head, the upper cervical spinal roots also contribute to the sensory innervation of cranial and cervical structures. Occipital and suboccipital structures, such as vessels and the dura mater of the posterior fossa, deep paraspinal neck muscles, and (zygapophysial) joints and ligaments, are innervated by the upper cervical roots and are recognized sources of neck and head pain (Anthony, 1992; Bogduk & Aprill, 1993; Bogduk, 2001). The nociceptive inflow from these suboccipital structures is also mediated by small-diameter afferent fibers in the upper cervical roots terminating in the dorsal horn of the cervical spine extending from the C2 segment up to the medullary dorsal horn (Scheurer et al., 1983; Bakker et al., 1984; Pfister & Zenker, 1984; Neuhuber & Zenker, 1989; Goadsby et al., 1997). The major afferent contribution is mediated by the spinal root C2 that is peripherally represented by the greater occipital nerve (GON) (Vital et al., 1989; Bovim et al., 1991; Becser et al.,

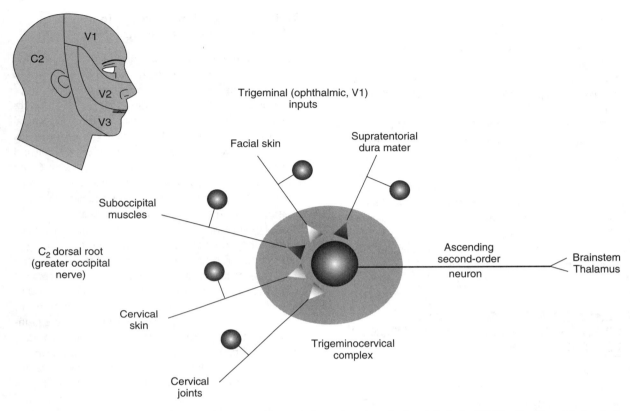

Figure 10.1 **The Convergence of Dura Mater and Skin Inputs from the Trigeminal (ophthalmic, V1) Distribution with Cervical (Muscle, Joints, Skin) Afferents onto the Same Nociceptive Second-Order Neuron in the Trigeminocervical Complex at the Level of C2.** These inputs ascend to brainstem modulatory sites, such as the periaqueductal gray matter, and for further processing in the sensory thalamus, including ventroposteromedial thalamus.

Source: Courtesy of Peter J. Goadsby.

1998). Similarly to the trigeminal sensory neurons, these cervical neurons show a convergence of input from neck muscles and skin (Bartsch & Goadsby, 2002). Indeed, stimulation specifically of occipital muscle afferents will also activate neurons across the anatomic extent of the trigeminocervical complex (Le Doare et al., 2006).

Physiologic Evidence for Convergence

Although an anatomic overlap of trigeminal and cervical afferents throughout the trigeminocervical complex from the level of the caudal trigeminal nucleus to at least the C2 segment was first suggested by Kerr and Olafson (1961), a direct coupling between meningeal afferents and cervical afferents in the spinal dorsal horn was not described until recently (Bartsch & Goadsby, 2002). A population of neurons in the C2 dorsal horn

was characterized receiving convergent input from the supratentorial dura mater and the GON. These neurons showed properties typical for dura-sensitive trigeminal neurons with a convergent input from the facial skin corresponding to the dermatome of the ophthalmic division of the trigeminal nerve including the cornea, but also showed a receptive field corresponding to the cervical skin of the C2/C3 dermatomes and to deep paraspinal muscles innervated by the GON. Interestingly, these trigeminocervical neurons showed convergent synaptic input not only from the supratentorial dura mater and from the ipsilateral GON, but also from the contralateral GON. Taken together with other studies that show similar contralateral projections of nociceptive afferents following labeling of the trigeminal and cervical dorsal root ganglia (Jacquin et al., 1982; Pfaller & Arvidsson, 1988) or after facial afferent stimulation (Ellrich & Messlinger, 1999) or GON stimulation

(Goadsby et al., 1997), it seems that bilateral or contralateral endings of nociceptive afferents of visceral and deep somatic tissues are more common than previously acknowledged (Cervero & Lumb, 1988). This anatomic arrangement may find its functional correlate in the dull and poorly localized quality of head and neck pain (Linderoth & Brodin, 1994).

The convergence of the GON and dural afferents in the trigeminocervical complex is noticeable because it is a convergence of a somatic spinal nerve (GON) and a visceral nerve (dura). Both systems show functional differences, as visceral nerves show a greater portion of unmyelinated C fibers (Cervero, 1987) and show no wind-up to repetitive noxious stimulation (Cervero & Laird, 1999; Herrero et al., 2000), suggesting a different neuroplastic potential to noxious stimulation (Bolton et al., 2005).

CENTRAL MECHANISMS OF PAIN PROCESSING: CENTRAL SENSITIZATION AND DESCENDING INHIBITION

After strong noxious inputs, nociceptive second-order neurons in the spinal cord can be subject to a transient or long-lasting hyperexcitability to afferent stimulation. The current concept of this central sensitization considers an increased afferent barrage from primary nociceptive afferents, especially C fibers, onto second-order neurons as crucial in the development of this hyperexcitability. In particular, stimulation of afferents from visceral and deep somatic tissues, such as muscle and joints, are more effective than cutaneous input in evoking such a central hyperexcitability (Schaible & Grubb, 1993; Mense, 1993). The hypersensitivity of the afferent synaptic input in the spinal cord is thought to be caused by the release of various neuropeptides (e.g., calcitonin gene-related peptide) or to glutamate release and action at the NMDA receptor in response to afferent stimulation, but may also be caused by decrease of local segmental spinal inhibition in response to the afferent stimulation (McMahon et al., 1993; Woolf & Salter, 2000). The hyperexcitability is reflected in a reduction of the activation threshold, an increased responsiveness to afferent stimulation, an enlargement of receptive fields or the emergence of new receptive fields, and the recruitment of "silent" nociceptive afferents. The clinical correlates of this central hypersensitivity include the development of spontaneous pain, hyperalgesia, and allodynia (McMahon et al., 1993; Koltzenburg, 2000).

Activity-Dependent Change in Trigeminocervical Neurons

Similar to the spinal cord, these activity-dependent changes in synaptic strength have been shown to take place also in dura-sensitive trigeminal neurons. Application of an "inflammatory soup" onto the dura mater can induce a central sensitization of trigeminal second-order neurons in the caudal trigeminal nucleus with a subsequent increased responsiveness to dural and cutaneous facial stimulation (Burstein et al., 1998). Some component of this response can be blocked by naproxen (Jakubowski et al., 2007), just as trigeminocervical transmission can be modulated by intravenous aspirin (Kaube et al., 1993b). We further analyzed this functional interaction and found that convergent neurons responding to both dural and GON stimulation showed a central sensitization to GON stimulation with an increased excitability to dural input (Bartsch & Goadsby, 2002). Interestingly, the stimulation of neck muscle afferents in the GON by the C-fiber activator mustard oil was significantly more effective in increasing dural input than stimulation of cutaneous afferents in the GON. Furthermore, stimulation of the dura mater led also to a sensitization of these convergent neurons with a subsequent increased excitability to neck muscle and GON stimulation (Bartsch & Goadsby, 2003).

Some Clinical Implications of Sensitization

It seems that this neuronal population is crucial for understanding the most common clinical patterns of pain referral between trigeminal and cervical dermatomes in migraine that does not necessarily involve a peripheral pathology in the cervical innervation territory (Bogduk, 2001). Interestingly, many headache forms benefit from a blockade of the greater occipital nerve, including migraine (Bovim & Sand, 1992; Peres et al., 2002; Afridi et al., 2006); perhaps more fascinating to readers of this volume, and a pointer to its pathophysiology, tension-type headache does not (May et al., 1998).

The clinical changes seen in primary headaches, such as increased cutaneous sensitivity, hyperalgesia, allodynia, and spread and referral of pain in the trigeminal and cervical dermatomes, are very suggestive of an altered trigeminocervical nociceptive system in terms of a facilitation or sensitization of central nociceptive neurons (Katsarava et al., 2002; Kaube et al., 2002). It could be shown that similar changes, such as extradural hypersensitivity and receptive field changes described in experimental models, can also be seen in headache patients, suggesting that a sensitization of central nociceptive neurons indeed takes place during migraine attacks (Selby & Lance, 1960; Burstein et al., 2000a, 2000b).

CENTRAL PAIN MODULATION

It is now well established that the nociceptive inflow to second-order neurons in the spinal cord and the trigeminocervical complex is subject to a modulation by descending inhibitory projections from brainstem structures such as the periaqueductal gray matter (PAG), nucleus raphe magnus (NRM), and the rostroventral medulla (RVM) (Fields & Heinricher, 1985; Sandkuhler et al., 1987; Behbehani, 1995), because stimulation of these regions produces profound antinociception (Fields et al., 1991). In particular, findings suggest that the ventrolateral division of the PAG (vlPAG) has a pivotal role in trigeminal nociception because stimulation of the vlPAG modulates dural nociception and selectively receives input from trigeminovascular afferents (Keay & Bandler, 1998; Hoskin et al., 2001; Knight & Goadsby, 2001; Knight et al., 2002).

In recent years it emerged that the pain-modulating circuits in the brainstem are not only involved in antinociception but also under certain conditions in the promotion of central sensitization and secondary hyperalgesia (Urban & Gebhart, 1999; Lin et al., 1999; Ren & Dubner, 2002). These findings suggest the possibility that the level of excitability of dura-sensitive neurons in the trigeminocervical complex could be increased by (possibly dysfunctional) brainstem pain-modulatory structures.

Central Modulation and Primary Headache

It was shown that about 55% of patients suffering from familial hemiplegic migraine (FHM), an autosomal-dominant hereditary of migraine, have a missense mutation in the *CACNA1A* gene (Ophoff et al., 1996). This mutation encodes for the α_1 subunit of the voltage-gated P/Q-type calcium channel, and the mutation produces important changes in its function in vivo (van den Maagdenberg et al., 2004). Human functional imaging data using positron emission tomography (PET) have shown activation of brainstem structures in both episodic (Weiller et al., 1995) and chronic migraine (Matharu et al., 2003) that is not seen in experimental head pain (May et al., 1998).

In an experimental model of dural nociception, pharmacologic blockade of P/Q-type calcium channels in the vlPAG facilitated nociceptive input with increased responses to dural stimulation, as well as increased spontaneous activity, of neurons in the trigeminocervical complex (Knight et al., 2002, 2003). This underlines the role of the vlPAG in dural antinociception and suggests that dysfunctional P/Q-type calcium channels in the PAG can increase the sensitivity and gain in dural-sensitive neurons in the trigeminocervical complex. Similarly increased spontaneous activity of dura-sensitive neurons in the trigeminocervical complex after blockage of P/Q-type calcium channels in the brainstem has been demonstrated (Richter et al., 2002). Given the generic importance of trigeminocervical complex neurons in primary headache, the interplay between brainstem modulatory systems and the trigeminocervical complex is likely to play an important role in the expression of many headache phenotypes.

CONCLUSIONS

Current data gleaned from both clinical and basic experimental studies suggest a pivotal role for the trigeminocervical complex in primary headache syndromes. The most important lesson to be learned initially in this general area is that intracranial nociceptive signals converge at the level of the second-order neuron. For this reason, conclusions from clinical history and trials of physical therapy must be very carefully evaluated because one generic hypothesis to advance from the anatomy and physiology of these systems is that they have been designed and evolved as warning, not localization, systems.

REFERENCES

Afridi SK, Shields KG, Bhola R, Goadsby PJ. Greater occipital nerve injection in primary headache syndromes: prolonged effects from a single injection. *Pain* 2006;122:126–129.

Anthony M. Headache and the greater occipital nerve. *Clin Neurol Neurosurg* 1992;94:297–301.

Bakker DA, Richmond FJ, Abrahams VC. Central projections from cat suboccipital muscles: a study using transganglionic transport of horseradish peroxidase. *J Comp Neurol* 1984;228:409–421.

Bartsch T, Goadsby PJ. Stimulation of the greater occipital nerve induces increased central excitability of dural afferent input. *Brain* 2002;125:1496–1509.

Bartsch T, Goadsby PJ. Increased responses in trigemino-cervical nociceptive neurons to cervical input after stimulation of the dura mater. *Brain* 2003;126: 1801–1813.

Bartsch T, Goadsby PJ. Anatomy and physiology of pain referral in primary and cervicogenic headache disorders. *Headache Currents* 2005;2:42–48.

Becser N, Bovim G, Sjaastad O. Extra-cranial nerves in the posterior part of the head. Anatomic variations and their possible clinical significance. *Spine* 1998;23:1435–1441.

Behbehani MM. Functional characteristics of the midbrain periaqueductal gray. *Prog Neurobiol* 1995;46:575–605.

Bogduk N. Headache and the neck. In: Goadsby PJ, Silberstein SD, eds. *Headache*. Oxford: Butterworth Heinemann; 1997:369–381. Asbury AK, Marsden CD, eds. *Blue Books in Practical Neurology*; Vol. 17.

Bogduk N. Cervicogenic headache: anatomic basis and patho-physiologic mechanisms. *Current Pain Head Rep* 2001;5:382–386.

Bogduk N, Aprill C. On the nature of neck pain, discography and cervical zygapophysial joint blocks. *Pain* 1993;54: 213–217.

Bolton S, O'Shaughnessy CT, Goadsby PJ. Properties of neurons in the trigeminal nucleus caudalis responding to noxious dural and facial stimulation. *Brain Res* 2005;1046: 122–129.

Bovim G, Sand I. Cervicogenic headache, migraine without aura and tension-type headache. Diagnostic blockade of the greater occipital and supra-orbital nerves. *Pain* 1992;51: 43–48.

Bovim G, Bonamico L, Fredriksen TA, et al. Topographical variations in the peripheral course of the greater occipital nerve. Autopsy study with clinical correlations. *Spine* 1991;16:475–478.

Burstein R, Yamamura H, Malick A, Strassman AM. Chemical stimulation of the intra-cranial dura induces enhanced responses to facial stimulation in brain stem trigeminal neurons. *J Neurophysiol* 1998;79:964–982.

Burstein R, Cutrer MF, Yarnitsky D. The development of cutaneous allodynia during a migraine attack. *Brain* 2000a; 123:1703–1709.

Burstein R, Yarnitsky D, Goor-Aryeh I, Ransil BJ, Bajwa ZH. An association between migraine and cutaneous allodynia. *Ann Neurol* 2000b;47:614–624.

Busch V, Jakob W, Juergens T, et al. Functional connectivity between trigeminal and occipital nerves revealed by occipital nerve blockade and nociceptive blink reflexes. *Cephalalgia* 2006;26:50–55.

Cervero F. Fine afferent fibres from viscera and visceral pain: anatomy and physiology of viscero-somatic convergence. In: Schmidt RF, Schaible HG, Vahle-Hinz C, eds. *Fine Afferent Nerve Fibres and Pain*. Weinheim, Germany: VCH; 1987:321–333.

Cervero F, Laird JM. Visceral pain. *Lancet* 1999;353: 2145–2148.

Cervero F, Lumb BM. Bilateral inputs and supraspinal control of viscero-somatic neurons in the lower thoracic spinal cord of the cat. *J Physiol* 1988;403:221–237.

Cremer P, Halmagyi GM, Goadsby PJ. Secondary cluster headache responsive to sumatriptan. *J Neurol Neurosurg Psychiatry* 1995;59:633–634.

Ellrich J, Messlinger K. Afferent input to the medullary dorsal horn from the contra-lateral face in rat. *Brain Res* 1999;826:321–324.

Feindel W, Penfield W, McNaughton F. The tentorial nerves and localization of intra-cranial pain in man. *Neurology* 1960;10:555–563.

Feinstein B, Langton JNK, Jameson RM, Schiller F. Experiments on pain referred from deep somatic tissues. *J Bone Joint Surgery* 1954;36A:981–997.

Fields HL, Heinricher MM. Anatomy and physiology of a nociceptive modulatory system. *Philos Trans Roy Soc Lond B Biol Sci* 1985;308:361–374.

Fields HL, Heinricher MM, Mason P. Neurotransmitters in nociceptive modulatory circuits. *Ann Review Neuroscience* 1991;14:219–245.

Goadsby PJ, Hoskin KL. The distribution of trigemino-vascular afferents in the nonhuman primate brain *Macaca nemestrina*: a c-fos immunocytochemical study. *J Anatomy* 1997;190:367–375.

Goadsby PJ, Oshinsky M. The patho-physiology of migraine. In: Silberstein SD, Lipton RB, Dodick D, eds. *Wolff's Headache and Other Head Pain*. 8th ed. New York: Oxford; 2007.

Goadsby PJ, Hoskin KL, Knight YE. Stimulation of the greater occipital nerve increases metabolic activity in the trigeminal nucleus caudalis and cervical dorsal horn of the cat. *Pain* 1997;73:23–28.

Herrero JF, Laird JM, Lopez-Garcia JA. Wind-up of spinal cord neurones and pain sensation: much ado about something? *Prog Neurobiol* 2000;61:169–203.

Hoskin KL, Zagami A, Goadsby PJ. Stimulation of the middle meningeal artery leads to Fos expression in the trigemino-cervical nucleus: a comparative study of monkey and cat. *J Anatomy* 1999;194:579–588.

Hoskin KL, Bulmer DCE, Lasalandra M, Jonkman A, Goadsby PJ. Fos expression in the midbrain periaqueductal grey after trigemino-vascular stimulation. *J Anatomy* 2001;197: 29–35.

Hunter CR, Mayfield FH. Role of the upper cervical roots in the production of pain in the head. *Am J Surgery* 1949;78: 743–749.

Hutchinson PJ, Pickard J, Higgins J. Vertebral artery dissection presenting as cerebellar infarction. *J Neurol Neurosurg Psychiatry* 2000;68:98–99.

International Headache Society. The International Classification of Headache Disorders: 2nd edition. *Cephalalgia* 2004;24(suppl 1):1–160.

Jacquin MF, Semba K, Rhoades RW, Egger MD. Trigeminal primary afferents project bilaterally to dorsal horn and ipsi-laterally to cerebellum, reticular formation, and cuneate, solitary, supra-trigeminal and vagal nuclei. *Brain Res* 1982;246:285–291.

Jakubowski M, Levy D, Kainz V, Zhang XC, Kosaras B, Burstein R. Sensitization of central trigemino-vascular neurons: blockade by intravenous naproxen infusion. *Neuroscience* 2007;148:573–583.

Katsarava Z, Lehnerdt G, Duda B, Ellrich J, Diener H-C, Kaube H. Sensitization of trigeminal nociception specific for migraine but not pain of sinusitis. *Neurology* 2002;59: 1450–1453.

Kaube H, Keay KA, Hoskin KL, Bandler R, Goadsby PJ. Expression of c-*Fos*-like immunoreactivity in the caudal medulla and upper cervical cord following stimulation of the superior sagittal sinus in the cat. *Brain Res* 1993a;629: 95–102.

Kaube H, Hoskin KL, Goadsby PJ. Intravenous acetylsalicylic acid inhibits central trigeminal neurons in the dorsal horn of the upper cervical spinal cord in the cat. *Headache* 1993b;33:541–550.

Kaube H, Katsarava Z, Kaufer T, Diener H-C, Ellrich J. A new method to increase the nociception specificity of the human blink reflex. *Clin Neurophysiol* 2000;111:413–416.

Kaube H, Katsarava Z, Przywara S, et al. Acute migraine headache. Possible sensitization of neurons in the spinal trigeminal nucleus? *Neurology* 2002;58:1234–1238.

Keay KA, Bandler R. Vascular head pain selectively activates ventro-lateral periaqueductal gray in the cat. *Neurosci Lett* 1998;245:58–60.

Kerr FWL. A mechanism to account for frontal headache in cases of posterior fossa tumors. *J Neurosurgery* 1961;18: 605–609.

Kerr FWL, Olafson RA. Trigeminal and cervical volleys. *Arch Neurol* 1961;5:69–76.

Knight YE, Goadsby PJ. The periaqueductal gray matter modulates trigemino-vascular input: a role in migraine? *Neuroscience* 2001;106:793–800.

Knight YE, Bartsch T, Kaube H, Goadsby PJ. P/Q-type calcium channel blockade in the PAG facilitates trigeminal nociception: a functional genetic link for migraine? *J Neurosci* 2002;22(RC213):1–6.

Knight YE, Bartsch T, Goadsby PJ. Trigeminal anti-nociception induced by bicuculline in the periaqueductal grey (PAG) is not affected by PAG P/Q-type calcium channel blockade in rat. *Neurosci Lett* 2003;336:113–116.

Koltzenburg M. Neural mechanisms of cutaneous nociceptive pain. *Clin J Pain* 2000;16:S131–S138.

Lance JW, Goadsby PJ. *Mechanism and Management of Headache*. 7th ed. New York: Elsevier; 2005.

Le Doare K, Akerman S, Holland PR, Lasalandra MP, Classey JD, Knight YE, et al. Occipital afferent activation of second order neurons in the trigemino-cervical complex in rat. *Neurosci Lett* 2006;403:73–77.

Levy D, Strassman A. Mechanical response properties of A and C primary afferent neurons innervating the rat intra-cranial dura. *J Neurophysiol* 2002;88:3021–3031.

Lin Q, Wu J, Peng YB, Cui M, Willis WD Jr. Nitric oxide-mediated spinal disinhibition contributes to the sensitisation of primate spinothalamic tract neurons. *J Neurophysiol* 1999;81:1086–1094.

Linderoth B, Brodin E. "Mirror pain" and indications of bilateral dorsal horn activation in response to unilateral nociception. *Pain* 1994;58:277–288.

Mackenzie J. *Symptoms and Their Interpretation*. London: Shaw and Sons; 1909.

Matharu MS, Bartsch T, Ward N, et al. Central neuro-modulation in chronic migraine with implanted suboccipital stimulators. *Neurology* 2003;60(suppl 1):A404–A405.

Matharu MS, Bartsch T, Ward N, et al. Central neuro-modulation in chronic migraine patients with suboccipital stimulators: a PET study. *Brain* 2004;127:220–230.

May A, Kaube H, Buechel C, et al. Experimental cranial pain elicited by capsaicin: a PET-study. *Pain* 1998;74:61–66.

McMahon SB, Lewin GR, Wall PD. Central hyper-excitability triggered by noxious inputs. *Curr Opin Neurobiol* 1993;3:602–610.

McNaughton FL. The innervation of the intra-cranial blood vessels and dural sinuses. *Proc Assoc Res Nervous Ment Dis* 1938;18:178–200.

Mense S. Nociception from skeletal muscle in relation to clinical muscle pain. *Pain* 1993;54:241–289.

Neuhuber WL, Zenker W. Central distribution of cervical primary afferents in the rat, with emphasis on proprioceptive projections to vestibular, peri-hypoglossal, and upper thoracic spinal nuclei. *J Comp Neurol* 1989;280: 231–253.

Ophoff RA, Terwindt GM, Vergouwe MN, et al. Familial hemiplegic migraine and episodic ataxia type-2 are caused by mutations in the Ca^{2+} channel gene CACNL1A4. *Cell* 1996;87:543–552.

Penfield W, McNaughton FL. Dural headache and the innervation of the dura mater. *Arch Neurol Psychiatry* 1940;44:43–75.

Peres MFP, Stiles MA, Siow HC, et al. Greater occipital nerve blockade for cluster headache. *Cephalalgia* 2002;22: 520–522.

Pfaller K, Arvidsson J. Central distribution of trigeminal and upper cervical primary afferents in the rat studied by anterograde transport of horseradish peroxidase conjugated to wheat germ agglutinin. *J Comp Neurol* 1988;268:91–108.

Pfister J, Zenker W. The splenius capitis muscle of the rat, architecture and histochemistry, afferent and efferent innervation as compared with that of the quadriceps muscle. *Anat Embryol (Berl)* 1984;169:79–89.

Piovesan EJ, Kowacs PA, Tatsui CE, et al. Referred pain after painful stimulation of the greater occipital nerve in humans: evidence of convergence of cervical afferents on trigeminal nuclei. *Cephalalgia* 2001;21:107–109.

Ray BS, Wolff HG. Experimental studies on headache. Pain sensitive structures of the head and their significance in headache. *Arch Surg* 1940;41:813–856.

Ren K, Dubner R. Descending modulation in persistent pain: an update. *Pain* 2002;100:1–6.

Richter F, Ebersberger A, Mikulik O, Schaible H-G. P/Q-type channels in the brainstem regulate activity of neurons with input from the dura by controlling GABA release from inhibitory interneurons. *Proc Soc Neurosci* 2002;28:349.13.

Ruch TC. Patho-physiology of pain. In: Ruch TC, Patton HD, eds. *Physiology and Biophysics*. Philadelphia: Saunders; 1965:345–363.

Sandkuhler J, Fu QG, Zimmermann M. Spinal pathways mediating tonic or stimulation-produced descending inhibition from the periaqueductal gray or nucleus raphe magnus are separate in the cat. *J Neurophysiol* 1987;58: 327–341.

Schaible HG, Grubb BD. Afferent and spinal mechanisms of joint pain. *Pain* 1993;55:45–54.

Schepelmann K, Ebersberger A, Pawlak M, Oppmann M, Messlinger K. Response properties of trigeminal brain stem neurons with input from dura mater encephali in the rat. *Neuroscience* 1999;90:543–554.

Scheurer S, Gottschall J, Groh V. Afferent projections of the rat major occipital nerve studied by transganglionic transport of HRP. *Anat Embryol (Berl)* 1983;168:425–438.

Selby G, Lance JW. Observations on 500 cases of migraine and allied vascular headache. *J Neurol Neurosurg Psychiatry* 1960;23:23–32.

Strassman AM, Mineta Y, Vos BP. Distribution of fos-like immunoreactivity in the medullary and upper cervical dorsal horn produced by stimulation of dural blood vessels in the rat. *J Neurosci* 1994;14:3725–3735.

Urban MO, Gebhart GF. Supraspinal contributions to hyperalgesia. *Proc Natl Acad Sci USA* 1999;96:7687–7692.

Van den Maagdenberg AMJM, Pietrobon D, Pizzorusso T, et al. A CACNA1A knock-in migraine mouse model with increased susceptibility to cortical spreading depression. *Neuron* 2004;41:701–710.

Vital JM, Grenier F, Dautheribes M, et al. An anatomic and dynamic study of the greater occipital nerve (n. of Arnold). Applications to the treatment of Arnold's neuralgia. *Surg Radiol Anat* 1989;11:205–210.

Weiller C, May A, Limmroth V, et al. Brain stem activation in spontaneous human migraine attacks. *Nature Medicine* 1995;1:658–660.

Wirth FP, van Buren JM. Referral of pain from dural stimulation in man. *J Neurosurg* 1971;34:630–642.

Wolff HG. *Headache and Other Head Pain*. New York: Oxford University Press; 1948.

Woolf CJ, Salter MW. Neuronal plasticity: increasing the gain in pain. *Science* 2000;288:1765–1769.

Cervicogenic Headache: Consideration of Pathogenesis

Fabio Antonaci, MD, PhD

The idea that headache may originate from the neck has been discussed over decades. Various terms have been used, and different underlying pathologic processes in the cervical spine have been postulated, such as vertebral ischemia caused by uncovertebral deformities at the C3-C6 levels (cervical migraine) (Bärtschi-Rochaix, 1968); chronic inflammatory lesions, causing a possible entrapment of the greater occipital nerve (occipital neuralgia) (Sigwald & Jamet, 1968); noxious stimulation of the cervical muscles (post-traumatic occipital myalgia-neuralgia syndrome) (Blume & Ungar-Sargon, 1986; Bodguk, 1981); or tender nodules in the posterior neck muscles, called fibrositis (rheumatic headache) (Patrick, 1913).

The term *cervicogenic headache* (CeH) was introduced by Sjaastad et al. (1983) to describe a distinct headache syndrome, indicating that the pain is believed to originate from the neck. The pathophysiologic model for this kind of pain was described by Kerr (1961) and has been used to explain the referred pain in CeH. Pain generated in any location within the trigeminocervical territory can be referred to the frontal region via the trigeminocervical nucleus (Kimmel, 1961; Taren & Kahn, 1962; Bodguk, 1982, 1984).

ROLE OF THE STRUCTURE IN SPINAL CORD IN CERVICOGENIC HEADACHE

Trigeminocervical Nucleus Caudalis

The neuroanatomic basis for CeH is in the trigeminocervical nucleus caudalis in the spinal gray matter of the spinal cord at the C1-C3 level, where there is a convergence on the nociceptive second-order neurons receiving both trigeminal and cervical input (see Figure 10.1). The nociceptive axons of the trigeminal nerve run caudally after entering the spinal tract of the trigeminal nerve, and continue into the dorsolateral tract of the cervicospinal cord into the C3 or C4 level. Sensory fibers of the C2-C3 roots ramify into the dorsal horn of the spinal cord, not only in their respective segments but also into adjacent segments (Bogduk, 1981, 1982, 1992). On this anatomic basis, it is possible to explain that cervical spinal root involvement at the lower level may also cause hemicrania (Michler et al., 1991).

The trigeminal nucleus caudalis descends as low as the C3 or C4 segments of the spinal cord. This nucleus is contiguous with the gray matter of the spinal dorsal horn at these levels. This column of gray matter has been called the *trigeminocervical nucleus*. Interneurons within the trigeminocervical nucleus allow for an exchange of sensory information between the upper cervical spinal nerves and the trigeminal nerve. It is through this exchange of sensory information that nociceptive signals from the anatomic structures and soft tissues of the upper region of the neck can be referred to the sensory receptive fields of the trigeminal nerve in the head and face.

The topographic arrangement of the trigeminal nucleus caudalis allows the interchange of nociceptive information with the ophthalmic division of the trigeminal nerve (V1 nerve); therefore, it is most common for pain from a cervical source to be referred to the forehead, temple, or orbit. There is also some interchange of sensory signals with the maxillary division of the trigeminal nerve that allows referral of neck pain to the face. Afferent sensory signals ascend or descend up to three spinal cord segments in the dorsolateral tract and substantia gelatinosa before entering the spinal dorsal horn. This could allow nociceptive signals from spinal segments as low as C6 or C7 the potential to interact with interneurons in the trigeminocervical nucleus, and thereby the referral of pain from anatomic structures or soft tissues in the middle and lower portion of the neck to the head and face (Fredriksen et al., 1999). Chapter 10 discusses in detail the anatomy and physiology of the trigeminocervical complex.

Upper Cervical Spinal Nerves

The first three cervical spinal nerves and their rami are the primary peripheral nerve structures that can refer pain to the head. The suboccipital nerve (dorsal ramus of C1) innervates the atlanto-occipital joint; therefore, a pathologic condition or injury affecting this joint is a potential source for head pain that is referred to the occipital region. The C2 spinal nerve and its dorsal root ganglion have a close relationship to the lateral capsule of the atlantoaxial (C1-C2) zygapophysial joint and innervate the atlantoaxial and C2-C3 zygapophysial joints. Therefore, trauma to or degenerative changes around these joints can be a source of referred head pain. Neuralgia of C2 is typically described as a deep or dull pain that usually radiates from the occipital to parietal, temporal, frontal, and periorbital regions. A paroxysmal sharp or shocklike pain is often superimposed over the constant pain. Ipsilateral eye lacrimation and conjunctival injection are common associated signs. Arterial or venous compression of the C2 spinal nerve or its dorsal root ganglion might also be a cause for C2 neuralgia in some cases (Jansen et al., 1989; Pikus & Phillips, 1996).

The third occipital nerve (dorsal ramus C3) has a close anatomic proximity to and innervates the C2-C3 zygapophysial joint. This joint and the third occipital nerve appear most vulnerable to trauma from whiplash injuries (Lord & Bogduk, 1996). Pain from the C2-C3 zygapophysial joint is referred to the occipital region but is also referred to the frontotemporal and periorbital regions. Injury to this region is a common cause of CeH. Of certain interest are reports that patients with chronic headache had experienced substantial pain relief after discectomy at spinal levels as low as C5-C6 (Michler et al., 1991; Fredriksen et al., 1999). Finally, although referred head pain most often originates in the upper cervical regions, it may also be originated from the middle to lower cervical regions (**Figure 11.1**).

Muscle Referred Pain

Finally, pain originating from muscles in the neck can also be referred to the head and face. Predictable patterns for referred pain from muscles in the neck and shoulders to the head and face have been identified (see Chapter 6).

Trigger points are discrete areas of contracted muscle that have a lowered pain threshold and are hyperirritable (Jaeger, 1989). Muscle trigger points, when manually compressed, refer pain to distant regions (Simons et al., 1999). An active trigger point is able to elicit spontaneous pain or pain after physical stimulation that is referred to distant sites in predictable and reproducible patterns. A latent trigger point can also produce a pattern of referred pain when it is manually compressed or when the involved muscle is stretched or stressed in some way (for further descriptions, see Chapter 6).

Pain can be elicited directly through an activation of sensory afferents in the upper spinal nerves or referred through an exchange of mechanical and nociceptive signals between the spinal accessory nerve and upper cervical sensory afferent nerves. This interchange and convergence of sensory information would allow for the referral of nociceptive sensory signals from the trapezius, sternocleidomastoid, and other cervical muscles to regions of the head and face. At the present time, there is no clear-cut clinical evidence that CeH might primarily originate from contracted muscles or the spinal accessory nerve.

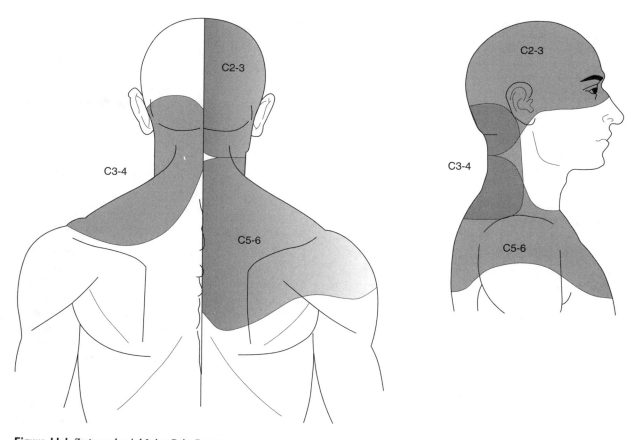

Figure 11.1 Zygapophysial Joint Pain Patterns
Source: Modified from Bogduk N, Marsland A. The cervical zygapophyseal joints as a source of neck pain. *Spine* 1988;13:610–617.

Role of the Extracranial Sensory Nerve

It is known that the scalp receives sensory fibers from the first and third branches of the trigeminal nerve and the C2-C3 spinal nerve. From the C2-C3 spinal dorsal rami originates the greater occipital nerve (GON), supplying the posterior medial part of the head with sensory branches. The ventral rami of the same spinal nerves form the lesser or minor occipital (MON) and the greater auricular nerve (GAN) supplying the posterolateral headache surface; the cranial surface of the auricle is supplied by both of the latter sensory nerves (Andersen Becser et al., 2001).

The frontal and periorbital regions receive sensory supply via the supraorbital nerve (SON) and supratrochlear nerve (STN), originated from the ophthalmic division of the trigeminal nerve. The temporal region of the scalp is supplied by the auriculotemporal nerve (ATN), stemming from the third branch of the trigeminal

nerve (Williams et al., 1980). All these extracranial sensory nerves ascend toward the vertex and have a rich intra- and interindividual topographic variability observed in morphologic studies in subjects without a known major headache syndrome (Bogduk, 1982; Bovim et al., 1991). Moreover, some communicative branches between the above-mentioned nerves might explain overlaps between these nerves' innervation areas.

Pathologic entrapment of the occipital extracranial nerves (GON, MON) has been considered as a possible source of neuropathic pain in CeH. So far, this has not been confirmed by morphologic studies of these nerves because patients with definite CeH have not been examined (Becser et al., 1998; Bovim et al., 1991; Lucas et al., 1994). The variation of occipital nerve topography, macroscopic signs of nerve compression, and a rich nerve network around the occipital artery surrounded by the fibrous aponeurosis contribute to the complexity

Table 11.1 The Possible Sources of Cervicogenic Headache, Listed According to Innervation and Type of Structure

	Innervation		
Structure	C1	C2	C3
Joints	Atlantoaxial	Median atlantoaxial, lateral atlantoaxial	C2-C3 zygapophysial, C2-3 disc
Ligaments		Transverse atlantoaxial and alar; membrane tectoria	
Muscles	Suboccipital	Prevertebral, SCM, trapezius, semispinalis, splenius	Multifidus, semispinalis
Dura		Upper spinal cord, posterior cranial fossa	
Arteries		Vertebral, internal carotid	

SCM, sternocleidomastoid.
Modified from Bogduk, 2001.

of the situation. These structures can still not be ruled out as possible pain sources in CeH. GON neurolysis in the trapezius muscle in patients with CeH provided only short-lasting pain relief in the majority of them (Bovim et al., 1992b). Also, during liberation operations apparent nerve compression has been found, but this does not indicate that this is the cause of the head pain. Further observations of nerve impairment of this type are needed on subjects with a diagnosis of certain CeH before final conclusions can be made. The trigeminocervical nucleus can be considered as a communication center with an extensive afferent area, that is, from both the trigeminal and C1-C3 spinal nerves. This means that any of the structures innervated by the latter nerves could be a source of CeH. Such a theory is still the main pathophysiologic model of CeH at the present time (Bodguk, 2001).

CLINICAL STUDIES

Clinical studies in normal volunteers and in patients with headache can provide better insight regarding particular structures innervated by the upper three cervical nerves either by stimulation to aggravate the headache or by selectively blocking structures in order to relieve the headache. These studies use highly selective, target-specific techniques to establish a cervical source of pain.

Two studies have reported that in some patients with headache, the pain can be reproduced by stimulation of the C2-C3 intervertebral disc, but not lower discs (Schellhas, 1996; Grubb & Kelly, 2000). This is evidence that this disc could be a source of CeH, but the problem arises of other possible inferences. Patients with pain can suffer hyperalgesia, such that noxious stimulation

of any structure in the painful area might reproduce or aggravate their pain. This observation does not necessarily implicate the stimulated structure as the singular or primary source of pain.

More relevant data are obtained from results of studies in which headache has been relieved by anesthetic blockade of certain cervical structures. In this regard, the criterion of complete relief of headache could be the proof that the anesthetized structure is the source of pain. Moreover, the responses to anesthetic blocks are more correct if the block is also performed in controls because of the possible placebo response. Ehni and Benner (1984) found complete relief of headache in patients with osteoarthritis of the lateral atlantoaxial joints following periarticular local anesthetic blocks of those joints. Busch and Wilson (1989) reported relief of headache in a small number of patients following intra-articular blocks of either the atlanto-occipital or the lateral atlantoaxial joints. Neither of these studies, however, used control blockades. Their results provide only preliminary evidence that these joints might be the source of CeH. If nerve blocks were used in the investigation of CeH, a complete relief of headache following anesthetization of either the C2 spinal nerve or the GON must be obtained (Sjaastad et al., 1986; Bovim et al., 1992a). A minor drawback of this study is the lack of control blocks, but the responses still constitute an evidence of a cervical source (Anthony, 1992). Moreover, nerve blocks cannot be considered specific in that they do not identify the actual source of pain but only show that the pain is mediated by a nerve that is anesthetized.

Other evidence on the possible source of CeH comes from studies in which the C2-C3 zygapophysial joint was anesthetized under controlled conditions (**Table 11.1**). Lord et al. (1994), in a double-blind study under highly selective conditions, used blocks of the third occipital nerve to anesthetize the C2-C3 zygapophysial joint. Anesthetic agents with different durations of action on separate occasions were used to compare local anesthetic blocks. They found that among patients with headache following whiplash, the headache could be completely abolished in over 50% of cases if the C2-C3 joint was anesthetized. In another study, the same group (Lord & Bogduk, 1996) reported that the C3-C4 zygapophysial joint could also be a source of CeH, but far less commonly than the C2-C3 joint.

CONCLUSIONS

There are controversies regarding whether the signs and symptoms of neck involvement represent a cervical source for the pain in the clinical condition that Sjaastad et al. (1983) denominated cervicogenic headache. For some authors, the relationship between some signs and symptoms and neck involvement is not so straightforward. According to Edmeads (2001), the evidence of neck involvement may be equivocal, because local pressure on cervical nerves or facet joints may demonstrate the existence of a cervical problem but does not establish the cervical origin of the headache. That author also says that when a nerve block is made and the pain is relieved, it does not necessarily mean that the pain is emanating from a structure innervated by the nerve.

Bogduk (1998) considers that demonstrating a cervical source for the pain is essential for the diagnosis. He disagrees that "symptoms and signs of neck involvement and confirmatory evidence by diagnostic anesthetic blockage" would be valid signs of a cervical disorder when radiographs and other procedures fail to reveal cervical lesions. He proposes strict criteria to establish a cervical source for headache; one such criterion is that "the location of the pain-producing focus should be specified in anatomic terms." Similar to the criteria proposed by Bogduk (1998), in the *International Classification of Headache Disorders*, second edition (ICHD-II) (International Headache Society, 2004), CeH (item 11.2.1) appears as a part of headache that is attributed to a neck disorder and demands "strict evidence that pain can be attributed to neck disorder." It may be observed that in the ICHD-II, the purpose of the criteria in Chapter 11 "is not to describe headaches in all their possible sub-forms, but rather to establish specific causal relationships between headaches and facial pain to disorders of cranium, neck etc."

Although many clinical studies do not follow the scientific rigor now required to identify a source of pain, the data from clinical studies agree with results of studies on normal healthy volunteers. They show that various joints in the upper cervical spine can be sources of headache. The studies of normal subjects have additionally implicated the upper cervical muscles, although no controlled studies have convincingly demonstrated whether or how often the muscles are the primary source of CeH. In all instances, however, the structures implicated as sources of headache are all ones innervated by the upper three cervical nerves. These data provide a foundation for the differential diagnosis and investigation of putative CeH.

The definition of CeH requires that a cervical source of pain be established (Antonaci et al., 2001). The experimental data indicate that the source will lie somewhere among the structures innervated by the upper three cervical nerves. The definitive diagnosis of CeH, therefore, rests on determining which of these structures is the source. This cannot be done reliably and validly by history and clinical examination, nor by medical imaging. At present, controlled diagnostic blocks of putative sources of pain are the only secure means of determining that source.

REFERENCES

Andersen Becser N, Bovim G, Sjaastad O. The fronto-temporal peripheral nerves. Topographic variations of the supra-orbital, supra-trochlear and auriculo-temporal nerves and their possible clinical significance. *Surg Radiol Anat* 2001;23:97–104.

Anthony M. Headache and the greater occipital nerve. *Clin Neurol Neurosurg* 1992;94:297–301.

Antonaci F, Torbjorn FA, Sjaastad O. Cervicogenic headache: clinical presentation, diagnostic criteria and differential diagnosis. *Curr Pain Headache Rep* 2001;5: 387–392.

Bärtschi-Rochaix W. Headaches of cervical origin. In: Vinken PJ, Bruyn GW, eds. *Handbook of Clinical Neurology*. Vol. 5. *Headache and Cranial Neuralgia*. Amsterdam: North Holland Publishing; 1968:192–203.

Becser N, Bovim G, Sjaastad O. Extra-cranial nerves in the posterior part of the head. Anatomical variations and their possible clinical significance. *Spine* 1998;23: 1435–1441.

Blume H, Ungar-Sargon J. Neurosurgical treatment of persistent occipital myalgia-neuralgia syndrome. *J Craniomand Pract* 1986;4:65–73.

Bogduk N. Local anaesthetic blocks of the second cervical ganglion: a technique with application in occipital headache. *Cephalalgia* 1981;1:41–50.

Bogduk N. The clinical anatomy of the cervical dorsal rami. *Spine* 1982;7:319–330.

Bogduk N. Headaches and the cervical spine. *Cephalalgia* 1984;4:7–8.

Bogduk N. The anatomical basis for cervicogenic headache. *J Manipulative Physiol Ther* 1992;15:67–70.

Bogduk N. "Is it my neck?" Cervicogenic headache. *Headache, the Newsletter of ACHE* 1998;9(3).

Bogduk N. Cervicogenic headache: anatomical basis and patho-physiological mechanisms. *Curr Pain Headache Rep* 2001;5:382–386.

Bovim G, Bonamico L, Fredriksen TA, Lindboe CF, Stolt-Nielsen A, Sjaastad O. Topographic variations in the peripheral course of the greater occipital nerve. Autopsy study with clinical correlations. *Spine* 1991;16:475–478.

Bovim G, Berg R, Dale LG. Cervicogenic headache: anaesthetic blockades of cervical nerves (C2-C5) and facet joint (C2/C3). *Pain* 1992a;49:315–320.

Bovim G, Fredriksen TA, Lindboe CF, Stolt-Nielsen A, Sjaastad O. Neurolysis of the greater occipital nerve in cervicogenic headache. A follow-up study. *Headache* 1992b;32:175–179.

Busch E, Wilson PR. Atlanto-occipital and atlanto-axial injections in the treatment of headache and neck pain. *Reg Anesth* 1989;14(suppl 2):45.

Edmeads JG. Disorders of the neck: cervicogenic headache. In: Silberstein SD, Lipton RB, Dalessio DJ, eds. *Wolff's Headache and Other Head Pain*. New York: Oxford University Press; 2001:447–458.

Ehni G, Benner B. Occipital neuralgia and the C1-2 arthrosis syndrome. *J Neurosurg* 1984;61:961–965.

Fredriksen T, Salvesen R, Stolt-Nielsen A, Sjaastad O. Cervicogenic headache: long-term postoperative follow-up. *Cephalalgia* 1999;19:897–900.

Grubb SA, Kelly CK. Cervical discography: clinical implications from 12 years of experience. *Spine* 2000;25:1329–1382.

International Headache Society. The International Classification of Headache Disorders: 2nd edition. *Cephalalgia* 2004;24(suppl 1):9–160.

Jaeger B. Are "cervicogenic" headaches due to myofascial pain and cervical spine dysfunction? *Cephalalgia* 1989;9: 157–164.

Jansen J, Bardosi A, Hildebrandt J, Lucke A. Cervicogenic, hemi-cranial attacks associated with vascular irritation or compression of the cervical nerve root C2. Clinical manifestations and morphological findings. *Pain* 1989;39:203–212.

Kerr PW. A mechanism to account for frontal headache in cases of posterior fossa tumours. *J Neurosurg* 1961;5: 171–178.

Kimmel DL. Innervation of spinal dura mater and dura mater of the posterior cranial fossa. *Neurology* 1961;11: 800–809.

Lord SM, Bogduk N. The cervical synovial joints as sources of post-traumatic headache. *J Musculoskeletal Pain* 1996;4: 81–94.

Lord S, Barnsley L, Wallis B, Bogduk N. Third occipital headache: a prevalence study. *J Neurol Neurosurg Psychiatry* 1994;57:1187–1190.

Lucas GA, Laudanna A, Clopard R, Raffaelli E. Anatomy of the lesser occipital nerve in relation to cervicogenic headache. *Clin Anatomy* 1994;7:90–96.

Michler RP, Bovim G, Sjaastad O. Disorders in the lower cervical spine. A cause of unilateral headache? *Headache* 1991;31:550–551.

Patrick H. Indurative or rheumatic headache. *JAMA* 1913;71:82–85.

Pikus HJ, Phillips J. Outcome of surgical decompression of the second cervical root for cervicogenic headache. *Neurosurgery* 1996;39:63–70.

Schellhas KP, Smith MD, Gundry CR, Pollei SR. Cervical discogenic pain: prospective correlation of magnetic resonance imaging and discography in asymptomatic subjects and pain sufferers. *Spine* 1996;21:300–312.

Sigwald J, Jamet F. Occipital neuralgia. In: Vinken PJ, Bruyn GW, eds. *Handbook of Clinical Neurology*. Vol. 5. *Headache and Cranial Neuralgia*. Amsterdam: North Holland Publishing; 1968:368–374.

Simons DG, Travell J, Simons L. *Myofascial Pain and Dysfunction: The Trigger Point Manual*. Vol. 1. 2nd ed. Baltimore: Williams & Wilkins; 1999.

Sjaastad O, Saunte C, Hovdal H, et al. Cervicogenic headache: a hypothesis. *Cephalalgia* 1983;3:249–256.

Sjaastad O, Fredriksen TA, Stolt-Nielsen A. Cervicogenic headache, C2 rhizopathy, and occipital neuralgia: a connection? *Cephalalgia* 1986;6:189–195.

Taren J, Kahn E. Anatomic pathways related to pain in face and neck. *J Neurosurg* 1962;19:116–119.

Williams PL, Warwick R, eds. *Grays' Anatomy*. 36th ed. Edinburgh: Churchill Livingston; 1980:1086–1092.

Motor Control Impairment in Cervicogenic Headache

Deborah Falla, PT, PhD

Cervicogenic headache is generated by excitation of cervical nociceptors and may be associated with trauma or pathology in the cervical spine (Sjaastad et al., 1983). Most commonly pain originates from structures in the upper cervical region; however, structures in the mid- and lower regions of the cervical spine may also refer pain to the head (Bovim et al., 1992; Biondi, 2000). Referral of pain to the head is attributed to convergence of afferents from the upper cervical spinal roots with afferents in the descending tract of the trigeminal nerve (Chapter 10). Convergence occurs within the trigeminocervical nucleus, a region of the upper cervical spinal cord where interneurons permit exchange of sensory information between upper cervical spinal nerves and the trigeminal nerve (Kerr & Olafson, 1961). Excitation of cervical nociceptors by trauma or pathology of structures such as the zygapophysial joints (Bogduk, 1992; Jull et al., 1999), cervical muscles (Jaeger, 1989), or intervertebral disc (Jansen et al., 1989; Bogduk, 1992) is perceived as neck pain. In addition, pain can be experienced in the head and face consistent with the sensory receptive fields of the trigeminal nerve (Bogduk, 2004). Moreover, it is possible that afferent information from structures in the mid- and lower regions of the cervical spine may arrive at the

trigeminocervical nucleus due to the bidirectional exchange of sensory information across spinal cord segments (Biondi, 2000).

Differential diagnosis of cervicogenic headache can be challenging because of symptomatic overlap with other intermittent headache types, such as migraine or tension-type headache. Nevertheless, there are some distinguishing characteristics that help to differentiate cervicogenic headache from other headache types, including (a) headache triggered by sustained neck postures or neck movements, (b) pain spreading to the occipital region, (c) tenderness in the suboccipital tissues, (d) decreased cervical range of motion, and (e) unresponsiveness to typical headache medication (Sjaastad et al., 1998; International Headache Society [IHS], 2004). A further characteristic that appears to be unique to cervicogenic headache is the presence of impaired cervical muscle function (Bansevicius & Sjaastad, 1996; Barton & Hayes, 1996; Jull et al., 1999, 2007; Dumas et al., 2001; Amiri et al., 2007; Zito et al., 2006). The notion that cervicogenic headache is associated with impaired motor function of the neck is not unexpected given that the source of nociception originates from structures in the cervical region and given the knowledge of impaired neuromuscular control in people with neck pain (Vernon et al., 1992; Jull, 2000; Falla et al., 2004a, 2004b, 2004c; Jull et al., 2004; Ylinen et al., 2004; Mörk & Westgaard, 2006; O'Leary et al., 2007).

This chapter reviews evidence of impairment of muscle function in people with cervicogenic headache and discusses the potential value of assessing neuromuscular control to assist in the differential diagnosis of intermittent headaches.

MOTOR IMPAIRMENT IN CERVICOGENIC HEADACHE

The concept that cervicogenic headache is associated with motor impairment is not new. Reduced range of motion is well documented in these patients, and current classification criteria of cervicogenic headache include restricted range of motion of the cervical spine (Sjaastad et al., 1998; IHS, 2004). However, in recent years there has been an increase in the investigation of cervical motor impairment associated with headache. It is now known that cervicogenic headache sufferers present with an array of neuromuscular changes that are not unexpectedly different from those observed in people with neck pain. This section reviews current evidence of restricted range of motion in cervicogenic headache and explores other aspects of neural and muscular changes observed in these patients, including muscle coordination and altered muscle properties.

Cervical Range of Motion

It is well established that cervical range of motion is reduced in cervicogenic headache. In particular, movement appears to be most restricted for flexion, extension, and rotation (Zwart, 1997; Dumas et al., 2001; Amiri et al., 2007; Jull et al., 2007), and preliminary evidence suggests that range of motion is most restricted in patients with cervicogenic headache associated with neck trauma (Dumas et al., 2001) (**Figure 12.1**). Impaired range of motion is consistent with cervical segmental dysfunction assessed on manual examination in these patients (Jull et al., 2007). On the contrary, range of cervical motion in migraine or tension-type headache patients is consistent with normative data (Zwart, 1997; Dumas et al., 2001; Jull et al., 2007).

Muscle Strength and Endurance

In agreement with observations in people with neck pain, cervicogenic headache sufferers demonstrate

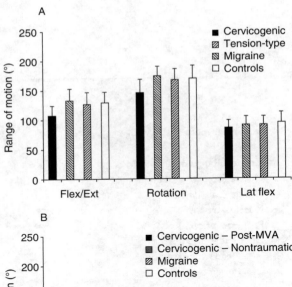

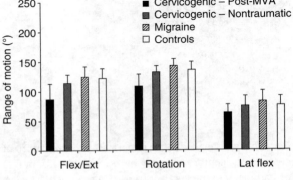

Figure 12.1 **Cervical Range of Motion. A:** People with cervicogenic headache show reduced range of cervical motion in the sagittal and transverse planes, whereas range of motion during lateral flexion is consistent with control data. People with migraine and tension-type headache show no differences from control subjects in the saggittal, coronal, and transverse plane. **B:** Preliminary findings suggest that range of motion in both the sagittal and transverse planes is most restricted for patients with cervicogenic headache originating from neck pain following a motor vehicle accident (MVA) compared with insidious onset. Again, no differences in range of motion are observed for people with migraine.

Source: **A:** Redrawn with permission from Zwart JA. Neck mobility in different headache disorders. *Headache* 1997;37:6–11. **B:** Redrawn with permission from Dumas JP, Arsenault A, Boudreau G, et al. Physical impairments in cervicogenic headache: traumatic vs. non-traumatic onset. *Cephalalgia* 2001;21:884–893.

deficits in the strength of their cervical flexor and extensor muscles (Watson & Trott, 1993; Dumas et al., 2001; Amiri et al., 2007; Jull et al., 2007) (**Figure 12.2**). Moreover, there is some evidence that suggests that neck extensor strength is more affected in cervicogenic headache originating from neck trauma following a motor vehicle accident (Dumas et al., 2001). There is conflicting evidence as to whether patients with migraine or tension-type headache have reduced strength

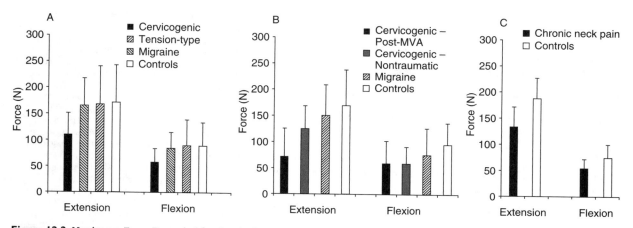

Figure 12.2 Maximum Force Recorded for Cervical Flexion and Extension. A: People with cervicogenic headache show reduced strength of the cervical flexor and extensor muscles compared with control subjects. Note that values obtained from both migraine and tension-type headache sufferers were consistent with the control data. **B:** People with cervicogenic headache following a motor vehicle accident (MVA) and nontraumatic cervicogenic headache showed reduced cervical flexor muscle strength compared with control subjects. However, only the patients with cervicogenic headache of traumatic onset showed reduced cervical extensor strength. Note, consistent with the findings of Jull et al. (2007), that no difference was observed for the patients with migraine. **C:** The reduction in neck muscle strength observed for people with cervicogenic headache is consistent with observations in people with chronic neck pain.

Source: **A:** Redrawn with permission from Jull G, Amiri M, Bullock-Saxton J, Darnell R, Lander C. Cervical musculo-skeletal impairment in frequent intermittent headache. Part 1: Subjects with single headaches. *Cephalalgia* 2007;27:793–802. **B:** Redrawn with permission from Dumas JP, Arsenault A, Boudreau G, et al. Physical impairments in cervicogenic headache: traumatic vs. non-traumatic onset. *Cephalalgia* 2001;21:884–893. **C:** Redrawn with permission from Ylinen J, Salo P, Nykanen M, Kautiainen H, Hakkinen A: Decreased isometric neck strength in women with chronic neck pain and the repeatability of neck strength measurements. *Arch Phys Med Rehabil* 2004;85:1303–1308.

compared with pain-free individuals (Dumas et al., 2001; Amiri et al., 2007; Jull et al., 2007; Fernández-de-las-Peñas et al., 2008), although the majority of studies indicates normal cervical muscle strength.

Cibulka (2006) reported ipsilateral weakness of the sternocleidomastoid muscle in a single case study of cervicogenic headache, albeit with manual muscle testing. Electromyographic studies may be useful for detecting side specificity of muscle impairment as documented in unilateral neck pain (Falla et al., 2004d). Additional evidence indicates that neck flexor endurance is limited in people with cervicogenic headache (Watson & Trott, 1993; Dumas et al., 2001), a finding that was not observed in migraine or tension-type headache. Additional studies are warranted to examine whether limited endurance is associated with greater myoelectric manifestations of neck muscle fatigue, a further finding in people with neck pain (Falla et al., 2003b).

Muscle Coordination

Electromyographic (EMG) studies have demonstrated an altered motor strategy when patients with cervicogenic headache perform the clinical test of craniocervical flex-

ion (Zito et al., 2006; Amiri et al., 2007; Jull et al., 2007). The craniocervical flexion muscle test (Jull et al., 1999) is designed to provide a clinical indicator of impaired activation of the deep cervical flexor muscles. The test requires the person to perform five progressive inner range positions of craniocervical flexion, the anatomic action of the deep longus capitis and colli muscles. As expected, a linear relationship exists between the amplitude of EMG activity of the longus capitis and longus colli muscles and the progressive stages of the test in pain-free individuals (Falla et al., 2003a). However, when patients with cervicogenic headache perform the craniocervical flexion test, greater activation of the sternocleidomastoid muscle is observed (Zito et al., 2006; Amiri et al., 2007; Jull et al., 2007), consistent with observations in idiopathic- and whiplash-induced neck pain (Jull, 2000; Falla et al., 2004c; Jull et al., 2004) (**Figure 12.3**). On the contrary, EMG studies assessing performance of migraine and tension-type headache groups show no difference from control subjects (Zito et al., 2006; Amiri et al., 2007; Jull et al., 2007).

Elevated sternocleidomastoid activity is associated with reduced activity of the longus colli and longus capitis in neck pain, and is considered to be a compensatory strategy to allow the motor output to be maintained

A

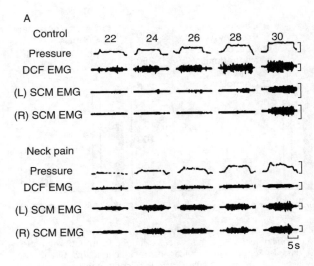

B

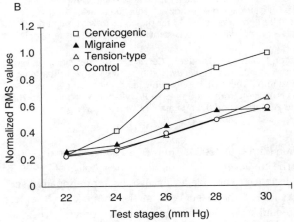

Figure 12.3 Craniocervical Flexion Test in Subjects with Neck and Head Pain. A: Representative raw electromyographic (EMG) data are shown for a control subject and person with neck pain during a task of staged craniocervical flexion. Data are shown for the deep cervical flexors (DCF) and left (L) and right (R) sternocleidomastoid (SCM) muscles. Note the incremental increase in EMG activity for all muscles with increasing craniocervical flexion (recorded as an increase in pressure in a pressure sensor under the cervical spine), but with lesser activity in the deep cervical flexors and greater activity in the superficial muscles for the neck pain patient, suggesting a reorganization of muscle activity to perform the task. EMG calibration: 0.5 mV.
Source: Redrawn with permission from Falla D, Bilenkij G, Jull G. Patients with chronic neck pain demonstrate altered patterns of muscle activation during performance of a functional upper limb task. *Spine* 2004a;29:1436–1440.
B: Consistent with observations in people with chronic neck pain, patients with cervicogenic headache display increased EMG activity (expressed as root mean square values: RMS) of the sternocleidomastoid muscle during the craniocervical flexion test compared with control subjects. Note that no differences were observed between people with migraine or tension-type headache compared with controls.
Source: Redrawn with permission from Jull G, Amiri M, Bullock-Saxton J, Darnell R, Lander C. Cervical musculo-skeletal impairment in frequent intermittent headache. Part 1: Subjects with single headaches. *Cephalalgia* 2007;27:793–802.

compared with healthy women (Fernández-de-las-Peñas et al., 2008). However, increased coactivation of antagonist musculature may reflect avoidance behavior, which would affect muscle use (Asmundson et al., 1999) and may explain altered motor control in tension-type headache patients in the absence of trauma or pathology in the cervical spine. In support of this notion, elevated upper trapezius activity was found both in cervicogenic and tension-type headache patients (Bansevicius & Sjaastad, 1996; Bansevicius et al., 1999) during a stressful task, suggesting that both patient groups react to a stressful situation in a similar way.

Muscle Atrophy

A study of real-time diagnostic ultrasound imaging revealed a reduced cross-sectional area of the semispinalis capitis measured at the level of the second cervical vertebrae on the symptomatic side in people with cervicogenic headache (Jull et al., 2007). No such atrophy was measured in association with migraine or tension-type headache, as there were no differences in cross-sectional areas between these and control subjects. Although atrophy of the semispinalis capitis muscle was observed ipsilateral to the side of headache in cervicogenic headache sufferers, there was no evidence of atrophy for the longissimus capitis or trapezius mus-

(Falla et al., 2004c). Although the deep cervical flexors have not been tested directly in cervicogenic headache sufferers, it is likely that their function would be impaired, consistent with observations in chronic neck pain patients. It would also prove interesting to identify whether other features of impaired motor control detected in people with neck pain are also present in people with cervicogenic headache, including altered activation of the cervical extensor muscles, reduced ability to relax muscles following activation, and reduced muscle rest periods during repetitive tasks (Veiersted et al., 1990; Hagg & Anstrom, 1997; Fredin et al., 1997; Nederhand et al., 2002; Falla et al., 2004a). There have been some observations that suggest changed motor control in tension-type headache. In one study, women with chronic tension-type headache displayed greater coactivation of cervical antagonist muscles during isometric cervical extension and flexion

cles. Selective atrophy of the semispinalis capitis was attributed to a localization of pain in the upper cervical segments in the participants with cervicogenic headache enrolled in this study and based on knowledge of the innervation of the semispinalis capitis, longissimus capitis, and trapezius at this level. That is, the semispinalis capitis in the upper cervical region is innervated by the dorsal rami of the upper cervical nerves (Strandring, 2005), consistent with the segmental levels that were symptomatic in the cervicogenic headache subjects. On the contrary, the upper trapezius is innervated by the accessory nerve, and the longissimus capitis by the dorsal rami of the lower cervical nerves (Strandring, 2005).

An observation in people with chronic neck pain is atrophy and connective tissue infiltration of the deep extensor muscles, notably, the rectus capitis minor and major and the multifidus (Hallgren et al., 1994; McPartland et al., 1997; Elliott et al., 2006). This finding has been also found in chronic tension-type headache (Fernández-de-las-Peñas et al., 2007a). Future magnetic resonance imaging analyses in people with cervicogenic headache may further clarify the proposal of Jull et al. (2007) of location-dependent muscle atrophy because the rectus capitis minor and major muscles are innervated solely by the dorsal ramus of C1 spinal nerve (Strandring, 2005). A study supported this hypothesis, albeit in a single case of cervicogenic headache (Fernández-de-las-Peñas et al., 2007b).

Proprioception

People with neck pain are known to have greater errors in positioning the head in neutral following voluntary movement (Revel et al., 1991; Heikkila & Astrom, 1996; Kristjansson et al., 2003; Treleaven et al., 2006). Alterations in proprioception are thought to reflect abnormal spindle afferent discharge either due to activation of chemo- or nociceptive sensory afferents (Pedersen et al., 1997; Wenngren et al., 1998; Thunberg et al., 2001; Hellstrom et al., 2002), direct trauma to cervical structures, or increased sympathetic drive (Roatta et al., 2002), resulting in a conflict of inputs from visual, vestibular, and somatosensory sources. Thus, it may be expected that people with cervicogenic headache also display deficits in proprioception. However, measures of repositioning accuracy in cervicogenic headache have failed to show differences from control populations (Dumas et al., 2001; Zito et al., 2006; Jull et al., 2007). One possible explanation for this

may be in the movements tested in these studies. Typically repositioning accuracy has been assessed during gross cervical rotation, extension, flexion, and lateral bending. Movements limited to the craniocervical region may yield different findings, especially if the subjects enrolled in the study have predominantly symptomatic upper cervical spine dysfunction. This should be explored in future studies.

DIFFERENTIAL DIAGNOSIS OF HEADACHE BASED ON MUSCULOSKELETAL IMPAIRMENTS

Current clinical diagnostic criteria for cervicogenic headache typically include unilateral headache without side shift; pain localized to the occipital, temporal, or orbital regions; deep, nonthrobbing pain; pain onset associated with awkward neck movement or sustained neck postures; and restricted range of cervical movement (Sjaastad et al., 1998; IHS, 2004). However, as mentioned earlier, there is considerable overlap in symptoms with other intermittent headaches, in particular, migraine and tension-type headache. It would seem that no one clinical sign or symptom is sufficient to define patients with cervicogenic headache (Jull et al., 2007). Thus, further quantitative measures that characterize cervicogenic headache may assist clinicians in making a differential diagnosis while avoiding the need for invasive diagnostic techniques. The presence of impaired neuromuscular control is a feature that shows promising potential to assist in the differential diagnosis of headache (Jull et al., 2007).

Even though people with migraine or tension-type headache may experience neck pain (Hagen et al., 2002; Bartsch & Goadsby, 2003), this can be attributed to convergence of afferent information at the trigeminocervical nucleus, which may give rise to the sensation of pain in the cervical region in the absence of actual pathology of the cervical structures or soft tissues of the neck region. Accordingly, signs of neuromuscular impairment that have been identified in people with chronic neck pain are also found in people with cervicogenic headache, but the majority of evidence shows that cervical musculoskeletal impairment is not present in people with migraine or tension-type headache (Zwart, 1997; Dumas et al., 2001; Zito et al., 2006; Amiri et al., 2007; Jull et al., 2007).

A study that assessed range of cervical movement, manual examination for symptomatic cervical segment dysfunction, the craniocervical flexion test, neck flexor and extensor strength, and the cross-sectional area of selected extensor muscles showed that all measures were impaired in the cervicogenic headache group when compared with the migraine, tension-type headache, and control groups (Jull et al., 2007). Furthermore, the presence of palpably painful upper cervical joint dysfunction associated with restricted range of cervical extension and with impaired performance on the craniocervical flexion test had 100% sensitivity and 94% specificity to differentiate cervicogenic headache from migraine and tension-type headache (Jull et al., 2007). The same features were also shown to distinguish cervicogenic headache as one of a multiple headache syndrome (Amiri et al., 2007). Although further research is required to validate the capacity of this pattern of cervical musculoskeletal impairment to differentially diagnose cervicogenic headache, incorporating measures of neuromuscular function in the physical examination of headache patients appears promising for the clinical diagnosis of cervicogenic headache.

CONCLUSIONS

Cervicogenic headache constitutes approximately 14% to 18% of chronic headaches (Pfaffenrath & Kaube, 1990; Nilsson, 1995), and only a minority of headache patients will have musculoskeletal dysfunction of the cervical spine. A clinical diagnosis of cervicogenic headache is essential for clinicians to differentiate this disorder from other benign frequent intermittent headache types. However, the current classification criteria of cervicogenic headache share considerable overlap with other headaches, particularly for migraine and tension-type headache. Recent studies have shown that altered neuromuscular control differentiates cervicogenic headache sufferers from other headache patients. The addition of measures of neuromuscular function may strengthen the current clinical diagnostic criteria.

REFERENCES

Amiri M, Jull G, Bullock-Saxton J, Darnell R, Lander C. Cervical musculoskeletal impairment in frequent intermittent headache. Part 2: Subjects with multiple headaches. *Cephalalgia* 2007;27:891–898.

Asmundson G, Norton PJ, Veloso F. Anxiety sensitivity and fear of pain in patients with recurring headaches. *Behav Res Ther* 1999;37:703.

Bansevicius D, Sjaastad O. Cervicogenic headache: the influence of mental load on pain level and EMG of shoulder-neck and facial muscles. *Headache* 1996;36:372–378.

Bansevicius D, Westgaard RH, Sjaastad O. Tension-type headache: pain, fatigue, tension, and EMG responses to mental activation. *Headache* 1999;39:419–425.

Barton PM, Hayes KC. Neck flexor muscle strength, efficiency, and relaxation times in normal subjects and subjects with unilateral neck pain and headache. *Arch Phys Med Rehabil* 1996;77:680–687.

Bartsch T, Goadsby P. The trigeminocervical complex and migraine. Current concepts and synthesis. *Curr Pain Headache Rep* 2003;7:371–376.

Biondi DM. Cervicogenic headache: mechanisms, evaluation, and treatment strategies. *J Am Osteopath Assoc* 2000;100: S7–S14.

Bogduk N. The anatomical basis for cervicogenic headache. *J Manipulative Physiol Ther* 1992;15:67–70.

Bogduk N. The neck and headaches. *Neurol Clin North Am* 2004;22:151–171.

Bovim G, Berg R, Dale LG. Cervicogenic headache: anesthetic blockades of cervical nerves (C2-C5) and facet joint (C2/C3). *Pain* 1992;49:315–320.

Cibulka MT. Sternocleidomastoid muscle imbalance in a patient with recurrent headache. *Man Ther* 2006;11:78–82.

Dumas JP, Arsenault A, Boudreau G, et al. Physical impairments in cervicogenic headache: traumatic vs. non-traumatic onset. *Cephalalgia* 2001;21:884–893.

Elliott J, Jull G, Noteboom JT, et al. Fatty infiltration in the cervical extensor muscles in persistent whiplash-associated disorders: a magnetic resonance imaging analysis. *Spine* 2006;31:847–855.

Falla D, Jull G, Dall'Alba P, Rainoldi A, Merletti R. An electromyographic analysis of the deep cervical flexor muscles in performance of cranio-cervical flexion. *Phys Ther* 2003a;83:899–906.

Falla D, Rainoldi A, Merletti R, Jull G. Myoelectric manifestations of sternocleidomastoid and anterior scalene muscle fatigue in chronic neck pain patients. *Clin Neurophysiol* 2003b;114:488–495.

Falla D, Bilenkij G, Jull G. Patients with chronic neck pain demonstrate altered patterns of muscle activation during performance of a functional upper limb task. *Spine* 2004a;29:1436–1440.

Falla D, Jull G, Hodges PW. Feed-forward activity of the cervical flexor muscles during voluntary arm movements is delayed in chronic neck pain. *Exp Brain Res* 2004b;157: 43–48.

Falla D, Jull G, Hodges PW. Patients with neck pain demonstrate reduced electromyographic activity of the deep cervical flexor muscles during performance of the cranio-cervical flexion test. *Spine* 2004c;29:2108–2114.

Falla D, Jull G, Rainoldi A, Merletti R. Neck flexor muscle fatigue is side specific in patients with unilateral neck pain. *Eur J Pain* 2004d;8:71–77.

Fernández-de-las-Peñas C, Bueno A, Ferrando J, Elliott JM, Cuadrado ML, Pareja JA. Magnetic resonance imaging of the morphometry of cervical extensor muscles in chronic tension type headache. *Cephalalgia* 2007a;27:355–362.

Fernández-de-las-Peñas C, Bueno A, Ferrando J, Cuadrado ML, Pareja JA. Unilateral atrophy of the rectus capitis posterior minor muscle in cervicogenic headache: a case report [abstract]. *Cephalalgia* 2007b;27:641–642.

Fernández-de-las-Peñas C, Falla D, Arendt-Nielsen L, Farina D. Cervical agonist-antagonist activity during isometric contractions in chronic tension type headache. *Cephalalgia* 2008 (in press).

Fredin Y, Elert J, Britschgi N, et al. A decreased ability to relax between repetitive muscle contractions in patients with chronic symptoms after whiplash trauma of the neck. *J Musculoskeletal Pain* 1997;5:55–70.

Hagen K, Einarsen C, Zwart J, Svebak S, Bovim G. The co-occurrence of headache and musculoskeletal symptoms amongst 51 050 adults in Norway. *Eur J Neurol* 2002;9: 527–533.

Hagg GM, Anstrom A. Load pattern and pressure pain threshold in the upper trapezius muscle and psychosocial factors in medical secretaries with and without shoulder/neck disorders. *Int Arch Occup Environ Health* 1997;69:423–432.

Hallgren RC, Greenman PE, Rechtien JJ. Atrophy of suboccipital muscles in patients with chronic pain: a pilot study. *J Am Osteopath Assoc* 1994;94:1032–1038.

Heikkila H, Astrom P. Cervico-cephalic kinesthetic sensibility in patients with whiplash injury. *J Rehab Med* 1996;28: 133–138.

Hellstrom F, Thunberg J, Bergenheim M, et al. Increased intra-articular concentration of bradykinin in the temporomandibular joint changes the sensitivity of muscle spindles in dorsal neck muscles in the cat. *Neurosci Res* 2002;42:91–99.

International Headache Society. The International Classification of Headache Disorders: 2nd edition. *Cephalalgia* 2004;24:1–151.

Jaeger B. Are "cervicogenic" headaches due to myofascial pain and cervical spine dysfunction? *Cephalalgia* 1989;9: 157–164.

Jansen J, Bardosi A, Hildebrandt J, Lucke A. Cervicogenic, hemicranial attacks associated with vascular irritation or compression of the cervical nerve root C2. Clinical manifestations and morphological findings. *Pain* 1989;39:203–212.

Jull GA. Deep cervical flexor muscle dysfunction in whiplash. *J Musculoskeletal Pain* 2000;8:143–154.

Jull G, Barrett C, Magee R, Ho P. Further clinical clarification of the muscle dysfunction in cervical headache. *Cephalalgia* 1999;19:179–185.

Jull G, Kristjansson E, Dall'Alba P. Impairment in the cervical flexors: a comparison of whiplash and insidious onset neck pain patients. *Man Ther* 2004;9:89–94.

Jull G, Amiri M, Bullock-Saxton J, Darnell R, Lander C. Cervical musculo-skeletal impairment in frequent intermittent headache. Part 1: Subjects with single headaches. *Cephalalgia* 2007;27:793–802.

Kerr FW, Olafson RA. Trigeminal and cervical volleys. Convergence on single units in the spinal gray at C1 and C2. *Arch Neurol* 1961;5:171–178.

Kristjansson E, Dall'Alba P, Jull G. A study of five cervico-cephalic relocation tests in three different subject groups. *Clin Rehabil* 2003;17:768–774.

McPartland JM, Brodeur RR, Hallgren RC. Chronic neck pain, standing balance, and suboccipital muscle atrophy—a pilot study. *J Manipulative Physiol Ther* 1997;20:24–29.

Mörk PJ, Westgaard RH. Low-amplitude trapezius activity in work and leisure and the relation to shoulder and neck pain. *J Appl Physiol* 2006;100:1142–1149.

Nederhand MJ, Hermens H, Ijzerman MJ, Turk D, Zilvold G. Cervical muscle dysfunction in the chronic whiplash associated disorder grade 2: the relevance of the trauma. *Spine* 2002;27:1056–1061.

Nilsson N. The prevalence of cervicogenic headache in a random population sample of 20–59 year olds. *Spine* 1995;20:1884–1888.

O'Leary S, Jull G, Kim M, Vicenzino B. Cranio-cervical flexor muscle impairment at maximal, moderate, and low loads is a feature of neck pain. *Man Ther* 2007;12:34–39.

Pedersen J, Sjolander P, Wenngren BI, Johansson H. Increased intramuscular concentration of bradykinin increases the static fusimotor drive to muscle spindles in neck muscles of the cat. *Pain* 1997;70:83–91.

Pfaffenrath V, Kaube H. Diagnostics of cervicogenic headache. *Funct Neurol* 1990;5:159–164.

Revel M, Andre Deshays C, Minguet M. Cervico-cephalic kinesthetic sensibility in patients with cervical pain. *Arch Phys Med Rehabil* 1991;72:288–291.

Roatta S, Windhorst U, Ljubisavljevic M, Johansson H, Passatore M. Sympathetic modulation of muscle spindle afferent sensitivity to stretch in rabbit jaw closing muscles. *J Physiol* 2002;540:237–248.

Sjaastad O, Saunte C, Hovdahl H, Breivik H, Gronbaek E. "Cervicogenic" headache. A hypothesis. *Cephalalgia* 1983;3:249–256.

Sjaastad O, Fredriksen TA, Pfaffenrath V. Cervicogenic headache: diagnostic criteria. The Cervicogenic Headache International Study Group. *Headache* 1998;38: 442–445.

Strandring S. *Gray's Anatomy.* 38th ed. Amsterdam: Elsevier; 2005.

Thunberg J, Hellstrom F, Sjolander P, et al. Influences on the fusimotor-muscle spindle system from chemo-sensitive nerve endings in cervical facet joints in the cat: possible implications for whiplash induced disorders. *Pain* 2001;91:15–22.

Treleaven J, Jull G, LowChoy N. The relationship of cervical joint position error to balance and eye movement disturbances in persistent whiplash. *Man Ther* 2006;11: 99–106.

Veiersted KB, Westgaard RH, Andersen P. Pattern of muscle activity during stereotyped work and its relation to muscle pain. *Int Arch Occup Environ Health* 1990;62:31–41.

Vernon HT, Aker P, Aramenko M, et al. Evaluation of neck muscle strength with a modified sphygmomanometer dynamometer: reliability and validity. *J Manipulative Physiol Ther* 1992;15:343–349.

Watson DH, Trott PH. Cervical headache: an investigation of natural head posture and upper cervical flexor muscle performance. *Cephalalgia* 1993;13:272–284.

Wenngren BJ, Pederson J, Sjolander P, Bergenheim M, Johansson H. Bradykinin and muscle stretch alter contralateral cat neck muscle spindle output. *Neurosci Res* 1998;32:119–129.

Ylinen J, Salo P, Nykanen M, Kautiainen H, Hakkinen A. Decreased isometric neck strength in women with chronic neck pain and the repeatability of neck strength measurements. *Arch Phys Med Rehabil* 2004;85: 1303–1308.

Zito G, Jull G, Story I. Clinical tests of musculoskeletal dysfunction in the diagnosis of cervicogenic headache. *Man Ther* 2006;11:118–129.

Zwart JA. Neck mobility in different headache disorders. *Headache* 1997;37:6–11.

Physical Examination of Patients with Headache

Clinical Reasoning in the Diagnosis: History Taking in Patients with Headache

Peter A. Huijbregts, PT, MSc, MHSc, DPT, OCS, MTC, FAAOMPT, FCAMT

ROLE OF HISTORY TAKING IN THE CLINICAL EXAMINATION

In physical therapy, as in other health-care professions, there are five elements to patient management. The examination is followed by evaluation of the examination findings, establishing a diagnosis, producing a prognosis and developing a plan of care, and, finally, performing the interventions (American Physical Therapy Association [APTA], 2001). The examination element of this process of care usually consists of history taking, systems review, and tests and measures. Unique to professions such as physical therapy with a limited scope of practice, a systems review is a brief history and physical examination specifically reviewing the cardiopulmonary, integumentary, musculoskeletal, and neuromuscular systems, but also meant to get an impression of a patient's communication ability, affect, cognition, language, and learning style (APTA, 2001).

Generally, the role of the examination process is twofold. First, intended to be comprehensive with regard to screening and specific testing, this process ideally leads to diagnostic classification. A second important role of the physical therapy examination and related to the limited neuromusculoskeletal scope of practice of physical therapy is the identification of problems outside this scope of practice that require a referral for medical or surgical diagnosis and, perhaps, co-management. The systems review component of the examination plays an important role in detecting indications for such referral (APTA, 2001).

Obtaining a comprehensive history is paramount to any diagnostic process but perhaps even more so in patients presenting with headache. Bartleson (2006) noted that in patients with complaint of headache, history taking in combination with the general and neurologic examinations constitutes the diagnostic gold standard. Indeed, the primary headache disorders defined in the *International Classification of Headache Disorders* (International Headache Society [IHS], 2004) have no available confirming diagnostic tests or procedures. Welch (2005) further emphasized the importance of history taking by noting that most patients presenting with headache often have few signs on physical examination. In children, the role of the history is perhaps even more important. Dooley et al. (2003) reported that the history provided the correct diagnosis and management in 100% of 150 children presenting with headaches.

Although there is some variation in a worldwide context, physical therapy interventions are generally limited to manual therapy, education, exercise, and modality-based treatments, thereby excluding pharmacologic and surgical interventions. In this aspect, physical therapy is similar to other professions that might be involved in the diagnosis and management of patients with headache, such as chiropractic and massage therapy. As discussed in this chapter, this makes the diagnostic process in such professions a bit easier.

There is mounting research evidence (or at the very least a plausible pathophysiologic rationale) that manual therapy interventions and other modalities within the scope of practice of physical therapy are effective in the management of five distinct types of headaches. Of the primary headaches, the scientific literature indicates that tension-type headache, and to a lesser extent migraine, may have an underlying neuromusculoskeletal contribution (Fernández-de-las-Peñas et al., 2006a, 2006b, 2006c; Tuchin et al., 2000; Simons et al., 1999; Tuchin, 1999). Secondary headaches with a neuromusculoskeletal etiology that are, therefore, potentially amenable to interventions within the physical therapy scope of practice include cervicogenic headache, occipital neuralgia, and headache associated with temporomandibular disorder (Issa & Huijbregts, 2006; Bronfort et al., 2001; Jull et al., 2002; Okeson, 1996; Bogduk, 1986). It should be noted here that these headache types—and especially migraine headache—all may benefit from pharmacologic management as well, indicating the (potential) need for medical comanagement.

This limited number of headache types potentially amenable to physical therapy management means that one of the main objectives of the examination will be to identify whether the presenting headache complaint can in fact be classified as one of these five headache types. **Tables 13.1 to 13.5** provide the diagnostic criteria for these headache types. We should note that for cervicogenic headache there are two different sets of diagnostic criteria (**Table 13.3**). In addition to the criteria in the *International Classification of Headache Disorders* (IHS, 2004), Sjaastad et al. and the Cervicogenic Headache International Study Group (1998) established criteria that are in fact used more frequently in the clinical situation.

Granella et al. (1994) demonstrated that diagnosis of primary headache types using the *International Classification of Headache Disorders* had adequate interrater reliability for clinical use ($\kappa = 0.74$). However, before we become too confident in our ability to diagnose headaches using this classification system, we have to realize that this system may seem simple to use but that the absence of confirming imaging, electrophysiologic, or laboratory tests for the primary headache disorders means that the clinician is frequently in the position of needing to consider or rule out a secondary headache type that may be similar in appearance to the primary headache disorder based on history and examination findings alone (Bartleson, 2006). For an extended outline of headache diagnosis, see Chapter 3.

Some of these secondary headache disorders mimicking the headache types that therapists can, in fact, manage may be serious or even life threatening and require urgent medical or surgical referral. Because the diagnostic procedures confirming such secondary headaches are outside the diagnostic scope of practice of the therapist, the second main objective of the history—and of the examination process in general—becomes not only the identification of a headache (or other undiagnosed) disorder not amenable to physical therapy intervention but also and more specifically the identification of those headache emergencies that require urgent referral (Chapter 3). Within the context of history taking, the clinician should seek to identify red flag symptoms indicating serious pathology. The history component of the systems review may also yield indications of pathology that may or may not be related to the presenting complaint of headache but that still require referral.

Table 13.1 Tension-Type Headache Criteria

Type	Diagnostic Criteria
Infrequent episodic tension-type headache (2.1)	A. At least 10 episodes occurring on <1 day per month on average (<12 days per year) and fulfilling criteria B–D B. Headache lasting from 30 minutes to 7 days C. Headache has at least two of the following characteristics: 1. Bilateral location 2. Pressing/tightening (nonpulsating) quality 3. Mild or moderate intensity 4. Not aggravated by routine physical activity such as walking or climbing stairs D. Both of the following: 1. No nausea or vomiting (anorexia may occur) 2. No more than one of photophobia or phonophobia E. Not attributed to another disorder
Frequent episodic tension-type headache (2.2)	A. At least 10 episodes of occurring on ≥1 but <15 days per month for at least 3 months and fulfilling criteria B–D B. Headache lasting from 30 minutes to 7 days C. Headache has at least two of the following characteristics: 1. Bilateral location 2. Pressing/tightening (nonpulsating) quality 3. Mild to moderate intensity 4. Not aggravated by routine physical activity such as walking or climbing stairs D. Both of the following: 1. No nausea and/or vomiting (anorexia may occur) 2. No more than one of photophobia and phonophobia E. Not attributed to another disorder
Chronic tension-type headache (2.3)	A. Headache occurring on ≥15 days per month on average for >3 months and fulfilling criteria B–D B. Headache lasts hours or may be continuous C. Headache has at least two of the following characteristics: 1. Bilateral location 2. Pressing/tightening (nonpulsating) quality 3. Mild to moderate intensity 4. Not aggravated by routine physical activity such as walking or climbing stairs D. Both of the following: 1. No more than one of photophobia, phonophobia, or mild nausea 2. Neither moderate or severe nausea nor vomiting E. Not attributed to another disorder
Chronic tension-type headache associated with pericranial tenderness (2.3.1)	A. Headache fulfilling criteria A–E for 2.3 (*chronic tension-type headache*) B. Increased pericranial tenderness on manual palpation
Chronic tension-type headache not associated with pericranial tenderness (2.3.2)	A. Headache fulfilling criteria A–E for 2.3 (*chronic tension-type headache*) B. No increased pericranial tenderness

Modified from International Headache Society, 2004.

In summary, although mirroring the two main goals of the examination in general as outlined earlier (APTA, 2001), the three main objectives of history taking in patients with headache disorders are more specific:

1. Confirm the diagnosis of tension-type headache, migraine headache, cervicogenic headache, occipital neuralgia, or headache associated with temporomandibular disorder, according to

Table 13.2 Migraine Headache Criteria

Type	Diagnostic Criteria

Migraine without aura (1.1)	A. At least five attacks fulfilling criteria B–D
	B. Headache attacks lasting 4–72 hours (untreated or unsuccessfully treated)
	C. Headache has at least two of the following characteristics:
	  1. Unilateral location
	  2. Pulsating quality
	  3. Moderate or severe pain intensity
	  4. Aggravation by or causing avoidance of routine physical activity (e.g., walking or climbing stairs)
	D. During headache at least one of the following:
	  1. Nausea and/or vomiting
	  2. Photophobia and phonophobia
	E. Not attributed to another disorder

Typical migraine with aura (1.2.1)	A. At least two attacks fulfilling criteria B–D
	B. Aura consisting of at least one of the following, but no motor weakness:
	  1. Fully reversible visual symptoms including positive features (e.g., flickering lights, spots or lines) and/or negative features (i.e., loss of vision)
	  2. Fully reversible sensory symptoms including positive features (i.e., pins and needles) and/or negative features (i.e., numbness)
	  3. Fully reversible dysphasic speech disturbance
	C. At least two of the following:
	  1. Homonymous visual symptoms and/or unilateral sensory symptoms
	  2. At least one aura symptom develops gradually over ≥5 minutes and/or different aura symptoms occur in succession over ≥5 minutes
	  3. Each symptom lasts ≥5 and ≤60 minutes
	D. Headache fulfilling criteria B–D for 1.1 (*migraine without aura*) begins during the aura or follows aura within 60 minutes
	E. Not attributed to another disorder

Chronic migraine (1.5.1)	A. Headache fulfilling criteria C and D for 1.1 (*migraine without aura*) on ≥15 days/month for >3 months B. Not attributed to another disorder
Probable migraine without aura (1.6.1)	A. Attacks fulfilling all but one of criteria A–D for 1.1 (*migraine without aura*) B. Not attributed to another disorder

Modified from International Headache Society, 2004.

established diagnostic classification systems (IHS, 2004; Okeson, 1996; Sjaastad et al., 1998).

2. Identify diagnostic indicators of headache types not amenable to physical therapy management, and specifically red flag symptoms indicating serious pathology requiring urgent referral.

3. Identify the presence—but not the exact nature—of pathology not necessarily related to the presenting headache complaint that requires referral for medical or surgical evaluation.

This chapter presents a suggested format for history taking in patients presenting with headache (**Table 13.6**) with specific attention to these three main objectives. The following sections discuss the various items in this format.

DEMOGRAPHICS

In patients older than 50, a new onset of migraine headache is unlikely (Gladstein, 2006). In fact, if a new headache suddenly appears in a patient older than 50, it should be considered a secondary headache until causes such as tumor, cerebrovascular disease, or temporal arteritis are excluded (Gentile, 2005). Temporal or

Table 13.3 Cervicogenic Headache Criteria

International Classification of Headache Disorders Criteria	Cervicogenic Headache International Study Group Criteria

A. Pain, referred from a source in the neck and perceived in one or more regions of the head and/or face, fulfilling criteria C and D
B. Clinical, laboratory, and/or imaging evidence of a disorder or lesion within the cervical spine or soft tissues of the neck known to be, or generally accepted as, a valid cause of headache
C. Evidence that the pain can be attributed to the neck disorder or lesion based on at least one of the following:
   1. Demonstration of clinical signs that implicate a source of pain in the neck
   2. Abolition of headache following diagnostic blockade of a cervical structure or its nerve supply using placebo or other adequate controls
D. Pain resolves within 3 months after successful treatment of the causative disorder or lesion
	I. Symptoms and signs of neck involvement:
	   a. Precipitation of head pain, similar to the usually occurring one:
	     1. By neck movement and/or sustained awkward head posturing, and/or
	     2. By external pressure over the upper cervical or occipital region on the symptomatic side
	   b. Restriction of the range of motion (ROM) in the neck
	   c. Ipsilateral neck, shoulder, or arm pain of a rather vague nonradicular nature or, occasionally, arm pain of a radicular nature
	
	II. Confirmatory evidence by diagnostic anesthetic blockades
	
	III. Unilaterality of the head pain, without side shift
	
	For a diagnosis of CGH to be appropriate, one or more aspects of Point I must be present, with Ia sufficient to serve as a sole criterion for positivity or Ib and Ic combined. For scientific work, Point II is obligatory, while Point III is preferably obligatory.

Modified from International Headache Society, 2004, and Sjaastad et al., 1998.

Table 13.4 Occipital Neuralgia Criteria

Type	Diagnostic Criteria
Occipital neuralgia (13.8)	A. Paroxysmal stabbing pain with or without persistent aching between paroxysms in the distribution(s) of the greater, lesser, and/or third occipital nerves B. Tenderness over the affected nerve C. Pain is eased temporarily by local anesthetic block of the involved nerve

Modified from International Headache Society, 2004.

Table 13.5 Criteria for Headache Attributed to Temporomandibular Disorder

Type	Diagnostic Criteria

Headache or facial pain attributed to temporomandibular joint (TMJ) disorder (11.7)	A. Recurrent pain in one or more regions of the head and/or face fulfilling criteria C and D
	B. X-ray, MRI, and/or bone scintigraphy demonstrates TMJ disorder
	C. Evidence that pain can be attributed to the TMJ disorder, based on at least one of the following:
	   1. Pain is precipitated by jaw movements and/or chewing of hard or tough food
	   2. Reduced range of or irregular jaw movements
	   3. Noise from one or both TMJs during jaw movements
	   4. Tenderness of the joint capsule(s) of one or both TMJs
	D. Headache resolves within 3 months, and does not recur, after successful treatment of the TMJ disorder

Modified from International Headache Society, 2004.

Table 13.6 Suggested Format for History Taking in Patients with Headache

Demographics
Location of pain
Onset and course of headache
Character and intensity of headache
Aggravating and easing factors
Neurologic symptoms
Otolaryngologic symptoms
Systemic symptoms
Medical history
Medication history
Family history
Previous diagnostic tests
Prognostic indicators
Systems review

giant cell arteritis can lead to blindness due to occlusion of the ocular arteries. Patients may report severe unilateral or bilateral throbbing pain in the temporal region that is worse at night. Patients may also report scalp tenderness, jaw claudication, visual complaints, fatigue or joint pain associated with polymyalgia rheumatica, weight loss, fever, and night sweats. They may also have noted a tender, red, thickened, and nonpulsatile temporal artery (Peters, 2004; Welch, 2005). The clinician should not get too fixated on an age limit of 50 years, because values reported in the literature as red flags for the onset of a new headache vary between 40 and 60 years (Bartleson, 2006).

Gender also plays a role in diagnosis in that various headaches are more prevalent in women. European and American studies have showed a 1-year prevalence of 6% to 8% in men but 15% to 18% in women for migraine headaches. In developed countries, tension-type headache affects two-thirds of men and over 80% of women (World Health Organization, 2004). Musculoskeletal pain due to temporomandibular disorder is nine times more common in women than in men (Türp et al., 2002). In contrast, cluster headaches are more common in men, most typically smokers in their late 20s (Welch, 2005).

LOCATION OF PAIN

Characteristic locations of pain for the five headache types amenable to physical therapy management are indicated to some extent in the diagnostic criteria provided in Tables 13.1 to 13.5. Myofascial trigger points have been suggested as a main etiologic factor in ten-

sion-type headache (Fernández-de-las-Peñas et al., 2006a, 2006b, 2006d, 2006e). This means that specific pain locations may be matched with established pain referral patterns from myofascial trigger points, which in turn will guide the subsequent palpatory examination. Headache location is matched to specific muscle trigger points in **Table 13.7** (Fernández-de-las-Peñas et al., 2005, 2006f; Simons et al., 1999).

Further, with cervical zygapophysial joints implicated as the major etiologic factor in cervicogenic headache, referral patterns of these joints as established by way of joint infiltration can also guide subsequent examination (Dwyer et al., 1990). **Figure 13.1** provides zygapophysial joint referral patterns.

Headache occurring exclusively on one side may indicate a need for referral. Note that unilateral headaches are also likely in patients with more innocuous headache types such as cervicogenic headache; occipital neuralgia; headaches due to temporomandibular disorder; cluster headaches; paroxysmal hemicrania; short-lasting, unilateral, neuralgiform headache attacks with conjunctival injection and tearing (SUNCT); and with migraine. However, in a patient with a new onset of unilateral headache that does not have the features of one of these headache disorders—and of course for all headache types not amenable to (sole) physical therapy management—referral for further medical diagnosis is required (Bartleson, 2006).

ONSET AND COURSE OF HEADACHE

Headache onset can be qualified as acute, subacute, and chronic. In addition, patients may report a course of intermittent, episodic, or continuous pain that is stable or progressive in intensity. The five headache types amenable to physical therapy intervention are generally insidious in their onset (with the exception of a first-ever migraine headache) and of an intermittent, nonprogressive nature. Cluster headaches are—as the name implies—episodic in nature. Especially if a constant headache is progressive and worsening or if the patient presents with an acute-onset, worst-ever headache, the clinician should be attentive to a serious underlying pathology. Mills et al. (1986) reported abnormal findings on computed tomography (CT) scan for 29% of patients presenting with sudden-onset, reported worst-ever, or severe persistent headaches.

Causes of acute-onset headache include intracranial or intracerebral hemorrhage, acute subdural or epidural hematoma, pituitary apoplexy, acute closed-angle

Table 13.7 Myofascial Trigger Point Pain Referral Areas

Location of Pain	Muscles Potentially Involved
Vertex of the head	Sternal portion of sternocleidomastoid Splenius capitis
Occipital headache	Trapezius Sternal and clavicular portions of sternocleidomastoid Semispinalis capitis Semispinalis cervicis Splenius cervicis Suboccipital muscles Occipitalis Digastric Temporalis
Temporal headache	Trapezius Sternal portion of sternocleidomastoid Temporalis Splenius cervicis Suboccipital muscles Semispinalis capitis Superior oblique Lateral rectus
Frontal headache	Sternal and clavicular portions of sternocleidomastoid Semispinalis capitis Frontalis Zygomaticus major Superior oblique Lateral rectus
Ear and temporomandibular joint pain	Lateral and medial pterygoid Masseter Clavicular portion of sternocleidomastoid
Eye and eyebrow pain	Sternal portion of sternocleidomastoid Temporalis Splenius cervicis Masseter Suboccipital muscles Occipitalis Orbicularis oculi Trapezius
Cheek and jaw pain	Sternal portion of sternocleidomastoid Masseter Lateral and medial pterygoid Trapezius Digastric Buccinator Platysma Orbicularis oculi Zygomaticus major

Modified from Simons et al., 1999; Fernández-de-las-Peñas et al., 2005, 2006f.

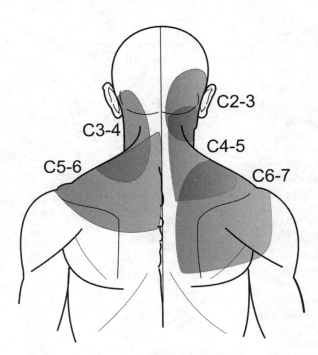

Figure 13.1 Zygapophysial Joint Pain Patterns
Modified from Lord SM, Barnsley L, Wallis BJ, Bogduk N.
Chronic cervical zygapophyseal joint pain after whiplash.
Spine 1996;21:1737–1745.

glaucoma, acute severe hypertension, internal carotid or vertebral artery dissection, head trauma causing a hemorrhage or cavernous sinus thrombosis, spontaneous low cerebrospinal fluid pressure headaches, acute obstructive hydrocephalus due to a tumor, benign central nervous system angiopathy, and idiopathic primary thunderclap headache. In contrast to all other causes listed here, primary thunderclap headache is innocuous, likely related to transient, and possibly recurrent, vasospasm (Bartleson, 2006; Peters, 2004).

Acute-onset headache, especially reported by the patient as a worst-ever headache, is also referred to as a thunderclap headache. Subarachnoid hemorrhage is the most common cause of this type of headache—usually located in the occipital region—and excluding this particular pathology takes priority in the diagnostic process (Bartleson, 2006; Gentile, 2005; Welch, 2005). Patients have compared the sensation of this type of headache to being hit across the back of the head with a blunt object (Welch, 2005). Thunderclap headache can also occur prior to aneurysmal subarachnoid hemorrhage in patients with an unruptured cerebral aneurysm (Bartleson, 2006). Relevant to the differential diagnosis from a first-ever migraine headache is that a thunderclap headache comes on within seconds, whereas a migraine builds up

for over an hour (Gladstein, 2006). However, even a headache fitting the diagnostic criteria of recent-onset migraine may be following a small subarachnoid hemorrhage, indicating the need to take into consideration the whole clinical picture, and particularly patient age as discussed earlier (Gentile, 2005). Subarachnoid hemorrhage can be accompanied by a low-grade fever and neck stiffness: blood in the subarachnoid space may act as a local irritant and endogenous pyrogen (Gladstein, 2006).

Glaucoma constitutes another acute-onset headache emergency, as does cavernous venous thrombosis. Patients with glaucoma will report eye pain and vision changes. In case of cavernous venous thrombosis, patients usually have a history of ear, nose, or throat surgery or localized nasal infection, or they may report using medications that could cause a hypercoagulable state (Gladstein, 2006).

Secondary headaches with a subacute onset that may worsen rapidly but not suddenly include headaches caused by meningitis, encephalitis, sinusitis, cerebral vein thrombosis, ischemic cerebrovascular disease, and cerebral vasculitis (Peters, 2004).

Secondary headaches with a more gradual buildup may be related to pathologies such as a brain tumor, chronic subdural hematoma, brain abscess, temporal arteritis, idiopathic intracranial hypertension or pseudotumor cerebri, intracranial infection (such as those caused by Lyme disease, AIDS, or other systemic infections), and chronic sinusitis (Peters, 2004). Chronic progressive headache increasing slowly but steadily over the course of weeks to months may indicate a space-occupying lesion such as a brain tumor. Coughing, straining in the bathroom, sneezing, bending forward, and physical activity may exacerbate the headache related to a brain tumor. Pain is often worse in the morning and then gets a little better as the day progresses (Gentile, 2005; Gladstein, 2006). Often headache due to an intracranial mass lesion is accompanied by vomiting that is not preceded by nausea, especially in children (Gentile, 2005). Chronic subdural hematoma often will manifest weeks to months after a precipitating but often forgotten injury. In addition to headache worsened by sudden head movements, symptoms may include apathy, confusion, and inappropriate behavior (Peters, 2004).

CHARACTER AND INTENSITY OF HEADACHE

The diagnostic relevance of worst-ever, acute-onset, or thunderclap headache was discussed earlier. In studies on patients presenting at the emergency room for this type of headache, the combined prevalence of significant intracranial pathology was 43% (95% CI: 20–68%) (Detsky et al., 2006).

The *International Classification of Headache Disorders* (IHS, 2004) classifies cluster headache as a primary headache. Cluster-type headaches are excruciating orbital and temporal headaches that come and go in a clusterlike pattern. Although this pattern is characteristic of the primary cluster headaches, it may also serve as an indicator of significant secondary headache types: the presence of cluster-type headaches carries a positive likelihood ratio (LR) of 10.7 (95% CI: 2.2–5.2) for the presence of serious intracranial abnormalities (Detsky et al., 2006).

Relevant to this portion of the history-taking process is that frequently headaches are of a mixed nature: migraine and tension-type headache frequently occur together, and they can be combined later in their course with headaches related to medication overuse. Of patients with migraine, 83% also have had tension-type headaches, whereas 23% of patients with tension-type headache also report migraine headaches (De Jongh et al., 2001). Every headache type requires a separate history (Welch, 2005). Tables 13.1 to 13.5 provide further details on the character and intensity of the headache types amenable to physical therapy management.

AGGRAVATING AND EASING FACTORS

Headaches amenable to physical therapy management should have underlying neuromusculoskeletal dysfunctions that can usually be aggravated or eased by mechanical factors such as those occurring with movement and position. Effects differ between these headache types: migraine may be differentiated from tension-type headache in that migraine headache is exacerbated by physical activity, whereas tension-type headache is not. Smetana (2000) established a positive LR of 3.7 (95% CI: 3.4–4.0) and a negative LR of 0.24 (95% CI: 0.23–0.26) for exacerbation by physical activity in the differential diagnosis of these two primary headache types. In fact, patients with tension-type headache may even seek out physical activity to decrease pain by way of distraction (Weeks & Weier, 2006). Patients with migraine tend to retreat to a dark and quiet environment, whereas patients with cluster headache are agitated and often will pace the room or rock back and forth holding their head (Gladstein, 2006; Weeks & Weier, 2006). However, some movement- and position-related effects on headache may be indicative of secondary headaches requiring (urgent) referral.

A more benign secondary headache is one related to cerebrospinal fluid hypotension. This type of headache is classically postural in that it occurs or worsens within 15 minutes of going from a lying to an upright position. It generally disappears within 30 minutes of again lying down. Usually bilateral and frontal in location, this headache is commonly associated with nausea, vomiting, dizziness, and tinnitus. One of the most common causes is a persistent cerebrospinal fluid leak after a lumbar puncture, but in the absence of such a medical history, it may be indicative of spontaneous low cerebrospinal fluid pressure syndrome (Bartleson, 2006; Peters, 2004).

Idiopathic intracranial hypertension usually causes a generalized frontal headache that may be unilateral or bilateral and is often worsened by bending over or straining. Patients may note a progressive loss of vision. This secondary headache is most common in obese women; average age of onset is 30 years (Peters, 2004).

It was noted earlier that the headache related to a brain tumor is exacerbated with coughing, straining in the bathroom, sneezing, bending forward, and physical activity. Pain is often worse in the morning and then gets a little better as the day progresses (Gentile, 2005; Welch, 2005; Gladstein, 2006). Coughing or posture changes may also cause the onset of headache if there is an underlying structural cause, such as Arnold-Chiari malformation type I, a colloid cyst of the third ventricle, or a tumor growing in the ventricular system (Gentile, 2005). Although exertional and cough headache can occur as an innocuous primary headache disorder, headache aggravated by exertion or a Valsalva-type maneuver carries a positive LR of 2.3 (95% CI: 1.4–3.8) for the presence of serious intracranial pathology (Detsky et al., 2006). In patients with a normal neurologic examination, headache aggravated by a Valsalva maneuver occurred significantly more often in those with secondary headaches than in patients with primary headaches (OR = 3.4) (Duarte et al., 1996). Bartleson (2006) noted that headache initiated by exertion or Valsalva maneuver (or cough) and associated neurologic symptoms or signs that are not consistent with the criteria for migraine with typical aura indicate the need to search for underlying intracranial disease.

Headache brought on by sexual activity can also occur as a relatively innocuous primary headache disorder. Similar to the exertional headache discussed earlier, it can be associated with migraine. Nevertheless, headache associated with sexual activity can also occur secondary to subarachnoid hemorrhage and arterial dissection and should always be considered a red flag warning symptom requiring urgent referral (Bartleson, 2006).

Nonmechanical triggers, such as headache brought on by consuming certain food substances (caffeine, monosodium glutamate, chocolate, cheese, sulfites, citrus fruits, or alcohol), headache when relaxing, or headache brought on by alterations in sleeping, exercising, and eating habits all suggest migraine. Cluster headache is often brought on during a cluster period by drinking alcoholic beverages (De Jongh et al., 2006; Gladstein, 2006; Welch, 2005). The role of nonmechanical triggers as prognostic indicators is discussed later in this chapter.

NEUROLOGIC SYMPTOMS

Headache with an aura carries a positive LR of 3.2 (95% CI: 1.6–6.6) for serious intracranial pathology (Detsky et al., 2006). Of course, a visual or sensory aura is also part of the diagnostic criteria of typical migraine with aura (IHS, 2004). These auras generally have a gradual onset and diffuse slowly, taking almost 20 minutes to reach their widest distribution. This slow diffusion helps to distinguish them from auras associated with transient ischemic attacks, which have a quicker diffusion (Gentile, 2005). Because most studies used to establish the above LR did not provide information regarding the type of aura, interpretation of the diagnostic utility of the presence of an aura is somewhat limited (Detsky et al., 2006).

Seizures can occur in patients with brain tumors, cerebral vein thrombosis, and other causes of raised intracranial pressure (Peters, 2004; Welch, 2005). They may also occur in patients with meningitis (Welch, 2005). Focal neurologic deficits can occur in patients with pathologies that cause raised intracranial pressure, including cerebral vein thrombosis and intracranial hemorrhage (Davenport, 2002; Welch, 2005). Transient vision deficits occur in cases of increased intracranial pressure (Welch, 2005). Drowsiness, apathy, confusion, altered consciousness, or inappropriate behavior may be related to raised intracranial pressure due to hemorrhage and chronic subdural hematoma (Davenport, 2002; Peters, 2004). A (pre)syncope starting off an acute-onset, worst-ever headache is usually associated with a subarachnoid hemorrhage (Gentile, 2005).

Meningism or stiffness on neck flexion can occur in patients with meningitis but also in patients with subarachnoid hemorrhage (Gladstein, 2006; Welch, 2005). Rotation of the neck is usually not affected by true meningism, but it is limited in patients with

Table 13.8 Brainstem Signs and Symptoms: Five D's and Three N's

---

Dizziness
Drop attacks
Diplopia (including amaurosis fugax and corneal reflux)
Dysarthria
Dysphagia (including hoarseness and hiccups)
Ataxia of gait
Nausea
Numbness (in ipsilateral face and/or contralateral body)
Nystagmus

Modified from Terrett, 2001.

cervical degenerative joint disease as implicated in cervicogenic headache, allowing for differential diagnosis (Davenport, 2002). However, it should be noted that nuchal rigidity has a sensitivity of only 30% for meningitis, making a negative test relatively meaningless when it comes to excluding serious causative pathology (Peters, 2004). In patients with brain tumors, the headache usually is preceded by neurologic symptoms, including, as noted earlier, seizure but also hemiparesis, ataxia, and cognitive or speech impairment (Peters, 2004).

Spinal manipulation has been associated with cervical artery dissection. Rubinstein et al. (2005) reported an OR of 3.8 for neck manipulation as a risk factor for cervical artery dissection. Perhaps this is why manual medicine practitioners, including physical therapists, chiropractors, medical and osteopathic physicians, and massage therapists, are hypervigilant with regard to the proposed ensuing classic brainstem signs and symptoms provided in **Table 13.8**. However, a variety of other pathologies can cause such symptoms. Specific to headache, during childhood and adolescence basilar migraine is a much more common cause than vertebral or internal carotid artery dissection (Gentile, 2005). **Table 13.9** summarizes the diagnostic criteria for basilar migraine (IHS, 2004).

With regard to a possible diagnosis of cervical artery dissection, it is important to realize that ischemic symptoms are not the only symptoms that may appear. Nonischemic symptoms usually develop first and are likely the result of deformation of nerve endings in the tunica adventitia of the affected artery and direct compression on local somatic structures (Kerry & Taylor, 2006). In fact, these nonischemic symptoms may occur hours to days and even a few weeks prior to the ischemic findings (Blunt & Galton, 1997). In the case of internal carotid artery dissection, this delay may even

Table 13.9 Diagnostic Criteria for Basilar Migraine

A. At least two attacks fulfilling criteria B–D
B. Aura consisting of at least two of the following fully reversible symptoms but no motor weakness: dysarthria, vertigo, tinnitus, hypoacusia, diplopia, visual symptoms simultaneously in both temporal and nasal fields of both eyes, ataxia, decreased level of consciousness, simultaneously bilateral paresthesia
C. At least one of the following: at least one aura symptom develops gradually over ≥5 minutes and/or different aura symptoms occur in succession over ≥5 minutes; each aura symptom lasts ≥5 and ≤60 minutes
D. Headache fulfilling criteria B–D from migraine without aura begins during the aura or follows the aura within 60 minutes
E. Not attributed to another disorder

Modified from International Headache Society, 2004.

be as long as years (Terrett, 2001). Ischemic findings develop in 30% to 80% of all dissections. Up to 20% of patients progress to a full cerebrovascular accident (Blunt & Galton, 1997). Nonischemic symptoms are unique to the exact pathology of the dissection, but ischemic neurologic symptoms can, of course, be expected to be similar for all underlying causes of cervical artery dysfunction.

In addition to the classic cardinal signs and symptoms summarized in Table 13.8, the literature has described further symptoms related to cervical artery dysfunction. **Table 13.10** provides ischemic and nonischemic signs or symptoms associated with cervical artery dissection (Albuquerque et al., 2002; Blunt & Galton, 1997; Guy et al., 2001; Kerry & Taylor, 2006; Taylor & Kerry, 2005; Terrett, 2001; Wojcik et al., 2003). Issues that are more relevant to the physical examination but that the patient may also report during the history taking

Table 13.10 Nonischemic and Ischemic Signs and Symptoms of Cervical Artery Dysfunction

	Vertebrobasilar System	Internal Carotid Artery
Nonischemic	Ipsilateral posterior neck pain Ipsilateral occipital headache Sudden onset and severe Described as stabbing, pulsating, aching, thunderclap, sharp, or of an unusual character: "a headache unlike any experienced before" Very rarely C5-C6 nerve root impairment (due to local neural ischemia)	Ipsilateral upper and midcervical spine pain Ipsilateral frontal-temporal or periorbital headache Sudden onset, severe, and of an uncommon character Horner syndrome Pulsatile tinnitus Cranial nerve palsies Ipsilateral carotid bruit Neck swelling Scalp tenderness Anhydrosis of face
Ischemic	Five **D**'s and three **N**'s (see Table 13.8) Vomiting Loss of short-term memory Vagueness Hypotonia and limb weakness affecting arm or leg Anhydrosis: lack of facial sweating Hearing disturbances Malaise Perioral dysesthesia Photophobia Clumsiness Agitation Cranial nerve palsies Hindbrain stroke: Wallenberg or locked-in syndrome	Transient ischemic attack Middle cerebral artery distribution stroke Retinal infarction Amaurosis fugax: temporary blindness Localized patchy blurring of vision: scintillating scotomata Weakness of extraocular muscles Protrusion of the eye Swelling of the eye or conjunctiva

Modified from Albuquerque et al., 2002; Blunt & Galton, 1997; Guy et al., 2001; Kerry & Taylor, 2006; Taylor & Kerry, 2005; Terrett, 2001; and Wojcik et al., 2003.

are the cranial nerve palsies that can occur with cervical artery dissection. Dissection of the internal carotid artery mainly causes cranial nerve IX to XII dysfunction, with the hypoglossal nerve initially affected and then the other three nerves; eventually, all cranial nerves except the olfactory can be affected (Blunt & Galton, 1997; Kerry & Taylor, 2006; Rubinstein et al., 2005).

Table 13.10 indicates that Horner syndrome is frequently associated with ipsilateral carotid artery dissection. The patient may have noted these physical signs and therefore may report these during the history taking. However, Horner syndrome is also common in cluster headaches. When the patient suffers symptoms and signs suggestive of a cluster headache, including Horner syndrome, but the pain is constant rather than intermittent and episodic, the possibility of arterial dissection needs to be considered, and, of course, more urgent referral is indicated (Gentile, 2005).

Arnold-Chiari type I malformation is a structural cause for headache with coughing or posture changes that requires surgical intervention once symptomatic (Gladstein, 2006). This pathology involves downward displacement of the cerebellar tonsils through the foramen magnum, causing symptoms of cerebellar involvement and brainstem compression. Ataxia in this malformation affects gait and is bilateral. Resultant hydrocephalus may also cause headache and vomiting. Brainstem compression can be associated with vertigo, nystagmus, and cranial nerve palsies (Simon et al., 1999). Other symptoms demonstrated in patients with compression at the level of the foramen magnum include suboccipital or neck pain (described as a tight collar) (in 65% of patients), often exacerbated by neck movement; pain in the hand (59%) or arm (55%), especially burning along the ulnar border of the contralateral arm in unilateral lesions; pain in the leg (26%) and face (7%); weak arm (40%) or leg (30%); hand clumsiness (27%); bladder dysfunction (22%); dysphagia (13%); dysarthria (3%); and paresthesia along the spine with trunk and neck flexion (positive Lhermitte sign) (3%). In addition to Horner syndrome occurring with internal carotid artery dissection and cluster headaches as discussed earlier, Arnold-Chiari malformation may also be the cause (Cross & Coles, 2002).

In summary, the neurologic symptoms associated with headaches can be varied and confusing. In general, we can state, though, that patients with nonmigrainous transient or persistent neurologic symptoms, seizures, or persistent neurologic signs most certainly require referral for medical diagnosis unless the neurologic symptoms and signs can be explained by another static and already medically diagnosed condition in the patient's medical history (Bartleson, 2006).

OTOLARYNGOLOGIC SYMPTOMS

Earlier we discussed how headache related to temporomandibular disorders could present with neuromusculoskeletal dysfunctions amenable to physical therapy. Temporomandibular disorders can present with any combination of headache, earache, or facial pain. The patient may also note limited opening of the jaw, joint noises, and localized muscle tenderness that is often unilateral (Cosenza, 2000; Türp et al., 2002). Patients may also report parafunctional habits such as teeth grinding, clenching, nail biting, and chewing gum (Royal College of Dental Surgeons of Ontario, 2002). This topic is addressed in detail in Chapter 17.

As discussed earlier, one of the pathologies resulting in a subacute-onset headache is acute sinusitis. Patients with sinusitis usually have purulent discharge from the nose, pain on palpation over the involved sinuses, cough, halitosis, and low-grade fever. However tempting to attribute all such symptoms to sinus pathology, we should assume that patients who present with lacrimation, rhinorrhea, sinus tenderness, and nasal congestion usually have migraine and not sinusitis (Gladstein, 2006; Peters, 2004). In case of autonomic symptoms and an acute and recurrent pattern, the likelihood of migraine headache is further increased. Of differential diagnostic importance is that sinus disease does not remit and return as migraine does (Gladstein, 2006).

SYSTEMIC SYMPTOMS

Nausea is a symptom helpful in distinguishing migraine from tension-type headache. Smetana (2000) reported a positive LR of 19 (95% CI: 15–25) and a negative LR of 0.19 (95% CI: 0.18–0.20). Photophobia and phonophobia also have good diagnostic utility for the purpose of distinguishing these two primary headache types, with a positive LR of 5.8 (95% CI: 5.1–6.6) and 5.2 (95% CI: 4.5–5.9) for the presence of migraine, respectively. The negative LR is 0.24 (95% CI: 0.23–0.26) and 0.38 (95% CI: 0.36–0.40) for photophobia and phonophobia, respectively (Smetana, 2000). Headache associated with vomiting has limited diagnostic utility for detecting serious intracranial pathology, with a positive LR of 1.8 (95% CI: 1.2–2.6) (Detsky et al., 2006). Vomiting, together with fatigue, diarrhea, and poor appetite, may also be the presenting picture of meningitis, especially in elderly patients and infants (Welch et al., 2005).

Up to 30% of acute headaches may be secondary to viral infections (Brna & Dooley, 2006). This may be even more relevant for children presenting with headaches. Burton et al. (1997) reported that viral illness accounted for 39% of headaches in children presenting to a U.S. emergency room. Fever and headache may indicate headache due to viral syndrome and need cause little concern. However, headache and fever associated with neck stiffness increases the suspicion of meningitis (Gladstein, 2006). The clinician should keep in mind the low sensitivity for meningism in the diagnosis of meningitis, as discussed previously. Usually meningitis is also associated with photophobia and a rash (Welch, 2005). Headache associated with fever and a change in mental status requires evaluation for encephalitis. A low-grade fever may also occur in a subarachnoid hemorrhage (Gladstein, 2006). This chapter has already discussed the fever, weight loss, and night sweats associated with temporal arteritis (Peters, 2004).

Night wakening due to headache has a high likelihood ratio (LR = 98) for serious intracranial pathology (Bartleson, 2006). Classically, headache associated with a brain tumor will disturb sleep (Peters, 2004). However, night wakening is also common with less worrisome headaches such as migraine, paroxysmal hemicrania, or cluster headache. Therefore, night wakening needs to be assessed in the context of the patient's total presentation. However, the clinician should keep in mind that waking from sleep because of headache is more worrisome in children (Bartleson, 2006). History-based indications for further diagnostic testing in children include recent onset of headache, seizures, and night wakening, especially in the absence of a family history of migraine (Bartleson, 2006).

MEDICAL HISTORY

Red flags in the medical history include history of human immunodeficiency virus (HIV) infection or cancer, because these diagnoses increase the chance of secondary headaches due to brain tumor, meningitis, and opportunistic infections (Bartleson, 2006; Clinch, 2001; Detsky et al., 2006). However, even a patient with cancer or HIV infection may require no further medical diagnosis if the presenting headache complaint is long-standing, stable, and consistent with a primary headache disorder (Bartleson, 2006).

Uncontrolled hypertension may lead to spontaneous intracerebral hemorrhage. Cerebral vein thrombosis should be considered in patients with hypercoagulable states, trauma, or rheumatologic disorders (Peters, 2004). In patients with headache due to cavernous venous thrombosis, there is usually a previous medical history of ear, nose, and/or throat surgery, localized nasal infection, or the use of medications that could cause a hypercoagulable state (Gladstein, 2006). Temporal arteritis is more common in patients with polymyalgia rheumatica (Welch, 2005). Cerebrospinal fluid hypotension headache is most commonly caused by a persistent leak after lumbar puncture (Peters, 2004).

A patient reporting a history of head and neck trauma indicates the need to look for epidural, subdural, subarachnoid, or other intracranial hemorrhage and posttraumatic dissection of the carotid and vertebral arteries (Bartleson, 2006). Acute subdural hematoma usually comes on after head trauma and is seen commonly in alcoholic patients who have frequent falls (Peters, 2004). With subdural hematoma and arterial dissection, there is often a delay between the precipitating trauma and the onset of headache. A relatively minor head injury, which may have occurred weeks or even months before the onset of the presenting headache, may be forgotten but significant in an older patient or a patient on anticoagulant medication (Bartleson, 2006). Prior facial injury, jaw fracture, or stressful life situations can all indicate the presence of headache related to temporomandibular disorders (Cosenza, 2000).

MEDICATION HISTORY

Collecting information on medications taken by the patient and on their effect allows the therapist to double-check the medical history provided for its comprehensiveness and accuracy. Asking about recreational or illicit substances may uncover underlying causes of headaches. Alcohol, caffeine, cannabis, and cocaine are examples of substances implicated with regard to producing headaches (Katsarava et al., 2006).

Medications that cause hypercoagulable states have been implicated in the etiology of cavernous venous thrombosis. In contrast, anticoagulant medications (e.g., warfarin, heparin, or aspirin) may lead to hemorrhage and hematoma even after minor trauma (Bartleson, 2006; Gladstein, 2006). Oral contraceptives; vitamin A; antibiotics, including tetracycline, minocycline, trimethoprim and sulfamethoxazole, and nalidixic acid; corticosteroids; and other drugs (e.g., isotretinoin or

Accutane, tamoxifen, cimetidine or Tagamet) have all been implicated in the etiology of idiopathic intracranial hypertension (Brna & Dooley, 2006; Clinch, 2001).

Perhaps most relevant to the etiology of chronic daily headache is the fact that overuse of analgesic medication—including most medications prescribed for acute attacks of migraine or tension-type headache—puts patients at risk of developing a daily, oppressive, dull headache that is worse in the mornings and is unrelieved by analgesics. This type of headache is known as a medication-overuse headache (Welch, 2005). In the context of medication-overuse headache, taking an acute attack medicine more than twice a week should be considered overuse. Usually patients have a headache that is improved by the acute attack medicine, only to return (rebound headache) as the effects of the analgesic wear off. Patients take the medicine again and thus start a vicious cycle. The main medications implicated with regard to medication-overuse headache are over-the-counter analgesics that combine Tylenol or aspirin with caffeine or codeine phosphate, or both. Relevant prescription analgesics include caffeine opiate agonists, ergotamine, and triptans (Goadsby & Boes, 2002).

Other medications can produce a headache mimicking either migraine or tension-type headaches. Nitrates, phosphodiesterase inhibitors, and histamine can cause a bilateral, frontotemporal headache that is aggravated by physical activity similar to migraine. In contrast, atropine, digitalis, imipramine, nifedipine, and nimodipine produce generalized headaches similar to tension-type headaches (Katsarava et al., 2006).

FAMILY HISTORY

Migraine headaches usually have a strong genetic component (Gladstein, 2006). In addition, taking a family history may reveal rheumatologic, collagenous tissue, and cardiovascular disorders that have been implicated in the etiology of secondary headaches.

PREVIOUS DIAGNOSTIC TESTS

Imaging findings and laboratory test results may indicate the presence of an underlying pathology responsible for a secondary headache disorder. The *International Classification of Headache Disorders* (IHS, 2004) notes imaging findings of a disorder or lesion within the cervical spine or soft tissues of the neck known to be, or generally accepted as, a valid cause of headache as one of the diagnostic criteria for cervicogenic headache.

PROGNOSTIC INDICATORS

Perhaps most relevant to physical therapists are symptoms that indicate a good prognosis (or absence thereof) with interventions within the physical therapy scope of practice. Although likely already collected as part of a comprehensive history taking, such prognostic indicators deserve to again be highlighted here.

Niere (1998) reported that patients noting diet as an aggravating factor, those who used affective and autonomic pain descriptors (i.e., *sickening, fearful, nauseating, punishing, splitting*), those who had unilateral headaches, and those with a low headache frequency all had a negative response to manipulative physiotherapy treatment, the content of which was left to the discretion of the treating clinician. In contrast, Niere found that high headache frequency predicted a positive outcome.

Jull and Stanton (2005) aimed to identify those patients with cervicogenic headache who did or did not achieve a 50% to 79% or 80% to 100% reduction in headache immediately and 12 months postintervention. Only the absence of lightheadedness indicated higher odds of achieving either a 50% to 79% (OR = 5.45) or 80% to 100% (OR = 5.7) reduction in headache frequency in the long term. Of note was that headaches of at least moderate intensity, patient age, and headache chronicity did not preclude a successful outcome with physical therapy consisting of combinations of manipulation and specific exercise.

Fleming et al. (2007) found that increased patient age, provocation or relief of headache with movement, and being gainfully employed were all patient factors that were significantly related to improved outcomes with physical therapy consisting of manual therapy and specific exercise aimed at specific impairments identified during the examination in patients with cervicogenic headache.

Clinical prediction rules are decision-making tools that contain predictor variables obtained from patient history, examination, and simple diagnostic tests. They can assist in making a diagnosis, establishing prognosis, or determining appropriate management (Laupacis et al., 1997). Fernández-de-las-Peñas et al. (2008) have developed a clinical prediction rule to identify patients with chronic tension-type headache apt to have short-term benefit from manual trigger point therapy consisting of varied combinations of pressure release, muscle energy, and soft-tissue techniques combined with progressive, low-load deep cervical flexor and extensor muscle strengthening exercises. Relevant improvement

Table 13.11 Suggested History Component for Systems Review

System	Questions
Cardiovascular	Do you ever experience chest pain (angina)?
	Do you experience excessive unexplained fatigue?
	Do you have shortness of breath?
	Do you ever note chest palpitations?
	Have you noted lightheadedness?
	Have you ever fainted?
	Do you experience widespread leg pains?
	Have you noted swelling in the feet, ankles, or perhaps the hands?
Pulmonary	Do you ever experience chest pain?
	Do you have shortness of breath?
	Have you been coughing more lately?
	Have you noticed a change in your breathing?
	Do you have difficulty catching your breath when lying flat; do you have to sleep propped up on multiple pillows?
Gastrointestinal	Have you had difficulty swallowing?
	Have you had abdominal pain?
	Has your stool been black?
	Has your stool been different in consistency (diarrhea, tarry stool)?
	Have you been constipated?
Genitourinary	Any difficulty urinating?
	Have you noted blood in your urine?
	Have you noted an increased frequency with regard to urination?
	Have you noted an increased urgency with regard to urination?
	Have you noted an increased difficulty with initiating urination?
	Have there been episodes of impotence?
	Have there been any changes with regard to menstruation?
	Have you experienced pain with intercourse?
	Have you noted incontinence for urine and/or stool?

was defined in this study as an at least 50% reduction in headache intensity, frequency, or duration and an increase of 5 or more points on a 15-point global rating of change or patient satisfaction scale. Four variables constituted the clinical prediction rule for benefit at 1 week after discharge: headache duration less than 8.5 hours per day, headache frequency less than 5.5 days per week, SF-36 bodily pain domain score less than 47, and SF-36 vitality domain score less than 47.5. If the patient had three of these four variables, the positive LR for short-term benefit at 1 week postdischarge was 3.4 (95% CI: 1.4–8.0). If all four variables were present, the positive LR increased to 5.9 (95% CI: 0.8–42.9). Two variables made up the clinical prediction rule for benefit 1 month postdischarge: headache frequency less than 5.5 days per week, and SF-36 bodily pain domain score less than 47. With one of these two variables present, the positive LR was 2.2 (95% CI: 1.2–3.8); two variables present yielded a positive LR of 4.6 (95% CI: 1.2–17.9).

SYSTEMS REVIEW

As discussed earlier, a systems review is part of the physical therapy examination and probably of the examination in all professions with a similarly limited scope of practice with regard to diagnosis and management. Partly consisting of a history component and partly of physical tests, this review of organ systems differs from the specific pathology-based diagnosis done by the physician or other health-care professional with a more comprehensive scope of practice and serves to alert the clinician to undiagnosed conditions that may affect patient management or that indicate the need for referral (Boissonnault, 1995). The clinician should keep in mind that such conditions may or may not be related to the presenting headache complaint. **Table 13.11** provides one example of a history component to the systems review process. Doing the history component and also—but to a lesser extent—the physical examination component of the systems review depends on the information obtained in the rest of the history-taking process, meaning that all questions are not mandatory but rather at the discretion of the clinician.

CLINICAL PREDICTION RULES FOR DIAGNOSIS

Research-based data on the diagnostic utility of the history-taking process in patients with headache is limited. Most of the evidence relevant to the diagnosis of patients with headaches comes from uncontrolled studies, case series, and expert opinion. The over 300 potential causes for headache and the benign nature of most headaches, especially the most common types of headache such as migraine and tension-type headache, may explain this dearth of research evidence (Bartleson, 2006). However, in their review of the literature, Detsky et al. (2006) identified one clinical prediction rule relevant to diagnosis. This clinical prediction rule consists of the following five questions:

1. Is it a pulsating headache?
2. Does it last between 4 and 72 hours without medication?
3. Is it unilateral?
4. Is there nausea?
5. Is the headache disabling (with disabling headaches defined as headaches that disrupt a patient's daily activities)?

When the patient answers yes to four or more of these five questions, the positive LR for a diagnosis of migraine headache is 24 (95% CI: 1.5–388). With a yes answer to three questions, the positive LR is 3.5 (95% CI: 1.3–9.2). For a yes answer to one or two of these criteria, the positive LR is 0.41 (95% CI: 0.32–0.52). The mnemonic POUNDing (*p*ulsating, *d*uration of 4–72 hours, *u*nilateral, *n*ausea, *d*isabling) may be helpful for clinicians when using this clinical prediction rule (Detsky et al., 2006).

OUTCOME MEASURES

The information discussed so far can serve to produce questions in the history-taking process that provide the therapist with diagnostic information. However, history taking also should include outcome measures. The intent of outcome measures is not the collection of data to help with diagnosis but rather to provide the therapist, the patient, and other interested parties (such as third-party payers) with a reliable, valid, and responsive gauge of the effect of treatment.

Pain Measures

The Numeric Pain Rating Scale (NPRS) and the Visual Analogue Scale (VAS) for pain both are reliable, valid, and easy-to-apply outcome measures with regard to headache pain parameters. The VAS may be the preferred measure because research into its responsiveness has greater external validity to headache patients than research available on responsiveness for the NPRS. Kelly (2001) determined the minimal clinically important difference (MCID) for the VAS in a varied population of patients presenting to the emergency department with pain as 10 to 12 (mm), depending on but not significantly different between groups for severity of reported pain.

Disability Measures

The Headache Disability Inventory (HDI) is a 25-item questionnaire that seeks to measure the self-perceived disabling effects of headache on daily life. The questionnaire contains two subgroups of questions, thereby creating emotional and functional subscale scores and a total score. Two additional items on the questionnaire ask patients to rate the severity of their headache as mild, moderate, or severe, and the frequency as less than or equal to one per month, more than one but less than four per month, or four or more times per month. The HDI has good internal consistency reliability; correlations between the emotional and functional subscale scores and the total score were both excellent ($r = 0.89$) (Jacobson et al., 1994). It also has good short-term (1-week) ($r = 0.93$–0.95) (Jacobson et al., 1995) and generally good long-term (2-month) test-retest reliability ($r = 0.83$) for the total scores. The HDI also exhibits good internal construct validity ($P <0.001$) (Jacobson et al., 1994). A minimal detectable change (MDC_{95}) score at 1-week retest is 16 points. This value for the MDC_{95} indicates that a clinician can be 95% confident that a true change has occurred with a change in the HDI score of 16 or more points (Jacobson et al., 1995). Similarly, a 29-point score improvement constitutes the MDC_{95} over a 2-month time period (Jacobson et al., 1994). The HDI test is simple to administer and takes little time to complete.

With physical therapy interventions for the five headaches amenable to physical therapy management

Table 13.12 Red Flag Indicators in the History Taking of Patients with Headaches That Indicate the Need for Urgent Referral

History-Taking Category	Red Flag Symptoms
Demographics	New onset of headache or change in existing headache pattern in patients over 50
Location of pain	Persistent unilateral location of headaches
Onset and course of headache	New-onset headache
	Onset of a new headache type
	Unexplained change for the worse in pattern of existing headache
	Progressively worsening headache
	Abrupt, split-second onset of headache: thunderclap headache
Character and intensity of headache	New pain level, especially when described as worst ever
	Cluster-type headache
Aggravating and easing factors	Headache aggravated or brought on by physical exertion, coughing, sneezing, straining, or sexual activity
	Noted effect of position changes on pain
	No response to seemingly appropriate treatment
Neurologic symptoms	Seizures, confusion, changes in alertness, apathy, clumsiness, unexplained inappropriate behavior, brainstem symptoms, bowel and bladder symptoms, neck flexion stiffness, aura preceding the headache (especially one with quick diffusion), or weakness (not consistent with an existing diagnosis of migraine headaches or other pathology explaining these symptoms)
	Presyncope or syncope starting off headache
Otolaryngologic symptoms	Associated eye pain and simultaneous vision changes
Systemic symptoms	Fever, weight loss, temporal artery tenderness, profuse vomiting (especially when not associated with nausea), photophobia, phonophobia, or developing rash (not consistent with an existing diagnosis of migraine headaches)
	Headache that awakens a patient from night sleep (especially in children)
Medical history	Medical history of cancer and human immunodeficiency virus infection
	Head or neck injury
	Uncontrolled hypertension
Medication history	Use of anticoagulant medication in combination with even minor trauma
Family history	Absence of a family history of migraine in children with migrainelike symptoms

largely geared to affecting underlying neuromusculoskeletal impairments in the cervical spine, the Neck Disability Index (NDI) is potentially a useful outcome measure in that this 10-item questionnaire aims to measure the self-perceived disabling effects of neck pain on daily life. Interpretation is possible through scoring intervals as follows: 0–4 = no disability, 5–14 = mild, 15–24 = moderate, 25–34 = severe, and above 34 = complete disability (Vernon & Mior, 1991). To arrive at a percentage disability, the total score is multiplied by two. The NDI has moderate test-retest reliability (ICC = 0.68) (Cleland et al., 2006). Construct validity of the NDI as an outcome measure for neck pain has been demonstrated by comparing it with other tests or measures. Cleland et al. (2006) showed that a 7-point (14%) change in the NDI constituted a minimally clinically important difference for the NDI, albeit only in patients

with cervical radiculopathy and not specifically in patients reporting headaches.

RED FLAGS

One of the main objectives of the physical therapy history-taking process in patients presenting with a complaint of headaches is to identify red flag findings that indicate the need for urgent referral. **Table 13.12** provides a list of such red flag indicators based on the information presented in this chapter.

CONCLUSIONS AND IMPLICATIONS OF HISTORY FINDINGS

The history-taking process in patients with headaches presents unique challenges, particularly to health-care providers with a limited scope of practice, such as physical therapists, chiropractors, and massage therapists. The information provided in this chapter should allow the clinician to develop a history-taking process that allows him or her to meet the three main objectives noted in the beginning of this chapter, namely, diagnosing those headaches amenable to physical therapy interventions, identifying diagnostic indicators of headache not amenable to sole physical therapy management or even those that require urgent referral, and, finally, identifying undiagnosed pathology that may or may not be related to the presenting complaint of headache but that requires referral nevertheless for further diagnosis and management. History taking and systems review as discussed here are only part of the examination process, and other chapters address the other and interrelated portions in more detail.

Potentially most relevant to history taking and the diagnostic process is the identification of red flag indicators. The relevance and implications of finding such red flag indicators should always be considered in the context of the whole presenting clinical picture. However, the principle of *primum non nocere* clearly indicates the need at all times for referral in case of even minimal diagnostic uncertainty.

ACKNOWLEDGMENTS

I would like to thank Eugene Barsky, MILS, at the Irving K. Barber Learning Center of the University of British Columbia, who serves as the outreach librarian for the Physiotherapy Association of British Columbia, for his help with collecting some of the more relevant up-to-date research references upon which this chapter is based.

REFERENCES

Albuquerque FC, Han PH, Spetzler RF, Zabramski JM, McDougall CG. Carotid dissection: technical factor affecting endovascular therapy. *Can J Neurol Sci* 2002;29:54–60.

American Physical Therapy Association. Guide to physical therapist practice: second edition. *Phys Ther* 2001;81:9–744.

Bartleson JD. When and how to investigate the patient with headache. *Semin Neurol* 2006;26:163–170.

Blunt SB, Galton C. Cervical carotid or vertebral artery dissection. *Br Med J* 1997;314:243.

Bogduk N. Cervical causes of headache and dizziness. In: Grieve G, ed. *Modern Manual Therapy of the Vertebral Column.* New York: Churchill Livingstone; 1986.

Boissonnault WG. *Examination in Physical Therapy Practice: Screening for Medical Disease.* New York: Churchill Livingstone; 1995.

Brna PM, Dooley JM. Headaches in the pediatric population. *Semin Pediatr Neurol* 2006;13:222–230.

Bronfort G, Assendelft WJ, Evans R, Haas M, Bouter L. Efficacy of spinal manipulation for chronic headache: a systematic review. *J Manipulative Physiol Ther* 2001;24:457–466.

Burton LJ, Quinn B, Pratt-Cheney JL, et al. Headache etiology in a pediatric emergency department. *Pediatr Emerg Care* 1997;13:1–4.

Cleland JA, Fritz JM, Whitman JM, Palmer JA. The reliability and construct validity of the Neck Disability Index and patient-specific functional scale in patients with cervical radiculopathy. *Spine* 2006;31:598–602.

Clinch CR. Evaluation of acute headaches in adults. *Am Fam Physician* 2001;63:685–692.

Cosenza MJ. Headache as a manifestation of otolaryngologic disease. *J Am Osteopath Assoc* 2000;100(suppl):S1–S5.

Cross J, Coles A. Foramen magnum. *Adv Clin Neurosci Rehabil* 2002;2:16–17.

Davenport R. Acute headache in the emergency department. *J Neurol Neurosurg Psychiatry* 2002;72(suppl II): ii33–ii37.

De Jongh TOH, Knuistingh-Neven A, Couturier EGM. Hoofdpijn. *Huisarts Wetenschap* 2001;44:615–619.

Detsky ME, McDonald DR, Baerlocher MO, et al. Does this patient with headache have a migraine or need neuroimaging? *JAMA* 2006;296:1274–1283.

Dooley JM, Gordon KE, Wood EP, et al. The utility of the physical examination and investigations in the pediatric neurology consultation. *Pediatr Neurol* 2003;28:96–99.

Duarte J, Sempere AP, Delgado JA, et al. Headache of recent onset in adults: a prospective population-based study. *Acta Neurol Scand* 1996;94:67–70.

Dwyer A, Aprill C, Bogduk N. Cervical zygapophyseal joint pain patterns. I: a study in normal volunteers. *Spine* 1990;15:453–457.

Fernández-de-las-Peñas C, Cuadrado ML, Gerwin RD, Pareja JA. Referred pain from the trochlear region in tension-type headache: a myofascial trigger point from the superior oblique muscle. *Headache* 2005;45:731–737.

Fernández-de-las-Peñas C, Alonso-Blanco C, Cuadrado ML, Gerwin R, Pareja J. Myofascial trigger points and their relationship to headache clinical parameters in chronic tension-type headache. *Headache* 2006a;46:1264–1272.

Fernández-de-las-Peñas C, Alonso-Blanco C, Cuadrado ML, Gerwin RD, Pareja JA. Trigger points in the suboccipital muscles and forward head posture in tension-type headache. *Headache* 2006b;46:454–460.

Fernández-de-las-Peñas C, Cuadrado ML, Pareja JA. Myofascial trigger points, neck mobility and forward head posture in unilateral migraine. *Cephalalgia* 2006c;26: 1061–1070.

Fernández-de-las-Peñas C, Arendt-Nielsen L, Simons DG. Contributions of myofascial trigger points to chronic tension-type headache. *J Manual Manipulative Ther* 2006d;14:222–231.

Fernández-de-las-Peñas C, Alonso-Blanco C, Cuadrado ML, Pareja J. Myofascial trigger points in the suboccipital muscles in episodic tension-type headache. *Man Ther* 2006e;11:225–230.

Fernández-de-las-Peñas C, Cuadrado ML, Gerwin RD, Pareja JA. Referred pain from the lateral rectus muscle in subjects with chronic tension-type headache [abstract]. *Headache* 2006f;46:880.

Fernández-de-las-Peñas C, Cleland JA, Cuadrado ML, Pareja JA. Predictor variables for identifying patients with chronic tension type headache who are likely to achieve short-term success with muscle trigger point therapy. *Cephalalgia* 2008;28:264–275.

Fleming R, Forsythe S, Cook C. Influential variables associated with outcomes in patients with cervicogenic headache. *J Manual Manipulative Ther* 2007;15:155–164.

Gentile S. Indications for the diagnosis and treatment of acute headaches correlated with neurological pathologies. *J Headache Pain* 2005;6:290–293.

Gladstein J. Headache. *Med Clin North Am* 2006;90:275–290.

Goadsby P, Boes C. Chronic daily headache. *J Neurol Neurosurg Psychiatry* 2002;72(suppl II):ii2–ii5.

Granella F, D'Alessandro R, Manzoni GC, Cerbo R, Colucci D'Amato C. International Headache Society classification: inter-observer reliability in the diagnosis of primary headaches. *Cephalalgia* 1994;14:16–20.

Guy N, Deffond D, Gabrillargues J, et al. Spontaneous internal carotid artery dissection with lower cranial nerve palsy. *Can J Neurol Sci* 2001;28:265–269.

International Headache Society. The International Classification of Headache Disorders: 2nd ed. *Cephalalgia* 2004;24(suppl):1–150.

Issa TS, Huijbregts PA. Physical therapy diagnosis and management of a patient with chronic daily headache: a case report. *J Manual Manipulative Ther* 2006;14:E88–E123.

Jacobson GP, Ramadan NM, Aggarwal SK, Newman CW. The Henry Ford Hospital Headache Disability Inventory (HDI). *Neurology* 1994;44:837–842.

Jacobson GP, Ramadan NM, Norris L, Newman CW. Headache Disability Inventory (HDI): short-term test-retest reliability and spouse perceptions. *Headache* 1995;35:534–539.

Jull GA, Stanton WR. Predictors of responsiveness to physiotherapy management of cervicogenic headache. *Cephalalgia* 2005;25:101–108.

Jull G, Trott P, Potter H, et al. A randomized controlled trial of exercise and manipulative therapy for cervicogenic headache. *Spine* 2002;27:1835–1843.

Katsarava Z, Bartsch T, Diener H. Der medikamenteninduzierte Kopfschmerz. *Akta Neurol* 2006;33:28–43.

Kelly AM. The minimum clinically significant difference in visual analogue scale pain score does not differ with severity of pain. *Emerg Med J* 2001;18:205–207.

Kerry R, Taylor AJ. Cervical arterial dysfunction assessment and manual therapy. *Man Ther* 2006;11:243–253.

Laupacis A, Sekar N, Stiell I. Clinical prediction rules: a review and suggested modification of methodological standards. *JAMA* 1997;277:488–494.

Mills ML, Russo LS, Vines FS, Ross BA. High-yield criteria for urgent cranial computed tomography scans. *Ann Emerg Med* 1986;15:1167–1172.

Niere KR. Can subjective characteristics of benign headache predict manipulative physiotherapy treatment outcome? *Aust J Physiother* 1998;44:87–93.

Okeson JP. *Orofacial Pain: Guidelines for Assessment, Classification, and Management*. Hanover Park, IL: Quintessence Publishing; 1996.

Peters KS. Secondary headache and head pain emergencies. *Prim Care* 2004;31:381–393.

Royal College of Dental Surgeons of Ontario. *Guidelines: Diagnosis and Management of Temporomandibular Disorders*. Toronto, ON: Author; 2002.

Rubinstein SM, Peerdeman SM, Van Tulder M, Riphagen I, Haldeman S. A systematic review of the risk factors for cervical artery dissection. *Stroke* 2005;36:1575–1580.

Simon RP, Aminoff MJ, Greenberg DA. *Clinical Neurology*. 4th ed. Stanford, CT: Appleton & Lange; 1999.

Simons DG, Travell J, Simons LS. *Travell and Simons' Myofascial Pain and Dysfunction: The Trigger Point Manual*. Vol. 1. *Upper Half of the Body*. 2nd ed. Baltimore, MD: Williams & Wilkins; 1999.

Sjaastad O, Fredriksen TA, Pfaffenrath V, for the Cervicogenic Headache International Study Group. Cervicogenic headache: diagnostic criteria. *Headache* 1998;38:442–445.

Smetana GW. The diagnostic value of historical features in primary headache syndromes. *Arch Intern Med* 2000;160: 2729–2737.

Taylor AJ, Kerry R. Neck pain and headache as a result of internal carotid artery dissection: implications for manual therapists. *Man Ther* 2005;10:73–77.

Terrett AGJ. *Current Concepts in Vertebrobasilar Complications Following Spinal Manipulation*. 2nd ed. Norwalk, CT: Foundation for Chiropractic Education and Research; 2001.

Tuchin PJ. A twelve-month clinical trial of chiropractic spinal manipulative therapy for migraine. *Australas Chiropractic Osteopathy* 1999;8:61–65.

Tuchin PJ, Pollard H, Bonello R. A randomized controlled trial of chiropractic spinal manipulative therapy for migraine. *J Manipulative Physiol Ther* 2000;23:91–95.

Türp JC, et al. Schmerzen im Bereich der Kaumuskulatur und Kiefergelenke. *Manuelle Medizin* 2002;40:55–67.

Vernon H, Mior S. The Neck Disability Index: a study of reliability and validity. *J Manipulative Physiol Ther* 1991;14:409–415.

Weeks R, Weier Z. Psychological assessment of the headache patient. *Headache* 2006;46(suppl 3):S110–S118.

Welch E. Headache. *Nursing Standard* 2005;19:45–52.

Wojcik W, Pawlak JK, Knaus R. Doctor! I can't stand the noise in my ear! *Can J Diagnosis* 2003;20:55–59.

World Health Organization. Headache disorders. 2004. Available at: http://www.who.int/mediacentre/factsheets/fs277/en/index.html. Accessed September 20, 2007.

Cervical Spine Assessment in Patients with Headache

Pieter Westerhuis, PT, OMT, SVOMP

Because of overlap of symptoms, cervicogenic headache can often be confused with other types of headache, such as tension-type headache and migraine. Differences in pain features may implicate different structures as being responsible for the nociceptive irritation of the trigeminal nucleus caudalis (Nillson, 2000). Because cervicogenic headache is characterized by unilateral nonlancinating pain that is increased by head movement, maintained neck postures, or pressure over the upper cervical joints (Sjaastad et al., 1998), joint dysfunctions in the upper cervical spine (C0 to C2) should be implicated in the etiology of cervicogenic headache (Jull, 1994).

In addition to pain features, the effectiveness of spinal manipulation or mobilization directed at the upper cervical spine in cervicogenic headache (Jull et al., 2002; Fernández-de-las-Peñas et al., 2005) supports the hypothesis that upper cervical joint dysfunctions can be relevant for the pathogenesis of cervicogenic headache. Therefore, manipulative physical therapy should only be applied to those patients who actually have a cervical component causing or contributing to their specific headache. There are two ways in which the cervical spine may be involved with headache. First, the cervical spine can be the main cause of the headache. In this case the headache would be a true cervicogenic headache. Second, the cervical spine can be a contributing factor in other types of headache, such as migraine or tension-type headache. In these cases a cervical dysfunction can trigger a migrainous attack (Westerhuis, 2001) or can contribute to a tension-type headache attack (Fernández-de-las-Peñas et al., 2006c).

Therefore, the goal of the physical examination is to assess whether the patient has dysfunctions (joint mobility or motor control) in joints that theoretically could be responsible for, or contribute to, the headache. To assess for mobility impairments, the therapist should assess the following aspects: (a) the available range of motion, (b) the behavior of the resistance (e.g., loss of or increased stiffness, neutral zone, protective muscle spasm), and (c) the occurrence of symptoms. Any abnormality in these factors constitutes a so-called *objective sign*, or mobility impairment. If this sign is found in a cervical joint, which theoretically can be linked with headaches, it is called a *comparable sign* (Maitland et al., 2005).

Because of the convergence of the afferent input of the upper three spinal nerves and the trigeminal nerve into the trigeminocervical nucleus, most scientists have concentrated upon dysfunctions in the upper cervical spine in relation to headache (Bogduk, 1994; Piovesan et al., 2001). This chapter therefore mainly concentrates on the upper three cervical motion segments. Although there is little literature supporting this, clinicians may also recall cases in which treating, for example, the cervicothoracic junction (down to the T4 region) or the first rib, or both, also improved the headache symptoms. Therefore this region should also be assessed, because it may be contributing to excessive strain on the upper cervical spine. Ideally, the clinician would be able to reproduce the symptoms of the patient upon specific physical examination. Quite commonly, however, this is not possible and the clinician has to base his or her reasoning upon the interpretation and treatment of comparable signs.

PLANNING OF THE PHYSICAL EXAMINATION

After finishing the subjective examination, the therapist should plan the physical examination (PE). Categorizing one's thoughts along the clinical reasoning categories, as originally described by Jones (1992), will help in the clinical decision making. This categories system of hypotheses reflects the interrelated components of a patient's problem that the therapist should consider and manage in addition to the initial diagnosis of the physical problem. The seven categories are as follows (Christensen et al., 2004):

1. Functional limitation or disability (according to the International Classification of Functioning, Disability and Health [ICF])
2. Pathobiological mechanisms
   a. In relation to the phases of tissue healing
   b. Pain mechanisms
3. Physical and psychosocial impairments and their associated sources
4. Contributing factors
5. Precautions and contraindications to physical examination and treatment
6. Management and treatment
7. Prognosis

As the patient is being assessed and treated, the therapist's thought processes are continuously referring to these hypotheses categories.

Before starting the physical examination, the therapist should determine the irritability of the condition. The therapist should have an initial hypothesis about the amount and type of testing needed to reproduce the symptoms. In problems with a high level of irritability, one should only test to the first onset of pain. The amount of testing should be minimal, differential testing is usually not necessary, and the tests should not be very stressful. In a nonirritable disorder, however, one can test beyond the first onset of symptoms, perform more tests, perform differential testing when applicable, and use tests that are more provoking.

It is also important to realize that one test in isolation is not sufficient for diagnosing a cervical involvement. Clinical diagnosis should be based on a sound analysis of all tests. As De Hertogh et al. (2007) found, it is the clustering of the test results that increases the diagnostic value of the PE. The findings with the active movements should be confirmed with the *passive physiologic intervertebral movement (PPIVM)* or the *passive accessory intervertebral movement (PAIVM)* tests. The final clinical proof of a cervical spine involvement is improvement of the symptoms after the dysfunctions have been appropriately treated. Therefore, the physical examination may include the following aspects:

- Present pain and symptoms at rest (PP)
- Inspection
- Functional demonstration
- Active movements (plus overpressure, or plus localization)
- "If necessary" tests
- Neurologic examination
- Neurodynamic tests

- Passive physiologic intervertebral movements (PPIVM)
- Passive accessory intervertebral movements (PAIVM)
- Motor control impairment tests
- Screening tests for other regions or joints

The present chapter focuses on joint assessment of the cervical spine. The remaining aspects of the PE are covered in other chapters of this book.

INSPECTION

After the symptoms at rest (PP) have been ascertained, inspection of the patient's posture may give a first indication of a cervical involvement. Even more, although most patients will not be able to describe specific movements that bring on their symptoms, they might be able to describe sustained positions, such as sitting in front of the computer, as an aggravating factor of their symptoms. A so-called protective deformity is rare in these patients. A forward head posture (FHP) has been associated with different types of headache (Watson & Trott, 1993; Fernández-de-las-Peñas et al., 2006a, 2006b). Nevertheless, other authors failed to find a clear relationship in cervicogenic headache (Zito et al., 2006). Clinically, it is important to assess whether the patient has the mobility to correct the FHP. Therefore, the therapist should perform a correction maneuver of upper cervical flexion and lower cervical extension. Because some authors have described an association between FHP and dysfunction in the deep cervical flexors (Falla, 2004; Watson, 1994), later on in the PE these aspects should be addressed. Examination of the deep flexor activity is detailed in Chapter 12.

FUNCTIONAL DEMONSTRATION

The principle of the so-called functional demonstration is that the patient is asked to perform the movement or posture that most specifically increases symptoms. The therapist should then perform tests to implicate a specific structure or region of the cervical spine. For instance, if the patient describes that looking over his or her shoulder while reversing his or her car elicits symptoms (**Figure 14.1**), the therapist should try to maintain the painful position and to make a differential diagnosis:

1. Increase the rotation of the trunk by pushing with your elbows against the shoulder girdle (**Figure 14.2**). This increases the rotation stress

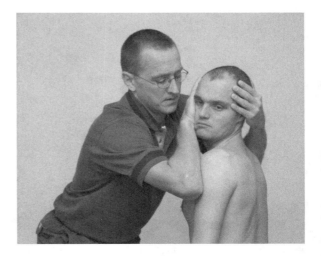

Figure 14.1 Cervical Rotation Stress

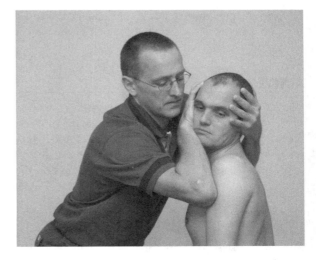

Figure 14.2 Cervical Rotation with Increased Rotation of the Trunk

of the upper thoracic spine while at the same time decreasing the stress of the cervical region. Therefore, if the symptoms decrease, an initial hypothesis of cervical spine involvement may be made.

2. The rotation stress of the trunk region should be decreased (**Figure 14.3**). If the hypothesis is correct, then the symptoms should now increase, because this maneuver increases the rotation stress of the cervical spine.

Although in the initial examination there are time constraints, it is also important at some point to

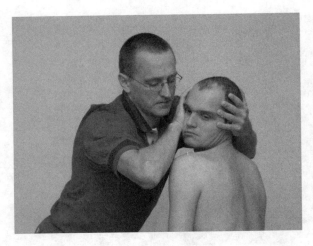

Figure 14.3 Cervical Rotation with Decreased Rotation of the Trunk

perform an ergonomic analysis of the patient's activities (e.g., an analysis of the working position of the patient at the computer).

ACTIVE MOVEMENTS

With all active movements, the therapist should analyze range of motion, quality of motion, and symptoms (increase, decrease, or no change). If there are no symptoms with the active movements, the therapist should apply gentle overpressure to increase the stress on the structure.

Cervical Range of Motion

Although for scientific purposes a cervical range of motion (CROM) goniometer is commonly used for accurate measurement, in clinical practice a visual approximation of the range of motion can be acceptable. For flexion-extension the frontal plane of the face may be used. Because the normal cervical range of motion is considerable, it is important to put the different movements in relationship to each other. A rough guideline for normal ranges of motion is as follows:

Flexion	80° ± 10°
Extension	80° ± 10°
Rotation	80° ± 10°
Side flexion	35° ± 10°

If a patient has 50° of flexion, and also 50° in extension and in rotation motions, this may reflect a general

hypomobility without any direct relationship with his or her headache. However, if the patient has 50° of flexion and 50° of rotation while having 80° of extension, this would reflect a segmental dysfunction.

It is also important to evaluate the relationship between the synergistic movements of the cervical spine: side flexion and rotation. For example, the clinician should assess whether the contralateral or ipsilateral side flexion is more restricted or painful or both.

Quality of Movement

The therapist should evaluate whether the movement that the patient performs is fluent and takes place in all motion segments, or whether specific regions are less mobile. Clinically, cervicogenic headache patients often show limitations in the upper cervical region: there is not enough movement of the head-on-neck motion.

Overpressure

Because it is usual that headache patients have only minimal symptoms with active movements, the therapist may need to apply overpressure at the end of range of motion. If symptoms do not appear, localized overpressure should be applied to increase the stress. For instance, a patient flexes the neck region to 50°, but without symptoms. Therefore, the therapist gently pushes the neck farther into range (**Figure 14.4**). Now the patient feels a pulling in the mid/upper cervical spine region. Then the therapist applies localized stress to the upper (**Figure 14.5**), middle (**Figure 14.6**), or lower (**Figure 14.7**) cervical spine, respectively, to differentiate the region from which the symptoms are being produced. The same procedure should be repeated applying localized overpressure for extension movement of the upper cervical (**Figure 14.8**), middle (**Figure 14.9**), or lower (**Figure 14.10**) cervical spine.

If there is a restriction with rotation motion, a quick differentiating test for the upper cervical spine should be used. For that purpose, the therapist grasps around and fixates the laminae and spinous process of C2 with the thumb and index finger of his or her left hand (**Figure 14.11**). The right hand is placed upon the crown of the patient's head and rotates toward the right. Normally there should be approximately 35° to 40° of

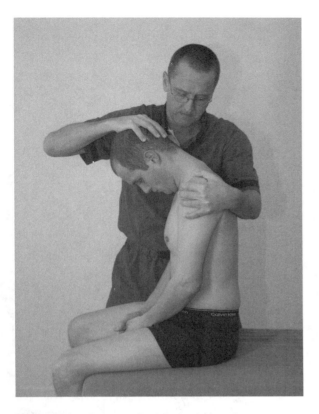

Figure 14.4 Full Range of Cervical Spine Motion

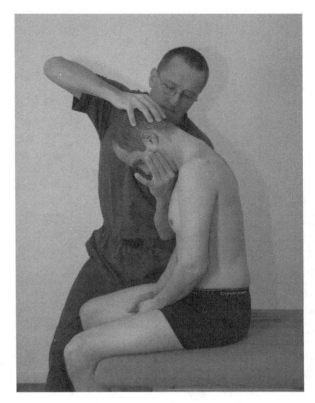

Figure 14.5 Manual Overpressure for Upper Cervical Spine Flexion

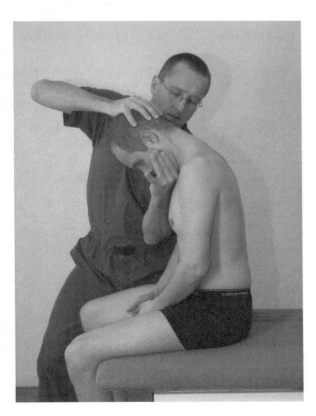

Figure 14.6 Manual Overpressure for Middle Cervical Spine Flexion

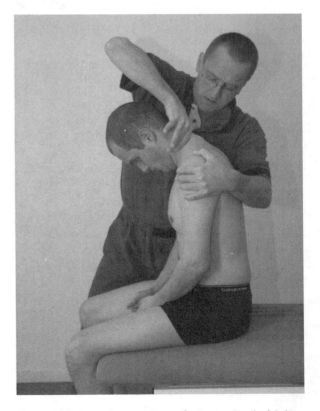

Figure 14.7 Manual Overpressure for Lower Cervical Spine Flexion

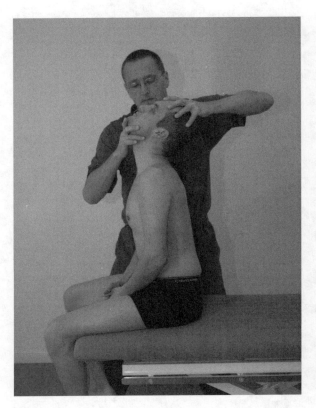

Figure 14.8 Manual Overpressure for Upper Cervical Spine Extension

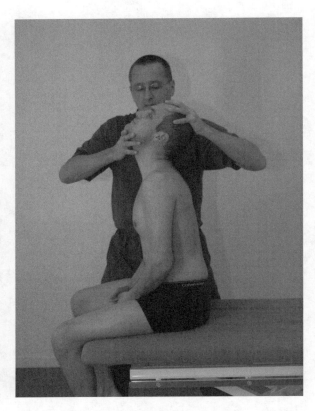

Figure 14.9 Manual Overpressure for Middle Cervical Spine Extension

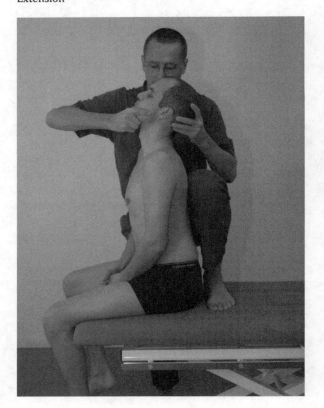

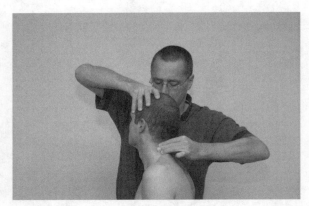

Figure 14.11 Manual Evaluation of Right Rotation of Occiput-C2 Vertebra

Figure 14.10 Manual Overpressure for Lower Cervical Spine Extension

rotation in the upper cervical spine (White & Panjabi, 1990).

"IF NECESSARY" TESTS

Quite commonly, standard active movements will not result in any reproduction of symptoms or production of comparable signs (Treleaven et al., 1994). In these cases it may be appropriate to increase the stress on the cervical spine region. This can be done by sustaining a certain end-of-range position or by combining movements. Commonly used tests are as follows.

- *Localized upper cervical flexion with lower cervical extension (**Figure 14.12**):* This test aims to stress both upper and lower cervical spine at the same time. The combination of upper cervical flexion and lower cervical extension simulates the joint correction of a forward head posture, since it involves upper cervical extension and lower cervical flexion (Chapter 8).

- *Localized upper cervical extension with lower cervical flexion (**Figure 14.13**):* This test is the opposite of the previous one. The aim is to stress the cervical joints simulating a forward head posture position (Chapter 8).

- *Combining flexion with either rotation or side flexion:* This test aims to stress the cervical spine with the combination of flexion with other movement in a different plane.

- *The so-called upper cervical quadrant:* For the upper cervical quadrant, the clinician initially performs an upper cervical extension (**Figure 14.14**), followed by upper cervical rotation (**Figure 14.15**) and finally side flexion (**Figure 14.16**) toward the same side. The combination of extension, rotation, and ipsilateral flexion will create a "close" stress in the upper cervical region. The objective of this test is to stress one side of the upper cervical spine in order to reproduce the headache pain of the patient.

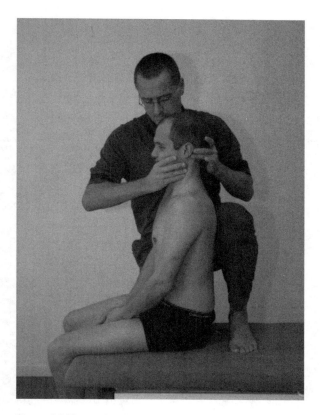

Figure 14.12 Localized Upper Cervical Flexion with Lower Cervical Extension

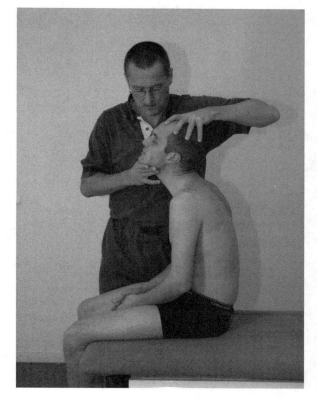

Figure 14.13 Localized Upper Cervical Extension with Lower Cervical Flexion

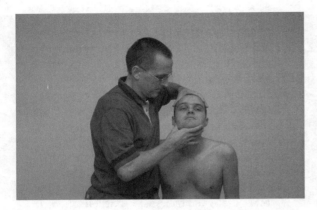

Figure 14.14 Upper Cervical Extension for the Upper Cervical Quadrant

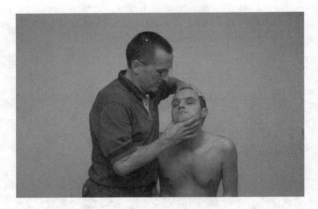

Figure 14.15 Upper Cervical Rotation for the Upper Cervical Quadrant

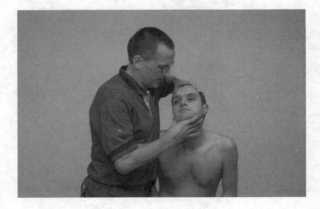

Figure 14.16 Upper Cervical Side Flexion for the Upper Cervical Quadrant

NEUROLOGIC EXAMINATION

Because most headaches are referred symptoms, a neurologic examination is usually not necessary (Jull, 1994). However, in rare cases headache may be the first symptom of a more serious disease such as a brain tumor. It is usually recommended that an experienced neurologist first examine a patient showing any red flag or a patient in whom the clinician has any doubt regarding the onset of the symptoms.

NEURODYNAMIC TESTS INVOLVING THE CERVICAL SPINE REGION

Neurodynamic structures such as the dura are also innervated by the upper three cervical segments (Bogduk, 1994). Further, they have to adapt to length changes by lengthening and shortening (Breig, 1978; Butler, 1991; Vital et al., 1989). Increased sensitivity or movement restrictions with these structure may also lead to headache, and therefore the neural structure should be assessed (Chapter 20). Standard tests that involve the cervical spine are the cervical slump, greater occipital nerve slump (Westerhuis & Von Piekartz, 2001), and upper limb neural test.

PASSIVE PHYSIOLOGIC INTERVERTEBRAL MOVEMENTS

PPIVM tests assess the passive intersegmental physiologic range of motion. Although patients with upper cervical spine instability may complain of headache, the typical headache patient is more likely to have hypomobile segments (Jull, 1994; Westerhuis, 2007; Zito et al., 2006). For these tests, the patient lies over the edge of the plinth. The head lies well supported in the therapist's hands and lower abdomen.

Occiput Versus C1 Vertebra (Atlas)

The therapist feels with his or her thumbs the space between the transverse process of C1 and the mastoid process (**Figure 14.17**). With *flexion* there should be a posterior sliding movement of mastoid on C1 vertebra. With *extension* there should be an anterior sliding movement. With *side flexion* to the left, there should be a separating movement on the right side and also a translatory movement of C1 toward the left (**Figure 14.18**). With *rotation* toward the right, the therapist tries to assess the relative anterior movement of the left mas-

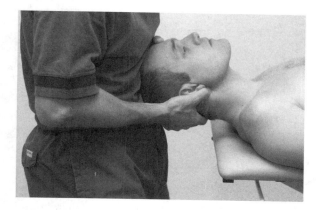

Figure 14.17 PPIVM: Occiput Atlas in Flexion

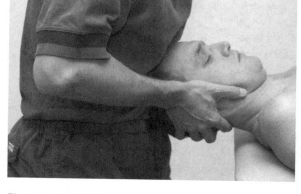

Figure 14.19 PPIVM: Occiput Axis in Flexion

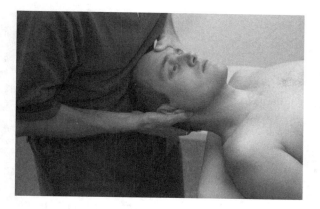

Figure 14.18 PPIVM: Occiput Atlas in Side Flexion

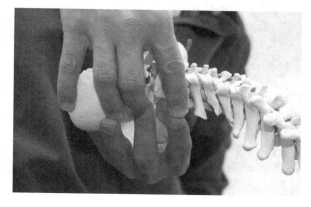

Figure 14.20 Manual Contact for PPIVM of Occiput Axis

toid process in relation to the left transverse process. Because occiput-C1 rotation mainly takes place at the end of the total range, this movement may be best appreciated at the end of rotation.

Occiput Versus C2 Vertebra (Axis)

With *flexion* the therapist assesses the separation of the spinous process of C2 (index finger) and the occipital (middle finger) (**Figures 14.19** and **14.20**). With *extension* the index finger and middle finger are placed bilaterally on the posterior ring of C1 vertebra. The therapist evaluates the approximation of occiput bone and C2 vertebra. With *rotation* to the right, the therapist fixates the spinous process and lamina of C2 with the left thumb and index finger. The right hand rotates the head toward the right. Range of motion may be measured by a visual estimation of the circular movement of the tip of the nose.

C2 Versus C3 Vertebrae

The clinician palpates with the index and middle fingers bilaterally between the laminae of the C2 and C3 vertebrae. The thumbs lie gently and anteriorly on the transverse process (**Figures 14.21** and **14.22**). From a clinical viewpoint, the most important movements are flexion, extension, and side flexion.

With *flexion and extension*, the opening and closing of the interlaminar space is evaluated. With *side flexion* to the right, there should be an opening on the left and a closing on the right. A restriction on side flexion to the right could be caused by either a closing-down movement dysfunction on the right or by an opening movement dysfunction on the left. To differentiate, the therapist should subsequently compare right side-flexion motion in extension with right side-flexion in flexion. If the movement is more restricted in flexion,

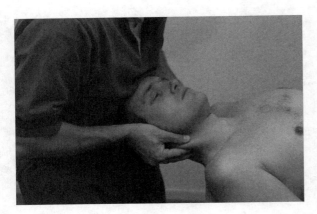

Figure 14.21 PPIVM: C2-C3 in Flexion

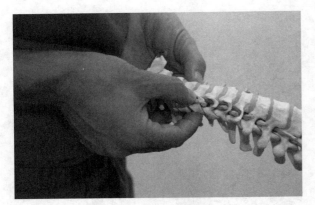

Figure 14.22 Manual Contact for PPIVM of C2-C3 in Flexion

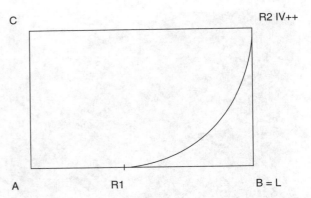

Figure 14.23 Movement Diagram of a Normal Unilateral Posterior-Anterior Movement on the Right Side

this would imply an opening movement dysfunction on the left, which is usually treated with techniques that emphasize the opening of the motion segment (e.g., side flexion or side flexion in flexion). However, if the movement is restricted in extension, this would imply a closing-down movement restriction. In these cases it is more appropriate to use treatment techniques that close down (e.g., PAIVM or side flexion in extension). The technique to assess the segments from C3 down to C7 is similar to that used for C2 versus C3.

PASSIVE ACCESSORY INTERVERTEBRAL MOVEMENTS

PAIVM tests assess the passive intersegmental accessory range of motion. In clinical practice, the PAIVM is much more likely to produce symptoms in the patient than the PPIVM. Tests that rely solely on the assessment of range of motion are much less reliable than those that also incorporate symptom response (Hanten et al.,

2002; Humpreys et al., 2004; Jull et al., 1988, 1997; Seffinger et al., 2004; Van Suijlekom et al., 1999). Therefore, the PAIVMs are the most important tests for implicating the cervical spine as contributing to headache. Although the therapist should continuously analyze the behavior of tissue resistance and symptoms with any examination procedure, it is especially with the PAIVMs that it may be useful to depict these findings in so-called movement diagrams.

From a scientific perspective, the reliability of a movement diagram in isolation is very poor. However, clinically it is not important whether the first resistance appears at 1 mm or at 4 mm. What is important is the following: Is there a movement restriction? Is the problem pain dominant or resistance dominant? How do the findings with the PAIVMs support other findings within the physical examination? Is the segmental impairment comparable to the patient's headache?

Movement Diagrams

- *Movement diagram of a normal unilateral posterior-anterior (PA) movement on the right side (Figure 14.23): The A–B line represents the range of movement. B stands for the average normal range of movement. L indicates the individual motion limit. In a normal movement diagram, L should equal B.*

The *A–C line* shows the intensity of various factors. *R* stands for resistance, *P* for pain, and *S* for protective muscular spasm. *C* indicates the maximum intensity the examiner is prepared to apply during the examination. The gradient of the resistance curve represents the stiffness of the movement segment. In this example of a

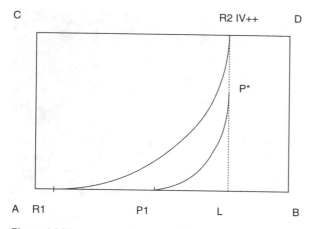

Figure 14.24 Movement Diagram of a Hypomobile Unilateral PA on the Right That Is Resistance Dominant

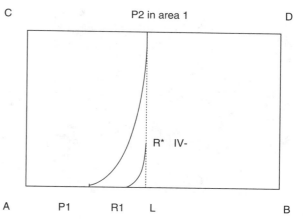

Figure 14.25 Movement Diagram of a Hypomobile Unilateral Posterior-Anterior Movement on the Right That Is Pain Dominant

unilateral PA movement on C2 vertebra, the normal average range of motion is only a few millimeters. (It is accepted that for a unilateral PA movement on C2 vertebra, the line A–B represents 10 mm.) The examiner perceives a first resistance at approximately 4 mm that increases gently, until it rises exponentially from 6 mm to the normal range of motion of approximately 10 mm. There is neither pain nor spasm.

- *Movement diagram of a hypomobile unilateral PA movement on the right, which is resistance dominant (**Figure 14.24**):* This movement diagram shows that the unilateral PA movement on the right side is limited by the intensity of the resistance at approximately 6 mm (*L*). The first resistance is felt by the examiner at approximately 1 mm. Pain is first perceived by the patient at 4 mm. It increases to 6 of 10 on the Visual Analogue Scale (VAS) at the end of range of motion. Although the intensity of the pain is 6 of 10, this still depicts a so-called resistance-dominant movement restriction.
- *Movement diagram of a hypomobile unilateral PA movement on the right, which is pain dominant (**Figure 14.25**):* This movement diagram shows that the unilateral PA movement on the right side is limited at approximately 4 mm. The patient feels the first onset of pain at 2 mm. It increases strongly; because of this, the therapist decides not to move any further. It is the intensity of the pain that limits the movement (P2 = limit = *L*). The therapist feels the first resistance at 3 mm. At the limit of the range of motion there is only minimal resistance.

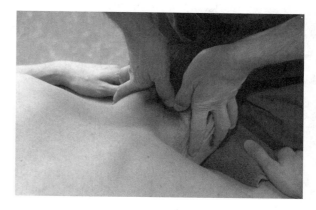

Figure 14.26 Unilateral Posterior-Anterior Pressure on the Articular Process of C1

The Most Commonly Used PAIVMs

The following PAIVMs are commonly used (Watson & Trott, 1993; Jull, 1994, Jull et al., 2002; Maitland et al., 2005).

- *Posterior-anterior pressure on the tip of the spinous process of C1 (central PA):* The therapist places the thumbs over the posterior process of the atlas under the occipital bone. Then, a gently posterior-anterior pressure over the vertebra is applied following the principles explained earlier in this chapter.
- *Unilateral PA pressure on the articular process of C1 (**Figure 14.26**):* The therapist places the thumbs over the zygapophysial joint (articular process) of the atlas. Then, a gently posterior-

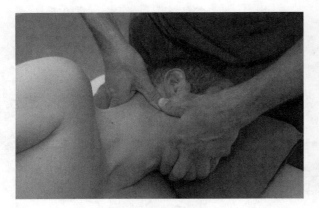

Figure 14.27 Transverse Pressure on the Tip of the Transverse Process of C1

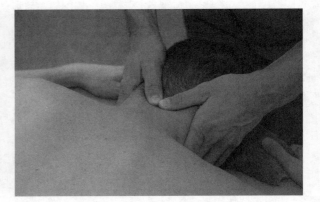

Figure 14.28 Central Posterior-Anterior Pressure on C2 Vertebra

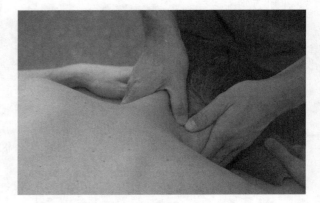

Figure 14.29 Unilateral Posterior-Anterior Pressure on C2 Vertebra

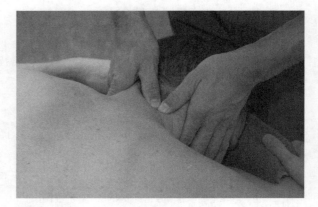

Figure 14.30 Unilateral Posterior-Anterior Pressure on C2 on the Right in 30° Rotation to the Right

anterior pressure over the vertebra is applied following the principles explained earlier in this chapter. The pressure can be applied in a perpendicular way or can be angulated, with the aim to reproduce the patient's pain.

- *Unilateral PA pressure on the most lateral aspect of the transverse process of C1:* The therapist places the thumbs over the most lateral aspect of the transverse process of the atlas vertebra. Then, a gently posterior-anterior pressure over the vertebra is applied.

- *Transverse pressure on the tip of the transverse process of C1 (**Figure 14.27**):* With the patient lying on the side, the therapist places the thumbs over the lateral aspect of the transverse process of the atlas. Then, a gently posterior-anterior pressure over the vertebra is applied. This pressure will induce a transverse movement of the atlas vertebra over the occipital bone.

- *Central PA pressure on C2 vertebra (**Figure 14.28**):* The therapist places the thumbs over the spinous process of the axis (this is the first spinous process of the cervical spine). A gently posterior-anterior pressure is also applied following the principles explained earlier in this chapter.

- *Unilateral PA pressure on C2 vertebra (**Figure 14.29**):* The therapist places the thumbs over the zygapophysial joint (articular process) of the axis vertebra. Posterior-anterior pressures over the vertebra, either perpendicular or angulated, are applied following the principles explained earlier in this chapter.

- *Unilateral PA pressure on C2 on the right in 30° rotation to the right (**Figure 14.30**):* If right

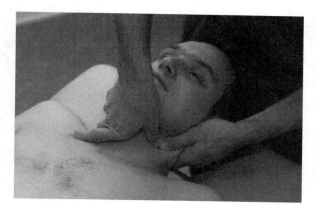

Figure 14.31 Unilateral Anterior-Posterior Pressure on C2 Vertebra

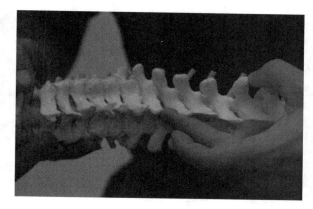

Figure 14.32 Manual Contact for Cervicothoracic PPIVM

unilateral PA pressure on C2 produces symptoms, this could either be caused by the C1-C2 or the C2-C3 motion segment. Rotation to the right increases the anterior stress of C1 on C2 on the right. Therefore the C1-C2 segment should be responsible for the patient's symptoms, since an increase of the symptoms would be expected in the rotated position.

- *Central PA pressure on C3 vertebra:* The therapist places the thumbs over the spinous process of the C3 vertebra. A gently posterior-anterior pressure is again applied.
- *Unilateral anterior-posterior pressure on C2 vertebra:* In addition to the above PAIVMs, it may also be useful to assess the unilateral anterior-posterior (AP) movements of the cervical spine. From a clinical viewpoint, the most important segments would be AP pressure on C2 vertebra (**Figure 14.31**) and AP pressure on C7. For that purpose, the therapist places the thumbs over the anterior aspect of the transverse process of the axis vertebra. Then, a gently anterior-posterior pressure is applied.

MOTOR CONTROL IMPAIRMENT TESTS

In an impressive series of studies, the group of researchers of the Brisbane University has shown the importance of assessing and treating dysfunctions of the deep cervical neck flexors in cervicogenic headache (Jull et al., 1999; Falla, 2004; Falla et al., 2004). This topic is dealt with in more detail in Chapter 12.

SCREENING TESTS FOR OTHER REGIONS: THE CERVICOTHORACIC REGION

In subsequent visits, it is absolutely essential to also screen other structures, such as the temporomandibular joint (Chapter 17) and the first rib and the thoracic spine (Chapter 15) for dysfunctions that could contribute to the headache. The present chapter includes the assessment of the cervicothoracic region, although readers are referred to Chapter 15 for a detailed discussion.

A forward head posture is usually associated with an extension restriction of the cervicothoracic region (Fernández-de-las-Peñas et al., 2006a). This position may lead to excessive extension strain on the upper cervical segments, which in turn may lead to an upper cervical flexion restriction. In these cases it is appropriate to assess the cervicothoracic PPIVM.

Cervicothoracic Passive Physiologic Intervertebral Movements

The patient lies on his or her left side. The therapist cradles the patient's head in his or her right arm with his or her biceps against the front of the head. The therapist's right hand with the little finger grasps around the C7 vertebra. The left lower arm stabilizes the patient's thoracic spine, with the tip of the middle finger palpating the interspinous space. The distal interphalangeal joint of the middle finger will stabilize the lower spinous process (it may need to be supported by the tip of the index finger) (**Figure 14.32**). By giving a slight pressure with the right hand and biceps, the therapist tries to

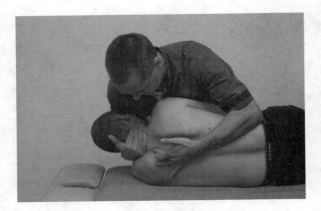

Figure 14.33 Cervicothoracic PPIVM in Flexion

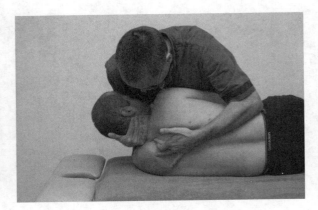

Figure 14.35 Cervicothoracic PPIVM in Rotation

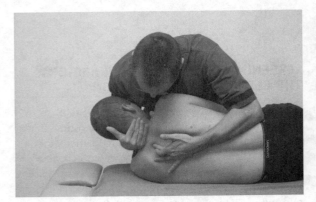

Figure 14.34 Cervicothoracic PPIVM in Lateral Flexion

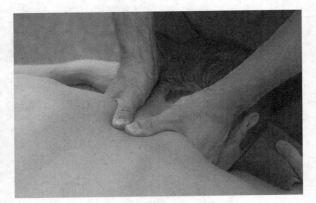

Figure 14.36 Central Posterior-Anterior Pressure on T1 Vertebra

stabilize the whole head and neck as one unit. This "unit" is subsequently moved in relationship to the upper thoracic segments. With *flexion-extension*, the therapist performs the movement by a retraction-protraction movement of his or her shoulder girdle (**Figure 14.33**). With *side flexion*, it is important to grasp around the side of the neck with the ulnar border of the right hand, and the movement is performed by doing a small trunk rotation (**Figure 14.34**). To assess *rotation*, the therapist tries to hook his or her little finger around the spinous process of the C7 vertebra (**Figure 14.35**). The therapist performs an elevation movement of his or her shoulder girdle.

Cervicothoracic Passive Accessory Intervertebral Movements

- *Central PA pressure on T1 vertebra (**Figure 14.36**):* The therapist places the thumbs over the spinous process of the first thoracic vertebra. A gently

posterior-anterior pressure is applied to the cervicothoracic region.

- *Unilateral PA pressure on T1 vertebra (**Figure 14.37**):* The therapist places the thumbs over the articular process of the first thoracic vertebra in the anatomic place where the vertebra joins with the first rib. Posterior-anterior pressures over the vertebra are applied following the principles explained earlier in this chapter.

- *Transverse pressure on T1 toward the right (**Figure 14.38**):* The therapist places the thumbs over the lateral part (lamina process) of the first thoracic vertebra. Transverse pressures over the lamina vertebra are applied.

First Rib Passive Accessory Intervertebral Movements

- *Unilateral AP pressure on the first rib (**Figure 14.39**):* With the patient lying supine, the

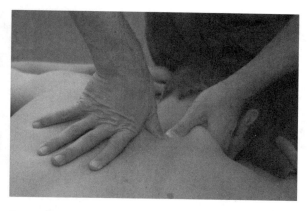

Figure 14.37 Unilateral Posterior-Anterior Pressure on T1 Vertebra

therapist places the thumbs over the anterior aspect of the first rib, under the clavicle bone. Then, a gently anterior-posterior pressure is applied.

- *Posterior-anterior movement of the first rib:* The therapist places the thumbs over the posterior process of the first rib. Then, posterior-anterior pressures over the rib are applied following the principles explained earlier in this chapter.
- *Longitudinal caudal pressure on the first rib:* With the patient lying supine, the therapist places the thumbs over the superior aspect of the posterior process of the first rib, behind the clavicle bone (**Figure 14.40**). Then, a gently caudal pressure is applied. This technique can also be done with the patient in a prone position (**Figure 14.41**).

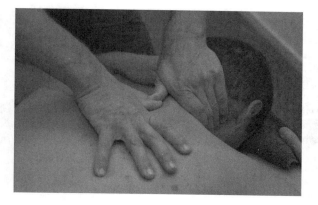

Figure 14.38 Transverse Pressure on T1 Toward the Right

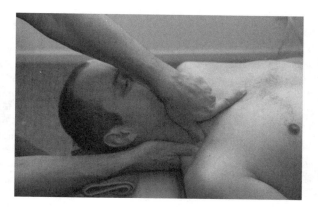

Figure 14.40 Longitudinal Caudal Pressure on the First Rib in Supine Position

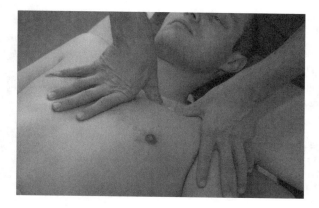

Figure 14.39 Unilateral Anterior-Posterior Pressure on the First Rib

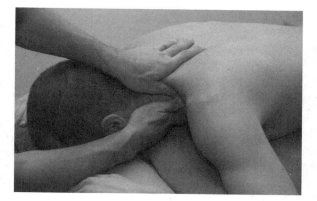

Figure 14.41 Longitudinal Caudal Pressure on the First Rib in Prone Position

ANALYSIS OF THE FINDINGS

Upon completion of the examination, a careful analysis of the separate findings is essential. The clinician should reflect whether the initial hypothesis of a cervical component to the patient's headache is supported or should be discarded. The clinician should search for clustering of individual findings that mutually support each other. Ideally, movement restrictions initially seen with the active movements should be confirmed with the PPIVM assessment. The most hypomobile segment with the PPIVM assessment would ideally also be the segment that has the most abnormal PAIVM findings.

CASE REPORT

A 44-year-old man complains of left-sided occipitofrontal headache that has a pulsating quality. The headache sometimes comes together with a left-sided suboccipital feeling of tightness. If the headache is severe, nausea and photophobia are also present. Typical aggravating factors are stress, lack of sleep, and wine. The patient has to use migraine medication at least three times per month. He has had these symptoms since he experienced a lot of stress to pass exams 20 years ago. The patient seeks physical therapy treatment because he is reluctant to keep on using so much migraine medication and because his neighbor was successfully treated for headache symptoms.

Table 14.1 Example of the Physical Examination of a Patient

PP:	None
Inspection:	Slight forward head posture that can be corrected without symptoms
Functional demonstration:	Not applicable
Active movements	
Flexion	60° no symptoms, but little head-on-neck movement
Extension	80° no symptoms
Left rotation	80° no symptoms
Right rotation	60° no symptoms
Left side-flexion	40° no symptoms
Right side-flexion	20° no symptoms
If necessary tests	Localized upper cervical flexion reproduced suboccipital tightness
	Left occiput–C2 rotation 40°
	Right occiput–C2 rotation 10°
	Because "opening" movements were most comparable, it was decided to:
	Combine flexion with side flexion toward the other side
	Combine flexion with right side-flexion
	Both tests caused a pulling sensation in the left occipital region
Neurologic:	Not necessary
Neurodynamic:	Greater occipital nerve test reproduces the headache
PPIVM	
Oc-C1	Flexion: Slightly restricted but otherwise normal
Oc-C2	Flexion: Limited by approximately 50%
	Extension: Normal
	Right rotation: 15°
	Left rotation: 40°
C2-C3	Normal
The pattern of movement with the PPIVM confirms the active movements.	
Conclusion:	**"Opening" hypomobility Oc-C2 on the left**
PAIVM	Left unilateral PA on C1 very limited with local pain
	Left unilateral PA on C2 very limited with local pain
	In left rotation, reproduction of the headache

The PAIVM confirms the PPIVM.

PA, posterior-anterior; PPIVM, passive physiologic intervertebral movement; PAIVM, passive accessory intervertebral movement.

Interpretation

At first sight, this seems to be a classic migraine without aura patient. However, indicators for a possible cervical contributing component could be that the pain is always on the left side; there is no side shift; the headache has an occipitofrontal development (Sjaastad and Bovim [1991] noted that vascular migraines usually have a frontal-occipital development); there are concomitant suboccipital symptoms; and the intensity of the associated symptoms is not very high (e.g., no vomiting, or photophobia plus phonophobia). **Table 14.1** depicts the initial physical examination of this patient.

Conclusions of the Physical Examination

The findings of the physical examination confirm the hypothesis of a mechanical hypomobile C1-C2 level dysfunction with a greater occipital nerve involvement. The greater occipital nerve is the direct continuation of the dorsal ramus of the second spinal nerve. The second spinal nerve passes directly posterior to the C1-C2 joint. Therefore, it was initially decided to treat the joint dysfunction and to reassess the effect both on the joint and on the neural mechanosensitivity.

REFERENCES

Bogduk N. Cervical causes of headache and dizziness. In: Boyling JD, Palastanga N, eds. *Grieves' Modern Manual Therapy*. London: Churchill Livingston; 1994:317–331.

Breig A. *Adverse Mechanical Tension in the Central Nervous System*. Stockholm: Almqvist and Wiksell; 1978.

Butler D. *Mobilisation of the Nervous System*. Melbourne: Churchill Livingston; 1991.

Christensen N, Jones M, Edwards I. Clinical reasoning in the diagnosis and management of spinal pain. In: Boyling JD, Jull GA, eds. *Grieves Modern Manual Therapy. The Vertebral Column*. Edinburgh: Churchill Livingstone; 2004:391–404.

De Hertogh WJ, Vaes PH, Vijverman V, de Cordt A, Duquet W. The clinical examination of neck pain patients: the validity of a group of tests. *Man Ther* 2007;12:50–55.

Falla D. Unravelling the complexity of muscle impairment in chronic neck pain. *Man Ther* 2004;9:125–133.

Falla D, Jull G, Hodges P. Patients with neck pain demonstrate reduced electromyographic activity of the deep cervical flexor muscles during performance of the craniocervical flexion test. *Spine* 2004;29:2108–2114.

Fernández-de-las-Peñas C, Alonso-Blanco C, Cuadrado ML, Pareja JA. Spinal manipulative therapy in the management of cervicogenic headache. *Headache* 2005;45:1260–1263.

Fernández-de-las-Peñas C, Alonso-Blanco C, Cuadrado ML, Pareja JA. Forward head posture and neck mobility in chronic tension type headache: a blinded, controlled study. *Cephalalgia* 2006a;26:314–319.

Fernández-de-las-Peñas C, Cuadrado ML, Pareja JA. Myofascial trigger points, neck mobility and forward head posture in unilateral migraine. *Cephalalgia* 2006b;26:1061–1070.

Fernández-de-las-Peñas C, Alonso-Blanco C, Miangolarra-Page JC. Referred pain elicited by posterior-anterior mobilization of the atlanto-axial joint in tension type and cervicogenic headache [abstract]. *Headache* 2006c;46:881.

Hanten WP, Olson SL, Ludwig GM. Reliability of manual mobility testing of the upper cervical spine in subjects with cervicogenic headache. *J Man Manipulative Ther* 2002;10:76–82.

Humpreys BK, Delahaye M, Peterson CK. An investigation into the validity of cervical spine motion palpation using subjects with congenital block vertebrae as a gold standard. *BMC Musculoskelet Disord* 2004;19:1471–1474.

Jones MA. Clinical reasoning in manual therapy. *Phys Ther* 1992;72:875–883.

Jull GA. Examination of the articular system. In: Boyling JD, Palastanga N, eds. *Grieves' Modern Manual Therapy*. 2nd ed. London: Churchill Livingston; 1994:511–528.

Jull GA, Bogduk N, Marsland A. The accuracy of manual diagnosis for cervical zygapophyseal joint pain syndromes. *Med J Aust* 1988;148:233–236.

Jull G, Zito G, Trott P, et al. Inter-examiner reliability to detect painful upper cervical joint dysfunction. *Aust Physiother* 1997;43:125–129.

Jull G, Barrett C, Magee R. Further characterization of muscle dysfunction in cervical headache. *Cephalalgia* 1999;19:179–185.

Jull G, Trott P, Potter H, et al. A randomized controlled trial of exercise and manipulative therapy for cervicogenic headache. *Spine* 2002;27:1835–1843.

Maitland GD, Hengeveld E, Banks K, English K. *Maitland's Vertebral Manipulation*. 7th ed. Edinburgh: Elsevier Health Sciences; 2005.

Nillson N. Evidence that tension-type headache and cervicogenic headache are distinct disorders. *J Manipulative Physiol Ther* 2000;23:288–289.

Piovesan EJ, Kowacs PA, Tatsui CE, et al. Referred pain after stimulation of the greater occipital nerve in humans: evidence of convergence of cervical afferences on trigeminal nuclei. *Cephalalgia* 2001;21:107–109.

Seffinger MA, Najm WI, Mishra SI. Reliability of spinal palpation for diagnosis of back and neck pain: a systematic review of the literature. *Spine* 2004;29:E413–E425.

Sjaastad O, Bovim G. Cervicogenic headache: the differentiation from common migraine, an overview. *Funct Neurol* 1991;6:93–100.

Sjaastad O, Fredriksen TA, Pfaffenrath V. Cervicogenic headache: diagnostic criteria. *Headache* 1998;38:442–445.

Treleaven J, Jull G, Atkinson L. Cervical musculoskeletal dysfunction in post-concussional headache. *Cephalalgia* 1994;14:273–279.

Van Suijlekom JA, de Vet HC, van der Berg SG, Weber WE. Inter-observer reliability of diagnostic criteria for cervicogenic headache. *Cephalalgia* 1999;19:817–823.

Vital JM, Grenier F, Dautheribes M, et al. An anatomic and dynamic study of the greater occipital nerve (Arnold). *Surg Radiol Anat* 1989;11:205–210.

Watson DH. Cervical headache: an investigation of natural head posture and upper cervical flexor muscle performance. In: Boyling JD, Palastanga N, eds. *Grieves' Modern Manual Therapy*. 2nd ed. London: Churchill Livingstone; 1994:349–359.

Watson DH, Trott PH. Cervical headache: an investigation of natural head posture and upper cervical flexor muscle performance. *Cephalalgia* 1993;13:272–284.

Westerhuis P. Zervikogener Kopfschmerz: Perspektive eines Klinikers. In: Von Piekartz HJM, ed. *Kraniofaziale Dysfunktionen und Schmerzen*. Stuttgart: Thieme; 2001:83–99.

Westerhuis P. Cervical instability. In: Von Piekartz HJM, ed. *Cranio-facial pain*. Edinburgh: Butterworth Heinemann; 2007:119–148.

Westerhuis P, von Piekartz HJM. Zervikogener Kopfschmerz: Körperliche Untersuchung und Behandlung. In: Von Piekartz HJM, ed. *Kraniofaziale Dysfunktionen und Schmerzen*. Stuttgart: Thieme; 2001:99–113.

White AA, Panjabi M. *Clinical Biomechanics of the Spine*. 2nd ed. Philadelphia: Lippincott; 1990.

Zito G, Jull G, Stoty I. Clinical tests of musculoskeletal dysfunction in the diagnosis of cervicogenic headache. *Man Ther* 2006;11:118–129.

Thoracic Spine Assessment in Patients with Headache

Bill Egan, PT, DPT, OCS, FAAOMPT, Josh Cleland, PT, DPT, PhD, OCS, FAAOMPT, and Paul Glynn, PT, DPT, OCS, FAAOMPT

Because of the intimate relationship between the thoracic spine, cervical mobility, and the overall posture of the upper quarter, clinicians should examine the mobility of the thoracic spine and rib cage region in patients presenting with cervicogenic or tension-type headache. Mapping studies have suggested that the thoracic spine does not appear to directly refer pain to the head region; however, dysfunction in this area may contribute indirectly to headaches (Dreyfuss et al., 1994; Fukui et al., 1997). Evidence exists suggesting that joint mobility impairments of the upper thoracic region are directly correlated with and are potential risk factors for neck pain, shoulder pain, and headaches (Norlander & Nordgren, 1998). Furthermore, there is emerging evidence that manual therapy treatment of the thoracic spine can decrease pain, improve range of motion, and decrease functional disability in patients with mechanical neck pain, cervical radiculopathy, postwhiplash-related pain, and cervical myelopathy (Browder et al., 2004; Cleland et al., 2005a, 2005b; Fernández-de-las-Peñas et al., 2004, 2007; Flynn et al., 2001; Savolainen et al., 2004). Additionally, preliminary evidence exists supporting the notion that interventions directed at the thoracic spine can improve symptoms in patients with headaches (Viti & Paris, 2000). Extrapolating the findings from these studies involving patients with neck pain, it is plausible that treatment of the thoracic spine can improve symptoms in patients with cervicogenic or tension-type headache. We are not suggesting assessment and treatment of the thoracic spine region in isolation. Rather, addressing impairments in the thoracic spine region should be part of a comprehensive treatment plan that involves evaluation and treatment of the cervical and other related upper quarter regions (Jull et al., 2002).

This chapter describes a comprehensive evaluation scheme of the thoracic spine tailored to the patient presenting with headaches. Identified thoracic spine impairments are classified and directly correspond to the interventions presented in Chapter 24.

EXAMINATION OF THE THORACIC SPINE

As previously mentioned, the examination of the thoracic spine should constitute part of a comprehensive upper quarter examination. What follows are those parts of the examination that focus specifically on the thoracic region. Readers are referred to Chapter 14 for information regarding examination of the cervical spine and subcranial region.

Seated Examination

Postural Scan

The examination of the thoracic spine begins with an overall assessment of the contour and posture of the region. While viewing the patient posteriorly, the shape of the thoracic curve is noted, as are any deviations in the front plane. From the lateral view the convexity of the normal kyphosis is noted. In particular, judgments of areas of increased or decreased kyphosis are made relative to what is considered a normal kyphotic curve. In the scientific literature there has been little to no relationship found between postural impairments of the thoracic spine and any specific upper quarter pain syndrome (Griegel-Morris et al., 1992; Refshauge et al., 1995). Nevertheless, the postural screen may indicate potential areas of movement impairment. For example, a common finding in patients with neck pain is the presence of a reduced kyphosis in the upper to midthoracic region (T3 to T5). **Figure 15.1** depicts a patient with a reduced T3-T5 kyphosis. This could indicate the presence of a restriction in thoracic flexion at that region due to the relative flattening or extension of this region compared with the usual, gradual kyphosis.

In a clinical study, Cleland et al. (2007) found that reduced kyphosis of the T3-T5 region was associated with

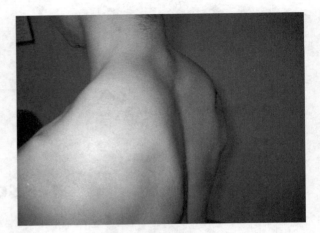

Figure 15.1 Postural Assessment Depicting Decreased Kyphosis of the T3-T5 Region

a positive response to thoracic spine thrust manipulation in patients with neck pain, many of whom also reported the presence of headaches. Cleland et al. (2006) studied the interrater reliability of postural assessment of the thoracic spine in patients with neck pain. They divided the spine into three regions: T1 to T2, T3 to T5, and T6 to T10. Judgment was made for the presence of increased or decreased kyphosis at each region. Good to excellent ICC values (0.58–0.9) were found for assessment of posture across all three regions.

Cervical Active Range of Motion

With the patient seated, cervical range of motion is tested next. Based on the opinion of several clinical experts and emerging evidence, we often use cervical range of motion and symptom reproduction with active cervical range of motion as a test-retest measure when using manual interventions directed toward the thoracic spine in patients with neck pain (Erhard, 1996; Flynn et al., 2001; Greenman, 1996). Flynn et al. (2001) found an immediate increase in cervical range of motion after thrust manipulation of the thoracic spine in 26 patients presenting with neck pain. Patients' cervical mobility was measured using a gravity inclinometer before and immediately following manipulation directed to the thoracic spine. Manipulative techniques were selected based on clinical examination findings. The results were as follows: mean flexion increased by 13°, mean total side bending increased by 8°, and mean extension increased by 3°.

The gravity inclinometer allows for accurate and efficient measurement of cervical range of motion. For

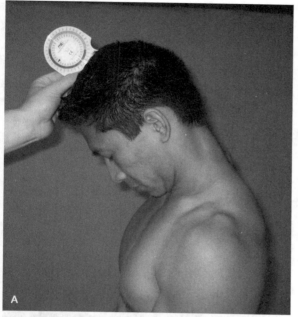

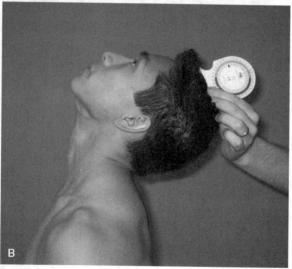

Figure 15.2 A: Cervical Flexion Range of Motion Measurement Utilizing the Gravity Inclinometer. B: Cervical Extension Range of Motion Measurement Utilizing the Gravity Inclinometer

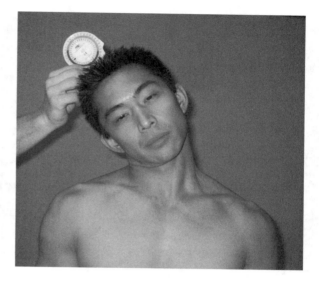

Figure 15.3 Cervical Side-Bending Range of Motion Measurement Utilizing the Gravity Inclinometer

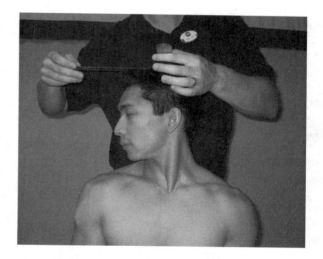

Figure 15.4 Cervical Rotation Range of Motion Measurement Utilizing a Standard Goniometer

flexion (**Figure 15.2A**) and extension (**Figure 15.2B**), the inclinometer is placed on the center of the patient's head in the sagittal plane. The clinician inquires about baseline symptoms, and the patient is instructed to actively flex and extend his or her neck. The clinician follows the motion with the inclinometer and records the motion at end range. Further, any change in the

patient's symptoms from baseline is recorded. A similar procedure is utilized for right and left side-bending, with the inclinometer placed on the center of the head in the frontal plane (**Figure 15.3**). For cervical rotation, a standard dual-armed goniometer is utilized (**Figure 15.4**). Several studies that have investigated the interrater reliability of the aforementioned range of motion procedures found good to excellent reliability for all measures of cervical range of motion (Cleland et al., 2006; Piva et al., 2006; Wainner et al., 2003). Reliability of the assessment of symptom reproduction during active cervical range of motion varies more widely, with some measures showing poor reliability whereas others are good to excellent (Cleland et al., 2006; Piva et al., 2006).

A biomechanical link between the upper thoracic and cervical spine has been proposed in the literature (Norlander & Nordgren, 1998). Further, research has shown that thoracic spine thrust manipulation can produce a short-term increase in cervical range of motion and decrease in pain (Cleland et al., 2005a, 2007; Fernández-de-las-Peñas et al., 2007; Flynn et al., 2001). For these reasons we would suggest that cervical range of motion and its effect on symptoms be reassessed after any manual therapy procedure directed to the thoracic spine in a patient presenting with a headache.

Thoracic Rotation

A functional test for the presence of thoracic spine restriction is conducted next. The patient is seated with his or her arms crossed. The patient is instructed to actively rotate his or her trunk to the right and to the left without changing the position of the head or neck (**Figure 15.5A**). If no symptoms are evoked, the examiner can then apply passive overpressure to end-range rotation in each direction (**Figure 15.5B**). The examiner notes both the change from baseline in symptoms, if any, and the relative amount of rotation occurring to each side.

Cleland et al. (2006) reported on the reliability of assessing for the presence of symptoms during thoracic rotation in patients with neck pain. They found an ICC of −0.03 for thoracic right rotation and 0.7 for thoracic left rotation. The low ICC for right rotation could be explained by the lower prevalence of symptoms reported with right rotation (63%) versus left rotation (73%) by patients in this study. This was the first study in which the reliability of the thoracic spine rotation test was assessed in patients with neck pain. Further research is required to examine the reliability of thoracic spine rotation in patients with neck pain. In a patient presenting with headache, it would be unusual to replicate headache symptoms with this test; however, asymmetrical motion or thoracic spine pain would not be unexpected.

Palpatory Examination

With the patient seated, a palpatory scan is next conducted. For the thoracic spine, running the fingertips

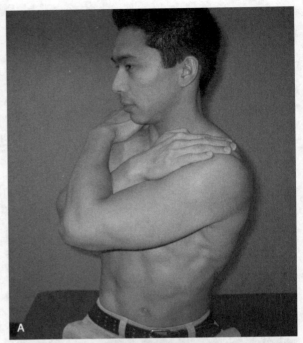

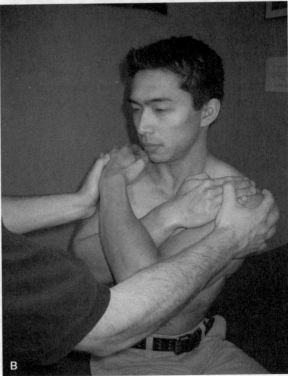

Figure 15.5 A: Seated Active Thoracic Rotation Test Without Overpressure. B: Seated Active Thoracic Rotation Test with Overpressure

down either side of the vertebral gutters just lateral to the spinous process can be useful to assess for the presence of soft-tissue texture changes, pain, or tenderness (**Figure 15.6**). Both tissue texture change and tenderness can indicate potential underlying segmental dysfunction. To assess for the presence of rib cage dysfunction, the contour of the rib angle is next palpated. The patient crosses his or her hand over the contralateral shoulder to protract the scapula out of the way. The clinician palpates over the rib angle, assessing the contour and the presence of pain or tenderness (**Figure 15.7**). Tenderness of the rib angle is a marker for potential underlying rib dysfunction.

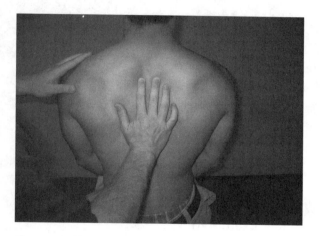

Figure 15.6 Palpation of the Soft Tissue of the Thoracic Spine Region

First Rib Examination

Because of its location, the first rib is palpated differently from the others. With the patient seated, the examiner gently pulls posteriorly on the upper trapezius muscle while palpating inferiorly for the superior shaft of the first rib (**Figure 15.8**). The clinician assesses for the presence of tenderness and the relative height of the first rib compared with the other side. A first rib shaft that is superior with respect to the contralateral side suggests the presence of an elevated first rib. Lindgren et al. (1992) devised a test, confirmed with cineradiology, for the presence of an elevated first rib. The cervical rotation lateral flexion test (CRLF) is conducted by passively rotating the patient's head away from the side to be tested and then laterally flexing the head toward the chest (**Figure 15.9**). The test is repeated with the neck rotated to the other side. The presence of restricted neck lateral flexion in this position suggests the presence of an elevated rib on the side contralateral to the neck rotation.

Similar to the other tests described so far, the reproduction of headache symptoms would not be expected. The test, as described by Lindgren et al. (1992), was devised for patients suffering from thoracic outlet syndrome. Nevertheless, the authors frequently use this test in patients with mechanical neck pain to assess for the presence of an elevated first rib. An elevated first rib could contribute to a patient's headache symptoms because of the hypertonicity of the scalene that is usually associated with a first rib impairment. The middle scalene attaches to the transverse processes of C1 to C6 segments. Hypertonicity of the scalene could contribute

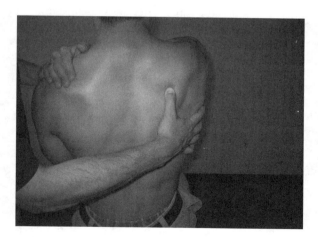

Figure 15.7 Palpation of the Rib Angle

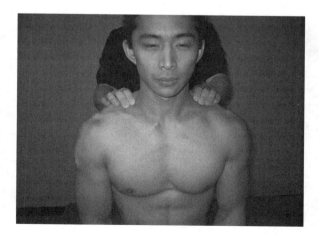

Figure 15.8 Palpation of the First Rib

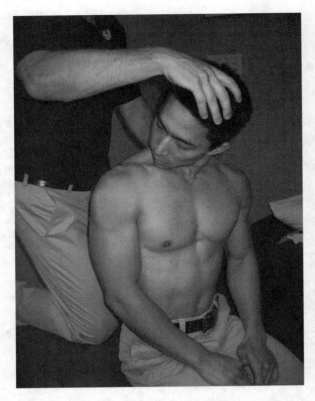

Figure 15.9 Cervical Rotation Lateral Flexion Test for First Rib Dysfunction

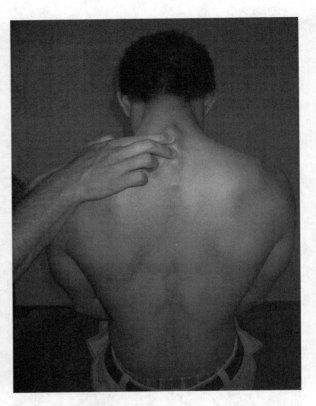

Figure 15.10 Upper Thoracic Flexion Passive Physiologic Intervertebral Motion Test

to dysfunction of the upper cervical spine (Greenman, 1996).

Upper Thoracic Passive Physiologic Intervertebral Movement Testing

While the patient is in the seated position, the next recommended procedure is the upper thoracic segmental examination. Using the fingertips, the C7-T1, T1-2, and T2-3 interspaces are palpated. The clinician passively flexes and extends the patient's neck, feeling for the relative amount of widening of the interspace during flexion and of closing during extension (**Figure 15.10**). Norlander and Nordgren (1998) found that a relative reduction in flexion between C7 and T1 compared with T1 and T2 was associated with patients who had neck/shoulder pain, some who also reported headaches. Therefore, in a patient with headache and limited cervical flexion mobility, assessment of the upper thoracic spine for potential restriction would be indicated.

Prone Examination

Thoracic Passive Accessory Intervertebral Movement Testing

Examination of the thoracic spine proceeds with the patient in a prone position. Previously identified areas of tenderness and soft-tissue hypertonicity can be assessed again. Accessory motion testing via posterior-to-anterior spring testing is commenced at each thoracic vertebral level in addition to the ribs. For the thoracic spine, the clinician places his or her hypothenar eminence over the thoracic spinous process and directs posterior-to-anterior force (**Figure 15.11**). The clinician may need to change the angle of his or her hand depending on the contour of the thoracic spine to maintain the forces in the true anterior-to-posterior plane. The clinician records the presence of hypomobility or hypermobility at each level and also the presence of local or referred symptoms. When examining patients with headaches, it is recommended that, at the least, thoracic segments T1 to T6 be screened. Cleland et al.

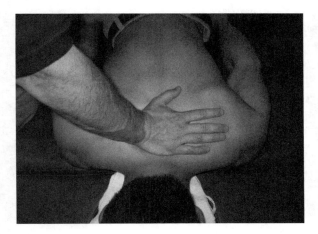

Figure 15.11 Prone Thoracic Passive Accessory Intervertebral Motion Test

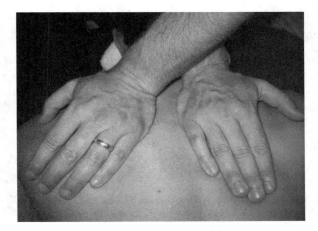

Figure 15.12 Prone Rib Spring Test

(2006) reported a weighted kappa of between 0.13 to 0.82 for interrater reliability of spring testing, assessing for hypomobility from T1 to T7. In the same study, weighted kappa for pain provocation with springing was −0.10 to 0.90.

Typical Rib Passive Accessory Intervertebral Movement Testing

Springing over the ribs is accomplished using a crossed-hand technique. Standing at the head of the prone patient, the clinician places his or her right hypothenar eminence over the patient's left rib just lateral to the transverse process. The clinician's left hypothenar eminence is used to stabilize the right transverse process of the same segment (**Figure 15.12**). The clinician springs the rib in an anterior-to-posterior direction along the posterior shaft of the rib. The clinician records the presence of hypomobility or hypermobility and the presence of local or referred symptoms. In patients with headaches, the second through sixth ribs, at the least, should be examined in this fashion. The first rib examination has already been described.

Assessment of Muscle Length and Strength

The following procedures are designed to assess the length and strength of various muscles that can potentially influence the thoracic spine and rib cage. This is not an exhaustive list but rather the muscles more commonly tested and thought to contribute to impairments

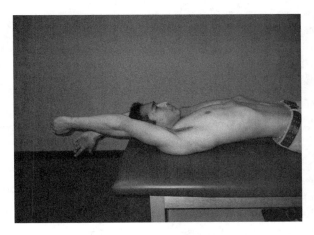

Figure 15.13 Muscle Length Testing of the Latissimus Dorsi Muscle

of the thoracic spine and rib cage (Flynn et al., 2000; Greenman, 1996). Cleland et al. (2006) studied the reliability of these assessment procedures.

Muscle Length: Latissimus Dorsi

The latissimus dorsi muscle is tested with the patient supine. The patient actively flexes both upper extremities to his or her end range. Normal length of the latissimus dorsi muscle is considered when the patient can lay his or her hands flat on the table (**Figure 15.13**). The examiner ensures that the patient does not compensate by extending the thoracolumbar spine or moving the upper extremity out of the sagittal plane. Reliability (κ) of the length of assessment for the right latissimus dorsi

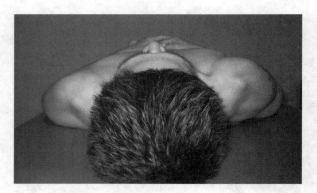

Figure 15.14 Muscle Length Testing of the Pectoral Minor Muscle

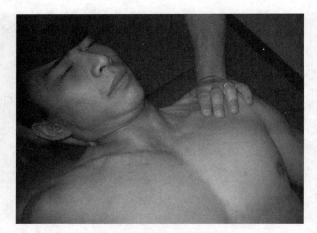

Figure 15.15 Muscle Length Testing of the Left Anterior and Middle Scalene Muscles

was 0.83 and for the left latissimus dorsi was 0.62 (Cleland et al., 2006). Unilateral or bilateral shortening of the latissimus dorsi is thought to contribute to thoracic spine extension restrictions.

Muscle Length: Pectoralis Minor

The pectoralis minor muscle is assessed with the patient supine. The examiner observes the height of the shoulders in the frontal plane (**Figure 15.14**). An anterior position of the shoulder girdle, either unilaterally or bilaterally, is considered to be due to impaired length of the pectoral minor muscle. Reliability (κ) of the pectoralis muscle length assessment was 0.81 for the right side and 0.71 for the left side (Cleland et al., 2006). According to Bookhout (2001), a tight shoulder posterior capsule can also cause this forward shoulder position. If caused by a tight posterior capsule, the anterior-to-posterior glide of the humerus would be restricted. Because of its attachment onto the anterior rib cage (ribs 2 to 5), reduced length of the pectoralis minor could contribute to dysfunction of the rib cage in addition to postural impairment of the shoulder girdle.

Muscle Length: Scalene

The scalene muscle's length is assessed with the patient supine with his or her head off the end of the treatment table. When assessing the left side, the clinician uses his or her right hand to support the patient's head under the occiput and right shoulder over the patient's forehead. With his or her left hand, the clinician stabilizes the patient's first rib and clavicle. With his or her right hand and shoulder, the clinician translates the patient's head into cervical retraction, right side-bending, and left

rotation until the patient reports a stretching sensation in the scalene region (**Figure 15.15**). Muscle length of the scalene muscle is compared with the opposite side. The reliability (κ) of scalene muscle length assessment was 0.81 for the right side and 0.62 for the left side (Cleland et al., 2006). As mentioned previously, shortening of the scalene muscles could contribute to an elevated first rib.

Muscle Strength: Middle and Lower Trapezius

To test the strength and motor control of the right middle and lower trapezius muscles, the patient is positioned prone with his or her right arm off the side of the table. With the upper extremity in external rotation (thumb toward the ceiling), the patient is instructed to horizontally abduct the upper extremity in approximately 90° of abduction for the middle trapezius (**Figure 15.16A**) and 120° to 130° of abduction for the lower trapezius muscle (**Figure 15.16B**). The clinician observes for scapular depression, adduction, and upward rotation. In the study by Cleland et al. (2006), reliability (κ) of the muscle strength test for the middle and lower trapezius was between −0.04 to −0.07. This was most likely due to the almost 100% prevalence of positive findings for both of these tests. Clinically, the most common substitution for weakness and impaired motor control of the middle and lower trapezius is excessive scapular elevation. Hypomobility of the mid- to lower thoracic spine is thought to contribute to inhibition of the lower trapezius (Bookhout, 2001). Two studies

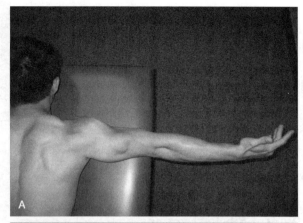

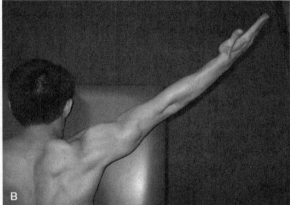

Figure 15.16 A: Manual Muscle Testing of the Middle Trapezius Muscle. B: Manual Muscle Testing of the Lower Trapezius Muscle

demonstrated improved activation of the lower trapezius muscle in a normal subject population following either nonthrust mobilization (Liebler et al., 2001) or thrust manipulation of the mid- to lower thoracic spine (Cleland et al., 2004).

Muscle Strength: Serratus Anterior

Assessment of the strength of the serratus anterior is conducted with the patient standing. The patient flexes his or her upper extremity to 120° to 130°, and the clinician observes for scapular winging (**Figure 15.17**). In the absence of winging, the clinician applies manual downward pressure to the upper extremity. The clinician observes or palpates for scapular winging or movement of the scapular inferior angle away from the rib cage. Reliability (κ) of the serratus anterior muscle strength assessment was 0.11 for the right side and 0.77

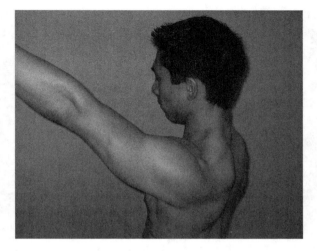

Figure 15.17 Manual Muscle Testing of the Serratus Anterior Muscle

for the left side (Cleland et al., 2006). Weakness and inhibition of the serratus anterior are thought to be associated with flexion restrictions of the upper to mid-thoracic spine, although this theory has not been researched at this time (Bookhout, 2001).

MOTION IMPAIRMENT–BASED DIAGNOSIS DERIVED FROM PHYSICAL EXAMINATION

From the physical examination of the thoracic spine and rib cage, movement impairments of the thoracic spine can be identified and matched with a manual therapy intervention. For example, a clinician could combine the findings of reduced cervical flexion range of motion, soft-tissue tenderness around the T3 to T5 area, hypomobility with spring of the T3 to T5 segments, and a reduced kyphosis from T3 to T5. Based on these findings, the clinician could select a thrust manipulation targeting the T3 to T5 region in an attempt to produce flexion to this area (Chapter 24). Some models of manual therapy espouse very specific biomechanical assessment with accompanying treatment for each specific biomechanical-based movement dysfunction. Although the authors do not desire to discredit these models and the pioneers who have helped develop them, emerging evidence suggests that the accuracy and reliability of many manual physical examination procedures that purport to identify specific biomechanical lesions are poor. Furthermore, evidence suggests that the specificity of treatment techniques directed toward these biomechanical-based restrictions is less than was previously thought. For example, in the thoracic spine, Ross et al. (2004) recorded audible cavitations during thrust manipulation procedures. They found that the audible cavitation occurred, on average, within 3.5 cm vertebral levels above or below the targeted segment. In most cases between two and six audible cavitations occurred during an individual manipulation.

In the manual therapy literature, much is made of the direction of the restriction and the subsequent direction of the manual therapy technique to correct the biomechanical lesion. In a study conducted by Bereznick et al. (2002), clinicians were unable to direct a force vector in a specific direction during a prone manipulative procedure to the thoracic spine. Using complex modeling, these researchers determined that friction does not exist at the thoracic-skin interface to allow for thrusting a thoracic segment in a cephalic direction during the manipulation. Further, the study also cast doubt on the ability to hook onto either a thoracic spinous or transverse process during the manipulation. Although this was an experimental model, the authors concluded that their study challenges the concept of directional specificity during spinal thrust manipulation. Keeping this evidence in mind, the authors believe that it is still useful to derive movement impairment–based diagnoses from the physical examination of the thoracic spine. The diagnosis will direct the clinician toward the level of the restriction and the direction of the movement impairment.

Flexion Restrictions

Limited thoracic flexion can occur throughout all regions of the thoracic spine. A flexion restriction is a limitation in the ability to forward bend in one or more thoracic segments. There are several physical examination findings that would direct the clinician toward diagnosing a flexion restriction at a particular region. The first is local tenderness and hypertonicity of the soft tissue surrounding a particular vertebral region. Tenderness and increased soft-tissue texture changes could indicate underlying segmental dysfunction at that region. Another finding is pain and hypomobility as assessed with posterior-to-anterior spring testing. Postural assessment could also indicate a region of relative flattening in the normally kyphotic thoracic spine. Finally, there should be restriction of gross cervical spine flexion mobility, especially with restrictions in the upper thoracic spine.

Extension Restrictions

Limitation of thoracic extension can occur throughout all thoracic regions. An extension restriction is the inability to bend backward at one or more thoracic segments. Similar to flexion restrictions, extension restrictions in the thoracic spine would also be expected to have soft-tissue tenderness and hypomobility with spring testing. Postural assessment may reveal an area of increased thoracic kyphosis in a particular region. Finally, gross cervical range of motion should be limited in extension.

Typical Rib Restrictions

Segmental restrictions of the ribs can occur at any level. Although the reliability of testing of segmental rib joint motion has not been studied, it is expected that the reliability and validity of such assessments would be comparable to other regions of the spine. Therefore, a more generalized diagnosis of hypomobility is described here. A typical rib restriction would include tenderness and soft-tissue hypertonicity at the rib angle. In addition, pain and hypomobility could be found with posterior-to-anterior spring testing over the rib. Clinically, the most common of the typical rib impairments found is a restriction of the fifth rib in association with a thoracic flexion restriction of the T4-5 (Flynn et al., 2000).

First Rib Restrictions

The particular case of an elevated first rib would have findings distinguishing it from other rib dysfunctions. Diagnosis of an elevated first rib is based on the findings of tenderness with palpation of the rib, the superior position of the rib in comparison with the other side, and a positive CRLF test with the head rotated to the contralateral side.

CONCLUSIONS

As mentioned previously, it would be unusual to reproduce a patient's headache symptoms during the assessment of the thoracic spine and rib cage; however, restriction of gross cervical range of motion and movement restrictions of the thoracic spine would not be unexpected. After the clinician identifies thoracic spine impairments, the final part of the thoracic spine assessment would be the treatment of the impairments with manual therapy techniques that can be augmented with exercise. Immediately following the intervention, key impairments would be retested and the patient's signs and symptoms reassessed. Chapter 24 describes manual therapy and exercise interventions that coincide with the thoracic spine and rib cage impairments identified in this chapter. At this time direct evidence for evaluation and treatment of the thoracic spine and rib cage in patients with headaches is limited. However, there is a growing body of evidence that manual therapy for the thoracic spine can be effective for patients with mechanical neck pain and radiculopathy. Following the concept of regional interdependence, the thoracic spine could potentially contribute to a patient's headaches because of its influence on the posture of the upper quarter, the contribution of the thoracic spine to gross cervical range of motion, and the muscular connections between the upper cervical and upper thoracic spines.

REFERENCES

Bereznick DE, Ross JK, McGill SM. The frictional properties at the thoracic skin-fascia interface: implications in spine manipulation. *Clin Biomech* 2002;17:297–303.

Browder DA, Erhard RE, Piva SR. Intermittent cervical traction and thoracic manipulation for management of mild cervical compressive myelopathy attributed to cervical herniated disc: a case series. *J Orthop Sports Phys Ther* 2004;34: 701–712.

Cleland JA, Selleck BS, Stowel T, et al. Short-term effects of thoracic manipulation on lower trapezius muscle strength. *J Man Manipulative Ther* 2004;12:82–90.

Cleland JA, Childs JD, McRae M, Palmer JA, Stowell T. Immediate effects of thoracic manipulation in patients with neck pain: a randomized clinical trial. *Man Ther* 2005a; 10:127–135.

Cleland JA, Whitman JM, Fritz JM, Palmer JA. Manual physical therapy, cervical traction, and strengthening exercises in patients with cervical radiculopathy: a case series. *J Orthop Sports Phys Ther* 2005b;35:802–811.

Cleland JA, Childs JD, Fritz JM, Whitman JM. Interrater reliability of the history and physical examination in patients with mechanical neck pain. *Arch Phys Med Rehabil* 2006;87:1388–1395.

Cleland JA, Childs JD, Fritz JM, Whitman JM, Eberhart SL. Development of a clinical prediction rule for guiding treatment of a subgroup of patients with neck pain: use of thoracic spine manipulation, exercise, and patient education. *Phys Ther* 2007;87:9–23.

Dreyfuss P, Tibiletti C, Dreyer SJ. Thoracic zygapophyseal joint pain patterns: a study in normal volunteers. *Spine* 1994; 19:807–811.

Erhard RE. *Manual Therapy in the Cervical Spine. Orthopedic Physical Therapy Home Study Course.* La Crosse, WI: American Physical Therapy Association; 1996.

Fernández-de-las-Peñas C, Fernández-Carnero J, Plaza-Fernández A, Lomas-Vega R, Miangolarra JC. Dorsal manipulation in whiplash injury treatment: a randomized controlled trial. *J Whiplash Related Disord* 2004;3:55–72.

Fernández-de-las-Peñas C, Palomeque-del-Cerro L, Rodríguez-Blanco C, et al. Changes in neck pain and active range of motion after a single thoracic spine manipulation in patients with mechanical neck pain: a case series. *J Manipulative Physiol Ther* 2007;30:312–320.

Flynn T, Whitman J, Magel J. *Orthopedic Manual Physical Therapy Management of the Cervico-thoracic Spine and Rib Cage.* Fort Collins, CO: Manipulations Inc.; 2000.

Flynn T, Wainner R, Whitman J. Immediate effects of thoracic spine manipulation on cervical range of motion and pain. *J Man Manipulative Ther* 2001;9:164.

Fukui S, Ohseto K, Shiotani M. Patterns of pain induced by distending the thoracic zygapophyseal joints. *Reg Anesth* 1997;22:332–336.

Greenman P. *Principles of Manual Medicine.* 2nd ed. Philadelphia: Lippincott Williams & Wilkins; 1996.

Griegel-Morris P, Larson K, Mueller-Klaus K, Oatis CA. Incidence of common postural abnormalities in the cervical, shoulder, and thoracic regions and their association with pain in two age groups of healthy subjects. *Phys Ther* 1992;72:425–431.

Jull G, Trott P, Potter H, Zito G, et al. A randomized controlled trial of exercise and manipulative therapy for cervicogenic headache. *Spine* 2002;27:1835–1843.

Liebler EJ, Tufano-Coors L, Douris P, Makofsky H, et al. The effect of thoracic spine mobilization on lower trapezius strength testing. *J Man Manipulative Ther* 2001;9: 207–212.

Lindgren K-A, Leino E, Manninen H. Cervical rotation lateral flexion test in brachialgia. *Arch Phys Med Rehabil* 1992;73: 735–737.

Norlander S, Nordgren B. Clinical symptoms related to musculoskeletal neck-shoulder pain and mobility in the cervico-thoracic spine. *Scand J Rehabil Med* 1998;30: 243–251.

Piva SR, Erhard R, Childs JD, Browder D. Inter-tester reliability of passive inter-vertebral and active movements of the cervical spine. *Man Ther* 2006;11:321–330.

Refshauge K, Bolst L, Goodsell M. The relationship between cervicothoracic posture and the presence of pain. *J Man Manipulative Ther* 1995;3:21–24.

Ross JK, Bereznick DE, McGill SM. Determining cavitation location during lumbar and thoracic spinal manipulation: is spinal manipulation accurate and specific? *Spine* 2004;29: 1452–1457.

Savolainen A, Ahlberg J, Nummila H, Nissinen M. Active or passive treatment for neck-shoulder pain in occupational health care? A randomized controlled trial. *Occup Med* 2004;54:422–424.

Viti JA, Paris SV. The use of upper thoracic manipulation in a patient with headache. *J Man Manipulative Ther* 2000;8:25–28.

Wainner RS, Fritz JM, Irrgang JJ, Boninger ML, Delitto A, Allison S. Reliability and diagnostic accuracy of the clinical examination and patient self-report measures for cervical radiculopathy. *Spine* 2003;28:52–62.

Manual Identification of Trigger Points in the Muscles Associated with Headache

César Fernández-de-las-Peñas, PT, DO, PhD, Hong-You Ge, MD, PhD, and Jan Dommerholt, PT, MPS

Simons et al. (1999) identified a muscle trigger point (TrP) as a hyperirritable spot associated with a taut band of a skeletal muscle that is painful on compression, stretch, overload, or contraction in the shortened position and responds with a referred pain pattern that is often distant from the spot. From a clinical point of view, active TrPs cause pain symptoms, and their local and referred pain resemble a usual or familiar pain for the

subject (Simons et al., 1999). In patients, the referred pain elicited by an active TrP reproduces at least part of their clinical pain pattern.

In patients presenting with headache, active TrPs are those TrPs in which the quality of the referred pain is similar to the sensations that the patients usually perceive during their spontaneous headache attacks, or those TrPs that reproduce the patient's headache upon examination. Latent TrPs also evoke referred pain upon mechanical stimulation, muscle contraction, or stretching, but this elicited pain is not a familiar or usual pain for the patient (Simons et al., 1999). Both active and latent muscle TrPs can provoke motor dysfunctions (e.g., muscle weakness) due to inhibition, increased motor irritability (spasm), muscle imbalance, or altered motor recruitment (Lucas et al., 2004) in either the affected muscle or in functionally related muscles (Simons et al., 1999).

Muscle TrPs are initially identified as requiring examination by manual palpation by a history of musculoskeletal or any enigmatic pain complaint. The diagnosis of a TrP for research purposes involves the identification of several features: (a) presence of a taut band in a skeletal muscle when accessible to palpation, (b) presence of a tender spot within the taut band, (c) palpable or visible local twitch response on snapping palpation (or needling) of the TrP, and (d) presence of referred pain elicited by stimulation or palpation of the sensitive spot (Simons et al., 1999).

TrP diagnosis requires adequate manual ability, training, and clinical practice to develop a high degree of reliability in the examination (Simons et al., 1999). For practical clinical purposes, Simons et al. (1999) and Gerwin et al. (1997) recommend that the *minimum* acceptable criteria for active muscle TrP diagnosis be the combination of the presence of a tender spot in a palpable taut band within a skeletal muscle and the patient's recognition of the referred pain elicited by pressure applied to the tender spot as a usual symptom. Latent TrPs are diagnosed in a similar way, but the difference is that the subject does not recognize the elicited referred pain as a familiar or usual symptom (Simons et al., 1999). Additional helpful clinical guides to which muscles need examination are painfully restricted stretch range of motion, muscle weakness, pain on contraction in the shortened position, and muscle tenderness to palpation. Nevertheless, there is no widely accepted clinical diagnosis of TrPs. Further research is needed to test the reliability and validity of TrP diagnostic criteria (Tough et al., 2007).

RELIABILITY OF MUSCLE TRIGGER POINT EXAMINATION

Interrater Reliability Studies of Muscle Trigger Point Diagnosis

Several studies published in the peer-reviewed literature have investigated the interexaminer reliability of muscle

TrP diagnosis. Wolfe et al. (1992), in a preliminary study, reported good concordance among rheumatologists when identifying tender points, but poor correlation for identification of muscle TrPs among experienced examiners. The examiners had 2 hours of practice prior to examination. During this time the rheumatologists were instructed in muscle TrP examination techniques, whereas the nonrheumatologists were instructed in tender point assessment. The instruction in palpation of TrPs included several muscles of both the upper and lower extremities. The study design allowed 15 minutes to evaluate muscle TrPs, which was clearly too short a time period for a correct TrP examination.

Nice et al. (1992) found poor agreement among examiners attempting to identify TrPs in the thoracolumbar erector muscles in patients presenting with low back pain by eliciting tenderness that reproduced both local and referred pain to the symptomatic region, but without attempting to identify taut band or local twitch responses. The identification of muscle TrPs was based on three features: local tenderness, reproduction of local pain, and referred pain in the symptomatic zone. Eleven percent of the responses were excluded because the elicited pain was referred outside the symptomatic area. Nevertheless, these points may still have fulfilled the definition of latent TrPs, which are also known to be clinically relevant (Simons et al., 1999; Lucas et al., 2004). Despite these limitations, the percent agreement for the three sites ranged from 76% to 79% (Nice et al., 1992).

Njoo and Van der Does (1994) found that palpation of the taut band, presence of local tenderness, and reproduction of pain symptoms were reliable signs among different examiners when studying TrPs in the quadratus lumborum or gluteus medius muscles in subjects suffering from low back pain. Insufficient numbers of positive responses limited the evaluation of local twitch responses and referred pain pattern. The examiners were either an experienced general practitioner or medical students at the end of their training, who spent 3 months working with the practitioner. These authors reported kappa values ranging from 0.09 to 0.7 (Njoo & Van der Does, 1994). Local tenderness (including the jump sign) and reproduction of symptoms were reliable signs in both muscles. Identification of taut bands was reliable in the gluteus medius muscle and approached reliability in the quadratus lumborum muscle (kappa = 0.47). However, the muscles selected in this study can be difficult to examine for all of the clinical features of

TrPs. The quadratus lumborum is a thin, deep muscle that presents problems in examination, especially for the identification of taut bands or local twitch responses (Simons et al., 1999). Further, the gluteus medius muscle was examined only for the presence of an anterior TrP, where local twitch responses are difficult to elicit.

Gerwin et al. (1997) reported good interexaminer reliability (kappa) ranging from 0.84 to 0.88 for the palpation of the tender spot within a taut band and for patients' recognition of the referred pain. Nevertheless, the reliability of identification of certain features of TrPs varies among muscles. In addition, they found that a taut band or local twitch response was very common in some muscles but not in others. For instance, taut bands were found in 100% of the extensor digitorum muscles, whereas the local twitch response was found in 98%. However, identification of the taut band in the infraspinatus muscle was less certain than in the extensor digitorum muscle. The authors concluded that the taut band and hypersensitive spot were the most reliable muscle TrP features to identify, and the minimal criteria for its identification, whereas the referred pain and local twitch responses were most useful as confirmatory signs for TrP diagnosis.

Lew et al. (1997) found that the agreement between two experienced clinicians in identifying the location of latent TrPs in the upper trapezius muscle by palpating for a taut band was poor despite effort to optimize the likelihood of agreement. One of the main limitations of this study was the inclusion of asymptomatic subjects.

Hsieh et al. (2000) found that referred pain was marginally reliable among nonexpert physicians with good training (kappa = 0.43), but not reliable without training (kappa = 0.32). However, both trained and untrained physicians did not show acceptable reliability when results were compared with those reported by an experienced assessor (Gerwin et al., 1997). It seems that training attempting to standardize the pressure for palpating referred pain would help to achieve a marginal interexaminer reliability for the nonexpert physicians and a higher reliability for the expert physicians.

Sciotti et al. (2001) confirmed that a group of four experienced, well-trained clinicians can diagnose and precisely locate latent TrPs within the trapezius muscle with a precision of 5.3, 5.3, and 4.6 millimeters in the mediolateral, superior-inferior, and anterior-posterior directions compared with a computer program. Additionally, these findings indicate that sufficient reliability (G coefficient >80%) can be obtained by averaging the results of two trained clinicians.

Bron et al. (2007) evaluated patients having subacromial impingement, rotator cuff disease, tendonitis, tendinopathy, or chronic subdeltoid-subacromial bursitis. Three examiners palpated the infraspinatus, the anterior deltoid, and the biceps brachii muscles for clinical characteristics of a total of 12 muscle TrPs. In this study, the most reliable features of TrPs were the referred pain sensation and the jump sign. Percentage of pairwise agreement (PA) was 70% or greater (range 63–93%) in all but three instances for the referred pain sensation. For the jump sign, PA was 70% or greater (range 67–77%) in 21 instances. Finding a nodule in a taut band (PA = 45–90%) and eliciting a local twitch response (PA = 33–100%) were shown to be least reliable. The best agreement regarding the presence or absence of TrPs was found for the infraspinatus muscle (PA = 69–80%).

Finally, there are a number of factors that may have contributed to the varying reliability of the results from different studies, including lack of identification of a taut band, which is one of the minimum acceptable muscle TrP diagnostic criteria (Simons et al., 1999); inexperience of the examiners in assessing muscle TrPs; incorrect positioning of the patient or the assessor; incorrect palpation techniques; and variation in the amount of manual force exerted on the palpated point and the duration of force applied.

Clinical Signs for Muscle Trigger Point Diagnosis

Based on published studies and clinical experiences, the reliability of each of the clinical signs used for TrP diagnosis is analyzed in this section.

Palpable Taut Band in a Skeletal Muscle

A palpable taut band in a skeletal muscle is a required sign for TrP diagnosis, although it may also occur in normal muscles without other clinical evidence of TrPs. Palpating for the taut band, however, requires manual skill. Palpation of a taut band in a deep muscle is especially difficult for a nonexperienced examiner. In addition, a study has examined the presence of muscle TrP taut bands with magnetic resonance imaging (Chen et al., 2007).

Hypersensitive Spot Within a Taut Band

A hypersensitive spot is an essential finding when examining for muscle TrPs (Gerwin et al., 1997; Simons et al., 1999). Spot tenderness is not, however, a specific sign of TrPs because it is also a defining characteristic of tender points of fibromyalgia syndrome (Wolfe et al., 1992), which are often located where TrPs are likely to occur. There is no published study investigating the correlation of tender areas used for the diagnosis of fibromyalgia syndrome (Wolfe et al., 1990) and the presence of muscle TrPs. In addition, hypersensitive spots of TrPs are found in a taut band of an accessible muscle, but not in all muscles. Finally, a tender spot (local pressure required to produce local pain) has higher reliability than referred pain.

Local Twitch Response

A local twitch response appears to show the lowest interexaminer reliability. It is considered that palpation for eliciting local twitch responses is the most difficult examination for TrP diagnosis, particularly in some muscles (Gerwin et al., 1997).

Referred Pain

Referred pain is thought to be a nonspecific finding by some authors or a confirmation sign of muscle TrPs by others (Gerwin et al., 1997). Therefore, the presence of referred pain is of limited diagnostic value unless observed in combination with other findings. The location of the referred pain is clinically useful as an initial guide as to which muscles might be harboring TrPs. The referred pain pattern should be checked as to whether or not it can be recognized by the patient as his or her usual pain symptoms. Pain recognition is a relatively easy test to perform and probably the most useful single diagnostic test for TrPs.

Summary

Palpation for a hypersensitive spot is usually considered the easiest examination, followed by pain recognition, palpable taut band, and referred pain. Simons et al. (1999) and Gerwin et al. (1997) recommend that the *minimum* acceptable criteria for active muscle TrP diagnosis be the combination of the presence of a tender spot in a palpable taut band within a skeletal muscle and the patient's recognition of the referred pain elicited by pressure applied to the tender spot as a usual symptom. These criteria have showed a reliability (kappa) ranging from 0.84 to 0.88.

MANUAL EXPLORATION OF MUSCLE TRIGGER POINTS RELATED TO HEADACHES

A detailed clinical history, examination of movement patterns, and consideration of referred pain patterns assist clinicians in determining which muscles may be clinically relevant for the development of headache symptoms. Muscle pain is perceived as aching and poorly localized (Chapter 4). There are no laboratory or imaging tests available that can confirm the presence of TrPs. Therefore, manual palpation is usually the key for the diagnosis of TrPs.

Methods for Manual Identification of Muscle Trigger Points

By definition, TrPs are located within a taut band of skeletal muscle, and palpating for TrPs starts with identifying this taut band by palpating perpendicular to the fiber direction. Once the taut band is located, the clinician moves along the taut band to find a discrete area of intense pain and hardness (hypersensitive spot). The presence of a local twitch response (sudden contraction of muscle fibers within a taut band when the taut band is strummed manually or needled), referred pain (not restricted to single segmental pathways or to peripheral nerve distributions), or reproduction of the patient's symptoms increases the certainty and specificity of TrP diagnosis.

Knowledge of both clinical anatomy and the direction of the muscle fibers along with the muscular attachments is essential for a correct TrP diagnosis. Contracting the muscle initially to locate the muscle's fiber direction may be helpful. The muscle needs to be placed in a position where the taut band can optimally be palpated. For patients with very tight and restricted muscles, the muscle may need to be placed in a relaxed position, whereas in hypermobile patients the muscle may need to be prestretched to allow the clinician to be able to identify taut bands. When the taut band has been located, the clinician moves along the taut band to identify an area of discrete tenderness with a nodular hardening and exquisite pain (the TrP). Finally, clinicians should avoid preconceived expectations regarding the location of muscle TrPs from referral diagrams, because the marks commonly used in TrP diagrams are for demonstration purposes only.

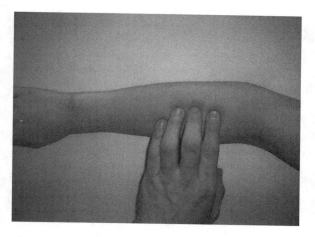

Figure 16.1 Flat Palpation of Muscle Trigger Points

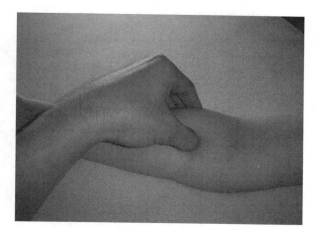

Figure 16.2 Pincer Palpation of Muscle Trigger Points

Flat Palpation

TrPs can be identified through a flat palpation technique, in which the therapist applies finger or thumb pressure to muscle against underlying bone tissue (**Figure 16.1**). When TrPs exist, taut bands; exquisite, focal tenderness; and a twitch response can be detected with flat palpation.

Pincer Palpation

The muscle is rolled between the tips of the digits to detect taut bands of fibers (**Figure 16.2**), to detect exquisite, focal tenderness, and to elicit local twitch responses.

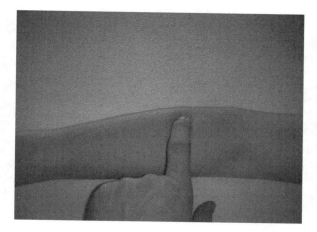

Figure 16.3 Snapping Palpation of Muscle Trigger Points

Snapping Palpation

Snapping palpation is usually conducted to elicit local twitch responses and is most effective when done near or on the TrP with the muscle slightly lengthened or at a neutral length. The clinician locates a taut band and places the fingertips at the side of the taut band. The clinician moves the fingers back and forth to roll the underlying muscle fibers under the fingers (**Figure 16.3**). This is similar to plucking a guitar string except that contact with the surface is maintained.

Manual Palpation of Trigger Points in the Muscles Related to Headaches

This section describes the palpation of those muscles from which referred pain can mimic head pain patterns of tension-type headache (Fernández-de-las-Peñas et al., 2005, 2006a, 2006b, 2007a, 2007b), cervicogenic headache (Roth et al., 2007), or migraine (Fernández-de-las-Peñas et al., 2006c, 2006d).

Trigger Point Examination of the Upper Trapezius Muscle

TrPs in the upper trapezius muscle commonly refer pain to the back of the neck, base of the skull, temple, or jaw (Simons et al., 1999; Fernández-de-las-Peñas et al., 2006b, 2007a).

To examine the upper trapezius muscle, TrPs can be examined in either the prone or supine position. With the patient supine, the upper trapezius muscle should be placed in a relaxed position. With a pincer palpation,

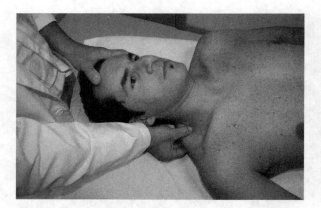

Figure 16.4 Pincer Palpation of Upper Trapezius Muscle Trigger Points

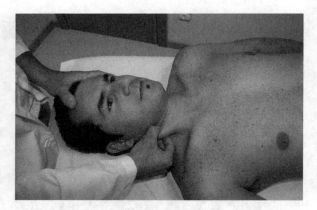

Figure 16.6 Pincer Palpation of Sternocleidomastoid Muscle Trigger Points

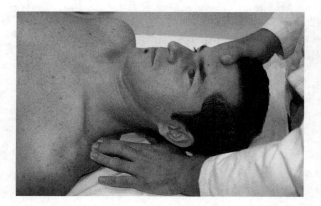

Figure 16.5 Flat Palpation of Upper Trapezius Muscle Trigger Points

any part of the upper trapezius muscle can be lifted off the underlying muscles or structures (**Figure 16.4**). Then, the muscle is firmly rolled between the fingers and thumb to palpate the taut band, locate the hypersensitive spot, and elicit local twitch responses. Finally, light compression of the TrP can be applied to elicit any referred pain (Simons et al., 1999). If a pincer palpation is too painful for the patient, examination of TrPs in the upper trapezius muscle can also be done with flat palpation (**Figure 16.5**).

It is important to repeat the manual examination technique along the entire upper trapezius muscle from its origin at the medial third of the superior nuchal line to its attachment at the outer third of the clavicle (Simons et al., 1999). In patients with bilateral headache (e.g., tension-type headache), the upper trapezius muscle on both sides should be examined (Fernández-de-las-Peñas et al., 2007a).

Trigger Point Examination of the Sternocleidomastoid Muscle

The referred pain elicited by TrPs located in the sternocleidomastoid muscle is perceived in the occiput, the vertex, the retroauricular area, the forehead, and the cheek (Simons et al., 1999; Fernández-de-las-Peñas et al., 2006b).

To examine the sternocleidomastoid muscle, the patient may be seated or supine. To examine the entire muscle belly, the examiner may ask the patient to turn his or her face slightly away from the muscle to be examined (contralateral rotation). Pincer palpation is best suited for this muscle (**Figure 16.6**). Nevertheless, for the distal section of the muscle (toward the mastoid process), flat palpation is the only possible way of palpation. The proximal sections (near the sternum and clavicle) cannot be palpated with a pincer palpation in many, if not most, subjects. The muscle is then grasped firmly between the thumb and index finger to search for the taut muscle bands, to identify spot tenderness, and to elicit local twitch responses. It is important to apply pincer palpation repeatedly to the entire muscle from its upper to lower attachments at all levels of the muscle. Both the sternal division and clavicular division should be examined.

Trigger Point Examination of the Suboccipital Muscles

The suboccipital muscles consist of four small muscles: rectus capitis posterior minor, rectus capitis posterior major, and inferior and superior oblique muscles (Chapter 7). TrPs in the suboccipital muscles refer pain in

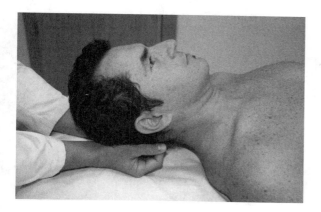

Figure 16.7 Flat Palpation of Suboccipital Muscle Trigger Points

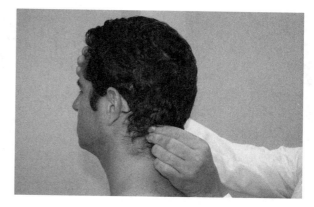

Figure 16.8 Flat Palpation of Inferior Oblique Capitis Muscle Trigger Points

a bandlike distribution along the side of the head in the occipital, temporal, and frontal region (Simons et al., 1999; Fernández-de-las-Peñas et al., 2006a).

One of the main limitations regarding the suboccipital muscles is that they are not directly accessible for palpation. Therefore, it is difficult to palpate TrPs individually in the deepest muscles, particularly the rectus capitis posterior minor and major muscles. Fernández-de-las-Peñas et al. (2006a) have proposed the following manual exploration of the suboccipital muscles for patients with headache: The patient lies supine with the cervical spine in a neutral position. The clinician palpates the suboccipital region, that is, the anatomic projection of the rectus capitis posterior major and minor muscles between the posterior arch of the atlas and the occiput bone (**Figure 16.7**), for 10 seconds. If referred pain is evoked upon slight compression, subjects are asked to extend their neck. This movement will produce a palpable contraction of the most superficial posterior cervical muscles, and conceivably a contraction of the suboccipital muscles, which are not directly palpable. Patients are asked to keep the neck straight and extend at the cervical-occipital junction to focus the contraction on both rectus capitis posterior muscles and other suboccipital extensor muscles. A TrP diagnosis is made when there is tenderness in the suboccipital region, referred pain evoked by maintained pressure for 10 seconds, and increased referred pain on contraction (Fernández-de-las-Peñas et al., 2006a).

In addition, TrPs in the inferior oblique muscle can be individually explored as follows (Gerwin, 2005): The patient is seated. The clinician locates the transverse process of C1 vertebra (atlas) and the spinous process of C2 vertebra (axis). The inferior oblique muscle lies

between these two anatomic points (**Figure 16.8**). The clinician performs a flat palpation of this muscle looking for the presence of a taut band, a tender spot, and reproduction of referred pain into the head.

Trigger Point Examination of the Temporalis Muscle

TrPs located in the temporalis muscle usually refer pain to the inside of the head in patients with chronic tension-type headache (Fernández-de-las-Peñas et al., 2007b). In patients with temporomandibular joint disorders, TrPs in the temporalis muscle can refer pain to the teeth or the mandible (Simons et al., 1999).

When examining TrPs in the temporalis muscle, the jaws can be partly open to slightly stretch the muscle, which in some patients may provide better information. The patient is supine. The examiner may ask the patient to bite his or her teeth slightly to locate the muscle belly. Snapping palpation may be applied to locate the taut bands, because muscle fibers of this muscle tend to be very thin. Flat palpation is used to find TrPs in the temporalis muscle and to induce referred pain. The clinician should explore the entire temporoparietal region looking for the presence of TrPs in any part of the muscle (**Figure 16.9**). The temporalis on both sides should be examined if the patient has bilateral headache, such as tension-type headache (Fernández-de-las-Peñas et al., 2007b).

Trigger Point Examination of the Masseter Muscle

TrPs in the masseter muscle refer pain above the ipsilateral eye, the ear, jaw, and teeth (Simons et al.,

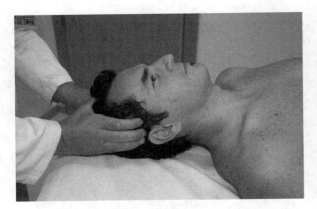

Figure 16.9 Flat Palpation of Temporalis Muscle Trigger Points

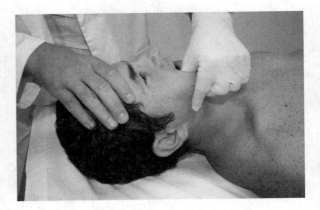

Figure 16.11 Pincer Palpation of Superficial Layer of Masseter Muscle Trigger Points

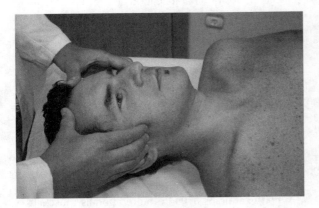

Figure 16.10 Flat Palpation of Deep Layer of Masseter Muscle Trigger Points

1999). TrPs in the deep layer of the masseter muscle usually refer pain to the ear and to the temporomandibular joints, whereas TrPs in the superficial layer of the muscle usually refer pain to the face (Simons et al., 1999).

The patient should be supine. The examiner can ask the patient to bite his or her teeth slightly to locate the masseter muscle. TrPs in the deep layer of the masseter muscle can be identified by flat palpation against the posterior portion of the ramus and along the base of the zygomatic buttress (**Figure 16.10**). For the superficial layer of the muscle, the clinician may use an intraoral pincer palpation between two digits (**Figure 16.11**).

Trigger Point Examination of the Splenius Capitis and Cervicis Muscles

TrPs in the splenius capitis muscle refer pain to the vertex, whereas TrPs in the splenius cervicis muscle refer pain along the side of the head in a band and behind the eye (Simons et al., 1999).

To examine TrPs in the splenius capitis muscle, the patient may be seated. This muscle attaches to the spinous processes of the lower half of the cervical spine and the first three or four thoracic vertebrae, and above and laterally to the mastoid process and to the adjacent occipital bone. To locate the splenius capitis muscle, the examiner may ask the patient to ipsilaterally rotate his or her neck. The clinician palpates the contraction of the splenius capitis muscle within the triangle formed by the trapezius posteriorly, the sternocleidomastoid anteriorly, and the levator scapulae inferiorly. Flat palpation is used to identify TrPs in this muscle.

To locate the splenius cervicis muscle, first ask the seated patient to flex his or her head and neck toward the side being examined in order to relax the upper trapezius and levator scapulae. The splenius cervicis muscle lies to the lateral side and caudal to the splenius capitis muscle. The clinician displaces the free border of the upper trapezius medially and presses the levator scapulae anterolaterally to permit palpation of the splenius cervicis muscle directly beneath the skin. Flat palpation is used for TrP examination in the splenius cervicis muscle. In patients with bilateral headache, the splenius capitis and splenius cervicis muscles on both sides should be examined.

Trigger Point Examination of the Frontalis Muscle

TrPs in the frontalis muscle refer pain to the forehead and to the supraorbital region (Simons et al., 1999). To examine TrPs in the frontalis muscle, the patient should be in the supine position. The examiner may ask the patient to raise an eyebrow and to frown. The examiner may feel the contraction of the muscle with the fingertips placed above the eyebrow (**Figure 16.12**). Flat palpation is used to identify TrPs in this muscle. An active TrP in the frontalis belly is identified mostly as spot tenderness above the medial end of the eyebrow (**Figure 16.13**).

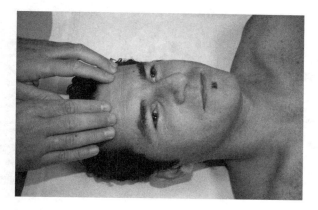

Figure 16.12 Flat Palpation of Frontalis Muscle Trigger Points

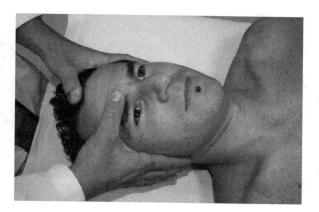

Figure 16.13 Flat Palpation of Frontalis–Eyebrow Muscle Trigger Points

Trigger Point Examination of the Superior Oblique Muscle

The superior oblique muscle is an extraocular muscle that has been related to tension-type headache (Fernández-de-las-Peñas et al., 2005) and migraine (Fernández-de-las-Peñas et al., 2006d). The referred pain is perceived as internal and deep pain located at the retro-orbital region, which can also extend to the supraorbital and to the homolateral forehead. Therefore, TrPs located in the superior oblique muscle may be an important cause of frontal and eye-related headache pain.

The exploration of TrPs in this muscle has been described by Fernández-de-las-Peñas et al. (2005) as follows: The patient is supine. The examiner palpates the trochlear region in the superior-internal corner of the orbit (upper medial canthus) (**Figure 16.14**). If local pain is evoked from palpation, moderate pressure on this region is applied by the thumb of the assessor for 30 seconds to elicit referred pain. Next, the patient is told to look in an inferior-medial direction (infra-adduction, contraction of the superior oblique muscle). Finally, the patient moves the eye in a superior and lateral direction (supra-abduction, active stretching of the superior oblique muscle). If both contraction and stretching of the muscle increase referred pain, a diagnosis of a TrP can be made; if only one of these maneuvers increases the referred pain, the diagnosis is a probable TrP. The clinical sequence for TrP examination is summarized in **Figure 16.15**.

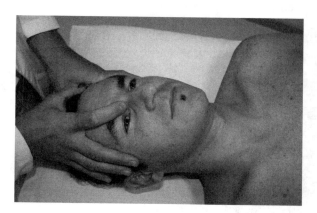

Figure 16.14 Location of the Superior Oblique Muscle

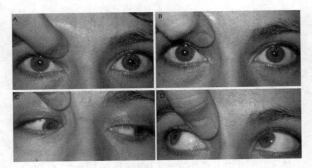

Figure 16.15 Exploration of Superior Oblique Muscle Trigger Points. A: Moderate pressure is applied with the second finger on the trochlear area in the superior-internal corner of the orbit. **B:** Moderate pressure is applied for 30 seconds with the thumb on the same location. **C:** Maintaining the pressure, the patient moves the right eye to downward-medial gaze (muscle contraction). **D:** Maintaining the pressure, the patient moves the right eye to upward-lateral gaze (active stretching).

Reprinted with permission from Fernández-de-las-Peñas et al. Referred pain from the trochlear region in tension-type headache: a myofascial trigger point from the superior oblique muscle. *Headache* 2005;45:731–737.

Trigger Point Examination of the Zygomaticus Major Muscle

The zygomaticus major muscle attaches to the malar surface of the zygomatic bone and to the angle of the mouth. The zygomaticus major insertion notch, which is a palpable landmark identified midway between the zygomaticus arch and the malar eminence, can be used to locate the upper insertion point of this muscle. The referred pain elicited by this muscle is perceived in the face (Simons et al., 1999). To examine TrPs in the zygomaticus major muscle, the patient may be supine. Because pincer palpation can be too painful for patients, we prefer to apply a flat palpation technique. Therefore, the zygomaticus major muscle will be palpated under the malar surface of the zygomatic bone (**Figure 16.16**).

Trigger Point Examination of the Scalene Muscles

The scalene muscles consist of four small muscles: scalene anterior, scalene medius, scalene posterior, and scalene minimus. Only the anterior and medial scalene muscles can be palpated. The referred pain elicited by TrPs in the scalene muscles is usually perceived in the upper extremity or in the chest. Fernández-de-las-Peñas et al. (2007c) have reported a new referred pain pattern

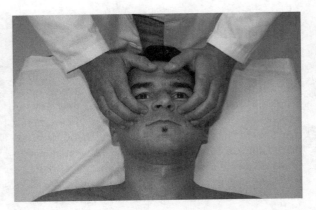

Figure 16.16 Flat Palpation of Zygomaticus Major Muscle Trigger Points

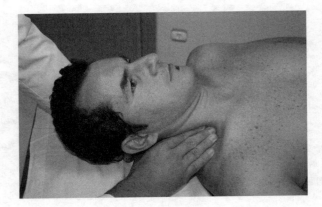

Figure 16.17 Flat Palpation of Scalene Muscle Trigger Points

to the head for the scalene anterior muscle in patients with tension-type headache.

To examine TrPs in the scalene muscles, the patient should be supine. The scalene muscles are located under and lateral to the posterior border of the clavicular division of the sternocleidomastoid muscle. The clinician may ask the patient to take a deep inspiration, while palpating the contraction of the scalene muscles with the fingertips. A flat palpation is used (**Figure 16.17**). For the identification of TrPs in the anterior scalene, the fingers of one hand straddle the muscle to establish its location, while the other hand palpates and locates the TrPs and finally induces referred pain with sustained pressure. The medial scalene lies deep to and anterior to the free border of the upper trapezius muscle. It can be palpated against the posterior tubercles of the transverse processes of the cervical vertebrae.

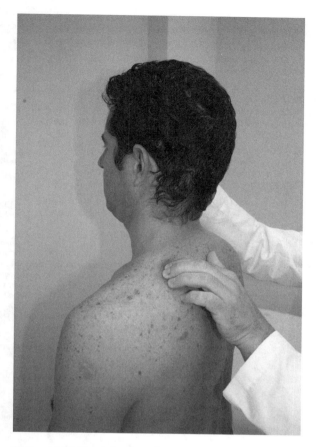

Figure 16.18 Flat Palpation of Levator Scapulae Muscle Trigger Points

Trigger Point Examination of the Levator Scapulae Muscle

The levator scapulae muscle is not associated with headache. Because patients with tension-type, cervicogenic, or migraine headache usually suffer from pain in the neck region, TrPs in the levator scapulae muscle may contribute to their symptoms.

To examine TrPs in the levator scapulae muscle, the patient may be seated. If the levator scapulae is taut, its muscle belly can be easily located with flat palpation on top of the superior angle of the scapula. Snapping palpation is repeated along the muscle belly to find the spot tenderness, and finally sustained pressure can be applied to induce referred pain. TrPs in the levator scapulae at the angle of the neck region can be reached by pushing the upper trapezius backward so as to uncover the levator scapulae muscle. TrPs located in the vicinity of the superior angle of the scapular can easily be identified by snapping palpation (**Figure 16.18**).

CONCLUSIONS

Clinicians should explore those muscles that may harbor TrPs that may feature referred pain contributing to head pain in both tension-type and cervicogenic headache. The diagnosis of TrPs requires adequate manual ability, training, and clinical practice. The current chapter reviewed the most common muscles related to headache, although in some patients other muscles may also be involved.

REFERENCES

Bron C, Franssen JL, Wensing M, Oostendorp AB. Inter-observer reliability of palpation of myofascial trigger points in shoulder muscles. *J Man Manipulative Ther* 2007;15:203–215.

Chen Q, Bensamoun S, Basford JR, Thompson JM, An KN. Identification and quantification of myofascial taut bands with magnetic resonance elastography. *Arch Phys Med Rehabil* 2007;88:1658–1661.

Fernández-de-las-Peñas C, Cuadrado ML, Gerwin RD, Pareja JA. Referred pain from the trochlear region in tension-type headache: a myofascial trigger point from the superior oblique muscle. *Headache* 2005;45:731–737.

Fernández-de-las-Peñas C, Alonso-Blanco C, Cuadrado ML, Gerwin RD, Pareja JA. Trigger points in the suboccipital muscles and forward head posture in tension type headache. *Headache* 2006a;46:454–460.

Fernández-de-las-Peñas C, Alonso-Blanco C, Cuadrado ML, Gerwin R, Pareja JA. Myofascial trigger points and their

relationship with headache clinical parameters in chronic tension type headache. *Headache* 2006b;46:1264–1272.

Fernández-de-las-Peñas C, Cuadrado ML, Pareja JA. Myofascial trigger points, neck mobility and forward head posture in unilateral migraine. *Cephalalgia* 2006c;26:1061–1070.

Fernández-de-las-Peñas C, Cuadrado ML, Gerwin RD, Pareja JA. Myofascial disorders in the trochlear region in unilateral migraine: a possible initiating or perpetuating factor. *Clin J Pain* 2006d;22:548–553.

Fernández-de-las-Peñas C, Ge H, Arendt-Nielsen L, Cuadrado ML, Pareja JA. Referred pain from trapezius muscle trigger point shares similar characteristics with chronic tension type headache. *Eur J Pain* 2007a;11:475–482.

Fernández-de-las-Peñas C, Ge H, Arendt-Nielsen L, Cuadrado ML, Pareja JA. The local and referred pain from myofascial trigger points in the temporalis muscle contributes to pain profile in chronic tension-type headache. *Clin J Pain* 2007b;23:786–792.

Fernández-de-las-Peñas C, De-la-Llave-Rincón AI, Miangolarra JC. Uncommon referred pain from scalene muscle trigger points in chronic tension type headache [abstract]. *J Musculoskeletal Pain* 2007c;15(suppl 13):21.

Gerwin R. Headache. In: Ferguson L, Gerwin R, eds. *Clinical Mastery in the Treatment of Myofascial Pain*. Philadelphia: Lippincott Williams & Wilkins; 2005:1–24.

Gerwin RD, Shannon S, Hong CZ, Hubbard D, Gevirtz R. Inter-rater reliability in myofascial trigger point examination. *Pain* 1997;69:65–73.

Hsieh CY, Hong CZ, Adams AH, et al. Inter-examiner reliability of the palpation of trigger points in the trunk and lower limb muscles. *Arch Phys Med Rehabil* 2000;81:258–264.

Lew PC, Lewis J, Story I. Inter-therapist reliability in locating latent myofascial trigger points using palpation. *Man Ther* 1997;2:87–90.

Lucas KR, Polus BI, Rich PA. Latent myofascial trigger points: their effects on muscle activation and movement efficiency. *J Bodywork Mov Ther* 2004;8:160–166.

Nice DA, Riddle DL, Lamb RL, et al. Inter-tester reliability of judgments of the presence of trigger points in patients with low back pain. *Arch Phys Med Rehabil* 1992;73: 893–898.

Njoo KH, Van der Does E. The occurrence and inter-rater reliability of myofascial trigger points in the quadratus lumborum and gluteus medius: a prospective study in non-specific low back pain patients and controls in general practice. *Pain* 1994;58:317–323.

Roth JK, Roth RS, Weintraub JR, Simons DG. Cervicogenic headache caused by myofascial trigger points in the sternocleidomastoid: a case report. *Cephalalgia* 2007;27:375–380.

Sciotti VM, Mittak VL, DiMarco L, Ford LM, Plezbert J, Santipadri E, Wigglesworth J, Ball K. Clinical precision of myofascial trigger point location in the trapezius muscle. *Pain* 2001;93:259–266.

Simons DG, Travell J, Simons LS. *Myofascial Pain and Dysfunction: The Trigger Point Manual*. Vol. 1. 2nd ed. Baltimore: Williams & Wilkins; 1999.

Tough EA, Write AR, Richards SS, Campbell J. Variability of criteria used to diagnose myofascial trigger point pain syndrome: evidence from a review of the literature. *Clin J Pain* 2007;23:278–286.

Wolfe F, Smythe HA, Yunus MB, et al. The American College of Rheumatology 1990 criteria for classification of fibromyalgia: report of the multicenter criteria committee. *Arthritis Rheum* 1990;33:160–170.

Wolfe F, Simons DG, Fricton J, et al. The fibromyalgia and myofascial pain syndromes: a preliminary study of tender points and trigger points in persons with fibromyalgia, myofascial pain syndrome and no disease. *J Rheumatol* 1992;19:944–951.

Clinical Examination of the Orofacial Region in Patients with Headache

Anton de Wijer, RPT, SCS, MT, PhD, and Michel H. Steenks, DDS, PhD

In the guidelines of the American Academy of Orofacial Pain (AAOP), the term *temporomandibular disorders* (TMD) is defined as a collective term embracing a number of clinical problems that involve the masticatory muscles, temporomandibular joint and associated structures, or both (Okeson, 1996). In the general population TMD are common clinical conditions. TMD is characterized by combinations of signs and symptoms in the locomotor system of the jaw, such as pain on mandibular movements, limitation and deviation in the range of motion of the mandible, and joint noises (Okeson, 1996). Because of the overlap of signs and symptoms in TMD, some cervical spine disorders, and tension-type headache, clinicians must evaluate the masticatory system in patients with persistent neck and head complaints in order to evaluate the condition of the masticatory system (Wijer de, 1995). Treatment directed toward functional disturbances of the masticatory system has a beneficial effect on mandibular dysfunction, and many patients who suffer from additional recurrent headaches experience a reduction of the frequency and severity of their headaches after this treatment (Magnusson & Carlsson, 1980). This chapter describes the clinical examination of the masticatory system, discusses some aspects of the overlap between TMD and cervical spine disorders, and presents a case report. After reading this chapter, the clinician should realize the necessity of including the masticatory system in the examination protocol in patients with headache. The examination protocol and the choices to be made are described, as well as the protocol's implementation in daily practice.

A nationwide survey of oral conditions, treatment needs, and attitudes toward dental health care was carried out in the Netherlands. The TMD study, using the Helkimo Index to rate the severity of the condition, found that 21.5% of the Dutch population reported dysfunction. Fifteen percent perceived a need for treatment, and 44.4% clinically had signs and symptoms of TMD (Kanter de et al., 1992, 1993). The actual level of treatment need for TMD has been analyzed and has been estimated as 3% of the population. The disorder is more prevalent in women in the age group between 20 and 40 years. This aspect is discussed extensively in the scientific literature, and the possible link between its pathogenesis and the female hormonal axis is described (Isselee et al., 2002; LeResche et al., 1997; Wijnhoven et al., 2007). Generally speaking, the etiologic concepts related to nonspecific TMD can be divided into functional theories (neuromuscular), structural theories (occlusive-anatomic), or psychophysiologic theories. Some well-described models are the trauma theory (Zarb et al., 1995), internal derangement theory (Farrar, 1978), osteoarthritic theory (Stegenga et al., 1989), and psychophysiologic theory (Laskin, 1969; Dworkin, 1994). Epidemiologic, neuromuscular, and neurophysiologic studies have been inconclusive regarding the theoretical concept of the etiology of TMD (Ververs et al., 2004; Suvinen et al., 2005).

In the scientific literature, the subclassification of TMD is well established: arthrogenous, myogenous, and combined temporomandibular joint (TMJ) and muscle problems (Lobbezoo-Scholte 1993; Steenks et al., 2007). There is general agreement that patients with TMD should be screened for biomedical (axis I) and psychosocial (axis II) dysfunctions (Dworkin & LeResche, 1992; Turner & Dworkin, 2004), for example, by utilizing methods described and endorsed by the International RDC/TMD Consortium (www.rdc-tmdinternational.org), AAOP (www.aaop.org), or European Academy of Craniomandibular Disorders (EACD; www.eacmd.org).

Suggestions for how to manage patients' orofacial pain or TMD in clinical settings can be found in the consensus guidelines of the professional organizations (AAOP, EACD) or, for example, the University Consensus Statements of the Netherlands (Projectgroep Musculoskelettale Stoornissen, 2003). The RDC/TMD states that for research purposes, criteria are offered to allow standardization and replication of research into the most common forms of muscle- and joint-related TMD. The aim to have a better insight into the characteristics of the group of patients included in a study is important and should make comparison of study results possible.

TMD, like lumbar and cervical spine problems, is classified as *specific* (signs and symptoms of TMD accompanying a specific disease, such as rheumatoid arthritis, fracture, cranial neuralgias, or Ehlers-Danlos syndrome) or *nonspecific* (arthrogenous, myogenous, and combination; signs and symptoms of TMD without a specific disease) (**Figure 17.1**) (Steenks, 2007). Specific conditions are caused by a well-known pathophysiologic mechanism or by disorder in anatomic structures, such as tumor, fracture, infection, or nerve root compression. Specific conditions are classified within the International Classification of Diseases (ICD) system of the World Health Organization (e.g., juvenile rheumatoid arthritis with signs and symptoms of TMD). Nonspecific locomotor problems are complaints for which no apparent specific cause can be found that offers an explanation for the symptoms, which means that the clarification of the condition, as far as we know now, is not related to a well-known pathophysiologic condition or pathology. In a patient classified as having nonspecific arthrogenous TMD, anterior disc displacement with reduction, the pathophysiologic condition seems to be clear; however, the alleged malposition of the disc is frequently present in healthy control subjects without further signs and symptoms of TMD or complaints. Many diseases are known to mimic TMD: dental or neurologic pathology, tumors, growth disturbances, and systemic diseases. Therefore, therapists working in this domain need to have knowledge of the probability of finding specific pathology in certain patient groups. Epidemiologic data (prevalence, incidence) and pathophysiologic knowledge will help the clinician judge the situation of each patient. When specific pathology is excluded, the condition is classified as nonspecific TMD.

It is important to include a comprehensive history, taking into account yellow flags (indicating psychosocial factors/axis II RDC/TMD) as well. When a patient has pain, it is also crucial to differentiate whether the condition is acute, subacute, or chronic; classify the type of the pain as neuropathic, inflammatory, or nociceptive; determine whether the symptoms are being caused by a known condition with a normal or abnormal presentation; determine which contextual factors or illness-impacting disorders (e.g., coping style, locus of control, emotional and social factors) are present; and deter-

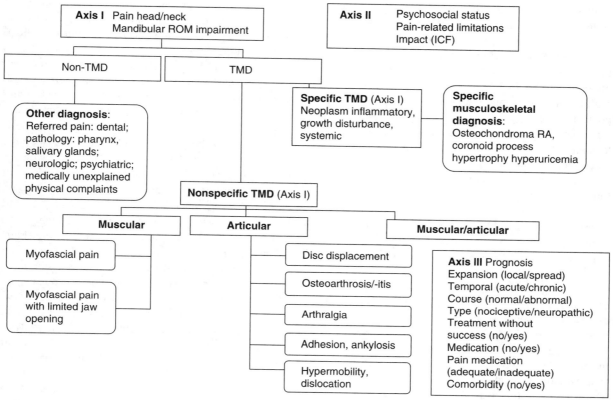

Figure 17.1 Flowchart of the Diagnostic Process in Suspected Painful Temporomandibular Disorders (TMD). Axis I represents the physical conditions. Non-TMD: other conditions presenting with pain in the head and the neck and limitations of mandibular range of motion. Specific TMD: conditions with a known substratum (e.g., neoplasms, growth disturbances, systemic disease). Nonspecific TMD: Conditions related to overloading or trauma surpassing the adaptation capacity. Generally divided into muscular and articular subgroups. Axis II represents psychosocial factors, which are increasingly important when chronicity plays a more prominent role. Axis III summarizes additional clinical considerations related to prognosis, such as pain characteristics, medication, and results of previous treatment. ROM, range of motion; RA, rheumatoid arthritis; ICF, International Classification of Functioning, Disability and Health of the World Health Organization.

mine what the consequences of these factors are for the level of functioning and disability. Other goals related to clinical history taking are to meet the patient; to clarify the reason for the visit and the main complaint; to determine signs and symptoms and their consequences on the ICF levels; to discuss the patient's beliefs about the condition and its consequences; and to tune one's hypotheses with the patient's ideas, exchange expectations, and discuss evaluation and treatment plans. Readers are referred to Chapter 13 for a discussion of the clinical reasoning during the clinical interview.

In the medical literature, *diagnosis* usually refers to a disease classification that contains knowledge about the signs, symptoms, test results, and underlying pathology. In physical therapy, the ICF model of functioning and disability is used (Steiner et al., 2002). This model is a

biopsychosocial model designed to provide a coherent view of various dimensions of health at biological, individual, and social levels. The traditional biomedical paradigm has its roots in the Cartesian division between mind and body and considers disease primarily as a failure within the soma. Currently, in clinical studies, authors include mental and social aspects in their definition of health.

TEMPOROMANDIBULAR DISORDERS AND CERVICAL SPINE DISORDERS

In physical therapy, postural abnormalities (forward head posture) and hypermobility are thought to be related to TMD and, therefore, are discussed as treatment indications. TMJ or orofacial pain in this construct is the result of muscle imbalance or poor posture. In the literature, however, there is no consensus on the exact role of posture in the development or perpetuation of TMD (Wijer de & Steenks, 1995; Olivo et al., 2006). Most of the studies are clinical observations and show several methodologic shortcomings. Forward head posture and rounded shoulders are frequently noticed in patient populations as well as in healthy people. In a conference statement in Milan in 1997, the EACD, SIDO (Società Italiana di Ortodonzia), and SIMFER (Società Italiana di Medicina fisica e riabilitazione) declared that a correlation between occlusal and postural pathophysiology under functional and morphologic aspects has yet to be scientifically shown. In the light of that fact, the proposal of reversible or irreversible therapy for the treatment of postural problems is not justified. Likewise, the proposal of physical or rehabilitative therapy for the treatment of occlusal problems is not justified.

Conflicting results were found in studies that have been performed to analyze the association between TMJ disorders and general joint hypermobility. At this moment the scientific evidence regarding the association between temporomandibular disorders and generalized hypermobility is scarce and conflicting. It is still not clear whether general joint hypermobility is associated with TMD (Dijkstra et al., 2002). Coster et al. (2005) found a positive relationship between generalized joint hypermobility due to inherited autosomal dominant connective tissue disease (Marfan syndrome and Ehlers-Danlos syndrome) and TMD. In their hypermobile population (n = 42), multiple TMD group diagnoses were found in 69% of the subjects; the greater proportion presented with both myofascial pain and disc displacement associated with unilateral or bilateral TMJ arthralgia. Recurrent TMJ dislocations for several seconds were a frequent finding in symptomatic patients compared with asymptomatic individuals, but their contribution to TMD development remains elusive.

Many authors agree that, in addition to complaints concerning the masticatory system, signs and symptoms related to cervical spine disorders (CSDs) are also observed and reported. In TMD patients, the location of pain may range from the suboccipital area or the sternocleidomastoid area to the temporal area or the cheek and angle of the jaw, with the most frequently cited pain location being the preauricular area, temple, and cheek (Leeuw de et al., 1994). CSDs are common chronic conditions affecting the cervical region and related structures with or without radiation of pain to the shoulder, arm, interscapular region, and/or head. Like TMD pa-

tients, who may show signs and symptoms related to CSD, CSD patients may also show signs and symptoms related to TMD (Wijer de et al., 1996a, 1996b, 1996c). Many authors have indicated the existence of neuroanatomic and biomechanical relationships and suggest that a dysfunction of the cervical spine may be the cause of signs and symptoms in the orofacial region (Sessle, 1999; Sjaastad, 1992; Wijer de & Steenks, 1995).

We assessed the prevalence of signs and symptoms related to CSD and TMD in order to determine whether CSD patients and subgroups of TMD patients differ with regard to specific signs, symptoms, and accompanying signs and symptoms (correlates) of TMD and CSD, and psychosocial factors or general health. In the diagnostic procedure, we use a standardized multidimensional self-administered questionnaire, Screen (Leeuw de 1993), and a functional examination of the stomatognathic system and the cervical spine (Lobbezoo-Scholte, 1993; Wijer de, 1995). In these Utrecht studies, the patient groups did not differ regarding correlates, with an exception of ear symptoms (more prevalent in TMD patients), as measured by the questionnaire. The mouth opening of CSD patients did not differ from that of the Dutch population and was in accordance with that of other studies with healthy controls. TMD patients with myogenous problems reported oral habits (i.e., grinding, clenching, or nail biting) more often than CSD patients, although no objective differences in oral habits between CSD and TMD patients were found. In spite of the biomechanical and anatomic relationship between the cervical spine and the stomatognathic system, the results of the studies show that CSD patients have signs and symptoms of TMD comparable to those of the adult Dutch population (Kanter de, 1990). Thus, the function of the masticatory system should be evaluated in patients with neck complaints in order to rule out the possible involvement of the masticatory system. Active and passive opening and palpation of the stomatognathic system can be used to discriminate between TMD and CSD patients (Wijer de, 1995). In contrast, orthopaedic tests of the cervical spine were of less importance in discriminating between patients with TMD and CSD (Wijer de et al., 1996b, 1996c).

EVIDENCE-BASED PRACTICE

There has been a progressive increase of controlled studies and systematic reviews in physical therapy. At this moment, clinical guidelines are part of the quality system for physiotherapists as well. More than 20 guidelines for physiotherapy practice are available in the Netherlands (www.kngf.nl), with up-to-date information regarding the most effective diagnostic procedures and treatments in some particular conditions. In orofacial pain, two systematic reviews have been published (Medlicott & Harris, 2006; McNeely et al., 2006).

Evidence-based medicine, including evidence-based patient information, is currently part of daily practice, and the World Confederation for Physical Therapy promotes evidence-based practice worldwide in order to improve the care of patients, to use evidence from the highest available authorities to inform physiotherapists by balancing known benefits and risks, to make decisions more transparent, and to integrate patient preferences into decision making. The issue today is how much of what is firmly evidence based is actually applied in the front lines of patient care.

PHYSICAL EXAMINATION

Diagnosis of a TMD can be simple or very complex. A well-known example of a simple diagnosis is a local preauricular pain caused by a functional painful anterior disc displacement with reduction, where relatively few data from the history and clinical and radiologic examination provide enough information to arrive at a diagnosis. A patient with subacute nociceptive, myofascial, unilateral pain localized in the masseter muscle, due to a sudden overload and temporary biomechanical stressors, with a normal course and no contextual factors (no red or yellow flags) can be simple as well.

However, when a patient presents with a persistent chronic pain in the temporal region or at the side of the face, with an abnormal course, treatment failure, and contextual factors (axis II, yellow flags), the diagnostic process is more complicated. In these cases, the clinician is strongly advised to follow a more or less fixed pattern of steps in order to arrive at the correct diagnosis. A quick diagnosis can be incorrect, and the clinician must be aware of pitfalls in diagnostic processes. This is also the case in the diagnostic process of apparently simple cases. The simultaneous existence of diseases can cause diagnostic confusion. Each therapist must be aware of the symptom overlap in this area due to different causes. The most prevalent cause of orofacial pain is dentoalveolar. Therefore, it is advisable to work in close cooperation with the dental profession, especially when

physical therapists have direct access. Nondental nociceptive pain caused by musculoskeletal conditions must not be mistaken for inflammation (sinusitis, otitis, parotitis) or neurovascular syndromes (trigeminal or glossopharyngeal neuralgia, postherpetic pain, arteritis temporalis, headache such as migraine, central sensitization).

Clinical History

Examples of knowledge organization used in clinical reasoning include illness scripts and pattern recognition. In making use of illness scripts or pattern recognition, the clinician recognizes certain features of a case almost instantly (Edwards et al., 2004). Lobbezoo-Scholte et al. (1995) and Leeuw et al. (1994) subdivided the TMD group of patients. Their studies give insight regarding the subgroup characteristics. In contrast with the forward reasoning of illness scripts, hypothetic-deductive reasoning moves from a generalization (multiple hypotheses) toward a specific conclusion. These two cognitively oriented methods are often referred to as *diagnostic reasoning*. The RDC criteria for research in TMD are also meant to increase the standardized classification criteria for defining clinical subtypes of TMD. In this system, both clinical TMD conditions (axis I) with muscle disorders, disc displacements and arthralgia, and inflammation or infection and psychosocial conditions (axis II) with pain-related disability and psychological status should be included. The AAOP classification is especially meant for daily practice.

Screen, a multidimensional standardized questionnaire, contains questions about five dimensions: (a) quantitative and qualitative aspects of pain in the head, neck, and shoulders, and factors influencing pain; (b) symptoms of TMD, such as pain, joint sounds, limited range of motion, and locking or luxation; (c) accompanying signs and symptoms of TMD; (d) psychosocial factors such as nervousness, depression, anxiety, and life events; and (e) general health factors, monitored by questions about symptoms in joints other than the TMJ (widespread pain), the limbs, circulatory system, digestive tract, and respiratory system (Steenks & Wijer de, 1989, 1991, 1996; Leeuw de et al., 1994). Screen is filled out before the first visit, and the result is studied before the consultation. At the start of the first visit, the clinician begins with history taking, checking the information of the referring clinician, including the patient's demand, reason for the visit and main complaint, prescribed medication, comorbidity, and the presence of relevant biopsychosocial factors that can influence the natural course of the disease.

Several other questionnaires can support the clinician as tools for judging the psychosocial aspects, such as the 4DKL, SCL-90, Fear-Avoidance Beliefs Questionnaire (FABQ), and Tampa Scale for Kinesiophobia. Personal factors, including lifestyle (e.g., sleeping habits, activities, eating, alcoholic beverages, drugs) and parafunctional and occupational habits (e.g., oral habits: clenching, grinding, nail biting, thumb sucking, or gum chewing), that may contribute to the origin or perpetuation of the problem will be evaluated with the patient. The therapist makes a survey of the actual health problem of the patient and determines prognostic factors and risk factors for treatment, called axis III by Steenks (Steenks et al., 2007) (Figure 17.1). On indication, the therapist includes other questionnaires, such as for patient-specific complaints, the Neck Disability Index, and headache or coping style. The Dutch Physiotherapy Association for TMD and Orofacial Pain has developed a toolkit with relevant information regarding diagnostic aids (www.NVFT.nl).

The history will guide the functional examination. This chapter focuses on the temporomandibular area. In general, the physiotherapist will judge the necessity of including the upper quarter (cervical spine, shoulder girdle, neurologic tests, and segmental tissue related to the face and head).

Intraoral and Extraoral Inspection and Orthopaedic Tests

Extraoral inspection or examination includes head, neck, and shoulder position; lymph nodes; skin condition; facial asymmetry; parafunctional habits; facial expression (mimic); oral behavior (tongue position in rest and while swallowing, speech); and breathing pattern (see Chapter 8).

The intraoral evaluation should focus on dental status, occlusal characteristics, restorations, hygiene, periodontal status, soft tissues (gingiva, tongue, floor of mouth, oropharynx), changes in occlusion, angle classification (I, II, III), overbite, wear facets, and guidance (canine, group) (**Figures 17.2, 17.3**). Orthopaedic tests commonly used to examine the function of the masticatory system are active and passive range of motion, palpation, traction and translation, and compression and resistance tests. During the tests, attention should be given to the presence, intensity, and location of pain; joint sounds, such as clicking and crepitation; and other

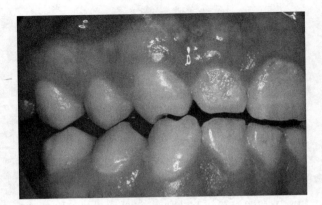

Figure 17.2 Wear Facets

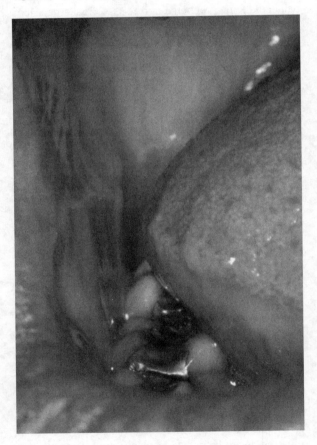

Figure 17.3 Ridging, Buccal Mucosa, and Scalopping of the Tongue

signs, such as restriction of movement and abnormal end-feel.

On active mouth opening, the range of motion is measured in millimeters with a ruler interincisally (**Figure 17.4**), corrected for the overbite (**Figure 17.5**).

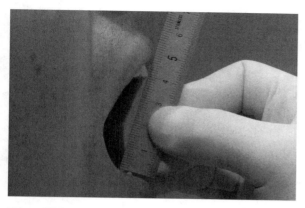

Figure 17.4 Assessment of Active Mouth Opening Range of Motion

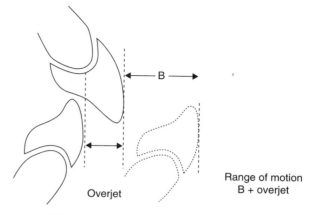

Figure 17.6 Evaluation of the Overjet

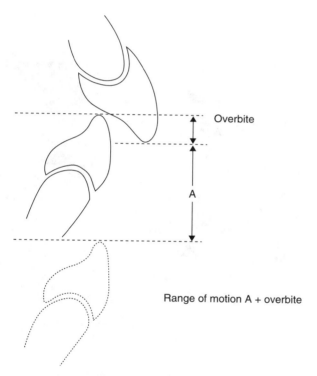

Figure 17.5 Overbite Correction for Active Mouth Opening Assessment

Horizontal movements are assessed by asking the patient to move the mandible in a lateral or anterior direction (protrusion). The distance of midline displacement in lateral movement is measured in millimeters and corrected for discrepancies in the starting position. In protrusion, the measurement will take place at the mesioincisal ridge of the right upper and lower central in-

cisors, and the forward displacement of the mandible will be corrected for the overjet (**Figure 17.6**). Normal jaw opening is usually considered to be about three finger widths at the knuckles of the patient's dominant hand. Normal range of motion in opening in the healthy population is between 50 and 60 mm. **Table 17.1** presents the distribution of range of motion on active and passive mouth opening in TMD and CSD patients. The average active opening in our TMD patient group was 50 mm (7.5 mm, SD); on passive opening, 53 mm (7 mm, SD). The horizontal movements had an average score of 10 mm (2 mm, SD). Ten percent of the TMD patients had a mouth opening of less than 40 mm. A mouth opening of less than 40 mm is usually considered as limited, and less than 35 mm is considered inconvenient (e.g., for taking a bite or chewing). TMD patients reported a limited mouth opening more frequently (44% to 72% depending on the subgroup classification) than CSD patients (4%). In healthy individuals we expect the horizontal movements to be between 7 and 12 mm (protrusion includes overjet). In patients, pain, limited jaw function, midline deviation on opening, protrusion, differences in mandible left and right excursions, a discrepancy between active and passive movements, and a discrepancy between horizontal and vertical movement can be predictive for TMD as well.

In passive movements the patient is asked to open the mouth. Then, a gentle pressure is exerted on the lower and upper incisors until the anatomic limit is reached (**Figure 17.7**). The end-feel distance—the difference (normally 2–3 mm) between the range of passive opening and active mouth opening—is measured, and signs and symptoms are documented.

Table 17.1 Range of Active and Passive Motion, Horizontal Overlap (Overjet), and Vertical Overlap (Overbite) in Patients with Temporomandibular Disorders and Patients with Cervical Spinal Disorders

Variables	TMD (n = 111)			CSD (n = 103)		
	μ	SD	Range	μ	SD	Range
Open active + overbite	50.0	7.5	31–65	53.7	7.8	38–80
Open passive + overbite	53.2	7.0	34–67	55.8	7.6	39–82
Laterotrusion right active	9.9	2.1	2–14	10.3	2.0	5–15
Laterotrusion left active	10.0	1.9	5–15	10.3	1.9	5–15
Protrusion active + overjet	10.2	2.0	6–14	10.6	1.9	7–18
Horizontal overlap (overjet)	4.1	2.0	1–11	4.2	1.7	1–11
Vertical overlap (overbite)	3.9	1.7	1–9	3.7	1.6	1–8

TMD, temporomandibular disorders; CSD, cervical spine disorders; μ, mean; SD, standard deviation.

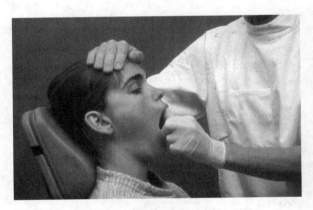

Figure 17.7 Application of Pressure on the Lower and Upper Incisors with the Mouth Open

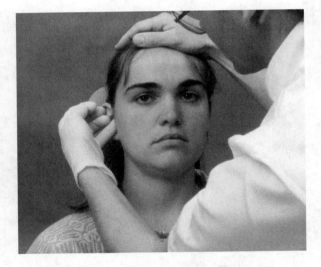

Figure 17.8 Palpation of the Temporomandibular Joint

The TMJ is palpated laterally slightly anterior to the tragus and posteriorly via the external meatus (**Figure 17.8**), with the mouth open or closed, with the mouth closed, and during opening and closing movements. The clinician should also palpate the masseter (**Figure 17.9**) and temporalis (**Figure 17.10**) muscles (including the insertion on the coronoid process intraorally) and the attachment of the medial pterygoid muscle extra-orally. Palpation gives an impression about pain, muscle tone, structural changes, contrast between contraction and relaxation, and other provoked signs and symptoms (e.g., feeling of stiffness, dizziness, ear tingling).

The results of the active and passive movement test will give the clinician a first impression about the condi-tion and the possible subgroup classification. Palpation will help to support this idea. It is important to realize that local pain can be the result of sensitization, with the cause being elsewhere (dental, throat, peripheral, or central). The close interaction of some structures can be confusing as well. After history taking, inspection, functional examination, and information from the panoramic radiograph (**Figure 17.11**), it should be clear whether nonspecific TMD is present, and its subclassifi-cation can be established. The decision regarding the kind of radiographic evaluation will depend on the aims

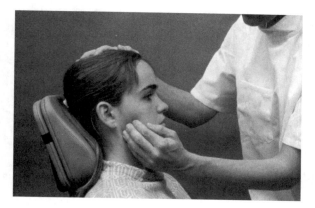

Figure 17.9 Palpation of the Masseter Muscle

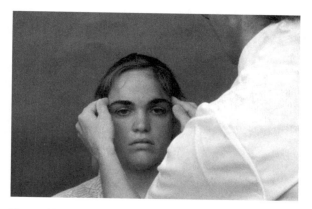

Figure 17.10 Palpation of the Temporalis Muscle

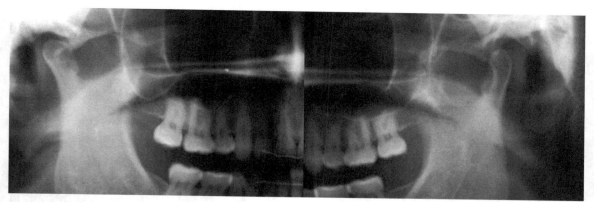

Figure 17.11 Panoramic Radiograph

and whether the imaging will influence the clinical course or treatment options. In the case of a specific TMD, magnetic resonance imaging and computed tomography can be indicated to obtain additional diagnostic information and weigh the treatment options.

On indication (e.g., closed lock), the clinician can get an impression of the joint function and local loading capacity by traction, translation, and compression techniques. For muscle loading, resistance tests can be helpful. Traction and translation tests will evaluate the passive accessory movement (joint play) and are executed with a thumb of the examiner placed on the occlusal surfaces of the molars (traction in caudal direction and translation in ventrodorsal direction) (**Figure 17.12**). The position of the thumb is changed to the lingual part of the molars for the mediolateral direction (**Figure 17.13**). Compression can be performed by a force in dorsocranial and ventrocranial directions, with the fixing hand providing a counterforce (**Figure 17.14**). Resistance tests are a static pain test with the mandible kept stationary and a gradually increasing force applied in each direction (**Figure 17.15**). Some masticatory and other relevant muscles cannot be directly palpated; an example is the lateral pterygoid muscle. These muscles are not incorporated in the examination protocol.

Measurement Properties

A basic requirement for a proper diagnosis is the reliability of the diagnostic procedure. The intra- and interexaminer reliability of the orthopaedic tests has been described extensively (Carlsson et al., 1980; Kopp & Wenneberg, 1983; Dworkin et al., 1990; Lobbezoo-Scholte et al., 1993; Steenks et al., 1996). The reliability of active and passive opening in all subgroups was high. The reliability scores for joint play tests were moderate (pain) to poor (end-feel). Physical

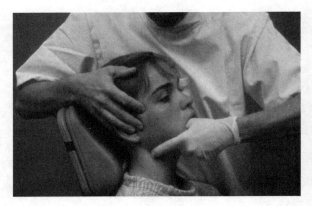

Figure 17.12 Traction in Caudal Direction and Translation in Ventrodorsal Direction

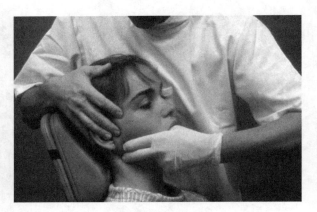

Figure 17.13 Translation in Mediolateral Direction

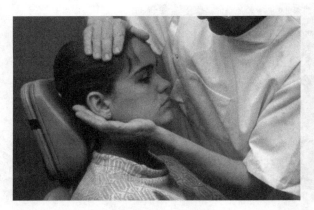

Figure 17.14 Compression in Dorsocranial or Ventrocranial Direction

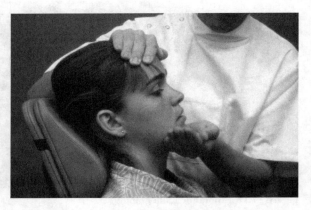

Figure 17.15 Resistance Test with the Mandible Stationary

therapists did not perform better than dentists (Vermeiren et al., 1995). The reliability scores for palpation were moderate.

Because the diagnostic process is based on combination of tests, and in some tests only a few signs and symptoms occur, multitest scores can be composed. The multitest scores for the combination of tests for the three main symptoms of TMD (i.e., pain, joint noises, and restriction of movement) are presented in **Table 17.2**. Multitest scores of combinations of tests are relevant because the establishment of the diagnosis is not based on single findings, but on multiple diagnostic tests (Haas, 1991a, 1991b). Because it is possible for two observers to disagree on the presence of pain in separate tests yet agree completely on the presence of pain during function, it seems that the presence or absence of musculoskeletal pain can be derived

more accurately from the combination of five tests (active, passive, palpation, joint play, and resistance). Movement restriction and the presence or absence of joint noises are determined to be reliable when based on active movements. Pain is obviously a symptom with high intrinsic variability and many possible influences, making it difficult to obtain a high interrater reliability score. The reliability of the combination of the active movements, passive opening, and palpation tests is satisfactory.

We determined the diagnostic value of the different orthopaedic tests to get an impression of the validity of the diagnostic procedure (**Table 17.3**). A functional examination consisting of active movements, passive opening, and palpation provided valuable diagnostic information (Lobbezoo-Scholte et al., 1993). Additional tests (compression, traction/translation, resistance)

Table 17.2 Interexaminer Reliability of the Multitest Scores for Combinations of Tests for the Three Main Symptoms of Temporomandibular Disorder

Multitest Score Categories	Agreement (%)	K	Presence of Signs and Symptoms (%)
Pain			
During active movements	65	0.3	49
During additional tests (passive opening, joint play, compression, static pain)	69	0.4	59
During function (active movements and/or additional tests)	89	0.7	69
During function and palpation	96	0.8	91
Noise			
During active movements	80	0.6	55
During additional tests	68	0.3	32
During function	77	0.5	60
Restriction of movement			
During active movements	92	0.6	10
During active movements and/or joint play tests	75	0.4	29

K, Coben κ, statistic in a temporomandibular disorders patient group ($n = 79$).
Modified from Lobbezoo-Scholte, 1993.

Table 17.3 Percentage of Subjects Correctly Classified by the Different Tests and Combination of Tests Selected by Stepwise Logistic Regression and Odds Ratio of the Myogenous Group Versus the Arthrogenous Group

	% Corrected Classified	% Corrected Classified M	% Corrected Classified A	OR
Active movements	78.6	84	74	15.36
Palpation	70.0	45	90	7.65
Combination of active movements and palpation	83.1	87	80	26.75
Passive opening	73.4	54	89	9.16
Joint play test	66.5	80	56	5.11
Compression	58.4	9	97	3.18
Static pain test	71.8	45	92	8.77
Combination of four tests	77.3	65	86	11.68
Combination of six tests	87.5	87	88	48.49

M, myogenous group ($n = 69$); A, arthrogenous group ($n = 91$); OR, odds ratio.
Modified from Lobbezoo-Scholte, 1993.

might be indicated if the subclassification is difficult (e.g., restricted mouth opening having an arthrogenous or myogenous origin); for example, disc displacement without reduction can be classified with a combination of active range of motion, passive opening, palpation, and translation tests. Our study showed that active movement was the most powerful test for distinguishing the different subgroups of patients, and passive opening and palpation were additionally useful for distinguishing between patients and control subjects and between the subgroups of arthrogenous and myogenous patients. Orthopaedic tests of the masticatory system can be used in patients with overlap of signs and symptoms to discriminate between CSD and TMD. In contrast, logistic regression analyses showed that orthopaedic tests of the cervical spine were of minor importance in discriminating between patients with TMD and CSD (Wijer de et al., 1996b, 1996c).

Conclusion

Because of the neurophysiologic and biomechanical interactions between the cervical spine and the stomatognathic system, overlap of signs and symptoms occurs. In TMD, patients will frequently perceive pain in the cervical area. CSD patients usually have signs and symptoms of TMD comparable with the epidemiologic data of the healthy population. This supports the idea that TMD can give rise to neck pain (sensitization). The physiotherapist must evaluate the masticatory system in patients with persistent head and neck pain.

CASE REPORT

Mrs. S.B., 31 years of age, visited our clinic with the following information from the oral surgeon. This patient had been seen in his office for more than 5 months with intermittent locking signs (closed lock) of the left TMJ (10 to 12 periods a day for a few minutes). She has had a history of clicking of the left joint for more than 4 years, related to diving. There has been a local pain in the preauricular area on the left side for more than 1 year. Besides the oral surgeon, S.B. also visited a dental specialist in orofacial pain and a physiotherapist for exercises. Splint therapy for more than 3 months was not successful. Because the response to treatment was inadequate, the patient had been referred.

Intake Questionnaire (Screen)

The main complaint is periodically closed lock of the left jaw, with pain and limited function. Question: What intervention will help restore normal jaw function and thereby eliminate locking and pain? The clinician can formulate the following question: Is an intervention available that will help restore normal jaw function in a diagnosed TMD patient already treated by counseling, exercises, and splinting?

The pain drawing in Screen shows a local pain in the preauricular area that is greater on the left than the right side. The intensity of the left-side preauricular pain is on average 4.5/10 cm (VAS), but can change between 4 and 8/10 cm. After exacerbation, the extra pain lasts for 15 to 30 minutes and decreases within 1 hour to the level of 2 to 3/10. The complaint has been present for more than 1 year; the frequency of pain and locking is increasing with time. There are no sleeping problems. The jaw frequently produces joint sounds during movements. There is pain on wide mouth opening and very inconvenient signs and symptoms of closed lock (mouth opening 20 mm). In the early morning, a stiff and tired feeling in the cheek area exists. She is aware of clenching but denies grinding activities. Other functional habits are nail biting and lip sucking. There is a reduction in functions such as biting an apple; eating soft, hard, and tough food; yawning; singing; and kissing. She has the impression that the occlusion has changed, and she had to change the mouthpiece for diving. There is no neck pain according to the questionnaire.

She experiences headache once a month related to the hormonal cycle, with vomiting and sharp pain. She works 22 hours a week as an office manager, can handle her work without problems, and has a good working environment without complaints. She is satisfied with her work and social life (mother with one child) and has no signs of depression, anxiety, or somatization. She avoids singing in the choir and long conversations at work. In the family history no problems are known.

Intraoral and Extraoral Inspection

There are no signs or symptoms of red flags, and no signs of forward head posture. Attrition is 13/43 (Figure 17.2). There is facial asymmetry (right side of the face more prominent) and intraoral signs of clenching activities. No signs or symptoms related to a Sunday face, speech problems, forward deviation on opening, or change in position of the tongue or jaw exist. There are no deviating occlusal characteristics.

Mandibular Range of Motion: Active

- *Opening:* 50 mm + 3 mm overbite; deviation on mouth opening of 5 mm to the left within 20 mm range of motion, clicking sound (left TMJ, moderate) on 20 mm opening. *Repetition:* local preauricular pain increases. Pain is rated a 6 on a numeric rating scale (NRS) of 0–10 (0 no pain at all; 10 the most pain imaginable).
- Closing not affected, normal intercuspal position.
- *Horizontal left:* 9 mm.
- *Horizontal right:* 6 mm, slight pain (NRS 4), click in the end position.
- *Protrusion:* 6 + 2 mm overjet (slight deviation to the left of 3 mm).

Mandibular Range of Motion: Passive

- *Opening:* 51 mm + 3 mm overbite; preauricular pain on wide opening, NRS 5 on the left and

NRS 2 on the right, with deviation to the left and clicking.

- *Horizontal movements:* 9 to 10 mm, no pain provocation anterior and to the left side. To the right side, clicking and pain in end position (NRS 4).

Palpation

- The temporalis muscle did not show hypertonus; no pain on palpation, no palpable changes. The coronoid process showed local pain, with NRS 7 on the left side.
- Masseter muscle: deep as well as superficial part was painful on the left (NRS 3, local pain).
- Attachments: medial pterygoid muscle (NRS 3, local pain) on the left side.

Conclusions

The oral surgeon referred a patient with an arthrogenous type of TMD on the left side due to an intermittent disc displacement without reduction. Muscle reactions were also noticed. Because the treatment result was negative, an arthrocentesis or intra-articular injection was considered. After the intake, we reached the following conclusion: a chronic orofacial, nonspecific pain in a 31-year-old woman with a clicking joint for more than 4 years, with clicking of the TMJ starting after the patient attended diving school. There are no red (medical comorbidity) or yellow (psychosocial) flags, and the character of the pain is nociceptive from the locomotor system (the TMJ or muscles). The time table shows an increasing frequency of locking and more periods of increased local preauricular pain. The objective part of the clinical examination reveals a moderate severity, and the subjective part reveals a moderate to high severity with periods of loss of control that trouble the patient. In such a period with no control, she fears to move. The way in which she copes with her complaints is adequate most of the time; only in an acute stage during a closed lock does she become insecure. She avoids singing and long conversations. The intraoral stabilization splint reduces the complaints during the evening and night so she can sleep, but the splint does not influence the complaints during the day.

Intervention

A physiotherapeutic intervention was successful and consisted of counseling with the help of video film, with information regarding the function of the TMJ, joint sounds due to disc displacement, closed lock, and normal tongue position. Massage techniques (control hypertonus, tender points, structural changes, muscle contraction or stretching pain) were used by the physiotherapist on the masseter and temporalis, including deep friction (2–4 minutes) on the attachment coronoid process. Auto massage instruction (homework, twice a day) was provided. Further, habit reversal techniques were taught, whereby the patient monitors the habits and related signs and symptoms (clenching, nail biting, lip sucking, and mouthpiece use when diving), and the circumstances in which they occur, with instructions to exercise behavior opposite to the dysfunctional behavior. Mobilization techniques of the joint with traction and translation techniques, starting with oscillation and followed by manipulation, were also applied.

Homework exercise on opening without repetitive clicking was as described by Yoda et al. (2003):

Open the mouth maximally with opening-click, close the mouth along the protrusive border movement path, contact the teeth at the protruded position, retrude to a contact position just before the click happens, open the mouth maximally again without the opening click and repeat this exercise for three [to] five minutes, three times a day.

In case of closed lock, a manipulation technique described by Minagi et al. (1991) was used: Place the thumb on the left side of the mandible and the fingers on the zygoma right side. Make a lateral excursion to the right side (nonaffected side) and open the mouth maximally through lateral right border path. Reciprocal clicking on the affected side occurs in the patient's case, and she could manage her closed lock in this way. The treatment was applied once a week for 4 weeks.

The postintervention evaluation revealed a pain-free active function and passive opening of the mandible, a decrease in frequency of the locks, less intense clicking, and more control in mandibular function. There was no need for further treatment, and the long-term follow-up (interview by phone after 6 months and 1 year) shows a good result on the level of impairment and function and no treatment demand.

REFERENCES

Carlsson GE, Ehgermark-Eriksson I, Magnusson T. Intra- and inter-observer variation in functional examination of the masticatory system. *Swed Dent J* 1980;4:187–194.

Coster de PJ, Berghe van den LI, Martens LC. Generalized joint hyper-mobility and temporomandibular disorders: inherited connective tissue disease as a model with maximum expression. *J Orofac Pain* 2005;19:47–57.

Dijkstra PU, Kropmans TJB, Stegenga B. The association between generalized joint hyper-mobility and temporomandibular joint disorder: a systematic review. *J Dent Res* 2002;81:158–163.

Dworkin SF. Perspectives on the interaction of biological, psychological and social factors in TMD. *J Am Dent Assoc* 1994;125:856–863.

Dworkin SF, LeResche L. Research diagnostic criteria for temporomandibular disorders: review, criteria, examinations and specifications, critique. *J Craniomandib Disord Facial Oral Pain* 1992;6:301–355.

Dworkin SF, LeResche L, DeRouen T, Korff von M. Assessing clinical signs of temporomandibular disorders: reliability of clinical examiners. *J Prosthet Dent* 1990;63:574–579.

Edwards I, Jones M, Carr J, Braunack-Mayer A, Jensen GM. Clinical reasoning strategies in physical therapy. *Phys Ther* 2004;84:312–320.

Farrar WB. Characteristics of the condylar path in internal derangements of the TMJ. *J Prosthet Dent* 1978;39:319–323.

Haas M. Inter-examiner reliability for multiple diagnostic test regimens. *J Manipulative Physiol Ther* 1991a;14:95–103.

Haas M. Statistical methodology for reliability studies. *J Manipulative Physiol Ther* 1991b;14:119–132.

Isselee H, De Laat A, De Mot B, Lysens R. Pressure-pain threshold variation in temporomandibular disorder myalgia over the course of the menstrual cycle. *J Orofac Pain* 2002;16:105–117.

Kanter de RJAM. *Prevalence and Aetiology of Cranio-mandibular Dysfunction: An Epidemiological Study of the Dutch Adult Population* [PhD thesis]. The Netherlands: University Nijmegen; 1990.

Kanter de RJ, Kayser AF, Battistuzzi PG, Truin GJ, Hof van't MA. Demand and need for treatment of cranio-mandibular dysfunction in the Dutch adult population. *J Dent Res* 1992;71:1607–1612.

Kanter de RJ, Truin GJ, Burgersdijk RC, Hof van't MA, Battistuzi PG, Kalsbeek H, Kayser AF. Prevalence in the Dutch adult population and a meta-analysis of signs and symptoms of temporomandibular disorder. *J Dent Res* 1993;72:1509–1518.

Kopp S, Wenneberg B. Intra- and inter-observer variability in the assessment of signs of disorder in the stomatognathic system. *Swed Dent J* 1983;7:239–246.

Laskin DM. Etiology of the pain-dysfunction syndrome. *J Am Dent Assoc* 1969;79:147–153.

Leeuw R. *Psychosocial Aspects and Symptom Characteristics of Cranio-mandibular Dysfunction* [thesis]. The Netherlands: Utrecht University; 1993.

Leeuw de R, Ros WJG, Steenks MH, Scholte AM, Bosman F, Winnubst JAW. Multidimensional evaluation of cranio-mandibular dysfunction II: pain assessment. *J Oral Rehabil* 1994;21:515–532.

LeResche L, Saunders K, Korff von MR, Barlow W, Dworkin SF. Use of exogenous hormones and risk of temporomandibular disorder pain. *Pain* 1997;69:153–160.

Lobbezoo-Scholte AM. *Diagnostic Subgroups of Cranio-mandibular Disorders* [thesis]. The Netherlands: Utrecht University; 1993.

Lobbezoo-Scholte AM, Steenks MH, Faber JAJ, Bosman F. Diagnostic value of orthopaedic tests in patients with cranio-mandibular disorders. *J Dent Res* 1993;72:1443–1453.

Lobbezoo-Scholte AM, de Leeuw JRJ, Steenks MH, Bosman F, Buchner R, Olthoff LW. Diagnostic subgroups of cranio-mandibular disorders. Part I: self-report data and clinical findings. *J Orofac Pain* 1995;9:24–36.

Magnusson T, Carlsson GE. Changes in recurrent headaches and mandibular dysfunction after various types of dental treatment. *Acta Odontol Scand* 1980;38:311–320.

McNeely ML, Olivo SA, Magee DJ. A systematic review of the effectiveness of physical therapy interventions for temporo-mandibular disorders. *Phys Ther* 2006;86:710–725.

Medlicott MS, Harris SR. A systematic review of the effectiveness of exercise, manual therapy, electrotherapy, relaxation training, and biofeedback in the management of temporomandibular disorder. *Phys Ther* 2006;86:955–973.

Minagi S, Nozaki S, Sato T, Tsuru H. A manipulation technique for treatment of anterior disk displacement without reduction. *J Prosthet Dent* 1991;65:686–691.

Okeson JP, ed. *Orofacial Pain: Guidelines for Assessment, Diagnosis, and Management.* Chicago: Quintessence Publishing; 1996.

Olivo SA, Bravo J, Magee DJ, Thie NMR, Major PW, Flores-Mir C. The association between head and cervical posture and temporomandibular disorders: a systematic review. *J Orofac Pain* 2006;20:9–23.

Projectgroep musculoskelettale stoornissen van het kauwstelsel. Consensus diagnostiek en therapie in de gnathologie. *Ned Tijdschr Tandheelkd* 2003;110:281–287.

Sessle BJ. The neural basis of temporomandibular joint and masticatory muscle pain. *J Orofac Pain* 1999;13:238–245.

Sjaastad O. Cervicogenic headache: the controversial headache. *Clin Neurol Neurosurg* 1992;94(suppl):S147–S149.

Steenks MH, Wijer de A. *Craniomandibulaire dysfuncties vanuit fysiotherapeutisch en tandheelkundig perpectief.* Lochem: De Tijdstroom; 1989.

Steenks MH, Wijer de A. *Kiefergelenkfehlfunktionen aus physiotherapeutischer und zahnmedizinischer sicht.* Berlin: Quintessenz bibliothek; 1991.

Steenks MH, Wijer de A. *Disfunções da Articulação temporomandibular, Ponto de Vista da Fisioterapia e da Odontologia.* São Paulo: Santos; 1996.

Steenks MH, Wijer de A, Bosman F. Orthopaedic diagnostic tests for temporo-mandibular and cervical spine disorders. *J Back Musculoskeletal Rehabil* 1996;6:135–153.

Steenks MH, Hugger A, Wijer de A. Painful arthrogenous temporomandibular disorders. In: Türp JC, Sommer C, Hugger A, eds. *The Puzzle of Orofacial Pain. Integrating Research into Clinical Management*. Basel: Karger; 2007.

Stegenga B, Bont de LGM, Boering G. Osteoarthritis as the cause of cranio-mandibular pain and dysfunction: a unifying concept. *J Oral Maxillofacial Surg* 1989;47: 249–256.

Steiner WA, Ryser L, Huber E, Uebelhart D, Aeschlimann A, Stucki G. Use of the ICF model as a clinical problem-solving tool in physical therapy and rehabilitation medicine. *Phys Ther* 2002;82:1098–1107.

Suvinen TI, Reade PC, Kemppainen P, Könönen M, Dworkin SF. Review of aetiological concepts of temporomandibular pain disorders: towards a bio-psycho-social model for integration of physical disorder factors with psychological and psychosocial illness impact factors. *Eur J Pain* 2005;9:613–633.

Turner JA, Dworkin SF. Recent developments in psychological diagnostic procedures: screening for psychological risk factors for poor outcomes. *J Am Dent Assoc* 2004;135: 1119–1125.

Vermeiren J, Heyrman A, Oostendorp RAB. Het joint-play onderzoek van het temporomandibulaire gewricht. *Ned Tijdschr Manuele Therapie* 1995;2:32–45.

Ververs MJB, Ouwerkerk JL, Heijden van der GJMG, Steenks MH, Wijer de A. Atiologie der kraniomandibulären dysfunktionen: eine Literaturübersicht. *Deutsche Zahnärztlische Zeitschrift* 2004;59:556–562.

Wijer de A. *Temporomandibular and Cervical Spine Disorders* [PhD dissertation]. The Netherlands: Universiteit Utrecht; 1995.

Wijer de A, Steenks MH. Cervical spine evaluation for the TMD patient, a review. In: Fricton J, Dubner R, eds. *Advances in Orofacial Pain and Temporomandibular Disorders*. New York: Raven Press; 1995:351–361.

Wijer de A, Leeuw de JRJ, Steenks MH, Bosman F. Temporomandibular and cervical spine disorders: self-reported signs and symptoms. *Spine* 1996a;21:1638–1646.

Wijer de A, Steenks MH, Bosman F, Helders PJ, Faber J. Symptoms of the stomatognathic system in temporomandibular and cervical spine disorders. *J Oral Rehabil* 1996b;23:733–741.

Wijer de A, Steenks MH, Leeuw de JR, Bosman F, Helders PJ. Symptoms of the cervical spine in temporomandibular and cervical spine disorders. *J Oral Rehabil* 1996c;23:742–750.

Wijnhoven HA, Vet de HCW, Picavet HSJ. Sex differences in consequences of musculoskeletal pain. *Spine* 2007;32: 1360–1367.

Yoda T, Sakamoto I, Imai H, Honma Y, Shinjo Y, Takano A, et al. A randomized controlled trial of therapeutic exercise for clicking due to disk anterior displacement with reduction in the temporomandibular joint. *J Craniomand Pract* 2003;21:10–16.

Zarb GA, Carlsson GE, Sessle BJ, Mohl ND. *Temporomandibular Joint and Masticatory Muscle Disorders*. 2nd ed. Copenhagen: Munksgaard; 1995.

Neurophysiologic Effects of Some Physical Therapy Interventions

Neurophysiologic Effects of Spinal Manipulation

Bill Vicenzino, PT, PhD, Tina Souvlis, PT, PhD, and Michele Sterling, PT, PhD

Spinal manipulation is clinically effective in the management of cervicogenic headaches (Hoving et al., 2002; Jull et al., 2002) and is frequently used by health-care practitioners. Spinal manipulation is the application of force of varying velocity and frequency profiles (e.g., sustained, oscillatory, or high-velocity thrust), usually manually applied, either to a vertebra or a number of vertebrae. Traditionally, spinal manipulation has been described as being passive (i.e., not involving any voluntary action by the patient), but there are more recent techniques that combine a sustained manual force applied to the spine with active movements of the neck and head, such as Mulligan's techniques (Hall et al., 2007; Mulligan, 1999).

Specific research on the neurophysiologic effects of manipulative techniques for headache treatment is scant, but there is some nascent research into manual therapy for other parts of the body that may be extrapolated to the treatment of the cervical spine, or more specifically to the upper cervical spine in cervicogenic headaches (Jull et al., 2002). There has been a long history of viewing the effects of manipulation in biomechanical terms, with a preoccupation on subluxations and conceptually related propositions. In relatively recent times, the emphasis has been to focus on the neurophysiologic mechanisms by which spinal manipulation may exert pain-relieving effects. In applying a spinal manual therapy technique to the cervical spine, the therapist perturbs the underlying skin, fascia, muscles, joints, and bones, which in turn likely activate afferent inputs into the central nervous system. Hence spinal manual therapy may be viewed as a physiologic stimulus that is used to bring about pain relief and improvements in movement and function by neurophysiologic mechanisms. These mechanisms are likely complex, with possible involvement from both local segmental and descending pain inhibitory mechanisms, as well as psychological influences (Wyke, 1985; Zusman et al., 1989; Wright, 1995; Wright & Vicenzino, 1995). This chapter presents a synthesis of relevant data pertaining to the neurophysiologic mechanisms of spinal manipulation by describing a proposed mechanism and presenting salient evidence.

A PROPOSED PHYSIOLOGIC MECHANISM FOR SPINAL MANIPULATION

A hypothetical model to explain the rapid hypoalgesic effect produced by spinal manipulation has been proposed by Wright (Wright, 1995; Wright & Vicenzino, 1995). The model posited a multifactorial basis in which a number of potential physiologic mechanisms for analgesia were included, such as assisting with healing, effects on connective tissues of the joints, alteration of the intra-articular milieu, modification of the chemical environment of peripheral nociceptors, and activation of both segmental pain inhibitory mechanisms and descending pain inhibitory systems. Psychologic influences were also considered. It has been suggested that the descending pain inhibitory system (DPIS) in particular could be responsible for mediating an immediate analgesic response. This suggestion arose from studies in both animals and humans that identified the midbrain periaqueductal gray matter (PAG) as a key center of control for mediation of descending inhibition of pain (Reynolds, 1969; Hosobuchi et al., 1977; Cannon et al., 1982; Depaulis & Bandler, 1991). The PAG has been shown to have an important integrative role for behavioral responses to pain, stress, and other stimuli in maintaining the organism's homeostasis, which it achieves through coordination of responses of a number of systems, including the nociceptive system, autonomic nervous system, and motor system (Fanselow, 1991; Lovick, 1991b; Morgan, 1991).

Somewhat in line with its functional role, the PAG has a columnar structure, with dorsomedial, dorsolateral, lateral, and ventrolateral columns being identified. The lateral (lPAG) and ventrolateral (vlPAG) subdivisions of the caudal PAG have been extensively investigated (Carrive, 1991; Lovick, 1991a, 1991b; Morgan, 1991; Bandler & Shipley, 1994; Farkas et al., 1998; Jansen et al., 1998), with emergence of an understanding that there is a complex but diverse set of responses following stimulation of the different PAG subdivisions. This research, performed in animals, demonstrated that stimulation of the vlPAG produced a tripartite effect that included opioid-mediated analgesia, sympatho-inhibition, and quiescence or immobility. In contrast, stimulation of the lPAG appears to result in a nonopioid analgesia accompanied by sympatho-excitation and motor excitation. Put simply, the functional behavioral consequences of the lPAG are summed up by the flight-or-fight response to threatening or nociceptive stimuli. As such, it appears that the PAG is responsible for coordinating responses that ensure survival rather than solely modulating pain perception (Fanselow, 1991).

It is of interest that low-threshold mechanoreceptors from joints and muscles project to the PAG and that therefore nonnoxious afferent input might also elicit components of this reaction (Yezierski, 1991). Consequently, the stimulus of spinal manipulation via activation of cutaneous, joint, and muscle afferents may be appropriate to activate key regions of the PAG. Experimental research conducted in humans has shown that some forms of spinal manipulation produce a tripartite response similar to that seen when the lPAG is stimulated in animal experiments, that is, there is a nonopioid form of hypoalgesia that is concomitant to sympatho-excitation and possibly motor excitation (Wright, 1995; Wright & Vicenzino, 1995; Vicenzino et al., 1998a; Souvlis et al., 2005).

Research Underpinning a DPIS Mechanism for Spinal Manipulation

Evidence contributing to a theoretical model that underpins a DPIS involvement in spinal manipulation is here addressed through sections on the evidence of immediate hypoalgesic effects, the characteristics of this effect (e.g., opioid involvement), and the possible meaning of a concomitant multisystem coordinated response to manipulation.

Spinal Manipulation Produces Immediate Hypoalgesia

Several studies have used quantitative sensory testing to investigate the effect of spinal manipulation in the cervical spine in both symptomatic and asymptomatic participants (Vicenzino et al., 1996, 1998a, 1998b, 2000; Souvlis et al., 1999; Sterling et al., 2001a). Within-subject controlled studies were performed in participants presenting with unilateral lateral epicondylalgia (Vicenzino et al., 1996; Souvlis et al., 2000) and nontraumatic neck pain (Sterling et al., 2001a). The spinal manipulation techniques studied were of the oscillatory type (not high-velocity thrusts), including posterior-anterior mobilization at the C5 segment and a lateral glide technique described by Elvey performed at the C5-C6 level (Elvey, 1986). The outcome measures included pressure and thermal pain threshold, pain-free grip force threshold, and neural tissue provocation test. To control for the non-specific effects related to manual contact and premanipulation joint set-up position, all studies in this series incorporated a placebo condition with no joint movement as well as a no-contact control condition.

This series of studies demonstrated that there was a rapid-onset hypoalgesic response with specific characteristics following intervention in both asymptomatic and symptomatic participants. In a study of 24 asymptomatic participants, there was 22% improvement in pressure pain thresholds but no concomitant change in thermal pain thresholds (Vicenzino et al., 1995a, 1995b). This finding suggested that there was a specificity of effect of spinal manipulation for mechanical pain but not thermal pain thresholds. These findings were confirmed in a study by Sterling et al. (2001a, 2001b), which also showed a specific effect of treatment in producing mechanical but not thermal hypoalgesia in treatment of neck pain. Using the lateral glide technique in 15 patients with unilateral elbow pain, Vicenzino et al. (1996) found improvements in pressure pain threshold (approximately 25%), pain-free grip threshold (30%), and neural tissue provocation test (approximately 40%). The technique produced clinically meaningful improvements of pain measured on a Visual Analogue Scale (VAS) (1.9 cm). These effects were deemed to be physiologic because the researchers recruited naïve subjects and implemented a placebo-control protocol, which was corroborated by results of the postintervention survey demonstrating that the participants were not able to distinguish treatment interventions from placebo or control conditions. Both asymptomatic and symptomatic groups were naïve to the effects of the treatment.

The above-mentioned studies on low-velocity techniques have reported findings in line with those reported for high-velocity thrust (Terrett & Vernon, 1984; Vernon

et al., 1990). For example, Terrett and Vernon (1984) reported an increase in pain tolerance of up to 130% on electrically induced cutaneous pain threshold at 10 minutes after a high-velocity-thrust manipulation of a painful spinal segment between T3 and T10 ($n = 50$; control was a premanipulation oscillatory palpation technique). Vernon et al. (1990) compared a rotational manipulation to premanipulation oscillatory mobilization in nine sufferers of chronic neck pain and reported a statistically significant increase in pressure pain thresholds (45%) in the manipulation group compared with the control group.

From these studies, it appears that manual therapy produces a robust hypoalgesic effect that is reproducible across a number of studies using different techniques and patient populations.

Role of Opioid Mechanisms

Attempts have been made to ascertain whether opioid mechanisms are involved in spinal thrust manipulation, with a number of methods having been employed in human research, such as measuring β-endorphin levels in plasma, using naloxone as an antagonist to block the hypoalgesic response of spinal thrust manipulation and tolerance to repeat exposure (Fields & Basbaum, 1994; Meyer et al., 2000; Vaccarino & Kastin, 2001).

The presence of the opioid β-endorphin following manipulation was assessed in a study by Sanders et al. (1990), who investigated the effect of manipulation of the lumbar spine with sham (light touch) and no-contact control conditions on VAS scores and β-endorphin levels. They demonstrated pain relief with manipulation compared with placebo and control conditions but were unable to detect a difference among the three conditions for β-endorphin level (Sanders et al., 1990). This finding was consistent with that from a study of manipulation of the cervical and thoracic spines in both symptomatic and asymptomatic populations, which showed no significant difference in β-endorphin levels between manipulation and a sham manipulation control (Christian et al., 1988). The only study to report counter to this trend was by Vernon et al. (1986), who measured the effect of cervical spine manipulation compared with sham and control. They found a small but statistically significant increase in β-endorphin level in the manipulation group 30 minutes postmanipulation. An issue with identifying an opioid mechanism through measuring plasma levels of circulating β-endorphin is that it may not be as sensitive to detecting change as would be expected if cerebrospinal fluid levels were monitored (Vernon, 2000).

A number of studies have administered naloxone in order to evaluate the role of opioids in spinal manipulation. Zusman et al. (1989) assessed the response to spinal manipulation by comparing the administration of naloxone with a saline control on the pain-relieving effect of a pragmatic spinal manipulation treatment session in 21 patients presenting with low back pain (10 naloxone, 11 saline). Pain provoked on movement was measured by the Visual Analogue Scale and shown to be reduced with manipulation, but this pain relief was not antagonized by naloxone, indicating that opioids were likely not involved (Zusman et al., 1989). In a more recent study by Vicenzino et al. (2000), the influence of naloxone on pain relief was compared with saline and with no-drug control conditions. In this study, a lateral glide technique to C5-C6 was performed in patients with lateral epicondylalgia ($n = 24$), and no influence of naloxone on the hypoalgesic response was demonstrated (Vicenzino et al., 2000). To further assess the possible contribution of opioid mechanisms to the analgesic response, the effect of repeated administration of lateral glide to C5-C6 in patients suffering from lateral epicondylalgia was undertaken to determine whether tolerance developed to the initial hypoalgesic effect of spinal manipulation (Souvlis & Wright, 1997; Souvlis et al., 1999). Results demonstrated that no tolerance developed to the initial effect when the technique was applied over six sessions.

The spinal manipulation research in humans has some support in a study that used rats to determine which spinal neurotransmitter receptors mediate the hypoalgesic effects (Skyba et al., 2003). Skyba et al. (2003) produced hyperalgesia, as measured with reduced mechanical withdrawal thresholds, by injecting the ankle joint of the rats with capsaicin. Once the ankle was inflamed and hyperalgesic, the investigators applied a range of neurotransmitter blocking agents and knee joint manipulation (vs. a no-manipulation control condition). The manipulation significantly reversed the hyperalgesia, showing that the treatment in this animal model mimics that in humans. The administration of naloxone and bicuculline did not alter the effects of manipulation, whereas the serotonin antagonists blocked the manipulation-induced effect, and the noradrenaline antagonism through yohimbine attenuated the manipulation effect. This pattern of effect with application of these spinal neurotransmitter blockers indicates that the effect of manipulation appears to involve a nonopioid DPIS that involves serotonin and noradrenaline (Skyba et al., 2003).

A Concomitant Multisystem Coordinated Response to Spinal Manipulation

Data from both basic animal studies and human studies support the premise that nonnoxious afferent stimulation of the neck can induce sympathetic nervous system responses. Studies from our laboratories have demonstrated that spinal manipulation is a sufficient stimulus to induce a sympathetic nervous system response. These excitatory responses appear to be reproducible independent of technique or subject population.

Based on the hypothesis that multisystem responses are evoked by spinal manipulation (Wright, 1995; Wright & Vicenzino, 1995), a series of studies have specifically investigated the effect of spinal manipulation on the sympathetic nervous system. Studies have investigated the effect of posterior-anterior and lateral glides of the cervical spine (C5-C6). Outcome measures for sympathetic nervous system function in these studies were sudomotor, cutaneous vasomotor, and cardiorespiratory functions (Petersen et al., 1993; Slater et al., 1994; Vicenzino et al., 1994, 1995a, 1995b, 1998a, 1998b; McGuiness et al., 1997; Simon et al., 1997; Souvlis et al., 2001; Paungmali et al., 2003). Both techniques produced a change in sympathetic nervous system function that was significantly different from that produced by placebo and control conditions in a suite of studies using a within-subject, controlled design. The changes in effects produced in these studies are indicative of an excitatory response of the peripheral indicators of sympathetic nervous system function (Vicenzino et al., 1998a, 1998b).

Nonnoxious stimulation of neck afferents by movements of the head and neck in animal models produced changes in sympathetic nerve activity, such as changes in heart rate, arterial pressure, vascular resistance, and limb blood flow (Bolton et al., 1998; Bolton & Ray, 2000), as also shown in human studies (Shortt & Ray, 1997; Fujimoto et al., 1999; Hume & Ray, 1999). Fujimoto et al. (1999) showed that innocuous movements of the neck, which are similar to those performed during spinal manipulation, may alter heart rate and arterial pressure. These effects have been reflected in human studies of spinal manipulation. Vicenzino et al. (1998a, 1998b) measured indices of sympathetic nervous system function, namely cardiovascular and respiratory function, during application of the lateral glide technique to C5-C6 in 24 asymptomatic subjects. A significant increase in heart rate and both diastolic and systolic blood pressure, on the order of approximately 14%, was observed in the treatment condition in comparison with 1% to 2% in the placebo and control conditions. The respiratory rate also showed an increase, of around 36%, that was significantly larger than the control conditions. Similar changes—that is, increase in heart rate, blood pressure (diastolic more than systolic), and respiratory rate—were shown following a posterior-anterior technique at C5 (McGuiness et al., 1997).

The premise that the PAG may be the locus of control of the initial analgesic effect of spinal manipulation (Wright, 1995; Wright & Vicenzino, 1995) is supported by findings from the above studies investigating sympathetic nervous system responses to treatment techniques of the cervical spine. Animal studies demonstrated that activation of lPAG produces a response incorporating nonopioid analgesia and excitation of sympathetic nervous systems (Lovick, 1991a, 1991b). Vicenzino et al. (1998a, 1998b) were able to demonstrate a significant relationship between the hypoalgesic and sympathetic nervous system responses to spinal manipulation using confirmatory factor analysis. The analgesia following spinal manipulation did not display opioid characteristics, because it was not reversed by naloxone (Vicenzino et al., 1998a, 1998b) and did not become tolerant to repeated application (Souvlis et al., 1999).

It would be anticipated that if the lPAG were involved in a DPIS following spinal manipulation, there would be an initial excitatory motor effect concurrent with the hypoalgesia and sympatho-excitation (Wright, 1995; Sterling et al., 2001a, 2001b). There is some evidence that the type of spinal manipulation techniques employed in these studies produce excitatory effects on the motor system concurrent with hypoalgesia and sympatho-excitation (Sterling et al., 2001a, 2001b). Sterling et al. (2001a, 2001b) used mobilization of C5-C6 segments in patients with neck pain to investigate the concurrent effects on motor, sympathetic nervous system function, and analgesia. The effect of a posterior-anterior glide technique on the craniocervical flexion test was assessed. A decreased activation of superficial musculature of the cervical spine, which was interpreted as facilitation of the deeper neck flexors, gives some confirmation that motor responses are altered following spinal manipulation. The patients in this study showed pain relief as measured by algometry, thus indicating concurrent hypoalgesic and motor effects.

The tripartite response in pain, sympathetic, and motor systems resulting from activation of the PAG has been explained behaviorally in terms of a flight-or-fight response to a perceived stress. Vicenzino et al. (1999) conducted a study to determine whether the sympatho-excitatory effects noted following spinal manipulation were related to stress and pain. The study surveyed participants to establish whether participants perceived that spinal manipulation produced stress and pain in comparison with placebo and control interventions. The results suggest that application of the technique was not linked with stress and pain and thus not an underlying reason for the observed changes in sympathetic nervous system function (Vicenzino et al., 1999).

Spinal Manipulation as a Physiologic Stimulus: Possible Afferent Pathways

Manipulation of the upper cervical spine resulting in displacement of the vertebra is accompanied by activation of primary and secondary afferents from the muscle spindles of the deep intervertebral muscle and to a much lesser extent from the zygapophysial joint afferents (Bolton & Holland, 1996; Bolton, 2000). The muscle spindle is the most common encapsulated nerve ending in both the human and animal neck (Amonoo-Kuofi, 1982; Richmond & Bakker, 1982). Spinal cord termini of the afferents from the muscles synapse in laminae IV to VI as well as the ventral horn, whereas those from zygapophysial joint afferents synapse in laminae I and II, and cutaneous afferents in laminae I through IV (Bolton & Holland, 1998).

Neurons in the lateral two-thirds of the lateral cervical nucleus in the upper cervical cord project strongly to the lateral part of the PAG, which is known to be involved in the fight-or-flight behavior in cats (Mouton & Holstege, 1994; Mouton et al., 1997). In addition, there are other cervical spine afferents that project to higher centers within the medulla, including the ipsilateral cuneate nucleus and vestibular nuclei, providing a relay for afferent information to the contralateral thalamus, cerebellum, and sensory-motor cortex (Bolton & Tracey, 1992), signaling both proprioceptive and nociceptive information. Thus, anatomically there exist both indirect and direct means by which manipulation-induced effects are mediated through the PAG and higher centers.

The afferent input from the cervical spine is likely only one possible element of the afferent input generated from spinal manipulation. Movement of the neck and head requires the central nervous system to integrate afferent information from a number of other systems (e.g., optical and vestibular systems) as well as from the structures of the cervical spine. Some spinal manipulation techniques may well stimulate many of these other systems, which will all contribute in a likely complex manner to the physiologic mechanisms of spinal manipulation.

CONCLUSIONS

Spinal manipulation is a physical treatment that has a role in the management of cervicogenic headache. Evidence to date lends support to several neurophysiologic mechanisms of spinal manipulation that involve a nonopioid-mediated descending pain inhibitory system with a locus of control within the PAG. The techniques studied in this research characteristically produce mechanical hypoalgesia and sympatho-excitation. Importantly, this evidence arises from a small proportion of the literature on manipulation (<1% has used physiologic measures) (Vernon, 2000), which urges caution in discarding the role of other mechanisms in the clinical effects of spinal manipulation in the management of neck and head pain. Treatment techniques with other characteristics (e.g., sympatho-inhibition, thermal hypoalgesia) (George et al., 2006) may well invoke other neurophysiologic mechanisms, yet to be determined.

REFERENCES

Amonoo-Kuofi HS. The number and distribution of muscle spindles in human intrinsic postvertebral muscles. *J Anat* 1982;135:585–599.

Bandler R, Shipley MT. Columnar organization in the midbrain periaqueductal gray: modules for emotional expression. *Trends Neurosci* 1994;17:379–389.

Bolton PS. The somatosensory system of the neck and its effect on the central nervous system. *J Manipulative Physiol Ther* 1998;21:553–563.

Bolton PS. Reflex effects of vertebral subluxations: the peripheral nervous system. An update. *J Manipulative Physiol Ther* 2000;23:101–103.

Bolton PS, Holland CT. Afferent signalling of vertebral displacement in the neck of the cat. *Neurosci Abstracts* 1996;22:1802.

Bolton PS, Holland TC. An in vivo method for studying afferent fibre activity from cervical paravertebral tissue during vertebral motion in anaesthetised cats. *J Neurosci Meth* 1998;85:211–218.

Bolton PS, Ray CA. Neck afferent involvement in cardiovascular control during movement. *Brain Res Bull* 2000;53:45–49.

Bolton PS, Tracey DJ. Neurons in the dorsal column nuclei of the rat respond to stimulation of neck mechanoreceptors and project to the thalamus. *Brain Res* 1992;595:175–179.

Bolton PS, Kerman IA, Woodring SF, Yates BJ. Influences of neck afferents on sympathetic and respiratory nerve activity. *Brain Res Bull* 1998;47:413–419.

Cannon JT, Prieto GJ, Lee A, Liebeskind JC. Evidence for opioid and non-opioid forms of stimulation produced analgesia in the rat. *Brain Res* 1982;243:315–321.

Carrive P. Functional organisation of PAG neurons controlling regional vascular beds. In: Depaulis A, Bandler R, eds. *The Midbrain Periaqueductal Gray Matter: Functional, Anatomical and Neuro-chemical Organisation.* London: Plenum Press; 1991:67–100.

Christian G, Stanton G, Sissons D, How H, Jamison J, Alder B, et al. Immuno-reactive ACTH, β-endorphin, and cortisol levels in plasma following spinal manipulative therapy. *Spine* 1988;13:1411–1417.

Depaulis A, Bandler R, eds. *The Midbrain Periaqueductal Gray Matter.* New York and London: Plenum Press in cooperation with NATO Scientific Affairs Division; 1991.

Elvey R. Treatment of arm pain associated with abnormal brachial plexus tension. *Aust J Physiother* 1986;32:225–230.

Fanselow M. The midbrain periaqueductal gray as a coordinator of action in response to fear and anxiety. In: Depaulis A, Bandler R, eds. *The Midbrain Periaqueductal Gray Matter.* New York: Plenum Press; 1991:151–173.

Farkas E, Jansen ASP, Loewy AD. Periaqueductal gray matter input to cardiac-related sympathetic pre-motor neurons. *Brain Res* 1998;792:179–192.

Fields HL, Basbaum AI. Central nervous system mechanisms of pain modulation. In: Wall PD, Melzack R, eds. *Textbook of Pain.* 3rd ed. Edinburgh: Churchill Livingstone; 1994:243–260.

Fujimoto T, Budgell B, Uchida S, Suzuki A, Meguro K. Arterial tonometry in the measurement of the effects of innocuous mechanical stimulation of the neck on heart rate and blood pressure. *J Auton Nerv Syst* 1999;75:109–115.

George SZ, Bishop MD, Bialosky JE, Zeppieri G, Robinson ME. Immediate effects of spinal manipulation on thermal pain sensitivity: an experimental study. *BMC Musculoskeletal Disord* 2006;7:68.

Hall T, Chan HT, Christensen L, Odenthal B, Wells C, Robinson K. Efficacy of a C1-C2 self-sustained natural apophyseal glide (SNAG) in the management of cervicogenic headache. *J Orthop Sports Phys Ther* 2007;37:100–107.

Hosobuchi Y, Adams JE, Linchitz R. Pain relief by electrical stimulation of the central gray matter in human and its reversal by naloxone. *Science* 1977;197:183–186.

Hoving JL, Koes BW, van der Windt D, Assendelft WJ, van Mameren H, et al. Manual therapy, physical therapy, or continued care by a general practitioner for patients with neck pain. *Ann Intern Med* 2002;136:713–722.

Hume KM, Ray CA. Sympathetic responses to head down rotations in humans. *J Appl Physiol* 1999;86:1971–1976.

Jansen ASP, Farkas E, Sams JM, Loewy AD. Local connections between the columns of the periaqueductal gray matter: a case for intrinsic neuro modulation. *Brain Res* 1998;784: 329–336.

Jull G, Trott P, Potter H, Zito G, Niere K, Shirley D, et al. A randomized controlled trial of exercise and manipulative therapy for cervicogenic headache. *Spine* 2002;27: 1835–1843.

Lovick T. Central nervous integration of pain and autonomic function. *News Physiol Sci* 1991a;6:82–86.

Lovick T. Interactions between descending pathways from the dorsal and ventrolateral periaqueductal gray matter in the rat. In: Depaulis A, Bandler R, eds. *The Midbrain Periaqueductal Gray Matter*. New York: Plenum Press; 1991b:101–120.

McGuiness J, Vicenzino B, Wright A. The influence of a cervical mobilisation technique on respiratory and cardiovascular function. *Man Ther* 1997;2:216–220.

Meyer T, Schwarz L, Kindermann W. Exercise and endogenous opiates. In: Warren MP, Constantini NW, eds. *Contemporary Endocrinology: Sports Endocrinology*. Totowa, NJ: Humana Press; 2000:31–42.

Morgan MM. Differences in anti-nociception evoked from dorsal and ventral regions of the caudal periaqueductal gray matter. In: Depaulis A, Bandler R, eds. *The Midbrain Periaqueductal Gray Matter*. New York: Plenum Press; 1991.

Mouton L, Holstege G. The periaqueductal gray in the cat projects to lamina VIII and the medial part of lamina VII throughout the length of the spinal cord. *Exp Brain Res* 1994;101:253–264.

Mouton LJ, VanderHorst VG, Holstege G. Large segmental differences in the spinal projections to the periaqueductal gray in the cat. *Neurosci Lett* 1997;238:1–4.

Mulligan B. *Manual Therapy: "NAGS," "SNAGS," "MWMS."* 5th ed. Wellington: Plane View Services; 1999.

Paungmali A, O'Leary S, Souvlis T, Vicenzino B. Hypoalgesic and sympatho-excitatory effects of mobilization with movement for lateral epicondylalgia. *Phys Ther* 2003;83: 374–383.

Petersen N, Vicenzino B, Wright A. The effects of a cervical mobilisation technique on sympathetic outflow to the upper limb in normal subjects. *Phys Theory Practice* 1993;9: 149–156.

Reynolds D. Surgery in the rat during electrical analgesia induced by focal brain stimulation. *Science* 1969;164: 444–445.

Richmond FJR, Bakker DA. Anatomical organisation and sensory receptor content of soft tissues surrounding upper cervical vertebrae in the cat. *J Neurophysiol* 1982;48:49–61.

Sanders GE, Reinert O, Tepe R, Maloney P. Chiropractic adjustive manipulation on subjects with acute low back pain: visual analogue pain scores and plasma beta-endorphin levels. *J Manipulative Physiol Ther* 1990;13: 391–395.

Shortt TL, Ray CA. Sympathetic and vascular responses to head-down neck rotation in humans. *Am J Physiol* 1997;272:1780–1784.

Simon R, Vicenzino B, Wright A. The influence of an anteroposterior accessory glide of the glenohumeral joint on measures of peripheral sympathetic nervous system functions in the upper limb. *Man Ther* 1997;2:18–23.

Skyba DA, Radhakrishnan R, Rohlwing JJ, Wright A, Sluka KA. Joint manipulation reduces hyperalgesia by activation of monoamine receptors but not opioid or GABA receptors in the spinal cord. *Pain* 2003;106:159–168.

Slater H, Vicenzino B, Wright A. "Sympathetic slump": the effects of a novel manual therapy technique on peripheral sympathetic nervous system function. *J Man Manipulative Ther* 1994;2:156–162.

Souvlis T, Wright A. The tolerance effect: its relevance to analgesia produced by physiotherapy interventions. *Phys Ther Rev* 1997;2:227–237.

Souvlis T, Kermode F, Williams E, Collins D, Wright A. Does the initial analgesic effect of spinal manual therapy exhibit tolerance? Paper presented at the 9th World Congress on Pain; Vienna; 1999.

Souvlis T, Pearce L, Vicenzino B, Jull GA, Wright A. Spinal manual therapy induced hypoalgesia is not naloxone reversible. Paper presented at the IFOMT; Perth; 2000.

Souvlis T, Vicenzino B, Wright A. Dose of spinal manual therapy influences change in SNS function. Paper presented at the MPA Biennial Conference; Adelaide; 2001.

Souvlis T, Vicenzino B, Wright A. Neurophysiological effects of spinal manual therapy. In: Boyling JD, Jull GA, eds. *Grieves' Modern Manual Therapy*. 3rd ed. Edinburgh: Churchill Livingstone; 2005:367–380.

Sterling M, Jull G, Wright A. Cervical mobilisation: concurrent effects on pain, sympathetic nervous system activity and motor activity. *Man Ther* 2001a;6:72–81.

Sterling M, Jull G, Wright A. The effect of musculoskeletal pain on motor activity and control. *J Pain* 2001b;2:135–145.

Terrett AC, Vernon H. Manipulation and pain tolerance. A controlled study of the effect of spinal manipulation on para-spinal cutaneous pain tolerance levels. *Am J Phys Med Rehabil* 1984;63:217–225.

Vaccarino AL, Kastin AJ. Endogenous opiates. *Peptides* 2001;22:2257–2328.

Vernon H. Qualitative review of studies of manipulation-induced hypoalgesia. *J Manipulative Physiol Ther* 2000;23: 134–138.

Vernon HT, Dhami MS, Howley TP, Annett R. Spinal manipulation and beta-endorphin: a controlled study of the effect of a spinal manipulation on plasma beta-endorphin levels in normal males. *J Manipulative Physiol Ther* 1986;9:115–123.

Vernon HT, Aker P, Burns S, Viljakaanen S, Short L. Pressure pain threshold evaluation of the effect of spinal manipulation in the treatment of chronic neck pain: a pilot study. *J Manipulative Physiol Ther* 1990;13:13–16.

Vicenzino B, Collins D, Wright T. Sudomotor changes induced by neural mobilisation techniques in asymptomatic subjects. *J Man Manipulative Ther* 1994;2:66–74.

Vicenzino B, Collins D, Wright A. Sudomotor changes induced by neural mobilisation techniques in asymptomatic subjects. *J Man Manipulative Ther* 1995a;2:66–74.

Vicenzino B, Gutschlag F, Collins D, Wright A. An investigation of the effects of spinal manual therapy on forequarter pressure and thermal pain thresholds and sympathetic nervous system activity in asymptomatic subjects: a preliminary report. In: Shacklock M, ed. *Moving In on Pain.* Adelaide: Butterworth-Heinemann Australia; 1995b: 185–193.

Vicenzino B, Collins D, Wright A. The initial effects of a cervical spine manipulative physiotherapy treatment on the pain and dysfunction of lateral epicondylalgia. *Pain* 1996;68:69–74.

Vicenzino B, Collins D, Benson H, Wright A. An investigation of the inter-relationship between manipulative therapy induced hypoalgesia and sympatho-excitation. *J Manipulative Physiol Ther* 1998a;21:448–453.

Vicenzino B, Collins D, Cartwright T, Wright A. Cardiovascular and respiratory changes produced by lateral glide mobilisation of the cervical spine. *Man Ther* 1998b;3:67–71.

Vicenzino B, Cartwright T, Collins D, Wright A. An investigation of stress and pain perception during manual therapy in asymptomatic subjects. *Eur J Pain* 1999;3:13–18.

Vicenzino B, O'Callaghan J, Kermode F, Wright A. The influence of naloxone on the initial hypoalgesic effect of spinal manual therapy. In: Devor M, Rowbotham M,

Wiesenfeld-Hallin Z, eds. *Proceedings of the 9th World Congress on Pain.* Seattle: IASP Press; 2000:1039–1044.

Wright A. Hypoalgesia post-manipulative therapy: a review of a potential neuro-physiological mechanism. *Man Ther* 1995;1:11–16.

Wright A, Vicenzino B. Cervical mobilisation techniques, sympathetic nervous system effects and their relationship to analgesia. In: Shacklock M, ed. *Moving In on Pain.* Adelaide: Butterworth-Heinemann Australia; 1995: 164–173.

Wyke BD. Articular neurology and manipulative therapy. In: Glasgow EF, ed. *Aspects of Manipulative Therapy.* Edinburgh: Churchill Livingstone; 1985:72–77.

Yezierski R. Somatosensory input to the periaqueductal gray: a spinal relay to a descending control centre. In: Depaulis A, Bandler R, eds. *The Midbrain Periaqueductal Gray Matter.* New York: Plenum Press; 1991:365–386.

Zusman M, Edwards B, Donaghy A. Investigation of a proposed mechanism for the relief of spinal pain with passive joint movement. *J Man Med* 1989;4:58–61.

Therapeutic Mechanisms Underlying Muscle Energy Approaches

Gary Fryer, PhD, BSc (Osteopathy), ND, and Christian Fossum, DO

Like many manual therapeutic approaches, the efficacy and effectiveness of muscle energy techniques (MET)—and related isometric stretching procedures such as proprioceptive neuromuscular facilitation (PNF)—are underresearched and poorly established, and the mechanisms underlying the possible therapeutic effects are largely speculative. Rationale for the mechanisms of therapeutic effects are drawn from research into connective tissue biomechanics and pain mechanisms, as well as inferences from studies that have investigated other manual techniques, but much research is required to establish the clinical effectiveness and the underlying mechanisms for therapeutic effect of this manual approach.

Authors in the field of osteopathy claim that MET can be used to lengthen a shortened muscle, mobilize a joint with restricted mobility, strengthen a physiologically weakened muscle, and reduce localized edema and passive congestion (Mitchell & Mitchell, 1995; Goodridge & Kuchera, 1997; Greenman, 2003; Chaitow, 2006). Although some texts have emphasized the role of MET for treatment of myofascial dysfunction (Chaitow, 2006), most have focused on the treatment

of spinal and pelvic articular dysfunctions (Mitchell & Mitchell, 1995; Goodridge & Kuchera, 1997; Greenman, 2003; DiGiovanna et al., 2005). In the field of osteopathy, segmental joint dysfunctions are referred to as *somatic dysfunction* and are characterized clinically by palpable tissue texture change, altered motion characteristics, and tenderness. Somatic dysfunction has been defined as impaired or altered function of related components of the somatic (body framework) system, including skeletal, arthroidal, and myofascial structures, and related vascular, lymphatic, and neural elements (American Association of Colleges of Osteopathic Medicine, 2003).

Somatic dysfunction is usually claimed to involve a functional disturbance of musculoskeletal elements and to be reversible following appropriate manipulation. The etiology—and very existence—of somatic dysfunction is speculative, and different models for dysfunction have been developed in response to evolving scientific evidence. It is likely that the clinical signs attributed to somatic dysfunction (palpable tissue texture change, altered motion characteristics, asymmetry, and tenderness) do not necessarily arise from a single clinical entity, but potentially involve a number of different tissues and physiologic processes, many of which may be related by a natural history of sprain and degeneration.

The following briefly outlines a hypothetical model for the etiology and clinical manifestations attributed to somatic dysfunction (**Figure 19.1**), drawn from elements in previous models (Van Buskirk, 1990; Fryer, 2003). Dysfunction may be initiated by external trauma, producing minor strain and inflammation of elements of the spinal unit. In acute spinal conditions, zygapophysial joint sprain and effusion could produce local pain and limited motion (active and passive), whereas more minor strains may be asymptomatic. Following strain and inflammation, activation of nociceptive pathways would potentially initiate a cascade of events, including the release of neuropeptides from involved nociceptors to promote further tissue inflammation ("neurogenic inflammation," which may outlast the tissue damage and create palpable tissue texture abnormality), and altering central nervous system motor strategies to affect deep (inhibition) and superficial (excitation) paraspinal muscles (producing altered quality of motion and tissue texture). Over time, degenerative changes to the intervertebral disc and zygapophysial facet joints would occur in response to repeated strain, periarticular connective tissue would undergo proliferation and shortening, and these degenerative changes would act as comorbid conditions that would continue to affect the mechanics of the spinal unit. Activated nociceptive pathways may interfere with proprioceptive processing, creating regional deficits in proprioception and further affecting segmental muscle control, which may disrupt the dynamic stability of the segment and predispose to ongoing mechanical strain and continuation of the cycle.

Given that the etiology of segmental somatic dysfunction is speculative, mechanisms underlying therapeutic action for the treatment of somatic dysfunction are also speculative, but may potentially involve a variety of neurologic and biomechanical mechanisms, depending on the exact nature of the tissues involved in an individual. It is also possible that MET may have physiologic effect in the absence of any theoretical dysfunction, as suggested by research conducted on asymptomatic subjects (Lenehan et al., 2003; Fryer & Ruszkowski, 2004). Traditional explanations for the therapeutic effects of MET relied on the concept of postisometric neurologic reflex muscle relaxation; however, there is little evidence to support this proposal (Fryer, 2006). The proposal of viscoelastic and plastic change to the myofascial connective tissue elements is appealing, but the evidence so far does not support lasting changes to the muscle property following isometric stretching, at least in healthy muscles. Although still speculative, it is possible that MET may chiefly produce therapeutic action by activating descending inhibitory systems and facilitating improved proprioception and motor control, as well as playing a limited mechanical role in promoting tissue fluid drainage.

MECHANISMS OF HYPOALGESIA

Several studies suggest that MET and related postisometric stretching reduce pain and discomfort when applied to the spine (Wilson et al., 2003) or myofascial structures (Magnusson et al., 1996a, 1996c; Ballantyne et al., 2003). The exact mechanisms for this are not known. This section proposes that possible mechanisms of MET-induced hypoalgesia include (a) the effect of rhythmic muscle contractions and mechanical stimulation of connective tissue fibroblasts on interstitial and tissue fluid flow, (b) the effect of stimulation of low-threshold mechanoreceptors on centrally mediated pain inhibitory mechanisms, and (c) the effect of stimulation of low-threshold mechanoreceptors in muscles on neuronal populations in the dorsal horn with possible gating effects (**Figure 19.2**).

Rhythmic muscle contractions will increase muscle blood and lymph flow rates (Schmid-Schonbein, 1990; Coates et al., 1993; Havas et al., 1997; Lederman, 2005). Mechanical forces (loading and stretching) acting on fibroblasts in connective tissues may have a substantial effect on their mechanical signal transduction processes (Langevin et al., 2004). Such loading has the potential to change the interstitial pressure and increase transcapillary blood flow (Langevin et al., 2005). These factors may play an important role in the tissue response to injury and inflammation. MET could potentially support these processes by reducing the concentrations of proinflammatory cytokines, resulting in decreased sensitization of peripheral nociceptors.

Low-threshold mechanoreceptors from joints and muscles project neurons to the periaqueductal gray matter (PAG) in the midbrain region (Yezierski, 1991). There is some evidence from animal and human studies that induced or voluntary muscle contraction results in sympatho-excitation and localized activation of the lateral and dorsolateral PAG (Li & Mitchell, 2003; Seseke et al., 2006). It has been suggested that stimulation of the lateral PAG through spinal manipulative therapy results in a

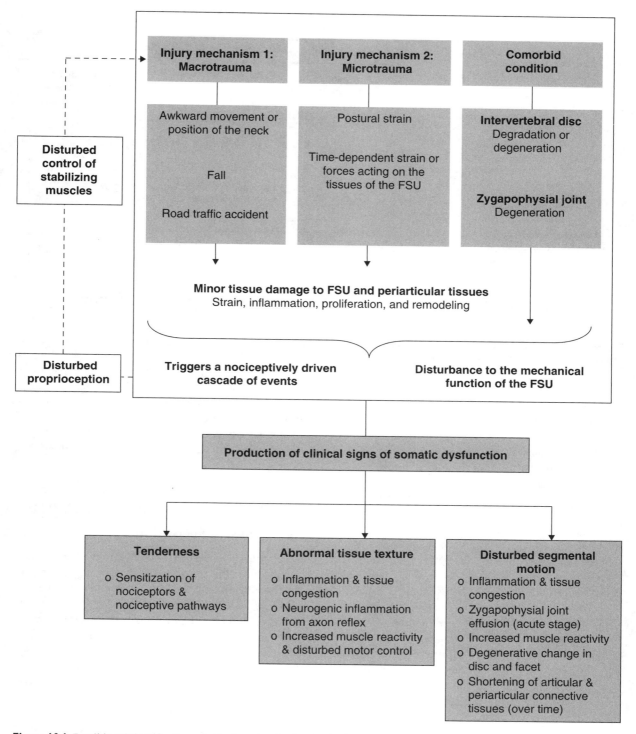

Figure 19.1 Possible Etiology for Somatic Dysfunction in the Cervical Spine. FSU, functional spinal unit.

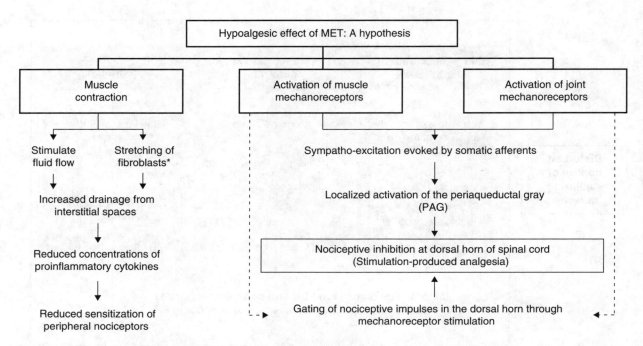

Figure 19.2 Hypoalgesic Effect of Muscle Energy Techniques: A Hypothesis. *In vivo mechanical stretching of fibroblasts has been shown to alter interstitial osmotic pressure and increase transcapillary blood flow.

nonopioid form of analgesia accompanied by sympatho-excitation (Souvlis et al., 2004). Activation of nonopioid descending inhibitory pathways (serotonergic and nor-adrenergic) following peripheral joint mobilization has been demonstrated in an animal model (Skyba et al., 2003). Spinal blockade of serotonin receptors (5-HT$_{1A}$ and 5-HT$_{2A}$) and noradrenalin receptors (α_2-adrenoreceptors) prevented the hypoalgesic effect produced by joint mobilization (Skyba et al., 2003; Hoeger Bement et al., 2007), suggesting the involvement of sero-tonergic and noradrenergic receptors and pathways. Furthermore, a study involving patients with lateral epi-condylitis showed that the administration of naloxone, which would antagonize an opioid analgesic effect, did not influence the hypoalgesic effect from the joint mobi-lization, suggesting nonopioid mechanisms (Paungmali et al., 2004). Using functional magnetic resonance imag-ing, Niddam et al. (2007) reported greater activation of the dorsal PAG in patients responding to electrostimula-tion of a myofascial trigger point in the trapezius muscle than those who did not respond, suggesting PAG involve-ment in the hypoalgesic effect.

It is therefore possible that MET acts to produce hypo-algesia both centrally and peripherally, through the activation of both muscle and joint mechanoreceptors

to involve centrally mediated pathways, such as the in-volvement of the PAG and nonopioid serotonergic and noradrenergic descending inhibitory pathways, and pro-ducing peripheral effects associated with increased fluid drainage.

OTHER NEUROPHYSIOLOGIC MECHANISMS
Reflex Muscle Relaxation

Reflex muscle relaxation is commonly cited as the ther-apeutic mechanism responsible for the length, range of motion (ROM), and tissue texture changes following MET (Kuchera & Kuchera, 1992; Mitchell & Mitchell, 1995; Greenman, 2003; Chaitow, 2006). Muscle relax-ation following isometric contraction has been pro-posed to be mediated by the golgi tendon organs, which have an inhibitory influence on the α-motor neuron pool, or by reciprocal inhibition produced by contrac-tion of a muscle antagonist (Kuchera & Kuchera, 1992). However, evidence supporting reflex muscle relaxation as an important mechanism for this technique is scarce (Fryer, 2006).

Support for the plausibility of postisometric muscle relaxation comes indirectly from studies that have examined the effect of muscle contraction on various electrophysiologic parameters. Several studies have reported a strong, brief inhibition of the H-reflex (an indicator of α-motor neuron pool excitability) following isometric muscle contraction (Etnyre & Abraham, 1986; Moore & Kukulka, 1991). The changes reported in these studies were very short-lived, lasting little more than a few seconds, which raises the question of their potential clinical relevance. Further, H-reflexes are very susceptible to repositioning artifact (Suter et al., 2005). Other researchers have reported decreases in electromyographic (EMG) activity in response to a sudden stretch (Carter et al., 2000) and reductions of responses to transcranial magnetic stimulation of the motor cortex (an assessment of motor neuron activity) following isometric contractions (Gandevia et al., 1999). Although these studies provide theoretical support for the potential of MET to produce reflex relaxation, evidence of a decrease in EMG activity following the use of MET is lacking.

Implicit in the proposal that MET acts by producing reflex muscle relaxation is the assumption that low-level motor activity plays a role in limiting the passive stretch of muscles and is elevated in dysfunctional muscle. Active motor activity, however, appears to have little role in producing resistance to passive stretch, and increases in muscle length following passive stretching have been reported to occur without any change to the low-level EMG activity of the muscle (Magnusson et al., 1996b).

Not only does motor activity appear not to play a role in passive resistance to stretching, but researchers also have found that MET and PNF techniques do not decrease the low-level EMG activity associated with stretching. Low-level EMG activity of the hamstring muscles was unchanged following both passive stretching and a PNF procedure using a 6-second forceful isometric contraction (Magnusson et al., 1996b). Osternig et al. (1987) reported that static stretching produced a small decrease (11%) in hamstring EMG response between initial treatment applications, whereas PNF techniques produced increases in EMG activity. At the end of five trials, the PNF techniques had produced considerably more EMG activity of the muscle when measured in its resting phase. Other studies have confirmed that whereas PNF stretching produces more muscle extensibility than passive stretching, it also produces more EMG activity (Osternig et al., 1990; Ferber et al., 2002). It appears clear that motor activity in hamstring muscles of healthy volunteers does not contribute to

resistance to passive stretching, and, although MET techniques produce greater ROM changes than static stretching, they paradoxically produce greater EMG activity in the muscle undergoing the stretch. It seems reasonable to conclude that other factors (such as a change in tolerance to stretch), rather than reflex muscle relaxation, appear to be responsible for the greater muscle extensibility and ROM following these techniques.

A small number of studies reported that application of MET produces increased ROM in the cervical, thoracic, and lumbar spine (Schenk et al., 1994, 1997; Lenehan et al., 2003; Fryer & Ruszkowski, 2004). Little can be concluded regarding the mechanisms behind the increased spinal range of motion, because none of these studies examined applied torque or EMG activity. Although there is evidence of EMG disturbance (increased, decreased, and delayed activity) in the paraspinal muscles of patients with low back pain (Fryer, 2004a), no study has investigated the effect on EMG activity of MET applied to the spine.

Proprioception

Spinal pain has been observed to produce disturbances in proprioception and motor control. Researchers have reported that patients suffering with pain display decreased awareness of direction of spinal motion and position (Gill & Callaghan, 1998; Taimela et al., 1999; Leinonen et al., 2002; Grip et al., 2007; Lee et al., 2008) and cutaneous touch perception (Voerman et al., 2000; Stohler et al., 2001). Evidence suggests that spinal pain also produces changes in motor strategies of paraspinal muscle activity, where deeper "stabilizing" paraspinal musculature is inhibited, and the more superficial spinal muscles overreact to stimuli at times when they should be relatively quiet (Fryer et al., 2004a, 2004b).

Although speculative, it is possible that MET may facilitate improvement in proprioception and motor control in patients with pain. The application of MET to the spine involves specific localization of motion to spinal articulations, and carefully controlled, purposeful isometric muscle contraction from the patient. This has been proposed to stimulate joint proprioceptors, highlight a different pattern of afferent activity from the proprioceptive-impaired region, and allow the central nervous system to normalize the proprioceptive and motor coordination from the involved region (Fryer, 2000).

No study has investigated the potential effect of MET on proprioception or motor control, but there is limited evidence to suggest that other manipulative treatments are of benefit. Cervical manipulation has been reported to improve head repositioning after active displacement in patients with chronic neck pain (Rogers, 1997; Palmgren et al., 2006) and in patients with vertigo and dizziness (Heikkila et al., 2000). Spinal manipulation has also been reported to affect motor recruitment strategies in low back pain patients (Ferreira et al., 2007). Cervical mobilization has been demonstrated to improve body sway in patients with whiplash trauma (Karlberg et al., 1991) and to decrease superficial neck muscle recruitment during staged cervical flexion (Sterling et al., 2001). Given that MET involves active and precise recruitment of muscles, there may be the potential for even greater changes in proprioceptive feedback, motor control, and motor learning; this is an area that deserves to be investigated.

BIOMECHANICAL MECHANISMS

Myofascial Extensibility

Application of MET to myofascial tissues for the purpose of stretching and increasing tissue extensibility may theoretically produce viscoelastic and structural change for lasting lengthening of the tissue. Changes to the connective tissue component of myofascial tissues, including viscoelastic and plastic (remodeling) changes and alteration of the water content of the ground substance, have been proposed as promising explanations for the therapeutic effect of MET and other soft-tissue modalities. Evidence of a change in human muscle property following stretching protocols, however, has so far been lacking.

Viscoelasticity refers to the mechanical properties that connective tissues display relating to their gel components and their elastic properties. Connective tissue elongation is time and history dependent, and if a constant stretching force is applied to a tissue, the tissue will respond with slow elongation or "creep." Additional loading may cause more permanent "plastic" change, produced by microtearing of collagen fibers and subsequent remodeling to a longer length (Lederman, 2005).

The addition of isometric contraction to a passive stretch may be more effective for producing viscoelastic change than passive stretching alone. Taylor et al. (1997) found that both muscle contraction and muscle stretching in the rabbit model resulted in passive

tension reductions of similar magnitude, indicating viscoelastic stress relaxation of the muscle-tendon unit. For a muscle to maintain the same length during an isometric contraction, the connective tissues must undergo lengthening to compensate for contractile element shortening, which suggests that isometric stretching procedures will more effectively load these connective tissues than passive stretching alone. Lederman (2005) proposed that passive stretching would elongate the parallel connective tissue fibers but have little effect on the tougher "in series" fibers, and the addition of an isometric contraction would more effectively load these in-series elements to produce lasting viscoelastic or plastic change.

Other possible influences on the mechanical property of myofascial connective tissue are a number of potential effects of stretching on fibroblast activity and the extracellular matrix. Stretch and isometric contraction may affect the water content of connective tissue to alter the stiffness and length of the tissue. Under high strain loads, collagen fiber bundles have been reported to initially reduce in diameter due to loss of water and glycosaminoglycan (GAG), and then swell beyond the initial diameter (Lanir et al., 1988). This mechanism may account for increased tissue stiffness after successive stretching (Yahia et al., 1993) and may play a role in tissue change following manual techniques. Schleip (2003) argued that there was a plausible rationale why stretching and tissue manipulation could stimulate interstitial mechanoreceptors to produce an autonomic mediated change in extracellular fluid dynamics, and that this mechanism should be investigated. Mechanical stimulation of fibroblasts has been demonstrated to result in changes to gene expression and growth factor production in addition to collagenase activity (MacKenna et al., 2000), which supports the possible influence of stretching and MET on fibroblast bioactivity and extracellular fluid dynamics. These proposals are speculative and it is not clear how some of these mechanisms would facilitate length changes in the muscle, but if manual therapy techniques are demonstrated to produce biomechanical changes in muscle property, they deserve to be thoroughly investigated.

Evidence of lasting changes to the biomechanical property of human muscle following stretching procedures has been scarce. Most studies that have reported length changes attributed to passive stretching or isometric stretching procedures have not measured the before and after torque (force) applied to produce the stretch, and therefore do not provide evidence that increases in muscle extensibility are attributed to change in the muscle property. Studies that have measured torque suggest that little lasting viscoelastic change occurs following application of either passive or isometric stretching, and that the increases in muscle extensibility are due to tolerance to increased stretching force (Magnusson et al., 1996a, 1996c; Ballantyne et al., 2003). This strongly suggests that short- and medium-term application of stretching and MET does not affect the biomechanics of the muscle, at least in the commonly studied hamstring muscles of healthy individuals.

In the only study found that has reported a change in muscle property following stretching (Reid & McNair, 2004), the subjects were school aged (mean age 15.8 years), and results may suggest that changes to muscle property can be more easily achieved in adolescents. Little is known concerning the benefit of treatment for the extensibility of injured and healing muscle; this would appear to be fertile ground for more research. Furthermore, anecdotal reports and observations of dancers, martial artists, and athletes who display above-average flexibility following dedicated stretching programs suggest that stretching can influence long-term muscle extensibility, and further investigation of the type and duration of stretching required to produce lasting changes should be undertaken.

Tissue Fluid Drainage

Authors of MET texts have proposed that MET can improve lymphatic flow and reduce edema (Mitchell et al., 1979; Mitchell & Mitchell, 1995), which is consistent with evidence that muscle contraction strongly influences interstitial tissue fluid collection and lymphatic flow (Schmid-Schonbein, 1990). Physical activity has been demonstrated to increase lymph flow peripherally in the collecting ducts, centrally in the thoracic duct, and within the muscle during concentric and isometric muscle contraction (Coates et al., 1993; Havas et al., 1997).

Minor injury to the spinal unit, periarticular tissues, or myofascial tissues may potentially result in inflammation and increased interstitial fluid. Increased tissue fluid may contribute to the production of clinical signs of somatic dysfunction, such as altered quality of joint motion and tissue texture. It is feasible that carefully applied MET, using intermittent isometric contraction and relaxation of the involved muscles, would assist lymphatic flow and clearance of excess tissue fluid and produce improvements evident to palpation. The role of MET in producing therapeutic benefit by increasing tissue drainage is speculative, but appears plausible given the established role of muscle contraction and lymphatic flow.

REFERENCES

American Association of Colleges of Osteopathic Medicine. Glossary of osteopathic terminology. In: Ward RC, ed. *Foundations for Osteopathic Medicine*. Baltimore: William & Wilkins; 2003:1138.

Ballantyne F, Fryer G, McLaughlin P. The effect of muscle energy technique on hamstring extensibility: the mechanism of altered flexibility. *J Osteopath Med* 2003;6: 59–63.

Carter AM, Kinzey SJ, Chitwood LF. Proprioceptive neuromuscular facilitation decreases muscle activity during the stretch reflex in selected posterior thigh muscles. *J Sport Rehabil* 2000;9:269–278.

Chaitow L. *Muscle Energy Techniques*. Edinburgh: Churchill Livingstone; 2006.

Coates G, O'Brodovich H, Goeree G. Hind limb and lung lymph flows during prolonged exercise. *J Appl Physiol* 1993;75:633–638.

DiGiovanna EL, Schiowitz S, Dowling D. *An Osteopathic Approach to Diagnosis and Treatment*. Philadelphia: Lippincott William & Wilkins; 2005.

Etnyre BR, Abraham LD. H-reflex changes during static stretching and two variations of proprioceptive

neuromuscular facilitation techniques. *Electroencephalogr Clin Neurophysiol* 1986;63:174–179.

Ferber R, Osternig LR, Gravelle DC. Effect of PNF stretch techniques on knee flexor muscle EMG activity in older adults. *J Electromyography Kinesiology* 2002;12:391–397.

Ferreira ML, Ferreira PH, Hodges PW. Changes in postural activity of the trunk muscles following spinal manipulative therapy. *Man Ther* 2007;12:240–248.

Fryer G. Muscle energy concepts—a need for change. *J Osteopath Med* 2000;3:54–59.

Fryer G. Inter-vertebral dysfunction: a discussion of the manipulable spinal lesion. *J Osteopath Med* 2003;6: 64–73.

Fryer G. Muscle energy technique: research and efficacy. In: Chaitow L, ed. *Muscle Energy Techniques*. Edinburgh: Churchill Livingstone; 2006:109–132.

Fryer G, Ruszkowski W. The influence of contraction duration in muscle energy technique applied to the atlanto-axial joint. *J Osteopathic Med* 2004;7:79–84.

Fryer G, Morris T, Gibbons P. Paraspinal muscles and inter-vertebral dysfunction. Part 1. *J Manipulative Physiol Ther* 2004a;27:267–274.

Fryer G, Morris T, Gibbons P. Paraspinal muscles and intervertebral dysfunction. Part 2. *J Manipulative Physiol Ther* 2004b;27:348–357.

Gandevia SC, Peterson N, Butler JE, Taylor JL. Impaired response of human motor-neurons to corticospinal stimulation after voluntary exercise. *J Physiol* 1999;521:749–759.

Gill KP, Callaghan MJ. The measurement of lumbar proprioception in individuals with and without low back pain. *Spine* 1998;23:371–377.

Goodridge JP, Kuchera ML. Muscle energy treatment techniques for specific areas. In: Ward RC, ed. *Foundations for Osteopathic Medicine*. Baltimore: William & Wilkins; 1997:697–761.

Greenman PE. *Principles of Manual Medicine*. Philadelphia: Lippincott William & Wilkins; 2003.

Grip H, Sundelin G, Gerdle B, Karlsson JS. Variations in the axis of motion during head repositioning: a comparison of subjects with whiplash-associated disorders or non-specific neck pain and healthy controls. *Clin Biomech* 2007;22:865–873.

Havas E, Parviainen T, Vuorela J, Toivanen J, Nikula T, Vihko V. Lymph flow dynamics in exercising human skeletal muscle as detected by scintography. *J Physiol* 1997;504:233–239.

Heikkila H, Johansson M, Wenngren BI. Effects of acupuncture, cervical manipulation and NSAID therapy on dizziness and impaired head positioning of suspected cervical origin: a pilot study. *Man Ther* 2000;5:151–157.

Hoeger Bement MK, Sluka KA. Pain: perception and mechanisms. In: Magee DJ, Zachazewski JE, Quillen WS, eds. *Scientific Foundations and Principles of Practice in Musculoskeletal Rehabilitation*. St. Louis, MO: Saunders Elsevier; 2007:217–237.

Karlberg M, Magnusson M, Malmstrom EM, Melander A, Moritz U. Postural and symptomatic improvement after physiotherapy in patients with dizziness of suspected cervical origin. *Arch Phys Med Rehabil* 1991;72:288–291.

Kuchera WA, Kuchera M. *Osteopathic Principles in Practice*. Kirksville, MO: Kirksville College of Osteopathic Medicine Press; 1992.

Langevin H, Cornbrookes CJ, Taatjes DJ. Fibroblasts form a body-wide cellular network. *Histochem Cell Biol* 2004;122:7–15.

Langevin H, Boulfard NA, Badger G, et al. Dynamic fibroblast cytoskeletal response to subcutaneous tissue stretch ex vivo and in vivo. *Am J Physiol Cell Physiol* 2005;288:C747–C756.

Lanir Y, Salant EL, Foux A. Physio-chemical and micro-structural changes in collagen fiber bundles following stretching in-vitro. *Biorheology* 1988;25:591–603.

Lederman E. *The Science and Practice of Manual Therapy*. Edinburgh: Elsevier Churchill Livingstone; 2005.

Lee HY, Wang JD, Yao G, Wang SF. Association between cervico-cephalic kinesthetic sensibility and frequency of subclinical neck pain. *Man Ther* 2008 (in press).

Leinonen V, Maatta S, Taimela S, et al. Impaired lumbar movement perception in association with postural stability and motor- and somatosensory-evoked potentials in lumbar spinal stenosis. *Spine* 2002;27:975–983.

Lenehan KL, Fryer G, McLaughlin P. The effect of muscle energy technique on gross trunk range of motion. *J Osteopath Med* 2003;6:13–18.

Li J, Mitchell JH. Glutamate release in midbrain periaqueductal grey by activation of skeletal muscle receptors and arterial baroreceptors. *Am J Physiol Heart Circ Physiol* 2003;285:H137–H144.

MacKenna D, Summerour SR, Villarreal FJ. Role of mechanical factors in modulating cardiac fibroblast function and extracellular matrix synthesis. *Cardiovasc Res* 2000;46:257–263.

Magnusson M, Simonsen EB, Aagaard P, Sorensen H, Kjaer M. A mechanism for altered flexibility in human skeletal muscle. *J Physiol* 1996a;497:293–298.

Magnusson M, Simonsen E, Dyhre-Poulsen P, et al. Visco-elastic stress relaxation during static stretch in human skeletal muscle in the absence of EMG activity. *Scand J Med Sci Sport* 1996b;6:323–328.

Magnusson SP, Simonsen EB, Aagaard P, et al. Mechanical and physiological responses to stretching with and without pre-isometric contraction in human skeletal muscle. *Arch Phys Med Rehabil* 1996c;77:373–377.

Mitchell FL Jr, Mitchell PKG. *The Muscle Energy Manual*. East Lansing, MI: MET Press; 1995.

Mitchell FL Jr, Moran PS, Pruzzo NA. *An Evaluation and Treatment Manual of Osteopathic Muscle Energy Procedures*. Valley Park, MO: Mitchell, Moran and Pruzzo; 1979.

Moore M, Kukulka C. Depression of Hoffman reflexes following voluntary contraction and implications for proprioceptive neuromuscular facilitation therapy. *Phys Ther* 1991;71:321–329.

Niddam DM, Chan RC, Lee SH, et al. Central modulation of pain evoked from myofascial trigger point. *Clin J Pain* 2007;23:440–448.

Osternig LR, Robertson R, Troxel RK, Hansen P. Muscle activation during proprioceptive neuromuscular facilitation (PNF) stretching techniques. *Am J Phys Med* 1987;66:298–307.

Osternig LR, Robertson RN, Troxel RK, Hansen P. Differential responses to proprioceptive neuromuscular facilitation (PNF) stretch techniques. *Med Sci Sports Exerc* 1990;22:106–111.

Palmgren PJ, Sandstrom PJ, Lundqvist FJ, Heikkila H. Improvement after chiropractic care in cervico-cephalic kinesthetic sensibility and subjective pain intensity in patients with non-traumatic chronic neck pain. *J Manipulative Physiol Ther* 2006;29:100–106.

Paungmali A, O'Leary S, Souvlis T, et al. Naloxone fails to antagonize initial hypoalgesic effect of a manual therapy treatment for lateral epicondylalgia. *J Manipulative Physiol Ther* 2004;27:180–185.

Reid DA, McNair PJ. Passive force, angle, and stiffness changes after stretching of hamstring muscles. *Med Sci Sports Exerc* 2004;36:1944–1948.

Rogers RG. The effects of spinal manipulation on cervical kinesthesia in patients with chronic neck pain: a pilot study. *J Manipulative Physiol Ther* 1997;20:80–85.

Schenk RJ, Adelman K, Rousselle J. The effects of muscle energy technique on cervical range of motion. *J Manual Manipulative Ther* 1994;2:149–155.

Schenk RJ, MacDiarmid A, Rousselle J. The effects of muscle energy technique on lumbar range of motion. *J Manual Manipulative Ther* 1997;5:179–183.

Schleip R. Fascial plasticity: a new neurobiological explanation. Part 1. *J Bodywork Movement Ther* 2003;7: 11–19.

Schmid-Schonbein GW. Microlymphatics and lymph flow. *Physiol Rev* 1990;70:987–1028.

Seseke S, Baudewig H, Kallenberg K, et al. Voluntary pelvic floor muscle control: an fMRI study. *Neuroimage* 2006;31: 399–407.

Skyba DA, Radhakrishnan R, Rohlwing JJ, et al. Joint manipulation reduces hyperalgesia by activation of monoamine receptors but not opioid or GABA receptors in the spinal cord. *Pain* 2003;106:159–168.

Souvlis T, Vicenzino B, Wright A. Neurophysiological effects of spinal manual therapy. In: Boyling JD, Jull GA, eds. *Grieves Modern Manual Therapy: The Vertebral Column.* Edinburgh: Elsevier Churchill Livingstone; 2004:367–380.

Sterling M, Jull GA, Wright A. Cervical mobilization: concurrent effects on pain, sympathetic nervous system activity and motor activity. *Man Ther* 2001;6:72–81.

Stohler CS, Kowalski CJ, Lund JP. Muscle pain inhibits cutaneous touch perception. *Pain* 2001;92:327–333.

Suter E, McMorland G, Herzog W. Short-term effects of spinal manipulation on H-reflex amplitude in healthy and symptomatic subjects. *J Manipulative Physiol Ther* 2005;28:667–672.

Taimela S, Kankaanpaa M, Luoto S. The effect of lumbar fatigue on the ability to sense a change in lumbar position. *Spine* 1999;24:1322–1327.

Taylor DC, Brooks DE, Ryan JB. Visco-elastic characteristics of muscle: passive stretching versus muscular contractions. *Med Sci Sports Exerc* 1997;29:1619–1624.

Van Buskirk RL. Nociceptive reflexes and the somatic dysfunction: a model. *J Am Osteopath Assoc* 1990;90: 792–794.

Voerman VF, Van Egmond J, Crul B. Elevated detection thresholds for mechanical stimuli in chronic pain patients: support for a central mechanism. *Arch Phys Med Rehabil* 2000;81:430–435.

Wilson E, Payton O, Donegan-Shoaf L, Dec K. Muscle energy technique in patients with acute low back pain: a pilot clinical trial. *J Orthop Sports Phys Ther* 2003;33: 502–512.

Yahia LH, Pigeon P, DesRosiers EA. Visco-elastic properties of the human lumbo-dorsal fascia. *J Biomed Eng* 1993;15: 425–429.

Yezierski RP. Somatosensory input to the periaqueductal grey: a spinal relay to a descending control center. In: Depaulis A, Bandler R, eds. *The Midbrain Periaqueductal Grey Matter.* New York: Plenum Press; 1991:365–386.

Neurophysiologic Effects of Neural Mobilization Maneuvers

Adriaan Louw, PT, MAppSc, CSMT, Paul Mintken, PT, DPT, OCS, FAAOMPT,
and Emilio "Louie" Puentedura, PT, DPT, GDMT, CSMT, OCS, FAAOMPT

The goal of this chapter is to review cervicogenic and tension-type headaches (TTH) from a neurodynamic perspective. The biological plausibility of a neurodynamic mechanism in patients with headache is discussed, followed by a review of the normal movement properties of the neural structures of the head and neck. The chapter then discusses how impairments in the movement of the neural structures combined with increased sensitivity to such movement may be a potential causative factor in patients with headache. Finally, it discusses how neurodynamic interventions may be of value to this patient population.

BIOLOGICAL PLAUSIBILITY OF A NEURODYNAMIC MECHANISM IN HEADACHE

It has been reported that some primary headaches can have a referred pain component, frequently from structures in the neck (Bogduk, 2001; Fernández-de-las-Peñas et al., 2007). The neurophysiologic mechanism behind this referral from the neck into the head lies in the convergence of afferent fibers from the upper three cervical nerve roots and the trigeminal nerve in the trigeminocervical nucleus (Bartsch & Goadsby, 2003b; Bogduk, 2004a). The spinal nucleus of the trigeminal nerve extends caudally to the dorsal horn of the upper three cervical spinal segments (**Figure 20.1**) (Narouze, 2007).

Kerr and Olafson (1961) demonstrated that afferents from the trigeminal nerve and the upper three cervical roots converge in the trigeminocervical nucleus in the upper cervical cord. The trigeminocervical nucleus resides in the upper part of the cervical spinal cord, where descending sensory fibers from the trigeminal nerve converge with sensory fibers from the upper cervical nerve roots (Shevel & Spierings, 2004). The convergence of these fibers suggested a mechanism by which pain may spread from the cervical region to the trigeminal area; this is often referred to as the *Kerr principle* (Kerr, 1961; Fredriksen & Sjaastad, 2000). C1 typically consists of three rootlets. Kerr (1961) showed that stimulating the upper rootlet caused pain in the orbit, stimulating the middle rootlet produced pain in the frontal area, and stimulating the lowest rootlet produced pain

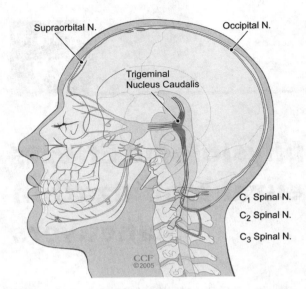

Figure 20.1 **The Trigeminocervical Complex**
Reprinted with the permission of The Cleveland Clinic Center for Medical Art & Photography © 2007. All Rights Reserved.

on the crown of the head. Bartsch and Goadsby (2002) demonstrated, in rat models, that a significant percentage of neurons in the trigeminocervical nucleus show convergent afferent input from both the dura, skin, and muscle of the upper cervical spine. As a result, nociceptive input from structures innervated by the upper three cervical nerve roots, including the joints, muscles, dura mater, nerves, bones, and vascular structures, may lead to the onset of headache (Bogduk, 2004a). This may lead to an overlapping of nociceptive processing in which afferent input from the dura and the cervical structures leads to head pain. More detailed data regarding the trigeminocervical complex can be found in Chapter 10 of the current textbook.

The challenge for the clinician is to attempt to differentially diagnose the cause of the patient's symptoms and provide the patient with an effective treatment based on current best evidence. This can be difficult, because on any given day a patient may have a slightly different trigger or mechanism for his or her headache. When reviewing the diagnostic criteria presented by the International Headache Society (IHS, 2004) for the various headache types, there is a considerable overlap of symptoms, and none of the criteria for diagnosing cervicogenic headache put forth by Sjaastad et al. (1998) is, in isolation, exclusive to cervicogenic headache. In fact, cervicogenic headache shares similar characteristics with TTH and migraine without aura (D'Amico et al.,

1994; Leone et al., 1995; Fishbain et al., 2003), and neck pain is a frequent symptom in patients with TTH and migraine (Solomon, 1997; Fishbain et al., 2001; Bartsch & Goadsby, 2003b). This is no doubt due to the convergence of afferents described previously in the trigeminocervical nucleus (Kerr & Olafson, 1961; Bartsch & Goadsby, 2002, 2003a, 2003b; Cady, 2007). Head pain may cause neck pain, and neck pain may cause head pain.

Breig (1978) contended that altered nervous system function plays a part in a wide variety of neuromuscular pain syndromes and described a "tissue-borrowing phenomenon" whereby lumbar nerve root tension results in displacement of the neighboring lumbosacral plexus, dura, and nerve roots toward the site of tension (Breig & Marions, 1963; Breig, 1978; Breig & Troup, 1979; Johnson & Chiarello, 1997). Put simply, an area of neural tissue with impaired mobility that is put under load may "borrow" resting slack or redundancy from neighboring meningeal tissues (Johnson & Chiarello, 1997). This results in a situation in which regional neural tissues have decreased redundancy and mobility (Breig, 1960, 1978; Reid, 1960; Breig & Marions, 1963; Breig & El-Nadi, 1966; Breig & Troup, 1979). The nervous system, as a structure, should be considered a continuous unit from the brain to the ends of the extremities (**Figure 20.2**).

Research by Breig and others has demonstrated that flexion of the cervical spine leads to tension in the dura and spinal cord resulting in a cephalad movement of the cauda equina. This ultimately limits the available mobility of the sciatic nerve (Breig, 1960, 1978; Reid, 1960; Breig & Marions, 1963; Breig & El-Nadi, 1966; Breig & Troup, 1979; Johnson & Chiarello, 1997). The nervous system can be affected by pathology inside the nervous tissue itself or in the tissues in which it resides and functions, and signs and symptoms may originate from local and distant neural and nonneural sources (Slater et al., 1994).

There are literally hundreds of different types of headaches per the Headache Classification Subcommittee of the International Headache Society (IHS, 2004). The mechanisms behind headaches are complex, and patients commonly present clinically with criteria for more than one type of headache (Rasmussen, 1992; Nelson, 1994; Niere, 2002).

Neural tissue may become sensitive to movement and hence be a pain generator in patients with headaches following trauma, compression, or inflammation (Hall & Elvey, 1999; Chen et al., 2004; Dilley

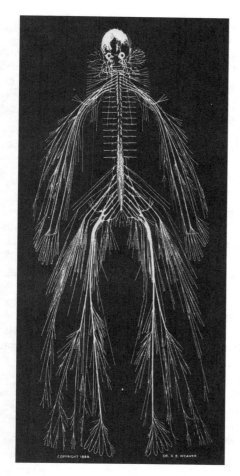

Figure 20.2 Hahnemann Anatomist Rufus B. Weaver's 1888 Dissection of a Complete Human Nervous System, Known as "Harriet," After Its Subject, Harriet Cole

Used with permission of the Archives and Special Collections on Women in Medicine and Homeopathy, Hahnemann Collection, Drexel University College of Medicine, Philadelphia, PA.

et al., 2005; Greening et al., 2005). Numerous neural structures in the head and upper cervical spine have the potential to cause head pain, including the dura mater, the greater occipital nerve, the upper cervical nerves, and the dorsal root ganglion (Alix & Bates, 1999; Jansen, 1999; Thakur et al., 2002; Bogduk, 2004b). Headaches have been reported following compression of the greater occipital nerve, the dorsal root ganglion, and the upper cervical nerve roots (Hildebrandt & Jansen, 1984; Jansen et al., 1989a, 1989b; Pikus & Phillips, 1995, 1996; Jansen, 2000). The upper cervical dura mater may be a potential headache generator because it has innervation from ventral rami of the upper

three cervical nerves, and the ligamentum nuchae and the rectus capitus posterior minor both have fibrous connections to the dura in this region (Hack et al., 1995; Mitchell et al., 1998; Bogduk, 2001, 2004a). The dura has also been shown to attach to the back of the body of the C2 vertebra and the cranial fossa (Hack et al., 1995). Flexion of the upper cervical spine is therefore important in structural differentiation and is used in provocation tests assessing the potential for contribution of upper cervical neural tissues in a patient with headache (Jull, 1997; Jull & Niere, 2004; Von Piekartz et al., 2007). From animal studies and research into mechanisms of nociception and neurogenic inflammation, it is thought that the movement of the dura mater may evoke pain, and neurogenically inflamed (craniocervical) dura may lead to changes in the contractile state of the blood vessels in the head, leading to a headache (Groen et al., 1988; Moskowitz & Macfarlane, 1993; Bove & Moskowitz, 1997).

There have been very few studies investigating the presence of neural tissue sensitivity in patients with headache. It has been reported that 7.4% to 10% of subjects with cervicogenic headaches exhibit neural mechanosensitivity (Jull et al., 2002; Jull & Niere, 2004; Zito et al., 2006). Mechanosensitivity of neural tissues was assessed maintaining the upper cervical spine in flexion while tensioning neural tissues in the upper and lower extremities via the brachial plexus provocation test and the straight leg raise test, respectively (Jull et al., 2002; Zito et al., 2006). A positive test was a perceived change in tissue resistance with provocation of neck pain or headache with the added movements. A study investigated the difference in cervical flexion and sensory responses (intensity and location) during the long sitting slump (LSS) test in 123 children aged 6 to 12 years (Von Piekartz et al., 2007). The test was performed on children with migraine, cervicogenic headache, and a control group. The results indicated that the intensities of the sensory response rate were highest in the migraine and cervicogenic headache groups compared with controls. The children with migraines predominantly had a sensory response in the legs (81.9%), whereas the cervicogenic group had a sensory response in the spine (80%). A total of 18% of the test subjects felt their responses in the head, five in the migraine group and seven in the cervicogenic headache group. The children with cervicogenic headaches showed cervical flexion ranges that differed significantly ($P < 0.001$) from both the control group and the migraine headache group. This may lend credence to

Breig's "tissue-borrowing" phenomenon. The reproducibility of the modified LSS test in the study by von Piekartz et al. (2007) was ICC 0.96 (95% CI: 0.89–0.99).

Clinically, the contribution of neural structures in patients with headache is often overlooked. In addition to the peripheral sensitization described earlier, we must also consider the role central sensitization plays in patients with headache. Many patients with headache disorders have had symptoms for a long time (Bronfort et al., 2006) and may have central sensitization, adding a layer to the complexity of clinical problem solving. *Central sensitization* is defined as a condition in which peripheral noxious inputs into the central nervous system lead to an increased excitability in which the response to normal inputs is greatly enhanced (Woolf, 2007). It has been proposed that central sensitization in migraines is induced by afferent input from the dura mater traveling on the trigeminovascular pain pathway (Malick & Burstein, 2000). The convergence of differing afferent signals in the trigeminal nucleus can then sensitize second-order neurons (Malick & Burstein, 2000; Cady, 2007). Repeated noxious stimuli may cause low-threshold neurons with very large receptive fields to depolarize with innocuous mechanical stimuli (Woolf, 2007). Injured neural tissue may actually alter its chemical makeup and reorganize synaptic contacts in the spinal cord such that innocuous inputs are directed to cells that normally only receive noxious inputs (Woolf, 2000). The central nervous system becomes hyperexcitable due to a combination of increased responsiveness and decreased inhibition (Woolf, 2000). This is analogous to the volume being turned up on the system such that normally innocuous stimuli generate painful sensations, and noxious stimuli cause an exaggerated pain response. Central sensitization has been described as a change in both the software and the hardware of the central nervous system (Woolf, 2000) such that the cellular depolarization threshold is reduced (Shevel & Spierings, 2004). Cellular activity continues after peripheral nociception stops, and this cellular activity spreads to neighboring cells (Woolf & Salter, 2000). In a person with headaches, nociceptive-specific cells in the trigeminal nucleus may begin to depolarize with input from primary afferent mechanoreceptors that are normally low threshold (Woolf et al., 1994). In other words, pain is then perceived in the presence of afferent input that is normally not perceived as noxious. In the centrally sensitized patient with chronic headaches, this may lead to the onset of a headache even in the presence of normal stimuli such as movement or pressure.

Mechanosensitive neural tissues in patients may be treated with specific controlled movements of the spine and extremities that move or slide the neural tissues relative to the surrounding tissues (Shacklock, 1995, 2005a; Elvey, 1997; Hall & Elvey, 1999; Coppieters & Butler, 2008). The effect of these treatments has not been investigated in patients with headache beyond a single case report (Rumore, 1989), yet many clinicians, including the authors of this chpater, have utilized these techniques successfully in patients with headaches.

NEURAL TISSUE AND HEADACHES

Most studies on cervicogenic headaches have focused on the joints of the upper cervical spine (Bogduk, 2004a) and muscle dysfunction (Jull et al., 1999, 2007; Petersen, 2003; Jull & Niere, 2004; Zito et al., 2006). Little is known about the role of the nervous system in cervicogenic headache (Jull, 1994). Any discussion of the potential influence of the nervous system on cervicogenic headaches requires a knowledge of normal nerve movement, or neurodynamics (Shacklock, 2005a). One of the main roles of the nervous system is electrochemical communication (Butler, 2000). The nervous system needs to perform these complex signaling processes while having to deal with movement issues (lengthening, sliding) (Coppieters & Butler, 2008), pressure (tunnels, pinch, surrounding tissues) (Breig, 1978; Butler, 1991, 2000; Shacklock, 2005a), and blood flow changes (increased/decreased blood flow, blood pressure changes) (Breig, 1978; Butler, 1991, 2000; Shacklock, 2005a).

Clinicians and researchers have therefore started investigating the physical properties of nerves, examination procedures aimed at detecting "normal" and "abnormal" nerve movement, and potential treatment strategies to improve neural tissue movement impairments (Butler, 1991, 2000; Elvey, 1997; Greening et al., 1999; Shacklock, 2005a). Neurodynamics is best described as the systematic assessment of the mechanics and physiology of a part of the nervous system (Shacklock, 2005a). From an anatomic and physiologic perspective, neural tissue has three important requirements: space, movement, and adequate blood supply (Butler, 1991, 2000). If any or all of these requirements are compromised, it may lead to clinical signs and symptoms.

Space

An easy way for clinicians to view the nervous system is to consider that the delicate nerves, spinal cord, and meninges all travel within containers or passageways. For nerves to properly function, they need to have the ability to "slide" and "glide" unhindered through different areas of the body (Butler, 2000; Shacklock, 2005a; Coppieters & Butler, 2008). As nerves travel through the body, they encounter many surrounding tissues, including muscle, bone, ligaments, and fascia (Breig, 1978; Butler, 1991, 2000; Shacklock, 2005a). Numerous studies have shown that if the interface is injured or damaged, it may have repercussions for the adjacent neural tissues. Examples include the cubital tunnel (Coppieters et al., 2004), carpal tunnel (Mackinnon, 1992; Nakamichi & Tachibana, 1995; Byl & Melnick, 1997; Coveney et al., 1997; Rozmaryn et al., 1998; Greening et al., 1999), intervertebral foramen (de Peretti et al., 1989; Fritz et al., 1998; Siddiqui et al., 2006; Chang et al., 2006), spinal canal (Fritz et al., 1998; Chang et al., 2006), and piriformis (Kuncewicz et al., 2006). When these spaces are compromised and nerves sustain unwanted pressure or irritation, it may lead to the onset of symptoms.

Direct mechanical pressure on a healthy nerve only causes paresthesia (Butler, 2000). If pressure is relieved, the nerve function should return to normal. If it is sustained, pressure will cause a vascular compromise of the nerve (Igarashi et al., 2005). Nerves are extremely "bloodthirsty," and if blood flow is altered to a nerve, it can evoke an ischemic reaction, which may lead to pain (Dommisse, 1994). This usually occurs when pressure on the nerve is sustained, but is also dependent on the severity of the compression, number of sites compressed, health of the patient's nervous system, and the general physical health of the individual (Butler, 2000). Direct compression of the upper cervical spine nerve roots, dorsal root ganglion, and greater occipital nerves has been documented (Hildebrandt & Jansen, 1984; Jansen et al., 1989a, 1989b; Pikus & Phillips, 1995, 1996; Jansen, 2000). Bogduk (2004a) describes the compression of these cervical spine structures as neuropathic pain and questions their relevance in "true" cervicogenic headaches, thus highlighting the controversy of the nervous system's role in headaches.

In recent years there has been an increased interest in the understanding of nerve pain and nerve sensitization. Although the process of nerve sensitization is not yet fully understood (Butler, 2000), it is believed to be associated with decreased myelin surrounding the nerve, resulting in exaggerated responses to mechanical, chemical, or thermal stimuli (Asbury & Fields, 1984; Devor & Seltzer, 1999; Hall & Elvey, 1999; Woolf & Mannion, 1999a). It is important to note that the dorsal root ganglion (DRG) has no myelin sheath and has been shown to be extremely mechanosensitive (Sugawara et al., 1996). It could therefore be argued that direct mechanical pressure on the DRG may, in fact, cause pain, which could be a contributing factor in headaches. Surgical studies have demonstrated direct pressure on the DRG, greater occipital nerve roots, and upper cervical spine nerve roots in patients with cervicogenic headaches (Hildebrandt & Jansen, 1984; Jansen et al., 1989a, 1989b; Pikus & Phillips, 1995, 1996; Jansen, 2000). This concept of "space" for nerves forms the basis of many therapeutic, medical, and surgical interventions such as laminectomy for lumbar radiculopathy and spinal stenosis, carpal tunnel surgery, cubital tunnel surgery, and more.

Movement

Closely linked to the previous discussion on the space requirements of the nervous system is the nervous system's ability to perform complex signaling processes during physiologic movement. For many years, medicine and physical therapy have been interested in the movement properties of joints, muscles, and even fascia, whereas the nervous system's movement capabilities had apparently been overlooked (Breig, 1978; Butler, 1991, 2000; Shacklock, 2005a). Under normal conditions nerves move quite well (Beith et al. 1995; Greening et al., 1999; Wright et al., 2001; Dilley et al., 2003; Shacklock, 2005a; Coppieters & Butler, 2008). Early cadaver studies showed that the nervous system is extremely well designed to handle movement. From a cervical spine neutral position to cervical spine flexion, the spinal cord lengthens approximately 10% (Margulies et al., 1992; Yuan et al., 1998), and from cervical spine extension to cervical spine flexion, the cervical cord lengthens approximately 20% (Breig, 1960) (**Figure 20.3**). It has also been shown that the spinal canal (the "container") can lengthen approximately 30% from spinal extension to spinal flexion (Troup, 1986) (**Figure 20.4**).

The peripheral nervous system must be able to lengthen as well, and research has shown that from a position of wrist and elbow flexion to a position of wrist and elbow extension, the median nerve must adapt to a

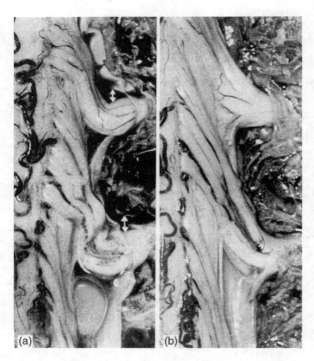

(a) (b)

Figure 20.3 Normal Deformation of the Dura, Cord, and Nerve Roots in the Cervical Canal in the Cadaver Caused by Full Extension and Flexion of the Cervical Spine. A total laminectomy has been performed and dura opened and retracted, although still able to transmit tension. In the image on the left **(A)**, the cervical spine is in extension, showing the nervous system slackened. In the image on the right **(B)**, the cervical spine is flexed, showing the nervous system's movement and tightening of the cervical spinal cord and nerve roots. Also note the effect of the movement on the adjacent blood vessels.

Reprinted with permission from Shacklock, 2008.

nerve bed that is almost 20% longer (Millesi et al., 1995). Although most of the original "movement studies" were performed on cadavers, newer research is utilizing real-time ultrasound to show that nerves not only have longitudinal movement but also significant lateral movement capabilities (Wiesler et al., 2006a, 2006b; Coppieters & Alshami, 2007a; Dilley et al., 2008). Furthermore, these ultrasound studies are showing that compared with normal populations, patients with pathology have decreased neural tissue movement (Wiesler et al., 2006a, 2006b; Coppieters & Alshami, 2007a; Dilley et al., 2008). The concept of neural tissue movement disorders has led to the development of structured neurodynamic tests to assess the movement capabilities of a specific nerve branch (Elvey, 1979; Butler, 1991, 2000; Shacklock, 2005a). These tests are

designed to identify physical dysfunction of the nervous system. After the development and refinement of these tests, clinicians began to use them in various forms of treatment, in essence trying to restore and maintain the normal anatomic and physiologic requirements of the nervous system (Shacklock, 2005b; Coppieters & Butler, 2008).

Because this is an emerging science, there are only a limited number of published research studies on neural tissue mobilization. Studies have shown that neural tissue mobilization is effective in the treatment of hamstring injuries (Kornberg & Lew, 1989), lateral epicondylitis (Drechsler et al., 1997), cervicobrachial neurogenic disorders (Coppieters et al., 2003a), hand pain (Sweeney & Harms, 1996), carpal tunnel syndrome (Rozmaryn et al., 1998; Coppieters & Alshami, 2007a), cubital tunnel syndrome (Coppieters et al., 2004), and ulnar nerve transposition (Weirich et al., 1998). In two studies conducted on cervicogenic headache, neurodynamics were assessed using passive upper cervical flexion along with either straight leg raise or placement of the upper limb in an upper limb neurodynamic position; 7.4% to 10% of subjects had a reproduction of a headache with the addition of the extremity movement (Jull et al., 2002; Zito et al., 2006). Another study found that 18% of children aged 6 to 12 with cervicogenic or migraine headaches felt a response in their head during the long sitting slump test (von Piekartz et al., 2007). In these three studies, 8% to 18% of the subjects experienced an increase in headache symptoms with the added neural tissue load. These findings suggest that a small percentage of headache patients may have a neurodynamic component to their headaches, which warrants additional research related to neurodynamic tests and treatment strategies.

Blood Flow

Neural tissue is extremely "bloodthirsty." The brain and spinal cord are estimated to only account for 2% of the total body mass, yet they consume 20% to 25% of the available oxygen in the circulating blood (Dommisse, 1994). Additionally, it has been shown that if a nerve is lengthened more than 6% to 8% of its length, blood flow in the peripheral nerve will slow (Lundborg & Rydevik, 1973; Ogata & Naito, 1986). If the nerve is elongated approximately 15%, blood flow may be completely occluded (Ogata & Naito, 1986). Adequate blood flow, nutrition, and movement (previous section) are therefore interdependent (**Figure 20.5**).

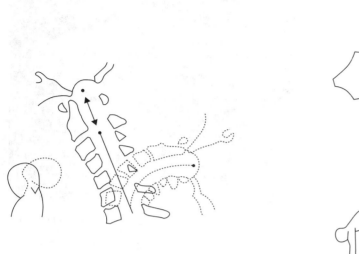
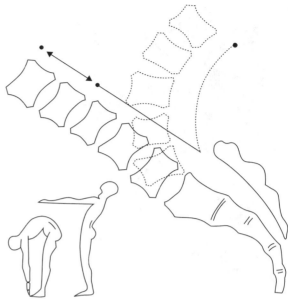

Figure 20.4 Change in Length of the Spinal Canal from Flexion to Extension. Images taken from tracing of X-rays. Reprinted with permission from Butler DS. *Mobilization of the Nervous System* (page 39). Copyright Churchill Livingstone (1991).

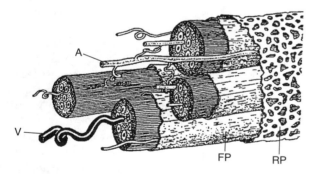

Figure 20.5 The Intrinsic Blood Supply to the Nerve Root. A, arteriole; FP, fascicular pia; RP, radicular pia; V, venule.

Reprinted with permission from Butler DS. *Mobilization of the Nervous System* (page 39). Copyright Churchill Livingstone (1991).

Significant, sustained pressure applied to a nerve may lead to demyelination (Dyck et al., 1990), which in turn may lead to peripheral sensitization, in which responses to mechanical, chemical, or thermal stimuli are exaggerated (Asbury & Fields, 1984; Devor & Seltzer, 1999; Hall & Elvey, 1999; Woolf & Mannion, 1999a). If blood flow to neural tissue is interrupted, it can lead to a hypoxic state, which may in turn lead to an ischemic-based pain state. Ischemic pain is a class of nociceptive pain in which lack of movement, sustained posturing, or decreased circulation creates an acidic environment (lower pH), which has been linked to pain (Butler, 2000). From the basic science literature, it seems clear that treatment techniques aimed at restoring movement, and thus blood flow, have the potential to decrease ischemic-based pain states as well as aid in maintaining normal movement and function of the nervous system (Rozmaryn et al., 1998; Coppieters & Butler, 2008).

DURAL HEADACHES

Many authors have implicated the dura mater as a potential source of headaches (Butler, 2000; Bartsch & Goadsby, 2002, 2003a; Bogduk, 2004a; Jull & Niere, 2004; Shacklock, 2005a). Three meninges surround the brain and spinal cord: the pia mater, the arachnoid, and the dura mater. From a purely mechanical perspective, the pia and arachnoid are extremely thin and fragile and are formed as a lattice of collagen fibers (Breig, 1978) (**Figure 20.6**).

The pia and arachnoid mater most likely have little to no mechanical properties and purportedly control fluid and ion channel flow (Haines et al., 1993). In comparison, the dura mater seems to have unique features emphasizing potential adaptations that allow for

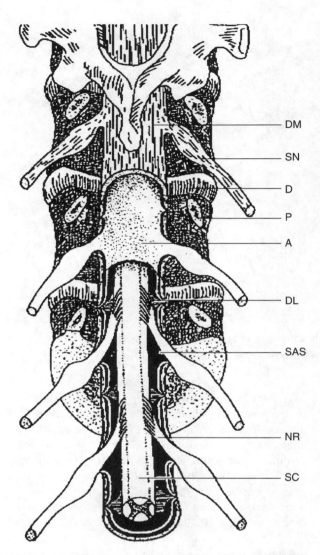

Figure 20.6 Diagrammatic Cutaway Section of the Spinal Canal, Meninges, and Spinal Cord. A, arachnoid; D, disc; DL, denticulate ligament; DM, dura mater; NR, nerve root; P, pedicle (cut); SAS, subarachnoid space; SC, spinal cord; SN, spinal nerve.

Reprinted with permission from Butler DS. *Mobilization of the Nervous System* (page 15). Copyright Churchill Livingstone (1991).

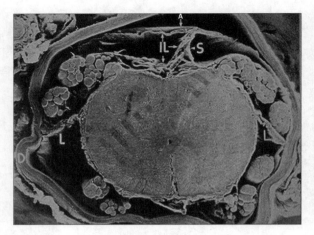

Figure 20.7 Scanning Electron Micrograph of the Lumbar Spinal Cord of a 15-Month-Old Child. L, denticulate ligaments; D, dura (note the layers); A, arachnoid; S, dorsal septum; IL, intermediate leptomeningeal layer.

Reprinted with permission from Butler DS. *Mobilization of the Nervous System* (page 15). Copyright Churchill Livingstone (1991).

movement. The cranial and spinal dura are continuous and are made up of both elastin and collagen fibers. The ventral dura is thinner than the dorsal dura. Furthermore, it is calculated that the ventral dura contains 7% elastin fibers, whereas the dorsal dura has about twice this amount (Nakagawa et al., 1994). The elastin content allows the cord and meninges to lengthen and remain functional during an almost 30%

increase in spinal canal length from spinal extension to spinal flexion (Troup, 1986) (**Figure 20.7**).

The dura mater of the upper cervical cord and the posterior cranial fossa are connected and receive innervation from branches of the upper three cervical nerves and, as such, are capable of being one of the causes of cervicogenic headache (Bogduk, 2004a). The fact that the dura is so richly innervated may make the best case for its potential role in headaches, particularly cervicogenic, tension type, or migraine (Moskowitz, 1993; Hu et al., 1995; Malick & Burstein, 2000; Turnbull & Shepherd, 2003). The best example of this occurs in post–dural puncture headaches. During an epidural steroid injection, the dura may be punctured. With the dural puncture, there is a leak of cerebrospinal fluid (CSF), which changes the overall pressure of the CSF. It is believed that this decreased pressure causes a downward pull on the cranial dura, which, due to its innervation, then produces the headache (Turnbull & Shepherd, 2003). These headaches have been shown to be posture dependent. When a patient lies down, the headache is eased by virtue of the decreased pressure. When the patient sits upright, there is a drop in CSF pressure, causing the downward (and thus potentially painful) pull of the spinal and cranial dura (Turnbull & Shepherd, 2003). These post–dural puncture headaches are often relieved with the delivery of a blood patch (Hess, 1991). The seal eliminates the CSF pressure change, thus decreasing the downward pull on the dura. Based on research investigating postepidural headaches, it seems plausible that any condition that causes a similar downward pull on the dura may also create such a "dural headache."

The dura may be implicated in the pathogenesis of several primary headaches because it receives its innervation from the upper cervical spine and has the potential, via afferent input into the trigeminal nerve in the trigeminocervical nucleus (Bartsch & Goadsby, 2003b; Bogduk, 2004a), to cause symptoms associated with many primary and secondary headaches (Bogduk, 2004a, 2005). This convergence of neural tissue in the trigeminocervical nucleus, as discussed in previous sections, allows for multiple tissues to become generators of head pain. Several authors have reported that pain with neck movement is characteristic of cervicogenic headache (Sjaastad et al., 1998; Hall & Robinson, 2004; Ogince et al., 2007), and others reported that neck pain is common in patients with migraine, TTH, and cervicogenic headaches (Bansevicius et al., 1999; Hall & Robinson, 2004; Jull et al., 2007; Ogince et al., 2007). Studies comparing range of motion between cervicogenic headache patients and nonheadache control groups have shown a significant decrease in cervical spine mobility—axial rotation, extension, and flexion (Zwart, 1997; Ogince et al., 2007; von Piekartz et al., 2007). Additionally, several authors have proposed the craniocervical flexion test (CCFT) as an important test in the examination of cervicogenic headaches (Jull et al., 2002, 2007; Hall & Robinson, 2004; Zito et al., 2006; Amiri et al., 2007). Passive neck flexion is a standard neurodynamic test (Breig, 1978; Butler, 1991, 2000; Shacklock, 2005a) as well as a screening test for upper cervical instability (Cattrysse et al., 1997), so this motion should be carefully examined prior to assessing the strength of the deep neck flexors. Anatomically, the CCFT tests upper cervical flexion, which may cause a downward pull on the dura. If the dura and other upper cervical spine neural structures are mechanosensitive, it is plausible that they may, via the trigeminocervical complex, initiate headache symptoms. Neurodynamic interventions aimed at maintaining or increasing the normal movement properties of the dura and other neural structures may be potentially beneficial for patients with headaches (Rumore, 1989; Butler, 2000; Shacklock, 2005a).

It is also important to consider the attachment of surrounding tissues that may potentially affect normal physiologic dural movement. Cadaveric studies have confirmed that there is a fibrous connection between the rectus capitus posterior minor (RCPM) muscle and the cervical dura (Hack et al., 1995). This pull on the dura may be further enhanced by the connection of the ligamentum nuchae and the posterior spinal dura at the C1 and C2 spinal levels (Mitchell et al., 1998). Changes in the length and pull of these tissues may thus also produce a potential painful reaction in the dura, similar to the post–dural puncture headache. In recent years, there has been a significant focus on muscle imbalances within the cervical spine showing altered recruitment patterns of the deep cervical spine flexors (Jull et al., 1999; Petersen, 2003; Sterling et al., 2003; Jull & Niere, 2004; Chiu et al., 2005; Zito et al., 2006) as well as increased fatigue rates (Gogia & Sabbahi, 1994; Falla et al., 2003). These impairments have been shown to occur in cervicogenic headache patients (Watson & Trott, 1993; Treleaven et al., 1994; Barton & Hayes, 1996; Placzek et al., 1999; Dumas et al., 2001). With weakening of the deep cervical flexors and increased fatigability, the patient may develop habitual postures of increased forward head posture with excessive upper cervical spine extension. These postures have been identified in office workers with neck pain (Watson & Trott, 1993; Grimmer, 1997; Szeto et al., 2002). In these forward head postures, the posterior neck musculature, such as the RCPM, may undergo adaptive shortening. Attempts at postural correction (e.g., verbal cues or via exercises) may lead to a direct pull on the dura, which may contribute to the development of a headache. Clinicians should be aware of this close relationship between the dura, the RCPM muscle, and ligamentum nuchae because it may have treatment implications. Caution is warranted because even gentle movement on sensitized neural tissue may potentially lead to the development or exacerbation of a headache.

When considering the dura as a potential initiator of cervicogenic headaches, it is important to realize that the cervical dura is continuous with the dura in the thoracic and lumbar spine, and also forms the peripheral nerve epineurium (Butler, 1991, 2000). If the concept of "space, movement, and blood flow" is followed, it would seem plausible that altered movement in regions other than the cervical spine may also influence the movement properties of the dura—such as thoracic spine hypomobility, postoperative lumbar laminectomy, and more. Studies have shown that impairments in the lower cervical or thoracic spine are associated with upper cervical spine dysfunction (Jensen et al., 1990; Griegel-Morris et al., 1992; Jull, 1997; Jull et al., 2002; Sizer et al., 2002; Jull & Niere, 2004). Whiplash-associated disorder (WAD) research has shown that patients with

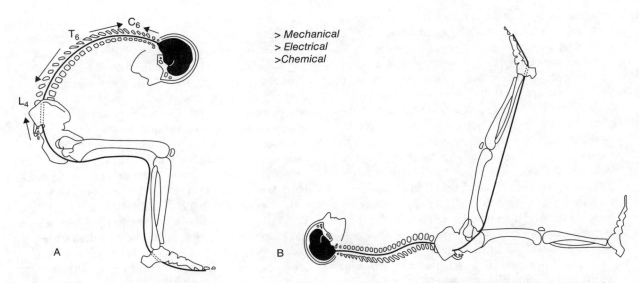

Figure 20.8 **The Dynamics of the Nervous System Both in Spinal Flexion or Slump (A) and Straight Leg Raise (B).** Notice the continuum of the nervous system.

Reprinted with permission from Butler DS. *Mobilization of the Nervous System* (page 31 and page 53). Copyright Churchill Livingstone (1991).

WAD (neck trauma) have restricted mobility and increased pain with upper limb neurodynamic tests, compared with asymptomatic subjects (Sterling et al., 2002). Additionally, research has shown decreased knee extension and ankle dorsiflexion range of motion during slump testing in patients with WAD compared with asymptomatic subjects (Yeung et al., 1997) (**Figure 20.8**).

These two whiplash studies suggest that neck trauma may lead to altered movement capabilities of the nervous system distant to the area of injury. Following Breig's "tissue borrowing" concept, the opposite might also be true: trauma, pain, or altered movement in the periphery and other spinal regions may lead to mechanical changes in the pull on the cervical and cranial dura, which, if sensitized, may contribute to the development of a headache. More research is obviously needed to further explore the movement properties of the nervous system in regard to headaches. It is worth noting that even the innervation of the meninges is designed for movement (Butler, 2000). Terminals are twisted and in coiled bundles (Groen et al., 1988), meaning that when a healthy, nonsensitized dura is stretched, there are minimal forces on the mechanosensitive nerve endings. This anatomic design feature further underscores the dura's movement capabilities in healthy individuals. It would therefore seem appropriate to extrapolate that when this normal movement is altered, the tissues may

become sensitized to movement and be a potential pain generator in patients with headache.

TREATMENT OF HEADACHES FROM A NEURAL PERSPECTIVE: NEURAL MOBILIZATION

To date, no randomized controlled trials have been conducted to assess the direct effect of neural tissue mobilization techniques compared with other interventions for headache patients. Some authors have advocated the use of neural tissue mobilization techniques for headache patients (Rumore, 1989; Butler, 1991, 2000; Shacklock, 2005a). There is growing evidence regarding the clinical use and efficacy of neural tissue mobilization techniques in other disorders (Kornberg & Lew, 1989; Kornberg & McCarthy, 1992; Sweeney & Harms, 1996; Drechsler et al., 1997; Rozmaryn et al., 1998; Weirich et al., 1998; Coppieters & Alshami, 2007b; Coppieters et al., 2004). These studies showed that active and passive neural tissue mobilization may facilitate a faster return to work and recreational activities (Kornberg & Lew, 1989; Weirich et al., 1998), increase the range of motion associated with the neurodynamic test (Sweeney & Harms, 1996; Vicenzino et al., 1996; Coppieters et al., 2003b, 2004; Coppieters & Alshami, 2007b), decrease the need for surgery (Rozmaryn et al., 1998), and decrease pain (Sweeney & Harms, 1996;

Vicenzino et al., 1996; Coppieters et al., 2003b, 2004; Coppieters & Alshami, 2007a). This research, combined with basic science evidence, suggests that improving the space, movement, and blood flow of the nervous system via gentle, nonthreatening movements may be of clinical value (Coppieters & Butler, 2008).

Current best evidence indicates that a multimodal approach consisting of manual therapy and specific exercise improves outcomes in patients with cervicogenic headaches (Jull et al., 2002; Gross et al., 2004, 2006). This is important because neural tissue mobilization involves both hands-on treatment and active exercises (Butler, 1991, 2000; Shacklock, 2005a). Although the focus of this chapter has been the potential effect of neural tissue mobilization in patients with headache, it is important to note that treatment techniques such as spinal manipulation and exercise may have indirect effects on the neurophysiology of the nervous system of a patient with headaches. Spinal manipulation's immediate effect on local muscle (Brodeur, 1995) may help decrease the tension in the RCPM muscle, and it also has been shown that thoracic manipulative procedures produce enough pressure to force 8 milliliters of CSF into the brain (Du Boulay et al., 1972). This may represent an indirect effect of spinal manipulation on headache patients, since a drop in CSF pressure has been linked to headaches (Turnbull & Shepherd, 2003). Cervical spine exercises that include large range of motion excursions could be viewed as a means of increasing circulation, but also as a potential neural mobilization maneuver (Butler, 1991, 2000; Shacklock, 2005a).

SUMMARY AND CONCLUSION

Very little is known about the role of neurodynamics in headaches. No randomized controlled trials have been performed investigating the effects of neurodynamic treatments in patients with headache, although there is an emerging base of evidence demonstrating the efficacy of such techniques in other musculoskeletal conditions. The basic science evidence (anatomy and physiology) would imply that the nervous system, especially the dura mater, may have a potential role in the development of headaches. Spinal manipulation and mobilization in combination with exercise represent the current best evidence-based conservative management of patients with cervicogenic headaches. The exact mechanisms of these beneficial techniques are often explained in regard to their effect on local joint and muscle. None of these claims is disputed. Could these techniques also have a direct or indirect effect, or both, on the neural structures responsible for causing headaches? This chapter should be seen as a first attempt at addressing a neurophysiologic link between the physical properties of the nervous system and headaches, particularly cervicogenic and tension-type headache. The field of neurodynamics now also encompasses pain science and neuroscience, including ion channel expression (Devor & Seltzer, 1999), central sensitization (Butler, 2000; Woolf, 2007), and changes in the central nervous system, including the brain—particularly in chronic pain states. These were not discussed as part of this chapter but are certainly important as we consider altering pain states and neural tissue sensitivity in patients with headache disorders. Is it possible that we may be able to change the "software" of the central nervous system via the gentle introduction of movement through the neural tissues, thus leading to a permanent change in this central pain state in patients with headache? This remains to be seen, and future research may give us some of these answers.

REFERENCES

Alix ME, Bates DK. A proposed etiology of cervicogenic headache: the neurophysiologic basis and anatomic relationship between the dura mater and the rectus posterior capitis minor muscle. *J Manipulative Physiol Ther* 1999;22:534–539.

Amiri M, Jull G, Bullock-Saxton J, Darnell R, Lander C. Cervical musculo-skeletal impairment in frequent intermittent headache. Part 2: subjects with concurrent headache types. *Cephalalgia* 2007;27:891–898.

Asbury AK, Fields HL. Pain due to peripheral nerve damage: an hypothesis. *Neurology* 1984;34:1587–1590.

Bansevicius D, Westgaard RH, Sjaastad OM. Tension-type headache: pain, fatigue, tension, and EMG responses to mental activation. *Headache* 1999;39:417–425.

Barton PM, Hayes KC. Neck flexor muscle strength, efficiency, and relaxation times in normal subjects and subjects with unilateral neck pain and headache. *Arch Phys Med Rehabil* 1996;77:680–687.

Bartsch T, Goadsby PJ. Stimulation of the greater occipital nerve induces increased central excitability of dural afferent input. *Brain* 2002;125:1496–1509.

Bartsch T, Goadsby PJ. Increased responses in trigeminocervical nociceptive neurons to cervical input after stimulation of the dura mater. *Brain* 2003a;126:1801–1813.

Bartsch T, Goadsby PJ. The trigeminocervical complex and migraine: current concepts and synthesis. *Curr Pain Headache Rep* 2003b;7:371–376.

Beith ID, Robins EJ, Richards PR. An assessment of the adaptive mechanisms within and surrounding the peripheral nervous system, during changes in nerve bed length resulting from underlying joint movement. In: Shacklock MO, ed. *Moving In on Pain.* Australia: Butterworth-Heinemann; 1995.

Bogduk N. Cervicogenic headache: anatomic basis and patho-physiologic mechanisms. *Curr Pain Headache Rep* 2001;5:382–386.

Bogduk N. The neck and headaches. *Neurol Clin* 2004a;22:151–171.

Bogduk N. Role of anesthesiologic blockade in headache management. *Curr Pain Headache Rep* 2004b;8:399–403.

Bogduk N. Distinguishing primary headache disorders from cervicogenic headache: clinical and therapeutic implications. *Headache Currents* 2005;2:27–36.

Bove GM, Moskowitz MA. Primary afferent neurons innervating guinea pig dura. *J Neurophysiol* 1997;77:299–308.

Breig A. *Biomechanics of the Central Nervous System.* Stockholm: Almqvist and Wiksell; 1960.

Breig A. *Adverse Mechanical Tension in the Central Nervous System.* Stockholm: Almqvist and Wiksell; 1978.

Breig A, El-Nadi FA. Biomechanics of the cervical spinal cord. *Acta Radiol* 1966;4:602–624.

Breig A, Marions O. Biomechanics of the lumbo-sacral nerve roots. *Acta Radiol* 1963;1:1141–1160.

Breig A, Troup J. Biomechanical considerations in the straight leg raising test. *Spine* 1979;4:242–250.

Brodeur R. The audible release associated with joint manipulation. *J Manipulative Physiol Ther* 1995;18:155–164.

Bronfort G, Nilsson N, Haas M, Evans R, Goldsmith CH, Assendelft WJJ, Bouter LM. Non-invasive physical treatments for chronic/recurrent headache. *Cochrane Library* 2006;(4):CD001878.

Butler DS. *Mobilization of the Nervous System.* London: Churchill Livingstone; 1991.

Butler DS. *The Sensitive Nervous System.* Adelaide: Noigroup Publications; 2000.

Byl NN, Melnick M. The neural consequences of repetition: clinical implications of a learning hypothesis. *J Hand Ther* 1997;10:160–174.

Cady RK. The convergence hypothesis. *Headache* 2007;47:S44–S51.

Cattrysse E, Swinkels RAH, Oostendorp RAB, Duquet W. Upper cervical instability: are clinical tests reliable? *Man Ther* 1997;2:91–97.

Chang SB, Lee SH, Ahn Y, Kim JM. Risk factor for unsatisfactory outcome after lumbar foraminal, and far lateral micro decompression. *Spine* 2006;31:1163–1167.

Chen C, Cavanaugh JM, Song Z, Takebayashi T, Kallakuri S, Wooley PH. Effects of nucleus pulposus on nerve root neural activity, mechanosensitivity, axonal morphology, and sodium channel expression. *Spine* 2004;29:17–25.

Chiu TTW, Law EYH, Chiu THF. Performance of the craniocervical flexion test in subjects with and without chronic neck pain. *J Orthop Sports Phys Ther* 2005;35:567–571.

Coppieters M, Alshami A. Longitudinal excursion and strain in the median nerve during novel nerve gliding exercises for carpal tunnel syndrome. *J Orthop Res* 2007a;25:972–980.

Coppieters MW, Butler DS. Do "sliders" slide and "tensioners" tension? An analysis of neurodynamic techniques and considerations regarding their application. *Man Ther* 2008 (in press).

Coppieters MW, Stappaerts KH, Wouters LL, Janssens K. Aberrant protective force generation during neural provocation testing and the effect of treatment in patients with neurogenic cervicobrachial pain. *J Manipulative Physiol Ther* 2003a;26:99–106.

Coppieters MW, Stappaerts KH, Wouters LL, Janssens K. The immediate effects of a cervical lateral glide treatment technique in patients with neurogenic cervicobrachial pain. *J Orthop Sports Phys Ther* 2003b;33:369–378.

Coppieters MW, Bartholomeeusen KE, Stappaerts KH. Incorporating nerve-gliding techniques in the conservative treatment of cubital tunnel syndrome. *J Manipulative Physiol Ther* 2004;27:560–568.

Coveney B, Trott P, Grimmer K. The upper limb tension test in a group of subjects with a clinical presentation of carpal tunnel syndrome. Presented at the Tenth Biennial Conference of the Manipulative Physiotherapists Association of Australia; Melbourne, Australia; 1997.

D'Amico D, Leone M, Bussone G. Side-locked unilaterality and pain localization in long-lasting headaches: migraine, tension-type headache, and cervicogenic headache. *Headache* 1994;34:526–530.

De Peretti F, Micalef J, Bourgeon A, Argenson C, Rabischong P. Biomechanics of the lumbar spinal nerve roots and the first sacral root within the inter-vertebral foramina. *Surg Radiol Anat* 1989;11:221–225.

Devor M, Seltzer Z. Pathophysiology of damaged nerves in relation to chronic pain. In: Wall PD, Melzack R, eds. *Textbook of Pain.* Edinburgh: Churchill Livingstone; 1999.

Dilley A, Lynn B, Greening J, DeLeon N. Quantitative in vivo studies of median nerve sliding in response to wrist, elbow, shoulder and neck movements. *Clin Biomech* 2003;18:899–907.

Dilley A, Lynn B, Pang SJ. Pressure and stretch mechanosensitivity of peripheral nerve fibres following local inflammation of the nerve trunk. *Pain* 2005;117:462–472.

Dilley A, Odeyinde S, Greening J, Lynn B. Longitudinal sliding of the median nerve in patients with non-specific arm pain. *Man Ther* 2008 (in press).

Dommisse GF. The blood supply of the spinal cord, and the consequences of failure. In: Boyling J, Palastanga N, eds. *Grieves Modern Manual Therapy.* Edinburgh: Churchill Livingstone; 1994.

Drechsler WI, Knarr JF, Snyder-Mackler L. A comparison of two treatment regimens for lateral epicondylitis: a randomized trial of clinical interventions. *J Sport Rehabil* 1997;6:226–234.

Du Boulay G, O'Connell J, Currie J, Bostick T, Verity P. Further investigations on pulsatile movements in the cerebrospinal fluid pathways. *Acta Radiol Diagnosis* 1972;13: 496–523.

Dumas JP, Arsenault AB, Boudreau G, Magnoux E, Lepage Y, Bellavance A, Loisel P. Physical impairments in cervicogenic headache: traumatic vs. non-traumatic onset. *Cephalalgia* 2001;21:884–893.

Dyck PJ, Lais AC, Giannini C, Engelstad JK. Structural alterations of nerve during cuff compression. *Proc Natl Acad Sci* 1990;87:9828–9832.

Elvey R. Brachial plexus tension test and the pathoanatomical origin of arm pain. In: Glasgow E, Twomey L, eds. *Aspects of Manipulative Therapy*. Melbourne: Lincoln Institute of Health Sciences; 1979:105–110.

Elvey RL. Physical evaluation of the peripheral nervous system in disorders of pain and dysfunction. *J Hand Ther* 1997;10: 122–129.

Falla D, Rainoldi A, Merletti R, Jull G. Myo-electric manifestations of sternocleidomastoid and anterior scalene muscle fatigue in chronic neck pain patients. *Clin Neurophysiol* 2003;114:488–495.

Fernández-de-las-Peñas C, Simons D, Cuadrado ML, Pareja J. The role of myofascial trigger points in musculoskeletal pain syndromes of the head and neck. *Curr Pain Headache Rep* 2007;11:365–372.

Fishbain DA, Cutler R, Cole B, Rosomoff HL, Rosomoff RS. International Headache Society headache diagnostic patterns in pain facility patients. *Clin J Pain* 2001;17: 78–93.

Fishbain DA, Lewis J, Cole B, Cutler RB, Rosomoff RS, Rosomoff HL. Do the proposed cervicogenic headache diagnostic criteria demonstrate specificity in terms of separating cervicogenic headache from migraine? *Curr Pain Headache Rep* 2003;7:387–394.

Fredriksen TA, Sjaastad O. Cervicogenic headache: current concepts of pathogenesis related to anatomical structure. *Clin Exp Rheumatol* 2000;18:S16–S18.

Fritz JM, Delitto A, Welch WC, Erhard RE. Lumbar spinal stenosis: a review of current concepts in evaluation, management, and outcome measurements. *Arch Phys Med Rehabil* 1998;79:700–708.

Gogia PP, Sabbahi MA. Electromyographic analysis of neck muscle fatigue in patients with osteoarthritis of the cervical spine. *Spine* 1994;19:502–506.

Greening J, Smart S, Leary R, Hall-Craggs M, O'Higgins P, Lynn B. Reduced movement of median nerve in carpal tunnel during wrist flexion in patients with non-specific arm pain. *Lancet* 1999;354:217–218.

Greening J, Dilley A, Lynn B. In vivo study of nerve movement and mechano-sensitivity of the median nerve in whiplash and non-specific arm pain patients. *Pain* 2005;115: 248–253.

Griegel-Morris P, Larson K, Mueller-Klaus K, Oatis CA. Incidence of common postural abnormalities in the cervical, shoulder, and thoracic regions and their association with pain in two age groups of healthy subjects. *Phys Ther* 1992;72:425–431.

Grimmer K. An investigation of poor cervical resting posture. *Aust J Physiother* 1997;43:7–16.

Groen GJ, Baljet B, Drukker J. The innervation of the spinal dura mater: anatomy and clinical implications. *Acta Neurochirurgica* 1988;92:39–46.

Gross AR, Hoving JL, Haines TA, et al. A Cochrane review of manipulation and mobilization for mechanical neck disorders. *Spine* 2004;29:1541–1548.

Gross AR, Hoving JL, Haines TA, et al. Manipulation and mobilization for mechanical neck disorders. *Cochrane Library* 2006;1:CD004249.

Hack GD, Koritzer RT, Robinson WL, Hallgren RC, Greenman PE. Anatomic relation between the rectus capitis posterior minor muscle and the dura mater. *Spine* 1995;20: 2484–2486.

Haines DE, Harkey HL, Al-Mefty O. The "subdural" space: a new look at an outdated concept. *Neurosurgery* 1993;32:111–120.

Hall TM, Elvey RL. Nerve trunk pain: physical diagnosis and treatment. *Man Ther* 1999;4:63–73.

Hall T, Robinson K. The flexion-rotation test and active cervical mobility: a comparative measurement study in cervicogenic headache. *Man Ther* 2004;9:197–202.

Hess JH. Postdural puncture headache: a literature review. *AANA J* 1991;59:549–555.

Hildebrandt J, Jansen J. Vascular compression of the C2 and C3 roots: yet another cause of chronic intermittent hemi-crania? *Cephalalgia* 1984;4:167–170.

Hu JW, Vernon H, Tatourian I. Changes in neck electromyography associated with meningeal noxious stimulation. *J Manipulative Physiol Ther* 1995;18: 577–581.

Igarashi T, Yabuki S, Kikuchi S, Myers RR. Effect of acute nerve root compression on endo-neural fluid pressure and blood flow in rat dorsal root ganglia. *J Orthop Res* 2005;23: 420–424.

International Headache Society. The International Classification of Headache Disorders: 2nd edition. *Cephalalgia* 2004;24(suppl):9–160.

Jansen J. Laminoplasty: a possible treatment for cervicogenic headache? Some ideas on the trigger mechanism of cervicogenic headache. *Funct Neurol* 1999;14:163–165.

Jansen J. Surgical treatment of non-responsive cervicogenic headache. *Clin Exp Rheumatol* 2000;18:S67–S70.

Jansen J, Bardosi A, Hildebrandt J, Lucke A. Cervicogenic, hemi-cranial attacks associated with vascular irritation or compression of the cervical nerve root C2: clinical manifestations and morphological findings. *Pain* 1989a;39:203–212.

Jansen J, Markakis E, Rama B, Hildebrandt J. Hemi-cranial attacks or permanent hemicrania: a sequel of upper cervical root compression. *Cephalalgia* 1989b;9:123–130.

Jensen OK, Justesen T, Nielsen FF, Brixen K. Functional radiographic examination of the cervical spine in patients with post-traumatic headache. *Cephalalgia* 1990;10: 295–303.

Johnson EK, Chiarello CM. The slump test: the effects of head and lower extremity position on knee extension. *J Orthop Sports Phys Ther* 1997;26:310–317.

Jull G. Headaches of cervical origin. In: Grant R, ed. *Physical Therapy of the Cervical and Thoracic Spine*. New York: Churchill Livingstone; 1994:261–285.

Jull G. Management of cervical headache. *Man Ther* 1997;2:182–190.

Jull G, Niere K. The cervical spine and headache. In: Boyling J, Jull GA, eds. *Grieves Modern Manual Therapy: The Vertebral Column.* London: Churchill Livingstone; 2004.

Jull G, Barrett C, Magee R, Ho P. Further clinical clarification of the muscle dysfunction in cervical headache. *Cephalalgia* 1999;19:179–185.

Jull G, Trott P, Potter H, et al. A randomized controlled trial of exercise and manipulative therapy for cervicogenic headache. *Spine* 2002;27:1835–1843.

Jull G, Amiri M, Bullock-Saxton J, Darnell R, Lander C. Cervical musculo-skeletal impairment in frequent intermittent headache. Part 1: subjects with single headaches. *Cephalalgia* 2007;27:793–802.

Kerr FWL. A mechanism to account for frontal headache in cases of posterior-fossa tumors. *J Neurosurgery* 1961;18:605–609.

Kerr FWL, Olafson RA. Trigeminal and cervical volleys: convergence on single units in the spinal gray at C-1 and C-2. *Arch Neurol* 1961;5:171–178.

Kornberg C, Lew P. The effect of stretching neural structures on grade one hamstring injuries. *J Orthop Sports Phys Ther* 1989;10:481–487.

Kornberg C, McCarthy T. The effect of neural stretching technique on sympathetic outflow to the lower limbs. *J Orthop Sports Phys Ther* 1992;16:269–274.

Kuncewicz E, Gajewska E, Sobieska M, Samborski W. Piriformis muscle syndrome. *Ann Academiae Medicae Stetinensis* 2006;52:99–101.

Leone M, D'Amico D, Moschiano F, Farinotti M, Filippini G, Bussone G. Possible identification of cervicogenic headache among patients with migraine: an analysis of 374 headaches. *Headache* 1995;35:461–464.

Lundborg G, Rydevik B. Effects of stretching the tibial nerve of the rabbit. A preliminary study of the intra-neural circulation and the barrier function of the peri-neurium. *J Bone Joint Surg (Br)* 1973;55:390–401.

Mackinnon SE. Double and multiple "crush" syndromes: double and multiple entrapment neuropathies. *Hand Clinics* 1992;8:369–390.

Malick A, Burstein R. Peripheral and central sensitization during migraine. *Funct Neurol* 2000;15:28–35.

Margulies SS, Meandey DF, Bilston LB, et al. In vivo motion of the human spinal cord in extension and flexion. Proceedings of the International Conference on the Biomechanics of Impacts; Verona, Italy; 1992.

Millesi H, Zoch G, Reihsner R. Mechanical properties of peripheral nerves. *Clin Orthop Rel Res* 1995;314:76–83.

Mitchell BS, Humphreys BK, O'Sullivan E. Attachments of the ligamentum nuchae to cervical posterior spinal dura and the lateral part of the occipital bone. *J Manipulative Physiol Ther* 1998;21:145–148.

Moskowitz MA. Neurogenic inflammation in the pathophysiology and treatment of migraine. *Neurology* 1993;43:S16–S20.

Moskowitz MA, Macfarlane R. Neurovascular and molecular mechanisms in migraine headaches. *Cerebrovasc Brain Metabol Rev* 1993;5:159–177.

Nakagawa H, Mikawa Y, Watanabe R. Elastin in the human posterior longitudinal ligament and spinal dura: a histologic and biochemical study. *Spine* 1994;19:2164–2169.

Nakamichi K, Tachibana S. Restricted motion of the median nerve in carpal tunnel syndrome. *J Hand Surg (Br)* 1995;20:460–464.

Narouze S. Cervicogenic headache: diagnosis and treatment. In: Schwartz AJ, Butterworth JF, Gross JB, eds. *ASA Refresher Courses in Anesthesiology.* Vol. 35. Philadelphia: Lippincott Williams & Wilkins; 2007:145–155.

Nelson CF. The tension headache, migraine headache continuum: a hypothesis. *J Manipulative Physiol Ther* 1994;17:156–167.

Niere KR. Pain descriptors used by headache patients presenting for physiotherapy. *Physiotherapy* 2002;88:409–416.

Ogata K, Naito M. Blood flow of peripheral nerve: effects of dissection, stretching and compression. *J Hand Surg (Am)* 1986;11:10–14.

Ogince M, Hall T, Robinson K, Blackmore AM. The diagnostic validity of the cervical flexion-rotation test in C1/2-related cervicogenic headache. *Man Ther* 2007;12:256–262.

Petersen SM. Articular and muscular impairments in cervicogenic headache: a case report. *J Orthop Sports Phys Ther* 2003;33:21–32.

Pikus HJ, Phillips JM. Characteristics of patients successfully treated for cervicogenic headache by surgical decompression of the second cervical root. *Headache* 1995;35:621–629.

Pikus HJ, Phillips JM. Outcome of surgical decompression of the second cervical root for cervicogenic headache. *Neurosurgery* 1996;39:63–71.

Placzek JD, Pagett BT, Roubal PJ, et al. The influence of the cervical spine on chronic headache in women: a pilot study. *J Manual Manipulative Ther* 1999;7:33–39.

Rasmussen BK. Migraine and tension-type headache in a general population: psychosocial factors. *Int J Epidemiol* 1992;21:1138–1143.

Reid JD. Effects of flexion-extension: movements of the head and spine upon the spinal cord and nerve roots. *J Neurol Neurosurg Psychiatry* 1960;23:214–221.

Rozmaryn LM, Dovelle S, Rothman ER, et al. Nerve and tendon gliding exercises and the conservative management of carpal tunnel syndrome. *J Hand Ther* 1998;11:171–179.

Rumore AJ. Slump examination and treatment in a patient suffering headache. *Aust J Physiother* 1989;35:262–263.

Shacklock M. Neurodynamics. *Physiotherapy* 1995;81:9–16.

Shacklock M. *Clinical Neurodynamics.* Edinburgh: Elsevier; 2005a.

Shacklock M. Improving application of neurodynamic (neural tension) testing and treatments: a message to researchers and clinicians. *Man Ther* 2005b;10:175–179.

Shevel E, Spierings EH. Cervical muscles in the pathogenesis of migraine headache. *J Headache Pain* 2004;5:12–14.

Siddiqui M, Karadimas E, Nicol M, Smith FW, Wardlaw D. Influence of X Stop on neural foramina and spinal canal area in spinal stenosis. *Spine* 2006;31:2958–2962.

Sizer PS Jr, Phelps V, Brismee J. Diagnosis and management of cervicogenic headache and local cervical syndrome with multiple pain generators. *J Manual Manipulative Ther* 2002;10:136–152.

Sjaastad O, Fredriksen TA, Pfaffenrath V. Cervicogenic headache: diagnostic criteria by the Cervicogenic Headache International Study Group. *Headache* 1998;38:442–445.

Slater E, Butler D, Shacklock M. The dynamic central nervous system: examination and assessment using tension tests. In: Boyling J, Palastanga N, eds. *Grieves Modern Manual Therapy: The Vertebral Column.* Edinburgh: Churchill Livingstone; 1994:587–606.

Solomon S. Diagnosis of primary headache disorders: validity of the International Headache Society criteria in clinical practice. *Neurol Clinics* 1997;15:15–26.

Sterling M, Treleaven J, Jull G. Responses to a clinical test of mechanical provocation of nerve tissue in whiplash associated disorder. *Man Ther* 2002;7:89–94.

Sterling M, Jull G, Vicenzino B, Kenardy J, Darnell R. Development of motor system dysfunction following whiplash injury. *Pain* 2003;103:65–73.

Sugawara O, Atsuta Y, Iwahara T, Muramoto T, Watakabe M, Takemitsu Y. The effects of mechanical compression and hypoxia on nerve root and dorsal root ganglia: an analysis of ectopic firing using an in vitro model. *Spine* 1996;21:2089–2094.

Sweeney J, Harms A. Persistent mechanical allodynia following injury of the hand: treatment through mobilization of the nervous system. *J Hand Ther* 1996;9:328–338.

Szeto GP, Straker L, Raine S. A field comparison of neck and shoulder postures in symptomatic and asymptomatic office workers. *Applied Ergonomics* 2002;33:75–84.

Thakur R, Hogan LA, Pannella-Vaughn J. Tension and cervicogenic headaches: keys to recognition, strategies for relief. *Consultant* 2002;42:1512–1515.

Treleaven J, Jull G, Atkinson L. Cervical musculoskeletal dysfunction in post-concussion headache. *Cephalalgia* 1994;14:273–279.

Troup JDG. Biomechanics of the lumbar spinal canal. *Clin Biomech* 1986;1:31–43.

Turnbull DK, Shepherd DB. Post-dural puncture headache: pathogenesis, prevention and treatment. *Br J Anaesth* 2003;91:718–729.

Vicenzino B, Collins D, Wright A. The initial effects of a cervical spine manipulative physiotherapy treatment on the pain and dysfunction of lateral epicondylalgia. *Pain* 1996;68:69–74.

Von Piekartz HJM, Schouten S, Aufdemkampe G. Neurodynamic responses in children with migraine or cervicogenic headache versus a control group: a comparative study. *Man Ther* 2007;12:153–160.

Watson DH, Trott PH. Cervical headache: an investigation of natural head posture and upper cervical flexor muscle performance. *Cephalalgia* 1993;13:272–28.

Weirich SD, Gelberman RH, Best SA, Abrahamsson SO, Furcolo DC, Lins RE. Rehabilitation after subcutaneous transposition of the ulnar nerve: immediate versus delayed mobilization. *J Shoulder Elbow Surg* 1998;7:244–249.

Wiesler ER, Chloros GD, Cartwright MS, Shin HW, Walker FO. Ultrasound in the diagnosis of ulnar neuropathy at the cubital tunnel. *J Hand Surg (Am)* 2006a;31:1088–1093.

Wiesler ER, Chloros GD, Cartwright MS, Smith BP, Rushing J, Walker FO. The use of diagnostic ultrasound in carpal tunnel syndrome. *J Hand Surg (Am)* 2006b;31:726–732.

Woolf CJ. Pain. *Neurobiol Dis* 2000;7:504–510.

Woolf CJ. Central sensitization: uncovering the relation between pain and plasticity. *Anesthesiology* 2007;106:864–867.

Woolf CJ, Mannion RJ. Neuropathic pain: etiology, symptoms, mechanisms, and management. *Lancet* 1999a;353:1959–1964.

Woolf CJ, Salter MW. Neuronal plasticity: increasing the gain in pain. *Science* 2000;288:1765–1769.

Woolf CJ, Shortland P, Sivilotti LG. Sensitization of high mechano-threshold superficial dorsal horn and flexor motor neurones following chemo-sensitive primary afferent activation. *Pain* 1994;58:141–155.

Wright TW, Glowczewski F Jr, Cowin D, Wheeler DL. Ulnar nerve excursion and strain at the elbow and wrist associated with upper extremity motion. *J Hand Surg (Am)* 2001;26:655–662.

Yeung E, Jones M, Hall B. The response to the slump test in a group of female whiplash patients. *Aust J Physiother* 1997;43:245–252.

Yuan Q, Dougherty L, Margulies SS. In vivo human cervical spinal cord deformation and displacement in flexion. *Spine* 1998;23:1677–1683.

Zito G, Jull G, Story I. Clinical tests of musculoskeletal dysfunction in the diagnosis of cervicogenic headache. *Man Ther* 2006;11:118–129.

Zwart JA. Neck mobility in different headache disorders. *Headache* 1997;37:6–11.

Neurophysiologic Effects of Needling Therapies

Jan Dommerholt, PT, MPS, and Robert D. Gerwin, MD

Needling therapies used in the treatment of individuals with active myofascial trigger points (TrPs) can be divided into injection and dry needling therapies. The most obvious distinction between the two categories is whether an injectable is used. TrP injections are administered with a syringe; TrP dry needling is administered with a solid filament needle. Trigger point injections are usually restricted to medical doctors and their professional support staff, including physician assistants and nurse practitioners, although in the state of Maryland physical therapists are allowed to perform myofascial trigger point injections as well (Dommerholt, 2004). Maryland is the only jurisdiction in the United States allowing this procedure to be performed by physical therapists. In the United Kingdom, physical therapists are allowed to perform joint and soft-tissue injections (Saunders & Longworth, 2006). A recent study of Canadian pain anesthesiologists showed that myofascial TrP injections are the second most common type of injection after epidural steroid injections (Peng & Castano, 2005).

During the 1940s, Dr. Janet Travell introduced injection techniques of muscle TrPs (Travell et al., 1942; Travell & Bobb, 1947; Travell, 1949). TrP dry needling interventions were not developed until the late 1970s, with nearly simultaneous publications in Canada and Czechoslovakia (the current Czech Republic), although one could argue that earlier acupuncture researchers and practitioners had already described TrP needling approaches even though they did not use the same terminology (Lewit, 1979; Gunn et al., 1980; Seem, 2007). Since those early publications, other health-care providers, including physical therapists, have embraced the dry needling techniques (Dommerholt, 2004; Dommerholt et al., 2006b). Currently, physical therapists around the world utilize TrP dry needling in their practices, for example, in Australia, Canada, Chile, Ireland, the Netherlands, New Zealand, South Africa, Spain, the United Kingdom, and the United States, among others (Dommerholt et al., 2006). Trigger point needling therapies are always part of a much broader treatment approach, which may include the assessment and treatment of metabolic and other perpetuating factors, postural training and core stabilization programs, and psychological and pharmacologic management (Gerwin, 2005; Gerwin & Dommerholt, 2006).

This chapter is mainly concerned with needling approaches of myofascial TrPs, which are defined as "hyperirritable spots in skeletal muscle that are associated with a hypersensitive nodule in a taut band" (Simons et al., 1999). By definition, muscle TrPs are located within a taut band, which is an endogenous localized contracture within the muscle without activation of the motor endplate (Mense, 1997). From a physiologic perspective, the term *contracture* is more accurate then *contraction* when describing chronic involuntary shortening of a muscle without electromyographic activity (Dommerholt et al., 2006). There is increasing evidence that TrPs are dysfunctional motor endplates (Chen et al., 1998a, 1998b; Couppé et al., 2001; Simons, 2001, 2004; Simons et al., 2002; Mense et al., 2003; Macgregor & Graf von Schweinitz, 2006; Hsieh et al., 2007; Kuan et al., 2007a, 2007b).

Myofascial TrPs can be divided into active and latent TrPs. Active TrPs are symptom-producing and feature local and referred pain or other paresthesia. A latent TrP does not cause pain without being stimulated. Both active and latent TrPs can be associated with disturbed motor function and motor planning, muscle weakness, muscle stiffness, and restricted range of motion. Active muscle TrPs are associated with local and referred pain, and with peripheral and central sensitization (Fernández-de-las-Peñas et al., 2007a). Migraine and tension-type headaches share many characteristics with referred pain patterns from muscle TrPs in the cervical and facial muscles (Graff-Radford, 1984; Fernández-de-las-Peñas et al., 2005, 2006a, 2006b, 2006c, 2006d, 2007b; Calandre et al., 2006; Giamberardino et al., 2007). Fernández-de-las-Peñas et al. (2008) defined clinical prediction rules to assist in identifying patients with chronic tension-type headaches who are likely to benefit from TrP therapy. Although both active and latent TrPs are painful on palpation, only active TrPs cause pain symptoms. Active myofascial TrPs feature a significant decrease of the pain threshold, not only in the muscular tissue, but also in the overlying cutaneous and subcutaneous tissues. In contrast, the sensory changes with latent TrPs do not involve the cutaneous and subcutaneous tissues (Vecchiet et al., 1990, 1994, 1998). The presence of a TrP causes a localized decrease in skin resistance regardless of whether a TrP is active or latent, although latent TrPs consistently featured a lower skin resistance than active TrPs (Giamberardino et al., 2007).

Shah et al. (2005) have demonstrated that the immediate biochemical milieu of active TrPs in the trapezius muscle differs significantly from the milieu of latent TrPs and normal muscle tissue, using immunocapillary electrophoresis and capillary electrochromatography. The biochemical milieu of active muscle TrPs had significantly higher levels of multiple inflammatory mediators, neuropeptides, cytokines, and catecholamines, including bradykinin, calcitonin gene-related peptide, substance P, tumor necrosis factor-α, interleukin-1β, serotonin, and norepinephrine, and the pH was always lower (Shah et al., 2005). In a follow-up study, the researchers examined the concentrations of other chemicals as well; they established that in subjects with active TrPs in the trapezius muscle, all concentrations differed quantitatively, even at a remote, uninvolved site in the gastrocnemius muscle (Shah et al., 2008).

Trigger points are thought to activate muscle nociceptors, which appear more effective at inducing neuroplastic changes in wide-dynamic-range dorsal horn neurons than pain associated with nociceptive stimulation of cutaneous receptors (Wall & Woolf, 1984). Muscle pain activates unique cortical structures, such as the anterior cingulate cortex, which is involved with the emotional, affective component of pain (Svensson et al., 1997). Niddam et al. (2007, 2008) have established that individuals with myofascial TrPs have abnormal central processing and hyperalgesia in response to electrical stimulation and compression of the TrPs. Enhanced brain activity was observed in somatosensory and limbic regions, and suppressed activity was noted in the hippocampus, which the authors speculated possibly indicated stress-related changes in relation to chronic pain (Niddam et al., 2008).

Clinicians need to develop excellent palpation skills and an outstanding kinesthetic sense, without which TrP dry needling would become a random process. Excellent anatomic knowledge is a prerequisite to develop the sensory-motor skill needed to be able to visualize the tip of the needle and the pathway the needle follows inside the patient's body (Noë, 2004; Dommerholt et al., 2006). With any needling procedure, the clinician needs to visualize a three-dimensional image of the exact location and depth of the TrP. The needle should not be used to locate the TrP, except in those muscles that cannot be palpated directly but are accessible with a needle only. The lateral pterygoid, parts of the subscapularis muscles, and the multifidi muscles are examples of such muscles (Brechner, 1982). In those cases, the needle is at the same time a tool for palpation, diagnosis, and treatment. Otherwise, TrPs are identified by manual palpation. Several studies have established the interrater reliability of locating myofascial TrPs (Gerwin et al., 1997; Hsieh et al., 2000; Sciotti et al., 2001; Bron et al., 2007).

Trigger point injections and deep dry needling often evoke patients' referred pain patterns and their primary pain complaint (Hong et al., 1997). Needling of TrPs in the sternocleidomastoid or upper trapezius muscles may trigger a patient's migraine or tension-type headache (Calandre et al., 2006). Needling of TrPs in the teres minor or gluteus minimus muscle may initiate pain resembling a C8 or L5 radiculopathy, respectively (Escobar & Ballesteros, 1988; Facco & Ceccherelli, 2005).

TRIGGER POINT INJECTIONS

A wide variety of injectables are used in the treatment of individuals with muscle TrPs, including local anesthetics (e.g., procaine, lidocaine, mepivacaine, bupivacaine, levobupivacaine, and ropivacaine), isotonic saline solutions, nonsteroidal anti-inflammatories, bee venom, botulinum toxin, corticosteroids, vitamin B_{12}, and serotonin antagonists, among others (Travell et al., 1942; Travell, 1949; Frost et al., 1980; Hameroff et al., 1981; Frost, 1986; Garvey et al., 1989; Davalos et al., 1994; Ettlin, 2004; Müller & Stratz, 2004; Rodriguez-Acosta et al., 2004; Ho & Tan, 2007; Menezes et al., 2007). Injections with botulinum toxin are discussed in detail in Chapter 32. Travell (1901–1997) treated patients with injections of procaine hydrochloride (Travell et al., 1942; Travell, 1949). In countries where procaine is not readily available anymore, as is the case in the United States, the recommendation is to use 0.25% lidocaine, which was found to be more effective than stronger lidocaine solutions (Iwama & Akama, 2000; Iwama et al., 2001). Nevertheless, stronger concentrations of 0.5%, 1%, or even 2% lidocaine solutions are commonly used in research studies and in clinical practice (Carlson et al., 1993; Hong, 1994a; Kamanli et al., 2005; Peng & Castano, 2005). A study of patients with severe migraine treated with TrP injections with ropivacaine concluded that the TrP injections were a useful prophylactic tool. The study did not include a control group (Garcia-Leiva et al., 2007). A comparison study of the effects of TrP injections with 0.25% levobupivacaine and 0.25% ropivacaine did not find any significant differences between the two substances for pain during injection, efficacy of the treatment, and duration of pain relief (Zaralidou et al., 2007). The injectables were equally effective, which is consistent with several obstetric and

pediatric injection studies that compared the two substances for non-TrPs (Alahuhta et al., 1995; Stienstra et al., 1995; Ala-Kokko et al., 2000). Ropivacaine is thought to have a slightly lower potency and half-life than bupivacaine (Brown et al., 1990; Van Kleef et al., 1994; Tuttle et al., 1995).

There is no evidence of any advantage of administering TrP injections with vitamin B_{12}, nonsteroidal anti-inflammatories, or steroids in the treatment of patients with myofascial pain. Intramuscular injections of steroids may actually lead to breakdown and degeneration of muscle fibers (Frost et al., 1980; Garvey et al., 1989; Fischer, 1997). Patients with widespread pain may have vitamin B_{12} deficiencies or insufficiencies and may require systemic vitamin B_{12} supplementation, but there is no evidence that injecting myofascial TrPs with vitamin B_{12} is beneficial (Gerwin, 2005). One study compared the effectiveness of diclofenac with lidocaine and found that injections with diclofenac reduced pain levels by a significantly greater degree (Frost, 1986). Injections with the serotonin antagonist tropisetron were found to be superior to injections with lidocaine in two German studies (Ettlin, 2004; Müller & Stratz, 2004). Injectable serotonin antagonists are not available everywhere in the world. Of interest is that a chemical analysis of the immediate environment of active myofascial TrPs found significantly elevated levels of serotonin, which may partially explain the effectiveness of tropisetron injections (Shah et al., 2005, 2008).

There is no direct evidence regarding injecting bee venom into muscle TrPs. However, some of the characteristics of bee venom suggest that there may be a future role in the treatment of myofascial TrPs. Bee venom is a commonly applied substance within the context of Chinese medicine. A few animal studies have demonstrated that bee venom has an antinociceptive and anti-inflammatory effect through activation of brainstem catecholaminergic neurons and activation of the alpha-2 adrenergic and serotonergic pathways of the descending inhibitory system (Kim et al., 2005; Kwon et al., 2001a, 2001b). Bee venom also involves activation of spinal cord circuits characterized by an increased release of spinal acetylcholine, which in turn is thought to stimulate sympathetic preganglionic neurons (Yoon et al., 2005). One of the active ingredients of bee venom is melitin, which has been shown to suppress lipopolysaccharide-induced nitric oxide and the transcription of cyclooxygenase-2 (COX-2) genes and proinflammatory cytokines, including interleukin-1β (IL-1β) and tumor necrosis factor alpha (TNF-α) in microglia (Han et al.,

2007). IL-1β and TNF-α have been found in increased concentrations in the direct milieu of active myofascial TrPs (Shah et al., 2005, 2008). The inhibition of c-Fos expression in the spinal cord by injection of bee venom may also be a possible mechanism of pain relief (Kim et al., 2003). In addition to melitin, bee venom contains several other peptides, including apamin, adolapin, mast cell degranulating peptide, enzymes, and biologically active amines such as histamine and epinephrine (Son et al., 2007a, 2007b). Injections of bee venom into specific acupuncture points in several animal and human studies of knee arthritis were beneficial and reduced pain levels significantly, but there are no studies that demonstrate the effectiveness of TrP injections with bee venom (Baek et al., 2006; Kwon et al., 2001a, 2001b; Lee et al., 2005a, 2005b; Son et al., 2007a). Clinicians who are considering using bee venom injections should always assess whether patients are allergic to bee venom to avoid unnecessary complications.

Many other clinical outcome studies confirm that TrP injections are effective in inactivating muscle TrPs and in reducing pain levels (Jaeger & Skootsky, 1987; Padamsee et al., 1987; Hong, 1993; Ling & Slocumb, 1993; McMillan & Blasberg, 1994; Fischer, 1995; Tschopp & Gysin, 1996). Fischer expanded the TrP model and developed the so-called spinal segmental sensitization model, which consists of preinjection blocks with lidocaine, needling and infiltration of tender spots and TrPs, somatic blocks, spray and stretch techniques, and relaxation exercises (Fischer & Imamura, 2000). Fischer speculated that injecting the supraspinous ligament may contribute to inactivating TrPs in the corresponding myotomes (Fischer, 1999). There are no studies comparing Fischer's spinal segmental sensitization approach to the TrP needling approaches.

TRIGGER POINT DRY NEEDLING

In 1944, Steinbrocker suggested that the effect of TrP injections was mostly due to mechanical stimulation of the TrP irrespective of the particular type of injectable used (Steinbrocker, 1944), but it was not until 1979 that Lewit published the first paper on dry needling of myofascial TrPs (Lewit, 1979). In a retrospective review, Lewit reported that dry needling of muscle TrPs caused immediate analgesia in almost 87% of the needle sites, which he referred to as the "needle effect." Nearly a third of subjects remained free of pain. About 20% of subjects experienced several months without pain;

22%, several weeks; 11%, several days; and approximately 14% had no pain relief. Lewit observed that the effectiveness of dry needling was directly related to the accuracy of needling (Lewit, 1979), which depends greatly on the ability to palpate myofascial TrPs accurately (Dommerholt et al., 2006). In 1980, Gunn et al. published a prospective dry needling study of injured workers with low back pain. They demonstrated that dry needling was an effective treatment for low back pain. Subsequently, Gunn (1997a) developed a theoretical concept that proposes that all myofascial pain is the result of peripheral neuropathy or radiculopathy, which he defined as "a condition that causes disordered function in the peripheral nerve." In his early work, Gunn did incorporate myofascial TrPs, but he soon abandoned the TrP model (Gunn & Milbrandt, 1977; Gunn, 1997b). The dry needling approach that Gunn developed is known as intramuscular stimulation (Gunn, 1997b).

Trigger point dry needling is divided into superficial and deep dry needling, based on the depth of needling (Dommerholt et al., 2006). Lewit and Gunn used deep dry needling techniques, similarly to injection techniques, in which the needle is placed directly into myofascial TrPs. One of the objectives of deep TrP needling and TrP injections is to elicit so-called local twitch responses, which are involuntary spinal cord reflex contractions of the muscle fibers in a taut band (Hong, 1994b). The sudden contractions can be observed visually, be recorded electromyographically, or be visualized with diagnostic ultrasound (Gerwin & Duranleau, 1997). When a muscle TrP is needled with a monopolar teflon-coated electromyography needle, local twitch responses appear as high-amplitude polyphasic discharges (Hong & Torigoe, 1994; Hong, 1994b). Eliciting local twitch responses is essential when using deep dry needling, not only to accomplish optimal treatment results, but also to confirm that the needle is placed into a taut band, which is critically important when needling close to peripheral nerves or internal organs, such as the lungs (Hong, 1994a; Mayoral del Moral, 2005). Eliciting local twitch responses in active TrPs appeared to normalize the biochemical milieu instantly (Shah et al., 2005, 2008). Shah et al. (2005, 2008) speculated that the drop in concentrations may be caused by a local increase in blood flow or by interference with nociceptor membrane channels, or by transport mechanisms associated with a briefly augmented inflammatory response. The concentrations of substance P and calcitonin gene-related peptide were significantly below their concentrations at baseline, which corresponds with the clinical observation of a reduction in pain following deep dry needling (Shah et al., 2008).

Superficial dry needling was developed by Baldry, who, after identifying muscle TrPs in a patient's anterior scalene muscle, was concerned about possibly causing a pneumothorax if he were to use deep dry needling techniques (Baldry, 2005b). Instead, Baldry placed the needle into the superficial tissues overlying the TrP, which reduced the exquisite tenderness and spontaneous pain (Baldry, 2005b). Encouraged by the successful treatment, Baldry started applying the superficial needling technique to other patients and to other muscles with equally good results. Baldry recommends inserting an acupuncture needle into the tissues overlying the myofascial TrP at a depth of approximately 5 to 10 mm for 30 seconds (Baldry, 2005b). In case of any residual pain, the needle is inserted for another 2 to 3 minutes. The intensity and duration of the stimulus are dictated by the responsiveness of the patients. Whether patients are so-called strong or weak responders may depend partially on the degree of available endogenous opioid peptide antagonist. Weak responders are thought to have excessive amounts of endogenous opioid peptide antagonists (Baldry, 2005b). Animal studies have shown that mice with deficient opioid peptide receptors did not respond well to needle-evoked nerve stimulation (Peets & Pomeranz, 1978).

In China, Fu developed a variation of superficial dry needling, which he refers to as Fu's subcutaneous needling (Fu & Xu, 2005; Fu et al., 2006, 2008). Fu does not use acupuncture needles, but a three-part needle system consisting of a 31-mm beveled-tip needle with a diameter of 1 mm, a soft plastic tube similar to an intravenous catheter, and a cap. The needle and the plastic tube are inserted into the subcutaneous tissue and moved from side to side for at least 2 minutes, after which the needle is removed from the tube. The tube is left in place until the patient returns to the clinic for a follow-up visit. For acute injuries, the tube is left in place for only a few hours. In chronic pain conditions, the tube is left in place for at least 24 hours, after which it is removed. Fu speculates that the tube stimulates connective tissues continuously, and he refers to the work of Langevin et al. (2006a, 2006b) to explain how mechanical stimulation of connective tissues may result in pain modulation through stretching of fibroblasts. Mechanical stimulation of fibroblasts is thought to trigger a cascade of cellular and molecular events, including cytoskeletal reorganization, cell contraction, a release of

growth factors, the stimulation of intracellular signaling pathways, variations in gene expression and extracellular matrix composition, and eventually the release of myokines and other substances in the immediate environment of the needle (Langevin et al., 2001, 2006a, 2006b). Langevin et al. have not studied the effects of mechanical stimulation on myofascial TrPs. However, based on their research, it may be beneficial to rotate the needle when performing superficial dry needling techniques (Dommerholt et al., 2006). Rotation of the needle is a painful stimulus, which may activate Aδ fibers and enkephalinergic, serotonergic, and noradrenergic inhibitory systems (Bowsher, 1998; Dommerholt et al., 2006).

Several studies have demonstrated that TrP dry needling is effective, and the results appear similar to injection therapies (Jaeger & Skootsky, 1987; Garvey et al., 1989; Hong, 1994a; Cummings and White, 2001; Furlan et al., 2005; Kamanli et al., 2005; Mayoral del Moral, 2005). Cummings and White (2001) concluded in their meta-analysis of needling therapies that dry needling of myofascial TrPs provides as much pain relief as injections of lidocaine. Two studies suggested that dry needling would cause more postneedling soreness, but they compared TrP injections to dry needling with a syringe (Hong, 1994a; Kamanli et al., 2005). A study comparing TrP injections with a syringe and TrP dry needling with acupuncture needles showed that TrP needling using an acupuncture needle does not cause more postneedling soreness than a TrP injection (Dommerholt et al., 2006; Ga et al., 2007a, 2007b).

TRIGGER POINT DRY NEEDLING AND ACUPUNCTURE

Dry needling techniques are performed with the same solid filament needles that acupuncture practitioners use, which triggers the question of whether TrP dry needling has similarities with acupuncture or perhaps could even be considered a form of acupuncture when it is administered by acupuncture practitioners. Dry needling does not require knowledge of the theoretical foundations of Chinese medicine and its ancient laws (Amaro, 2007). Travell, Simons, and Lewit were not familiar with the acupuncture literature when they published their observations and suggested management strategies of TrPs, and there are no indications that earlier medical practitioners who described TrP phenomena were familiar with the acupuncture literature (Strauss, 1898; Stockman, 1904; Lange & Eversbusch,

1921; Lange, 1931). Yet, there are some earlier publications in the medical literature that share similarities with the TrP dry needling literature. Baldry (2005a) reported that early in the 19th century, British physicians Campbell and Elliotson published books and articles about acupuncture without considering the concepts of traditional acupuncture (Churchill, 1821, 1828; Elliotson, 1827). Instead, they inserted needles in points of maximum tenderness, which resembles the current practice of TrP dry needling (Baldry, 2005a). In 1912, the prominent physician Sir William Osler recommended inserting ladies' hat pins at tender points in the treatment of low back pain (Osler, 1912).

Whether dry needling should be considered a form of acupuncture depends greatly on how acupuncture is defined. Seem, an eminent U.S. acupuncture practitioner, argued that American acupuncturists usually do not "treat tender or tight spots and, hence, never really achieve myofascial release in their recurrent and chronic pain patients" (Seem, 2007). Occasionally, the definition of acupuncture is so broad that any needling procedure would fall within the scope of acupuncture practice. For example, the New Mexico Acupuncture and Oriental Medicine Practice Act used to define acupuncture as "the use of needles inserted into and removed from the human body and the use of other devices, modalities, and procedures at specific locations on the body for the prevention, cure, or correction of any disease, illness, injury, pain, or other condition by controlling and regulating the flow and balance of energy and functioning of the person to restore and maintain health" (New Mexico Board of Acupuncture and Oriental Medicine, 1978). Interestingly, the current New Mexico statutes no longer define the practice of acupuncture, but they do suggest that acupuncture practice would be limited to doctors of oriental medicine, who are also authorized to include physical medicine modalities, including spray and stretch techniques using prescription vapocoolants (New Mexico Board of Acupuncture and Oriental Medicine, 1996).

A wide range of acupuncture approaches exists, based on different philosophies, opinions, and techniques. Even acupuncture societies and associations do not necessarily agree whether dry needling is a form of acupuncture. Whereas one U.S. acupuncture society insists that "dry needling is not acupuncture" when administered by physical therapists, another U.S. acupuncture association maintains that "dry needling is acupuncture" (Hobbs, 2007; Virginia Board of Physical Therapy Task Force on Dry Needling, 2007). When

acupuncture is defined as an effort to control energy flow, there are few if any correlations with TrP dry needling. Traditional Chinese medicine is based on prescientific ideas rather than the neurophysiologic and anatomic principles underlying dry needling (Amaro, 2007). Baldry (2005b) described the ancient views of traditional Chinese acupuncture as "not of any practical importance" within the context of TrP dry needling. On the other hand, in more modern biomedical neurophysiology-based applications of acupuncture, there may be significant overlap (Hong, 2000; Audette & Blinder, 2003; Campbell, 2006; Ma et al., 2005; Seem, 2007).

Opinions vary as to whether TrPs are the same as acupuncture points. Melzack et al. suggested a 71% overlap between acupuncture points and muscle TrPs based on anatomic location (Melzack et al., 1977; Melzack, 1981). Birch countered the arguments of Melzack et al. and concluded that they erroneously had assumed that local pain indications of acupuncture points would be sufficient to establish a correlation (Birch, 2003). Instead, Birch concluded that at best there is only an 18% to 19% overlap between acupuncture points and myofascial TrPs. He and others have suggested that myofascial TrPs are similar to the so-called *ashi* points in Chinese acupuncture or *kori* in Japanese acupuncture (Hong, 2000; Audette & Blinder, 2003; Birch, 2003; Cardinal, 2004; Ma et al., 2005; Campbell, 2006; Cardinal, 2007; Seem, 2007). *Ashi points* are defined as points where the patient expresses pain and discomfort in response to pressure. *Kori* is defined as a tight myofascial constriction that may or may not elicit discomfort with palpation, but which can be felt by the practitioner (Seem, 2007).

In 2006, Dorsher revisited the issue with an extensive study of the acupuncture and trigger point literature. Dorsher (2006) disagreed with Birch and concluded that most acupuncture points have pain indications and can be directly compared to TrPs. He concluded that of a total of 255 TrPs, 92% had anatomically corresponding acupuncture points. Nearly 80% of these acupuncture points had local pain indications similar to their corresponding TrPs (Dorsher, 2006). Dorsher (2006) compared acupuncture point locations with the depicted locations of TrPs in the TrP manuals, which may be an inaccurate assessment because those locations are only indications of Travell's observations (Simons & Dommerholt, 2007). In clinical practice there are many other TrP locations (Simons & Dommerholt, 2007). Seem (2007) and Amaro (2007) offered that TrP dry needling may be similar to treatment of the so-called musculotendinous meridians. There are also close similarities between the pathways of acupuncture meridians and the referred pain patterns of muscle TrPs (Cardinal, 2004, 2007; Dorsher, 2006; Seem, 2007). Dorsher (2006) found similar patterns for as many as 76% of corresponding points.

Medical and acupuncture practitioners may indeed be treating similar conditions with similar minimally invasive needling procedures regardless of how they refer to the treatment approach. Amaro (2007) recommended that practitioners of acupuncture "absorb the philosophy and procedure of dry needling as an adjunct for musculoskeletal pain control." Of interest is the growing evidence against the notion that acupuncture points would have distinct and reproducible clinical indications (Campbell, 2006). Several studies demonstrated that needling of known acupuncture points and sham points was more effective than no treatment, but there was no statistical difference between acupuncture and sham acupuncture (Linde et al., 2005; Melchart et al., 2005; Scharf et al., 2006).

To avoid any legal or statutory complications, the term *TrP acupuncture* may be the most appropriate term for the techniques that acupuncture practitioners use to treat myofascial TrPs. When nonacupuncture practitioners, such as physical therapists or physicians, treat TrPs with solid filament needles, the term *dry needling* may be preferable. It would seem that patients would only benefit if practitioners representing different disciplines were skilled in treating myofascial TrPs. In contrast, the American Association of Acupuncture and Oriental Medicine (AAAOM) issued a position statement in October 2007 opposing the practice of dry needling by physical therapists and suggested that physical therapists would be infringing upon the rights of acupuncture practitioners (McGee & Herbkersman, 2007). The AAAOM considered "dry-needling to fall squarely within the range of acupuncturist practice" and the "use of needles both an invasive procedure beyond the professional scope of physical therapy and directly related to the practice of acupuncture" (McGee & Herbkersman, 2007).

PROPOSED MECHANISMS OF TRIGGER POINT DRY NEEDLING

The exact mechanisms of TrP injections and dry needling remain elusive. It is likely that needling therapies directed at TrPs involve central pain mechanisms, as

has been demonstrated for needling of acupuncture points and nonacupuncture points, but to date there is no direct evidence (Dommerholt et al., 2006). Hui et al. (2000) reported specific changes in the limbic system and subcortical gray structures following acupuncture needling. Several other studies have implicated the limbic system (Wu et al., 1999, 2002; Biella et al., 2001; Hsieh et al., 2001). Takeshige et al. (1991, 1992a, 1992b) confirmed that needling of acupuncture and nonacupuncture points involved the descending inhibitory system.

Baldry (2005b) has suggested that superficial dry needling stimulates Aδ sensory afferent fibers for up to 72 hours following the needling procedure. As Bowsher (1998) has confirmed, stimulation of Aδ nerve fibers may activate enkephalinergic, serotonergic, and noradrenergic inhibitory systems, which suggests that superficial dry needling of muscle TrPs would cause opioid-mediated pain suppression. However, Aδ nerve fibers are only activated by nociceptive mechanical stimulation for type I high-threshold Aδ fibers, or by cold stimuli for type II Aδ fibers (Millan, 1999). Because superficial dry needling is neither a painful mechanical nor a cold stimulus, it is unlikely that Aδ fibers would be activated with this technique (Dommerholt et al., 2006). When superficial dry needling is combined with rotating the needle after it has been inserted, the stimulus would become a nociceptive stimulus, and as such may activate the pain inhibitory system associated with Aδ fibers through segmental spinal and propriospinal, heterosegmental inhibition, possibly involving stretching of fibroblasts in connective tissues (Sandkühler, 1996; Langevin et al., 2005, 2006a, 2006b). On the other hand, light touch of the skin has been shown to stimulate mechanoreceptors coupled to slow-conducting unmyelinated C-fiber afferents, which in turn can activate the insular region, but not the somatosensory cortex (Olausson et al., 2002). Superficial dry needling may activate these C-fiber tactile afferents and stimulate the anterior cingulate cortex with emotional and hormonal reactions representing a sense of progress, reduction of pain, and well-being (Olausson et al., 2002; Mohr et al., 2005; Lund & Lundeberg, 2006). The reduction of pain following superficial dry needling may also be partially due to the central release of oxytocin (Uvnas-Moberg et al., 1993; Lundeberg et al., 1994). Cutaneous and muscle stimulation of Aδ and C fibers was capable of producing an increase in cerebral blood flow in rodents and in patients with chronic pain (Alavi et al., 1997; Uchida et al., 2000).

As outlined previously, one of the objectives of deep dry needling and TrP injections is to elicit local twitch responses, which are thought to be critical in inactivating TrPs. Local twitch responses can instantly alter the chemical milieu of active TrPs, but can also diminish endplate noise associated with TrPs (Chen et al., 2001; Shah et al., 2005, 2008). It is conceivable that deep dry needling and TrP injections destroy motor endplates and cause distal axon denervations, which may trigger changes in the endplate cholinesterase and acetylcholine receptors as part of the normal muscle regeneration process (Sadeh et al., 1985; Gaspersic et al., 2001). Muscle regeneration involves the migration of satellite cells, which are activated not only following actual muscle damage, but also after light compression (Teravainen, 1970; Sadeh et al., 1985). Deep dry needling may cause a mechanical disruption of the contraction knots and stretch the contractured sarcomere assemblies and reduce the overlap between actin and myosin filaments (Simons et al., 1999; Dommerholt, 2004). Deep dry needling can also be combined with rotation of the needle, after which the needle is left in place until relaxation of the muscle fibers has occurred (Dommerholt et al., 2006). The mechanical pressure exerted with the needle may electrically polarize muscle and connective tissue and transform mechanical stress into electrical activity, which is required for tissue remodeling (Liboff, 1997).

Deep dry needling can easily be combined with electrical stimulation (Mayoral & Torres, 2003; Mayoral del Moral, 2005; Dommerholt et al., 2006). Although little is known about the optimal treatment parameters, Niddam et al. (2007) observed that an electrical current applied directly to a myofascial TrP may activate the periaqueductal gray matter in some subjects. One of the obvious advantages of percutaneous electrical stimulation is that the skin resistance encountered with cutaneous electrodes is eliminated. Stimulation frequencies between 2 and 4 Hz are thought to trigger the release of endorphins and enkephalins, whereas frequencies between 80 and 100 Hz may release gamma-aminobutyric acid, galanin, and dynorphin (Lundeberg & Stener-Victorin, 2002). Several rodent studies have shown that electrical acupuncture can modulate the expression of N-methyl-D-aspartate in primary sensory neurons (Choi et al., 2005; Wang et al., 2006). Unfortunately, there are few researched guidelines for needle-electrode placement and treatment parameters, such as optimal amplitude, frequency, and duration, when electrotherapy is used in combination with muscle TrP needling. One study recommended placing the needle-electrodes within the same dermatomes as the location of the lesion (White et al., 2000).

SUMMARY

Trigger point needling therapies should be considered an integral part of a comprehensive management approach to treat patients with acute and chronic pain problems. Although the exact mechanisms of TrP dry needling are largely unknown, a growing number of clinical outcome studies support the use of TrP needling in the management of patients.

REFERENCES

Alahuhta S, Rasanen J, Jouppila P, et al. The effects of epidural ropivacaine and bupivacaine for cesarean section on uteroplacental and fetal circulation. *Anesthesiology* 1995;83:23–32.

Ala-Kokko TI, Partanen A, Karinen J, Kiviluoma K, Alahuhta S. Pharmaco-kinetics of 0.2% ropivacaine and 0.2% bupivacaine following caudal blocks in children. *Acta Anaesthesiol Scand* 2000;44:1099–1102.

Alavi A, LaRiccia PJ, Sadek AH, et al. Neuroimaging of acupuncture in patients with chronic pain. *J Altern Complement Med* 1997;3(suppl 1):S47–S53.

Amaro JA. When acupuncture becomes "dry needling." *Acupuncture Today* November 2007;33:43.

Audette JF, Blinder RA. Acupuncture in the management of myofascial pain and headache. *Curr Pain Headache Rep* 2003;7:395–401.

Baek YH, Huh JE, Lee JD, Choi do Y, Park DS. Antinociceptive effect and the mechanism of bee venom acupuncture (apipuncture) on inflammatory pain in the rat model of collagen-induced arthritis: mediation by alpha2-adrenoceptors. *Brain Res* 2006;1073–1074:305–310.

Baldry P. The integration of acupuncture within medicine in the UK—the British Medical Acupuncture Society's 25th anniversary. *Acupunct Med* 2005a;23:2–12.

Baldry PE. *Acupuncture, Trigger Points and Musculoskeletal Pain*. Edinburgh: Churchill Livingstone; 2005b.

Biella G, Sotgiu M, Pellegata G, Paulesu E, Castiglioni I, Fazio F. Acupuncture produces central activations in pain regions. *Neuroimage* 2001;14:60–66.

Birch S. Trigger point–acupuncture point correlations revisited. *J Altern Complement Med* 2003;9:91–103.

Bowsher D. Mechanisms of acupuncture. In: Filshie J, White A, eds. *Western Acupuncture: A Western Scientific Approach.* Edinburgh: Churchill Livingstone; 1998.

Brechner VL. Myofascial pain syndrome of the lateral pterygoid muscle. *J Craniomandibular Pract* 1982;1: 42–45.

Bron C, Franssen J, Wensing M, Oostendorp RAB. Interrater reliability of palpation of myofascial trigger points in three shoulder muscles. *J Man Manipulative Ther* 2007;15: 203–215.

Brown DL, Carpenter RL, Thompson GE. Comparison of 0.5% ropivacaine and 0.5% bupivacaine for epidural anesthesia in patients undergoing lower-extremity surgery. *Anesthesiology* 1990;72:633–636.

Calandre EP, Hidalgo J, Garcia-Leiva JM, Rico-Villademoros F. Trigger point evaluation in migraine patients: an indication of peripheral sensitization linked to migraine predisposition? *Eur J Neurol* 2006;13:244–249.

Campbell A. Point specificity of acupuncture in the light of recent clinical and imaging studies. *Acupunct Med* 2006;24:118–122.

Cardinal S. *Points détente et acupuncture: approche neurophysiologique.* Montreal: Centre collégial de développement de matériel didactique; 2004.

Cardinal S. *Points-détente et acupuncture: techniques de puncture.* Montréal: Centre collégial de développement de matériel didactique; 2007.

Carlson CR, Okeson JP, Falace DA, Nitz AJ, Lindroth JE. Reduction of pain and EMG activity in the masseter region by trapezius trigger point injection. *Pain* 1993;55:397–400.

Chen JT, Chen SM, Kuan TS, Chung KC, Hong CZ. Phentolamine effect on the spontaneous electrical activity of active loci in a myofascial trigger spot of rabbit skeletal muscle. *Arch Phys Med Rehabil* 1998a;79:790–794.

Chen SM, Chen JT, Kuan TS, Hong CZ. Effect of neuromuscular blocking agent on the spontaneous activity of active loci in a myofascial trigger spot of rabbit skeletal muscle. *J Musculoskeletal Pain* 1998b;6(suppl 2):25.

Chen JT, Chung KC, Hou CR, et al. Inhibitory effect of dry needling on the spontaneous electrical activity recorded from myofascial trigger spots of rabbit skeletal muscle. *Am J Phys Med Rehabil* 2001;80:729–735.

Choi BT, Lee JH, Wan Y, Han J. Involvement of ionotropic glutamate receptors in low frequency electroacupuncture analgesia in rats. *Neurosci Lett* 2005;377:185–188.

Churchill JM. *A Treatise on Acupuncturation, Being a Description of a Surgical Operation Originally Peculiar to the Japanese and Chinese, and by Them Denominated Zin-King, Now Introduced into European Practice, with Directions for Its Performance and Cases Illustrating Its Success.* London: Simpkins & Marshall; 1821.

Churchill JM. *Cases Illustrative of the Immediate Effects of Acupuncturation in Rheumatism, Lumbago, Sciatica, Anomalous Muscular Diseases and in Dropsy of the Cellular Tissues, Selected from Various Sources and Intended as an Appendix to the Author's Treatise on the Subject.* London: Simpkins & Marshall; 1828.

Couppé C, Midttun A, Hilden J, Jørgensen U, Oxholm P, Fuglsang-Frederiksen A. Spontaneous needle electromyographic activity in myofascial trigger points in the infraspinatus muscle: a blinded assessment. *J Musculoskeletal Pain* 2001;9(3):7–17.

Cummings TM, White AR. Needling therapies in the management of myofascial trigger point pain: a systematic review. *Arch Phys Med Rehabil* 2001;82:986–992.

Davalos A, Fernandez-Real JM, Ricart W, et al. Iron-related damage in acute ischemic stroke. *Stroke* 1994;25: 1543–1546.

Dommerholt J. Dry needling in orthopedic physical therapy practice. *Orthop Phys Ther Practice* 2004;16:15–20.

Dommerholt J, Bron C, Franssen JLM. Myofascial trigger points; an evidence-informed review. *J Manual Manipulative Ther* 2006a;14:203–221.

Dommerholt J, Mayoral O, Gröbli C. Trigger point dry needling. *J Manual Manipulative Ther* 2006b;14:E70–E87.

Dorsher P. Trigger points and acupuncture points: anatomic and clinical correlations. *Med Acupunct* 2006;17:21–25.

Elliotson J. The use of the sulphate of copper in chronic diarrhoea together with an essay on acupuncture. *Medicochirurigical Transactions* 1827;13:451–467.

Escobar PL, Ballesteros J. Teres minor: source of symptoms resembling ulnar neuropathy or C8 radiculopathy. *Am J Phys Med Rehabil* 1988;67:120–122.

Ettlin T. Trigger point injection treatment with the 5-HT3 receptor antagonist tropisetron in patients with late whiplash-associated disorder. First results of a multiple case study. *Scand J Rheumatol* 2004;119:49–50.

Facco E, Ceccherelli F. Myofascial pain mimicking radicular syndromes. *Acta Neurochir Suppl* 2005;92:147–150.

Fernández-de-las-Peñas C, Cuadrado ML, Gerwin RD, Pareja JA. Referred pain from the trochlear region in tension-type headache: a myofascial trigger point from the superior oblique muscle. *Headache* 2005;45:731–737.

Fernández-de-las-Peñas C, Alonso C, Cuadrado ML, Pareja JA. Myofascial trigger points in the suboccipital muscles in episodic tension-type headache. *Man Ther* 2006a;11: 225–230.

Fernández-de-las-Peñas C, Alonso C, Cuadrado ML, Gerwin RD, Pareja JA. Myofascial trigger points and their relationship to headache clinical parameters in chronic tension-type headache. *Headache* 2006b;46:1264–1272.

Fernández-de-las-Peñas C, Alonso C, Cuadrado ML, Gerwin RD, Pareja JA. Trigger points in the suboccipital muscles and forward head posture in tension-type headache. *Headache* 2006c;46:454–460.

Fernández-de-las-Peñas C, Cuadrado ML, Gerwin RD, Pareja JA. Myofascial disorders in the trochlear region in unilateral migraine: a possible initiating or perpetuating factor. *Clin J Pain* 2006d;22:548–553.

Fernández-de-las-Peñas C, Cuadrado ML, Simons D, Arendt-Nielsen L, Pareja JA. Myofascial trigger points and sensitization: an updated pain model for tension-type headache. *Cephalalgia* 2007a;27:383–393.

Fernández-de-las-Peñas C, Ge HY, Arendt-Nielsen L, Cuadrado ML, Pareja JA. Referred pain from trapezius muscle trigger points shares similar characteristics with chronic tension type headache. *Eur J Pain* 2007b;11:475–482.

Fernández-de-las-Peñas C, Cleland JA, Cuadrado ML, Pareja JA. Predictor variables for identifying patients with chronic tension-type headache who are likely to achieve short-term success with muscle trigger point therapy. *Cephalalgia* 2008;28:264–275.

Fischer AA. Local injections in pain management: trigger point needling with infiltration and somatic blocks. In: Kraft GH, Weinstein SM, eds. *Injection Techniques: Principles and Practice*. Vols. 851–870. Philadelphia: WB Saunders; 1995.

Fischer AA. New developments in diagnosis of myofascial pain and fibromyalgia. In: Fischer AA, ed. *Myofascial Pain: Update in Diagnosis and Treatment*. Vol. 8. Philadelphia: WB Saunders; 1997:1–21.

Fischer AA. Treatment of myofascial pain. *J Musculoskeletal Pain* 1999;7(1/2):131–142.

Fischer AA, Imamura M. New concepts in the diagnosis and management of musculoskeletal pain. In: Lennard TA, ed. *Pain Procedures in Clinical Practice*. Philadelphia: Hanley & Belfus; 2000:213–229.

Frost A. Diclofenac versus lidocaine as injection therapy in myofascial pain. *Scand J Rheumatol* 1986;15:153–156.

Frost FA, Jessen B, Siggaard-Andersen J. A control, double-blind comparison of mepivacaine injection versus saline injection for myofascial pain. *Lancet* 1980;1:499–501.

Fu ZH, Xu JG. A brief introduction to Fu's subcutaneous needling. *Pain Clinical Updates* 2005;17:343–348.

Fu ZH, Chen XY, Lu LJ, Lin J, Xu JG. Immediate effect of Fu's subcutaneous needling for low back pain. *Chin Med J (Engl)* 2006;119:953–956.

Fu ZH, Wang JH, Sun JH, Chen XY, Xu JG. Fu's subcutaneous needling—possible clinical evidence of the subcutaneous connective tissue in acupuncture. *J Altern Complement Med* 2008 (in press).

Furlan A, Tulder M, Cherkin D, et al. Acupuncture and dry-needling for low back pain: an updated systematic review within the framework of the Cochrane Collaboration. *Spine* 2005;30:944–963.

Ga H, Choi JH, Park CH, Yoon HJ. Acupuncture needling versus lidocaine injection of trigger points in myofascial pain syndrome in elderly patients—a randomised trial. *Acupunct Med* 2007a;25:130–136.

Ga H, Koh HJ, Choi JH, Kim CH. Intramuscular and nerve root stimulation vs lidocaine injection to trigger points in myofascial pain syndrome. *J Rehabil Med* 2007b;39:374–378.

Garcia-Leiva JM, Hidalgo J, Rico-Villademoros F, Moreno V, Calandre EP. Effectiveness of ropivacaine trigger points inactivation in the prophylactic management of patients with severe migraine. *Pain Med* 2007;8:65–70.

Garvey TA, Marks MR, Wiesel SW. A prospective, randomized, double-blind evaluation of trigger-point injection therapy for low-back pain. *Spine* 1989;14:962–964.

Gaspersic R, Koritnik B, Erzen I, Sketelj J. Muscle activity-resistant acetylcholine receptor accumulation is induced in places of former motor endplates in ectopically innervated regenerating rat muscles. *Int J Dev Neurosci* 2001;19:339–346.

Gerwin RD. A review of myofascial pain and fibromyalgia—factors that promote their persistence. *Acupunct Med* 2005;23:121–134.

Gerwin RD, Dommerholt J. Treatment of myofascial pain syndromes. In: Boswell MV, Cole BE, eds. *Weiner's Pain Management: A Practical Guide for Clinicians*. Boca Raton, FL: CRC Press; 2006:477–492.

Gerwin RD, Duranleau D. Ultrasound identification of the myofascial trigger point. *Muscle Nerve* 1997;20:767–768.

Gerwin RD, Shannon S, Hong CZ, Hubbard D, Gevirtz R. Interrater reliability in myofascial trigger point examination. *Pain* 1997;69:65–73.

Giamberardino MA, Tafuri E, Savini A, et al. Contributions of myofascial trigger points to migraine symptoms. *J Pain* 2007;8:869–878.

Graff-Radford B. Myofascial trigger points: their importance and diagnosis in the dental office. *J Dent Assoc S Afr* 1984;39:249–253.

Gunn CC. Radiculopathic pain: diagnosis, treatment of segmental irritation or sensitization. *J Musculoskeletal Pain* 1997a;5:119–134.

Gunn CC. *The Gunn Approach to the Treatment of Chronic Pain*. 2nd ed. New York: Churchill Livingstone; 1997b.

Gunn CC, Milbrandt WE. Utilizing trigger points. *Osteopathic Physician* 1977:29–52.

Gunn CC, Milbrandt WE, Little AS, Mason KE. Dry needling of muscle motor points for chronic low-back pain: a randomized clinical trial with long-term follow-up. *Spine* 1980;5:279–291.

Hameroff SR, Crago BR, Blitt CD, Womble J, Kanel J. Comparison of bupivacaine, etidocaine, and saline for trigger-point therapy. *Anesth Analg* 1981;60:752–755.

Han S, Lee K, Yeo J, et al. Effect of honey bee venom on microglial cells nitric oxide and tumor necrosis factor-alpha production stimulated by LPS. *J Ethnopharmacol* 2007;111:176–181.

Ho KY, Tan KH. Botulinum toxin A for myofascial trigger point injection: a qualitative systematic review. *Eur J Pain* 2007;11:519–527.

Hobbs V. Dry needling and acupuncture emerging professional issues. *Qi Unity Report* September/October 2007. Available at: http://www.aaaomonline.info/qiunity/07/10/2a.html.

Hong CZ. Myofascial trigger point injection. *Crit Rev Phys Med Rehabil* 1993;5:203–217.

Hong CZ. Lidocaine injection versus dry needling to myofascial trigger point. The importance of the local twitch response. *Am J Phys Med Rehabil* 1994a;73:256–263.

Hong CZ. Persistence of local twitch response with loss of conduction to and from the spinal cord. *Arch Phys Med Rehabil* 1994b;75:12–16.

Hong CZ. Myofascial trigger points: pathophysiology and correlation with acupuncture points. *Acupunct Med* 2000;18:41–47.

Hong CZ, Torigoe Y. Electrophysiological characteristics of localized twitch responses in responsive taut bands of rabbit skeletal muscle. *J Musculoskeletal Pain* 1994;2:17–43.

Hong CZ, Kuan TS, Chen JT, Chen SM. Referred pain elicited by palpation and by needling of myofascial trigger points: a comparison. *Arch Phys Med Rehabil* 1997;78:957–960.

Hsieh CY, Hong CZ, Adams AH, et al. Interexaminer reliability of the palpation of trigger points in the trunk and lower limb muscles. *Arch Phys Med Rehabil* 2000;81: 258–264.

Hsieh JC, Tu CH, Chen FP, et al. Activation of the hypothalamus characterizes the acupuncture stimulation at the analgesic point in human: a positron emission tomography study. *Neurosci Lett* 2001;307:105–108.

Hsieh YL, Kao MJ, Kuan TS, Chen SM, Chen JT, Hong CZ. Dry needling to a key myofascial trigger point may reduce the irritability of satellite MTrPs. *Am J Phys Med Rehabil* 2007;86:397–403.

Hui KK, Liu J, Makris N, et al. Acupuncture modulates the limbic system and subcortical gray structures of the human brain: evidence from fMRI studies in normal subjects. *Hum Brain Mapping* 2000;9:13–25.

Iwama H, Akama Y. The superiority of water-diluted 0.25% to near 1% lidocaine for trigger-point injections in myofascial pain syndrome: a prospective, randomized, double-blinded trial. *Anesth Analg* 2000;91:408–409.

Iwama H, Ohmori S, Kaneko T, Watanabe K. Water-diluted local anesthetic for trigger-point injection in chronic myofascial pain syndrome: evaluation of types of local anesthetic and concentrations in water. *Reg Anesth Pain Med* 2001;26:333–336.

Jaeger B, Skootsky SA. Double blind, controlled study of different myofascial trigger point injection techniques. *Pain* 1987;4:S292.

Kamanli A, Kaya A, Ardicoglu O, Ozgocmen S, Zengin FO, Bayik Y. Comparison of lidocaine injection, botulinum toxin injection, and dry needling to trigger points in myofascial pain syndrome. *Rheumatol Int* 2005;25:604–611.

Kim HW, Kwon YB, Ham TW, et al. Stimulation using bee venom attenuates formalin-induced pain behavior and spinal cord fos expression in rats. *J Vet Med Sci* 2003;65: 349–355.

Kim HW, Kwon YB, Han HJ, Yang IS, Beitz AJ, Lee JH. Antinociceptive mechanisms associated with diluted bee venom acupuncture (apipuncture) in the rat formalin test: involvement of descending adrenergic and serotonergic pathways. *Pharmacol Res* 2005;51:183–188.

Kuan TS, Hong CZ, Chen JT, Chen SM, Chien CH. The spinal cord connections of the myofascial trigger spots. *Eur J Pain* 2007a;11:624–634.

Kuan TS, Hsieh YL, Chen SM, Chen JT, Yen WC, Hong CZ. The myofascial trigger point region: correlation between the degree of irritability and the prevalence of endplate noise. *Am J Phys Med Rehabil* 2007b;86:183–189.

Kwon YB, Kim JH, Yoon JH, et al. The analgesic efficacy of bee venom acupuncture for knee osteoarthritis: a comparative study with needle acupuncture. *Am J Chin Med* 2001a;29: 187–199.

Kwon YB, Lee JD, Lee HJ, et al. Bee venom injection into an acupuncture point reduces arthritis associated edema and nociceptive responses. *Pain* 2001b;90:271–280.

Lange F, Eversbusch G. Die Bedeutung der Muskelhärten für die allgemeine Praxis. *Münch Med Wochenschr* 1921;68: 418–420.

Lange M. *Muskelhärten (Myogelosen)*. Munich: J.F. Lehmann's Verlag; 1931.

Langevin HM, Churchill DL, Cipolla MJ. Mechanical signaling through connective tissue: a mechanism for the therapeutic effect of acupuncture. *FASEB J* 2001;15:2275–2282.

Langevin HM, Bouffard NA, Badger GJ, Iatridis JC, Howe AK. Dynamic fibroblast cytoskeletal response to subcutaneous tissue stretch ex vivo and in vivo. *Am J Physiol Cell Physiol* 2005;288:C747–C756.

Langevin HM, Bouffard NA, Badger GJ, Churchill DL, Howe A. Subcutaneous tissue fibroblast cytoskeletal remodeling induced by acupuncture: evidence for a mechanotransduction-based mechanism. *J Cell Physiol* 2006a;207:767–774.

Langevin HM, Storch KN, Cipolla MJ, White SL, Buttolph TR, Taatjes DJ. Fibroblast spreading induced by connective tissue stretch involves intracellular redistribution of alpha- and beta-actin. *Histochem Cell Biol* 2006b;125: 487–495.

Lee JD, Park HJ, Chae Y, Lim S. An overview of bee venom acupuncture in the treatment of arthritis. *Evid Based Complement Alternat Med* 2005a;2:79–84.

Lee JY, Kang SS, Kim JH, Bae CS, Choi SH. Inhibitory effect of whole bee venom in adjuvant-induced arthritis. *In Vivo* 2005b;19:801–805.

Lewit K. The needle effect in the relief of myofascial pain. *Pain* 1979;6:83–90.

Liboff AR. Bioelectromagnetic fields and acupuncture. *J Altern Complement Med* 1997;3(suppl 1):S77–S87.

Linde K, Streng A, Jurgens S, et al. Acupuncture for patients with migraine: a randomized controlled trial. *JAMA* 2005;293:2118–2125.

Ling FW, Slocumb JC. Use of trigger point injections in chronic pelvic pain. *Obstet Gynecol Clin North Am* 1993;20:809–815.

Lund I, Lundeberg T. Are minimal, superficial or sham acupuncture procedures acceptable as inert placebo controls? *Acupunct Med* 2006;24:13–15.

Lundeberg T, Stener-Victorin E. Is there a physiological basis for the use of acupuncture in pain? *Int Congress Series* 2002;1238:3–10.

Lundeberg T, Uvnas-Moberg K, Agren G, Bruzelius G. Antinociceptive effects of oxytocin in rats and mice. *Neurosci Lett* 1994;170:153–157.

Ma YT, Ma M, Cho ZH. *Biomedical Acupuncture for Pain Management: An Integrative Approach*. St. Louis: Elsevier; 2005.

Macgregor J, Graf von Schweinitz D. Needle electromyographic activity of myofascial trigger points and control sites in equine cleidobrachialis muscle: an observational study. *Acupunct Med* 2006;24:61–70.

Mayoral del Moral O. Fisioterapia invasiva del síndrome de dolor miofascial. *Fisioterapia* 2005;27:69–75.

Mayoral O, Torres R. Tratamiento conservador y fisioterápico invasivo de los puntos gatillo miofasciales. In: *Patología de partes blandas en el hombro*. Madrid: Fundación MAPFRE Medicina; 2003.

McGee L, Herbkersman M. Letter: To whom it may concern. Unpublished manuscript, Sacramento; 2007.

McMillan AS, Blasberg B. Pain-pressure threshold in painful jaw muscles following trigger point injection. *J Orofacial Pain* 1994;8:384–390.

Melchart D, Streng A, Hoppe A, et al. Acupuncture in patients with tension-type headache: randomised controlled trial. *BMJ* 2005;331:376–382.

Melzack R. Myofascial trigger points: relation to acupuncture and mechanisms of pain. *Arch Phys Med Rehabil* 1981;62:114–117.

Melzack R, Stillwell DM, Fox EJ. Trigger points and acupuncture points for pain: correlations and implications. *Pain* 1977;3:3–23.

Menezes C, Rodrigues B, Magalhaes E, Melo A. Botulinum toxin type A in refractory chronic migraine: an open-label trial. *Arq Neuropsiquiatr* 2007;65:596–598.

Mense S. Pathophysiologic basis of muscle pain syndromes. In: Fischer AA, ed. *Myofascial Pain: Update in Diagnosis and Treatment*. Philadelphia: WB Saunders; 1997:23–53.

Mense S, Simons DG, Hoheisel U, Quenzer B. Lesions of rat skeletal muscle after local block of acetylcholinesterase and neuromuscular stimulation. *J Appl Physiol* 2003;94:2494–2501.

Millan MJ. The induction of pain: an integrative review. *Prog Neurobiol* 1999;57:1–164.

Mohr C, Binkofski F, Erdman C, Buchel C, Helmchen C. The anterior cingulate cortex contains distinct areas dissociating external from self-administered painful stimulation: a parametric fMRI study. *Pain* 2005;114:347–357.

Müller W, Stratz T. Local treatment of tendinopathies and myofascial pain syndromes with the 5-HT3 receptor antagonist tropisetron. *Scand J Rheumatol Suppl* 2004;119:44–48.

New Mexico Board of Acupuncture and Oriental Medicine. New Mexico Administrative Code, Title16, Occupational and Professional Licensing; Chapter 2, Acupuncture and Oriental Medicine Practitioners; 1996.

New Mexico Board of Acupuncture and Oriental Medicine. New Mexico Statutes Annotated, Chapter 61, Professional and Occupational Licenses; Article 14A, Acupuncture and Oriental Medicine Practice; §3, Definitions; 1978.

Niddam DM, Chan RC, Lee SH, Yeh TC, Hsieh JC. Central modulation of pain evoked from myofascial trigger point. *Clin J Pain* 2007;23:440–448.

Niddam DM, Chan RC, Lee SH, Yeh TC, Hsieh JC. Central representations of hyperalgesia from myofascial trigger point. *Neuroimage* 2008;39:1299–1306.

Noë A. *Action in Perception*. Cambridge: MIT Press; 2004.

Olausson H, Lamarre Y, Backlund H, et al. Unmyelinated tactile afferents signal touch and project to insular cortex. *Nature Neurosci* 2002;5:900–904.

Osler W. *The Principles and Practice of Medicine*. New York: Appleton; 1912.

Padamsee M, Mehta N, White GE. Trigger point injection: a neglected modality in the treatment of TMJ dysfunction. *J Pedod* 1987;12:72–92.

Peets JM, Pomeranz B. CXBK mice deficient in opiate receptors show poor electroacupuncture analgesia. *Nature* 1978;273:675–676.

Peng PW, Castano ED. Survey of chronic pain practice by anesthesiologists in Canada. *Can J Anaesth* 2005;52:383–389.

Rodriguez-Acosta A, Pena L, Finol HJ, Pulido-Mendez M. Cellular and subcellular changes in muscle, neuromuscular junctions and nerves caused by bee (*Apis mellifera*) venom. *J Submicrosc Cytol Pathol* 2004;36:91–96.

Sadeh M, Stern LZ, Czyzewski K. Changes in end-plate cholinesterase and axons during muscle degeneration and regeneration. *J Anat* 1985;140:165–176.

Sandkühler J. The organization and function of endogenous antinociceptive systems. *Prog Neurobiol* 1996;50:49–81.

Saunders S, Longworth S. *Injection Techniques in Orthopaedics and Sports Medicine: A Practical Manual for Doctors and Physiotherapists*. 3rd ed. Edinburgh: Churchill Livingstone; 2006.

Scharf HP, Mansmann U, Streitberger K, et al. Acupuncture and knee osteoarthritis: a three-armed randomized trial. *Ann Intern Med* 2006;145:12–20.

Sciotti VM, Mittak VL, DiMarco L, et al. Clinical precision of myofascial trigger point location in the trapezius muscle. *Pain* 2001;93:259–266.

Seem M. *A New American Acupuncture: Acupuncture Osteopathy*. Boulder, CO: Blue Poppy Press; 2007.

Shah JP, Phillips TM, Danoff JV, Gerber LH. An in-vivo microanalytical technique for measuring the local biochemical milieu of human skeletal muscle. *J Appl Physiol* 2005;99:1980–1987.

Shah JP, Danoff JV, Desai MJ, et al. Biochemicals associated with pain and inflammation are elevated in sites near to and remote from active myofascial trigger points. *Arch Phys Med Rehabil* 2008;89:16–23.

Simons DG. Do endplate noise and spikes arise from normal motor endplates? *Am J Phys Med Rehabil* 2001;80:134–140.

Simons DG. Review of enigmatic MTrPs as a common cause of enigmatic musculoskeletal pain and dysfunction. *J Electromyogr Kinesiol* 2004;14:95–107.

Simons DG, Dommerholt J. Myofascial pain syndrome—trigger points. *J Musculoskeletal Pain* 2007;15(1):63–79.

Simons DG, Travell JG, Simons LS. *Travell and Simons' Myofascial Pain and Dysfunction: The Trigger Point Manual*. Vol. 1. 2nd ed. Baltimore: Williams & Wilkins; 1999.

Simons DG, Hong CZ, Simons LS. Endplate potentials are common to midfiber myofascial trigger points. *Am J Phys Med Rehabil* 2002;81:212–222.

Son DJ, Kang J, Kim TJ, et al. Melittin, a major bioactive component of bee venom toxin, inhibits PDGF receptor beta-tyrosine phosphorylation and downstream intracellular signal transduction in rat aortic vascular smooth muscle cells. *J Toxicol Environ Health* 2007a;70:1350–1355.

Son DJ, Lee JW, Lee YH, Song HS, Lee CK, Hong JT. Therapeutic application of anti-arthritis, pain-releasing, and anti-cancer effects of bee venom and its constituent compounds. *Pharmacol Ther* 2007b;115:246–270.

Steinbrocker O. Therapeutic injections in painful musculoskeletal disorders. *JAMA* 1944;125:397–401.

Stienstra R, Jonker TA, Bourdrez P, Kuijpers JC, van Kleef JW, Lundberg U. Ropivacaine 0.25% versus bupivacaine 0.25% for continuous epidural analgesia in labor: a double-blind comparison. *Anesth Analg* 1995;80:285–289.

Stockman R. The causes, pathology, and treatment of chronic rheumatism. *Edinburgh Med J* 1904;15:107–116.

Strauss H. Ueber die sogenannten "rheumatische Muskelschwiele." *Klin Wochenschr* 1898;35:121–123.

Svensson P, Minoshima S, Beydoun A, Morrow TJ, Casey K. Cerebral processing of acute skin and muscle pain in humans. *J Neurophysiol* 1997;78:450–460.

Takeshige C, Tsuchiya M, Zhao W, Guo S. Analgesia produced by pituitary ACTH and dopaminergic transmission in the arcuate. *Brain Res Bull* 1991;26:779–788.

Takeshige C, Kobori M, Hishida F, Luo CP, Usami S. Analgesia inhibitory system involvement in nonacupuncture point-stimulation-produced analgesia. *Brain Res Bull* 1992a;28:379–391.

Takeshige C, Sato T, Mera T, Hisamitsu T, Fang J. Descending pain inhibitory system involved in acupuncture analgesia. *Brain Res Bull* 1992b;29:617–634.

Teravainen H. Satellite cells of striated muscle after compression injury so slight as not to cause degeneration of the muscle fibres. *Z Zellforsch Mikrosk Anat* 1970;103:320–327.

Travell J. Basis for the multiple uses of local block of somatic trigger areas (procaine infiltration and ethyl chloride spray). *Miss Valley Med* 1949;71:13–22.

Travell J, Bobb AL. Mechanism of relief of pain in sprains by local injection techniques. *Fed Proc* 1947;6:378.

Travell JG, Rinzler S, Herman M. Pain and disability of the shoulder and arm: treatment by intramuscular infiltration with procaine hydrochloride. *JAMA* 1942;120:417–422.

Tschopp KP, Gysin C. Local injection therapy in 107 patients with myofascial pain syndrome of the head and neck. *ORL* 1996;58:306–310.

Tuttle AA, Katz JA, Bridenbaugh PO, Quinlan R, Knarr D. A double-blind comparison of the abdominal wall relaxation produced by epidural 0.75% ropivacaine and 0.75% bupivacaine in gynecologic surgery. *Reg Anesth* 1995;20:515–520.

Uchida S, Kagitani F, Suzuki A, Aikawa Y. Effect of acupuncture-like stimulation on cortical cerebral blood flow in anesthetized rats. *J Physiol* 2000;50:495–507.

Uvnas-Moberg K, Bruzelius G, Alster P, Lundeberg T. The antinociceptive effect of non-noxious sensory stimulation is mediated partly through oxytocinergic mechanisms. *Acta Physiol Scand* 1993;149:199–204.

Van Kleef JW, Veering BT, Burm AG. Spinal anesthesia with ropivacaine: a double-blind study on the efficacy and safety of 0.5% and 0.75% solutions in patients undergoing minor lower limb surgery. *Anesth Analg* 1994;78:1125–1130.

Vecchiet L, Giamberardino MA, Dragani L. Latent myofascial trigger points: changes in muscular and subcutaneous pain thresholds at trigger point and target level. *J Manual Medicine* 1990;5:151–154.

Vecchiet L, Giamberardino M, de Bigontina P. Comparative sensory evaluation of parietal tissues in painful and nonpainful areas in fibromyalgia and myofascial pain syndrome. In: Gebhart GF, Hammond DL, Jensen TS, eds. *Proceedings of the 7th World Congress on Pain: Progress in Pain Research and Management.* Vol. 2. Seattle: IASP Press; 1994:177–185.

Vecchiet L, Pizzigallo E, Iezzi S, Affaitati G, Vecchiet J, Giamberardino MA. Differentiation of sensitivity in different tissues and its clinical significance. *J Musculoskeletal Pain* 1998;6(1):33–45.

Virginia Board of Physical Therapy Task Force on Dry Needling. Meeting minutes. Richmond, VA; March 30, 2007.

Wall PD, Woolf CJ. Muscle but not cutaneous C-afferent input produces prolonged increases in the excitability of the flexion reflex in the rat. *J Physiol* 1984;356:443–458.

Wang L, Zhang Y, Dai J, Yang J, Gang S. Electroacupuncture (EA) modulates the expression of NMDA receptors in primary sensory neurons in relation to hyperalgesia in rats. *Brain Res* 2006;1120:46–53.

White PF, Crai WF, Vakharia AS, Ghoname E, Ahmed HE, Hamza MA. Percutaneous neuromodulation therapy: does the location of electrical stimulation effect the acute analgesic response? *Anesth Analg* 2000;91:949–954.

Wu MT, Hsieh JC, Xiong J, et al. Central nervous pathway for acupuncture stimulation: localization of processing with functional MR imaging of the brain–preliminary experience. *Radiology* 1999;212:133–141.

Wu MT, Sheen JM, Chuang KH, et al. Neuronal specificity of acupuncture response: a fMRI study with electroacupuncture. *Neuroimage* 2002;16:1028–1037.

Yoon SY, Kim HW, Roh DH, et al. The anti-inflammatory effect of peripheral bee venom stimulation is mediated by central muscarinic type 2 receptors and activation of sympathetic preganglionic neurons. *Brain Res* 2005;1049:210–216.

Zaralidou AT, Amaniti EN, Maidatsi PG, Gorgias N, Vasilakos D. Comparison between newer local anesthetics for myofascial pain syndrome management. *Methods Find Exp Clin Pharmacol* 2007;29:353–357.

Conservative Management of Tension-Type and Cervicogenic Headache

Cervical Joint Mobilization Techniques in Patients with Headache

Pieter Westerhuis, PT, OMT, SVOMP

As more and more information about a patient's impairment is gathered during the physical examination, the initial hypothesis (that there is a cervical component to the patient's headache) should be strengthened, confirmed, modified, or replaced. Based on the outcome, an initial treatment strategy will be developed. According to Maitland et al. (2005), the clinical proof that the outcome hypothesis is correct is if after appropriate treatment the reassessment or reevaluation of the comparable movements shows clinically relevant change. This would be further strengthened if the patient describes on the subsequent visit that his or her functioning in daily life has improved. The International Headache Society (2004) has also stated that one of the criteria that needs to be fulfilled for the diagnosis of cervicogenic headache is that there is an improvement of the symptoms after appropriate treatment of the underlying dysfunction. The continuing examination and assessment of the dysfunction of the headache patient on subsequent visits will be guided by the reassessment after the initial treatment.

The management plan (**Table 22.1**) should incorporate all biopsychosocial components of the patient's problem (Chapter 13) (Westerhuis & Von Piekartz, 2001; Gifford, 2002; Butler & Moseley, 2003). When planning treatment, the therapist will need to analyze individual findings and prioritize them. In some patients, postural issues may need to be addressed first, whereas in other patients it may be

Table 22.1 Management or Treatment Plan

1. Overall treatment aspects:
   A. Explanation
   B. Further diagnostic testing necessary
   C. Referral back to the doctor
   D. Postural advice
   E. Ergonomics
   F. Advice about sleeping habits (Diamond & Freitag, 1988)
   G. Intake of medication (Edmeads, 1990)
   H. Dietary restrictions (Diamond & Freitag, 1988)
   I. Overall fitness/endurance, etc.
2. Muscular reeducation (Chapter 12)
3. Neurodynamic mobilization (Chapter 30)
4. Joint mobilization (Grant & Niere, 2000; Biondi, 2005)
   A. Symptomatic joint
   B. Predisposing joints
   C. Direct techniques
   D. Indirect techniques
5. Home program

necessary to initially mobilize stiff motion segments. In most patients, it is essential to use a multidimensional approach incorporating all aspects.

Gross et al. (2002) conducted a systematic literature review regarding the effectiveness of manipulative physiotherapy on mechanical neck disorders. From this they drew the following conclusions:

- There is inconclusive evidence to support or refute the use of manipulation or mobilization alone in the management of patients with neck disorders.
- There seems to be some indication that when used in combination, the results favor this intervention. Therefore, the clinician should try to incorporate passive treatment within a multimodal management strategy.
- The best combination element seems to be exercise.
- A single session of spinal manipulation is not recommended. Nevertheless, it is unclear how many sessions of manipulation achieve the best benefit.

These findings agree with those previously found by Hurwitz et al. (1996). A review of spinal manual therapy in cervicogenic headache concluded that spinal manipulation showed strong evidence of effectiveness for reducing headache intensity, headache duration, and medication intake (Fernández-de-las-Peñas et al., 2005).

One of the best studies on cervicogenic headache was conducted by Jull et al. (2002), who showed that passive mobilization of the appropriate joint dysfunctions and muscle reeducation of the deep cervical flexors is beneficial in the management of cervicogenic headache.

Because the neural component (Chapter 29) and the muscle control aspect (Chapter 12) are covered in other chapters of the present book, this chapter limits itself to the joint mobilization component of the management plan.

SELECTION OF TECHNIQUE

Intensity of the Mobilization Procedure

When selecting the technique, the therapist has to make the following important decisions: (a) to what degree it is allowed to produce or reproduce the patient's symptoms, and (b) to what degree it is necessary to mobilize into resistance. Part of the answer to these two questions comes from analysis of the movement diagrams of the comparable movements. For example, if the movement diagram is pain dominant (Figure 14.25 in Chapter 14), the therapist does not need to move beyond the first onset of resistance, and there should not be any production of discomfort. The patient would be positioned in the most comfortable pain-free position, and the therapist would perform very gentle oscillatory mobilizations at the beginning of the range of joint motion (e.g., treatment technique of side flexion with a pillow, **Figure 22.1**) without pain.

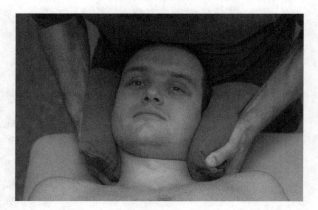

Figure 22.1 Treatment Technique: Side Flexion Grade II with a Pillow

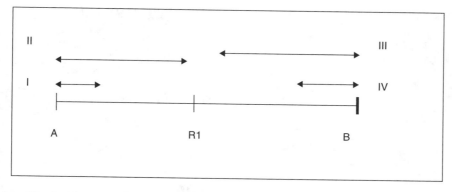

Figure 22.2 Grades of Passive Movement for Mobilization Procedures

If the movement diagram is resistance dominant (Figure 14.24), the therapist should move beyond the first onset of resistance. If there is only a minimal amount of pain at the limit, one should reproduce pain in an "on-off" oscillatory way.

Maitland usually performs treatment techniques in an oscillatory manner (Maitland et al., 2005). These oscillations can be performed with different amplitudes in different positions in the range of movement. He has described four different standard oscillatory grades of movement, which can be graphically depicted as shown in **Figure 22.2**.

The mobilizations with grades I and II are usually used in dysfunctions that are pain dominant, whereas grades III and IV are usually done in impairments that are resistance dominant. If the pain at the end of range is strong, the therapist would not want to produce discomfort (grades III and IV).

Direct Versus Indirect

As far as the technique is concerned, a division between direct and indirect techniques could be made. With direct techniques, the mobilizing fingers or thumbs of the therapist are in contact with the area he or she wants to mobilize (e.g., passive accessory intervertebral movement [PAIVM], as described in Chapter 14). With indirect techniques, the mobilizing part of the therapist's hand is not in direct contact. Examples of indirect techniques are cervical side flexion (Figures 22.3 to 22.5) and cervical rotation (Figures 22.6 and 22.7).

Direct techniques are hypothesized to have a more localized effect. A big advantage of the indirect techniques is that they are usually physiologic movements and are therefore more functional. Further, they will also stretch other polyarticular structures, such as mus-

cles, tendons, or the nervous system, which may be more efficacious.

In some patients the local tissue is very sensitive to local pressure. In these cases indirect techniques may be more appropriate. Other patients may have difficulty with relaxing. In these cases it may be more appropriate to use PAIVMs. In many cases, the therapist will use a combination of both direct and indirect techniques.

Local Versus Remote

The therapist should not restrict himself or herself to only mobilizing the symptomatic joint. Quite commonly, dysfunctions in neighboring regions are contributing to perpetuation of the symptomatic dysfunction. These regions would have to be examined and treated appropriately on subsequent visits. It has also been shown that mobilizing the joint dysfunctions of the thoracic spine may be beneficial in neck pain (Cleland et al., 2005). It may therefore be useful in very painful upper cervical spine impairments to initially treat the upper thoracic spine, because this may decrease upper cervical sensitivity (Chapter 24).

CERVICAL JOINT MOBILIZATION PROCEDURES FOR HEADACHE PATIENTS

This section describes the most frequently used mobilization techniques in the management of cervicogenic headache patients (Grant & Niere, 2000; Biondi, 2005).

Cervical Mobilization in Side Flexion Toward the Left

The patient lies supine facing the left side of the plinth with his or her head well over the edge. The therapist's

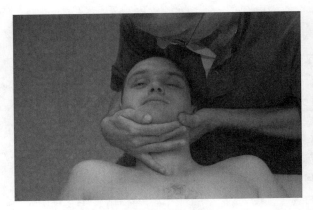

Figure 22.3 Manual Contact for the Cervical Mobilization in Side Flexion

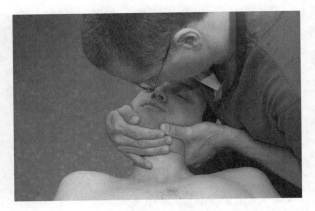

Figure 22.5 Cervical Mobilization in Side Flexion Toward the Left

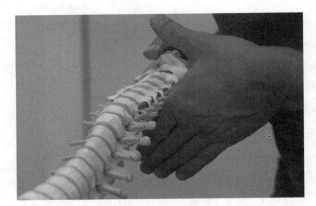

Figure 22.4 Joint Contact for the Cervical Mobilization in Side Flexion

right lower arm cradles the patient's head (**Figure 22.3**). His or her elbow lies behind the patient's ear. The thrusting knuckle of the therapist's left hand lies posterolaterally against the articular pillar of the segment he or she wants to mobilize (**Figure 22.4**). The segment is placed in the midposition between flexion and extension. Subsequently, the therapist performs a slight displacement of the head toward the right while at the same time side-flexing to the left at the level required (**Figure 22.5**).

If the patient has a very *pain-dominant closing-down dysfunction* on the right side (extension more painful than flexion; side flexion and rotation toward the right more painful than toward the left), the initial treatment should be side flexion toward the left. It may even be necessary to initially perform the technique in a flexed position. As the symptoms decrease, a possible progression could be as follows:

1. In some cervical flexion, apply side flexion to the left, grade II.
2. In some cervical flexion, apply side flexion to the left, grade III.
3. In neutral cervical position, apply side flexion to the left, grade III.
4. In some cervical flexion, apply side flexion to the right, grade II.
5. In neutral cervical position, apply side flexion to the right, grade II.
6. In neutral cervical position, apply side flexion to the right, grade III.
7. In neutral cervical position, apply side flexion to the right, grade IV.
8. In some cervical extension, apply side flexion to the right, grade IV.

As is the case with most techniques, this one has some advantages and disadvantages.

Advantages

- The technique can be localized better toward one segment.
- There is less stress on the vertebral artery.
- There is less stress on the vestibular organ.
- There is more mobilizing effect on the nervous system.

Disadvantages

- There is stressful closing down on the ipsilateral side.
- There is more lengthening stress on the nervous system.

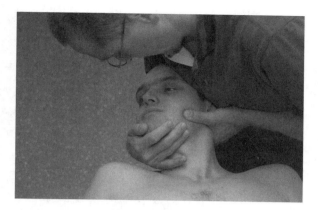

Figure 22.6 Manual Contact for the Cervical Mobilization in Rotation

- Although side-flexion mobilization will result in an increase of rotation, there is less stretching on the muscles that may be secondarily shortened with a rotation restriction.

Cervical Mobilization in Rotation Toward the Left

The patient lies supine facing the left side of the plinth with his or her head well over the edge. The therapist's right lower arm cradles the patient's head. His or her elbow lies behind the patient's ear (**Figure 22.6**). The left hand grasps around the occiput bone. The segment is placed in the midposition between flexion and extension. The therapist rotates the neck like a chicken on a spit by moving simultaneously with both arms. The left hand pulls cranially with an elevation of the left shoulder girdle, whereas the right elbow moves anteriorly to the therapist's body. The further into rotation the mobilization is performed, the more the therapist has to turn his or her body parallel to the longitudinal axis (**Figure 22.7**).

In some patients who are very pain sensitive to contact, it may be necessary to perform the technique with the patient's head on a soft, pliable pillow. The therapist folds the pillow like a collar around the cervical spine and rotates with the pillow. Another important variation is in those cases where it is important to be more localized. The therapist may grasp with the left hand around the spinous process and laminae of the cranial vertebra of the segment he or she wants to mobilize. Finally, the same type of progression as described with side flexion may be used.

Again, there are some advantages and disadvantages of the rotation mobilization technique.

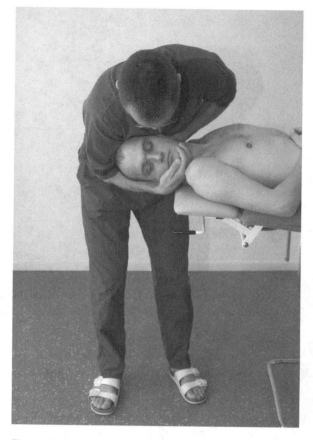

Figure 22.7 Cervical Mobilization in Rotation Toward the Left

Advantages

- There is less stressful closing down on the opposite side.
- There is less stress on the nervous system.
- There is more range of motion with rotation than with side flexion.
- Rotation is functionally more important than side flexion.

Disadvantages

- There will always be mobilizing stress on the caudal segments.
- There is more stress on the vertebral artery.
- There is more stress on the vestibular organ.

Therefore, depending upon the individual patient's dysfunction, the therapist should make a conscious decision regarding which technique is most appropriate.

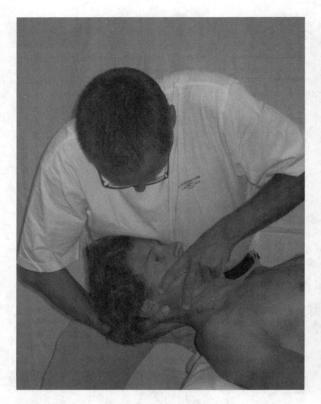

Figure 22.8 Upper Cervical Flexion Mobilization

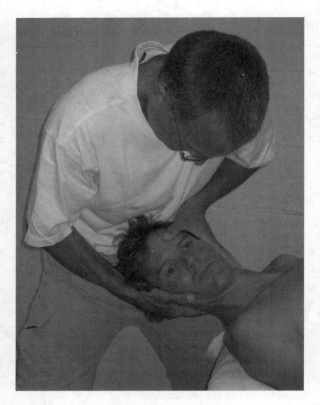

Figure 22.9 Cervical Mobilization in Side Flexion Toward the Left with 30° Rotation Toward the Right

Upper Cervical Flexion Mobilization

In those patients who have a hypomobility of upper cervical flexion (perhaps in combination with short suboccipital muscles), the following technique may be useful. The patient lies supine facing the left side of the plinth with his or her head well over the edge (**Figure 22.8**). The therapist stands on the left side of the patient's head. The therapist's right hand grasps around the occipital bone. The head is cradled in his or her right lower arm. The web space of the left hand grasps around the maxillary bone. By pulling with the right hand in a cranial direction and pushing with the left hand in an anterior-posterior cranial direction, an upper cervical flexion mobilization is induced. To emphasize one side, the neck may be prepositioned in some side flexion.

Cervical Mobilization in Side Flexion Toward the Left with 30° Rotation Toward the Right

The goal of this technique is to "open up" the right C2-C3 joint. For that purpose, the patient lies supine facing

the left side of the plinth with his or her head well over the edge (**Figure 22.9**). The therapist stands on the left side of the patient's head. The therapist's right hand grasps around the occipital bone. The head is rotated approximately 30° toward the right. The therapist places his or her left hand with the metacarpophalangeal joints on the left zygomatic arch. In this position the therapist performs a left side-flexion movement of "head on neck" by using his or her left hand as a fulcrum. This movement should normally create a stretching sensation on the opposite side.

Anterior-Posterior Mobilization of the Thoracic Spine (T2-T3 Segment) Through the Sternum in Extension

This technique is especially useful in those patients who have an exaggerated upper thoracic kyphosis and have stiffness in extension of this region. The patient lies supine with the spinous process of T3 at the edge and T2 over the edge of the plinth, and his or her left hand lying on the sternum (**Figure 22.10**). The therapist cradles the

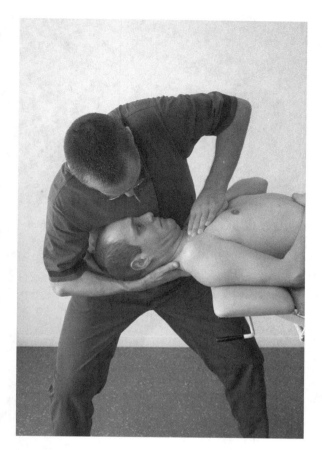

Figure 22.10 Anterior-Posterior Mobilization of the Thoracic Spine (T2-T3 Segment) Through the Sternum in Extension

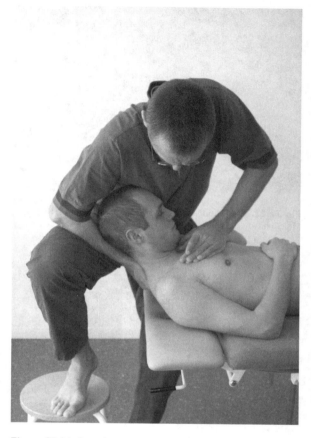

Figure 22.11 Anterior-Posterior Mobilization of the Thoracic Spine (T2-T3 Segment) Through the Sternum in Flexion

patient's head and neck with his or her right arm, and places his or her left hand on the hand of the patient that lies on the sternum. The whole head and neck is moved into extension upon the upper thoracic spine. With the left hand, the therapist reinforces the anterior-posterior movement through the sternum in a slightly cranially angulated direction.

Anterior-Posterior Mobilization of the Thoracic Spine (T2-T3 Segment) Through the Sternum in Flexion

This technique is especially useful in those patients who have a flattened upper thoracic kyphosis and have stiffness in flexion of this region. The patient lies supine with the spinous process of T3 at the edge and T2 over the edge of the plinth, and his or her hand lying on the sternum (**Figure 22.11**). The therapist cradles the pa-

tient's head and neck with his or her right arm, and places his or her left hand on the hand of the patient that lies on the sternum. The whole head and neck is moved into flexion upon the upper thoracic spine with the right arm. The therapist's right foot may be placed upon a chair. This enables the therapist to facilitate this flexion movement with his or her right knee; otherwise, the movement may be fatiguing for the elbow flexors. Simultaneous with the flexion movement, the therapist pushes with the left hand in an anterior-posterior direction with a slight cranial angulation. This creates a fulcrum around which the flexion occurs.

Lateral Glide Mobilization Toward the Left of the Midcervical Spine

The cervical lateral glide mobilization has been extensively studied in relation to its effect on neurodynamic

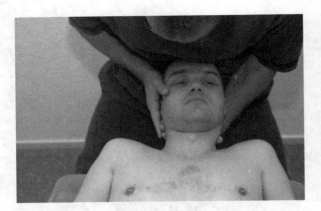

Figure 22.12 Manual Contact for the Lateral Glide Mobilization

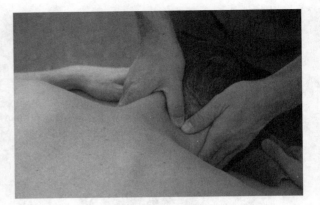

Figure 22.14 Unilateral Posterior-Anterior Mobilization of C2 Vertebra

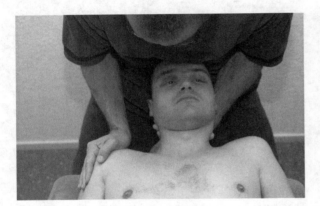

Figure 22.13 Lateral Glide Mobilization Toward the Left of the Midcervical Spine

dysfunction. Nevertheless, if a patient with headache shows a restriction in this movement in the midcervical spine, the technique may also be clinically useful. For that purpose, the patient lies supine with the head positioned just beyond the edge of the bed. The therapist holds the patient's head with his or her left hand and supports it with his or her abdomen. The patient's hands are rested on the abdomen (**Figure 22.12**).

The therapist stands behind the patient. The left hand holds C4 from dorsal. The left index finger is placed on the right side of the patient's neck. The right hand is at the side of the neck as far down as the C4 segment (**Figure 22.13**). The clinician needs to take care not to apply pressure on the spinal nerves. By transferring his or her weight toward the left leg, the therapist moves his or her upper body, and with it the patient's head,

sideways to the left. This transverse movement should be performed slowly, with large amplitude. As symptoms decrease, a possible progression could be as follows:

1. Initially the movement should stop before any resistance is felt.
2. To increase the intensity, one might then decide to move into resistance. To control the elevation of the right shoulder of the patient, the therapist can put his or her right hand onto the acromion of the patient.
3. A further increase in intensity of the technique can be achieved by positioning the right arm of the patient in elbow extension and slight abduction of the shoulder.

Unilateral Posterior-Anterior Mobilization of C2 Vertebra

Every PAIVM that is painful or restricted may be used as a mobilization technique. For instance, if the unilateral posterior-anterior movement of C2 vertebra is restricted, the therapist could adapt the grade of the technique appropriately to the impairment and mobilize with exactly the same grip (**Figure 22.14**). Further, with the differentiation maneuvers (Figures 14.28 to 14.30 in Chapter 14) that implicate the C1-C2 zygapophysial joint, it would be possible to progress the technique by placing the joint in slight ipsilateral rotation. If the differentiation wants to implicate the C2-C3 zygapophysial joint, it would be more appropriate to progress the technique by angulating in a more medial direction.

TREATMENT OF THE CASE REPORT FROM CHAPTER 14

Because the physical examination of this headache patient revealed an involvement of the upper cervical segments, a treatment plan aimed at restoring the joints' function was planned as follows. In the first session, the patient was treated with cervical side-flexion mobilization toward the right. In the second session, the temporomandibular joint was examined, and revealed to have no comparable joint impairment. The side-flexion mobilization was repeated, but it was done in some cervical flexion. Also, the patient was shown a home exercise to improve upper cervical side flexion toward the right. In the third session, the cervicothoracic region was screened and the graded craniocervical flexion test was evaluated. The chin-tuck exercise was taught as a home exercise. This patient continued to improve with joint mobilizations to improve the opening of the left upper cervical segments and specific training of the deep cervical neck flexors. In later sessions, other aspects, such as the patient's working position behind the computer and stress management, were also addressed.

REFERENCES

Biondi DM. Cervicogenic headache: a review of diagnostic and treatment strategies. *J Am Osteopath Assoc* 2005;100(9 suppl):S7–14.

Butler D, Moseley GL. *Explain Pain*. Adelaide, Australia: NOI Group Publications; 2003.

Cleland JA, Childs JD, McRae M, Palmer JA, Stowell T. Immediate effects of thoracic manipulation in patients with neck pain: a randomized clinical trial. *Man Ther* 2005;10:127–135.

Diamond S, Freitag FG. The mixed headache syndrome. *Clin J Pain* 1988;4:67–74.

Edmeads J. Analgesic-induced headache: an un-recognized epidemic. *Headache* 1990;30:614–615.

Fernández-de-las-Peñas C, Alonso-Blanco C, Cuadrado ML, Pareja JA. Spinal manipulative therapy in the management of cervicogenic headache. *Headache* 2005;45:1260–1263.

Gifford L, ed. *Topical Issues in Pain 3*. Falmouth, England: CNS Press; 2002.

Grant T, Niere K. Techniques used by manipulative physiotherapists in the management of headaches. *Aust J Physiother* 2000;46:215–222.

Gross AR, Kay TM, Kennedy C, et al. Clinical practise guidelines on the use of manipulation or mobilization in the treatment of adults with mechanical neck disorders. *Man Ther* 2002;7:193–205.

Hurwitz EL, Aker PD Adams AH, Meeker WC, Shekelle PG. Manipulation and mobilisation of the cervical spine: a systematic review of the literature. *Spine* 1996;21:1746–1760.

International Headache Society. The International Classification of Headache Disorders: 2nd edition. *Cephalalgia* 2004;24(suppl):9–160.

Jull G, Trott P, Potter H, et al. A randomized controlled trial of exercise and manipulative therapy for cervicogenic headache. *Spine* 2002;27:1835–1843.

Maitland GD, Hengeveld E, Banks K, English K. *Maitland's Vertebral Manipulation*. 7th ed. Oxford, England: Elsevier Butterworth-Heinemann; 2005.

Westerhuis P, Von Piekartz HJM. Zervikogener Kopfschmerz: Körperliche Untersuchung und Behandlung. In: Von Piekartz HJM, ed. *Kraniofaziale Dysfunktionen und Schmerzen*. Stuttgart, Germany: Thieme; 2001:99–113.

Cervical Joint Manipulation Procedures Applied to Patients with Headache

Christian Fossum, DO, and Gary Fryer, PhD, BSc (Osteopathy), ND

BASIC CONCEPTS

Manual treatment of the cervical region for patients with headaches has been performed by the osteopathic profession since the late 19th century (Barber, 1898). Since then, there has been increasing awareness and use of manual medicine approaches for a number of health problems and by practitioners from many disciplines (Haldeman, 2004; Cook, 2007; Seffinger & Hruby, 2007). As a nonpharmacologic treatment modality, manual therapy has become a popular choice for patients with common and benign forms of headaches, such as cervicogenic headache (CeH) and tension-type headaches (TTH). Because these two conditions are often associated with mechanical neck pain, they are commonly seen by clinicians who treat the spine, rather than those who treat headache (Haldeman & Dagenais, 2001). High-velocity, low-amplitude thrust (HVLA) techniques can be very useful in the treatment of musculoskeletal structures and mechanical pain in the axial spine, pelvis, and extremities. In the cervical region, HVLA procedures are commonly used in the management of patients presenting with cervicothoracic pain, neck pain, and certain types of primary headaches, such as CeH and TTH.

It is theorized that HVLA techniques act on the deeper somatic structures, such as the joint complex with its capsuloligamentous structures, connective tissues, and deep paraspinal muscles (Triano, 2000, 2001, 2003; Evans, 2002: Bolton & Budgell, 2006), producing hypoalgesia, altering motor excitability, and increasing range of motion through the neurophysiology of receptor-mediated events (Triano, 2001; Souvlis et al., 2004; Herzog, 2006). Furthermore, it is thought that this form of technique may also influence intra-articular biomechanics to restore range of motion and reduce pain, possibly by releasing entrapped meniscoid or synovial folds. It is a technique that requires highly developed psychomotor skills and manual dexterity and should be used only after any pathologic conditions that may jeopardize the safety of the patient have been ruled out. Therefore, the practitioner must be knowledgeable concerning relative and absolute contraindications to these techniques. In addition to satisfactory technical skill and knowledge of contraindications, a practitioner should also have a good understanding of when, how often, and how much the manual technique should be performed. A technique applied to the wrong subject, irrespective of how well executed, may be counterproductive and potentially produce undesirable adverse results (Hartman, 1998).

The Manipulable Lesion

At any time, 30% of American adults are affected by joint pain, swelling, and limitation of movement (Woolf & Pfleger, 2003), which have been described as the cardinal signs of joint dysfunction (Denslow, 1975). This "manipulable lesion," or somatic dysfunction, is characterized by the palpatory discrimination of tissue texture changes or abnormalities (including swelling and edema), limitation of movement, asymmetry, and tenderness (Greenman, 2003). The term *somatic dysfunction* broadly encompasses a variety of clinical descriptors used in the manual medicine literature (Kuchera, 2006), including *osteopathic spinal lesion* (Stoddard, 1959), *minor intervertebral derangements* (Maigne, 1996), *hypomobility* (Krauss et al., 2006), *subluxation* (Gatterman, 2005), *joint blockage* (Lewit, 1999), *loss of joint play* (Mennell, 1960), *manipulative lesion* (Mennell, 1992), and *restriction* (Stoddard, 1969). In fact, there are close to 300 terms identified in the literature as being more or less synonymous with each other to describe this clinical phenomenon (Rome, 1996).

Table 23.1 Characteristics (TART) of Somatic Dysfunction

"Somatic dysfunction is impaired or altered function of related components of the somatic (body framework) system: skeletal, arthrodial and myofascial structures; and related vascular, lymphatic and neural elements" (Educational Council on Osteopathic Principles, 2003).

T Tissue texture abnormalities or changes palpable in the paravertebral region associated with the somatic dysfunction
A Asymmetry of anatomic landmarks of structures involved in the somatic dysfunction
R Restricted range of motion, both quality and quantity, in the involved joint or motion segment
T Tenderness in the paravertebral and vertebral tissues to probing palpation

Somatic dysfunction is claimed to be a reversible condition, for which manual therapy is considered appropriate and effective treatment (Mitchell, 1979; Seffinger & Hruby, 2007). Thus, somatic dysfunction is considered to be a functional entity in which the range of motion of a joint, or accessory joint motion, has been reduced (**Table 23.1**). Once pathologic or degenerative changes have become established, some authors no longer consider the lesion as purely a somatic dysfunction (Stoddard, 1969). This claim notwithstanding, a joint with degenerative changes may still benefit from graded manual treatment because the techniques may help reduce swelling and pain and improve function.

There are several theoretical models regarding the mechanisms involved in the development of somatic dysfunction, with the proprioceptive and the nociceptive models being the most cited in the osteopathic literature (Howell & Willard, 2005). Direct evidence for such models remains elusive, and they are mostly based on speculation from indirect evidence for feasible mechanisms (Triano, 2001). Korr's proprioceptive model proposed that discrepancy between intrafusal and extrafusal muscle fiber activity creates aberrant afferent input into the spinal cord, resulting in facilitation or sensitization with efferent motor and autonomic effects (Korr, 1948, 1975). The nociceptive model is based on a nociceptively driven cascade of events resulting from tissue injury leading to inflammation, tissue proliferation, and remodeling (Van Buskirk, 1990; Howell & Willard, 2005), where somatic dysfunction is speculated to develop from ongoing inappropriate demand on injured tissues (Van Buskirk, 2007). Other models have emphasized the nociceptively driven disturbance to proprioception and motor control, and the

Table 23.2 Elements of the Musculoskeletal and Structural Evaluation

Global Screening	Regional Screening	Local Screening
General overview of the musculoskeletal system to answer the question: Is there a musculoskeletal problem? May include inspection, gait analysis, postural assessment, static asymmetry, and active and gross passive motion testing	Palpation and evaluation of soft tissues and joint function in a region to answer the question: Where is the problem? May include palpatory evaluation for tissue texture abnormalities (changes in muscle tension, presence of myofascial trigger points, tissue bogginess, and edema) and temperature changes, and active and passive regional motion testing	Evaluation of the specific tissue and joint to answer the question: What is the problem? May include the segment-specific palpatory evaluation of motion restriction, both range (quantity) and end-feel (quality), pain provocation to identify pain generators, and tissue characteristics that may accompany the alteration in motion

Modified from Seffinger & Hruby, 2007.

contribution of injury to the functional spinal unit to mechanical impairment of the motion segment (Fryer, 1999, 2003).

Diagnosing Somatic Dysfunction

It is a widely held belief in manual medicine that somatic dysfunction, directly or indirectly, can be a potential pain generator (Murphy, 2000; Kuchera, 2006). Furthermore, it has been proposed that somatic dysfunction in one region (which may be asymptomatic) may disturb the biomechanical equilibrium to create strain and secondary somatic dysfunction in a distant region, which may then present as the primary complaint (Sammut & Searle-Barnes, 1998; Lewit, 1999, 2007; Lewit & Kolar, 2000; Greenman, 2003; Murphy & Morris, 2004; Parsons & Marcer, 2006). In the manual medicine literature, it is often proposed that somatic dysfunctions in the thoracic spine and ribs may act as perpetuators causing strain and biomechanical alterations in the upper cervical spine (Isaac & Bookhout, 2006), the latter acting as pain generators in neck pain and headache. Postural alterations, especially the forward head posture as a consequence of muscular imbalances in the upper thorax and cervical region (also known as the *upper crossed syndrome*), have also been suggested to be key to biomechanical alterations or somatic dysfunctions in the upper cervical spine (Lewit, 1999; Liebenson, 2007; Chaitow, 2007). In treating patients, especially previous nonresponders to a local or symptomatic approach, it is suggested to treat the area of greatest restriction first (Lewit, 2007).

Somatic dysfunction is identified using visual and palpatory assessment of asymmetry of anatomic or structural landmarks, altered range and quality of regional and segmental joint motion, localized tissue texture abnormalities, tenderness, and possible temperature changes and is performed as a part of a complete history and physical examination (Seffinger & Hruby, 2007). For reasons mentioned earlier in this section, this process usually involves evaluating the whole patient before treatment is undertaken, starting with a global screening before proceeding to the regional and segmental evaluation (**Table 23.2**). The purpose of this process is to identify the potential somatic dysfunction(s) contributing to the presenting complaint (possible tissue-specific pain generators), and the overall pattern(s) of contributing factors.

The ability to reliably detect the clinical or cardinal signs of somatic dysfunction using manual methods has been questioned (Huijbregts, 2007; King et al., 2007). A review concluded that the interexaminer reliability of passive intervertebral motion testing in the cervical spine was low (van Trijffel et al., 2005). However, many of the reviewed studies had substantial shortcomings, including inadequate reporting of study design and protocol, inappropriate patient selection for the study, lack of internal and external validity, inadequate reporting of statistical data, and failure to follow the standards for reporting of diagnostic accuracy (STARD) criteria (van Trijffel et al., 2005). Pain provocation tests appear to be the most reliable criteria, whereas soft-tissue paraspinal palpatory diagnostic tests have not been shown to be reliable. Regional range of motion is more reliable than segmental range of motion. In the cases of soft-tissue palpatory diagnostic tests and range of motion, intraexaminer reliability is generally better than interexaminer reliability (Seffinger et al., 2004; Stochkendahl et al.,

Table 23.3 Predictor Variables for Clinical Prediction Rules (CPRs)

CPR to identify patients with immediate response to cervical manipulation (Tseng et al., 2006)

Initial Neck Disability Index <11.5
Bilateral involvement pattern
Not performing sedentary work >5 hours per day
Feeling better while moving the neck
Diagnosis of spondylosis without radiculopathy

CPR to identify patients with neck pain likely to respond to thoracic manipulation (Cleland et al., 2007)

Symptom duration <30 days
No symptoms distal to the shoulder
Looking up does not aggravate symptoms
Fear Avoidance Beliefs Questionnaire–Physical Activity
  Subscale score <12
Diminished upper thoracic kyphosis
Cervical extension range of motion <30°

Modified from Huijbregts, 2007.

2006). These reviews have concluded that more well-designed studies are needed to address the methodologic shortcomings of previous studies in this area.

Manual palpatory diagnosis is a multidimensional process that does not just involve testing for a single clinical sign of somatic dysfunction. The ability to arrive at an accurate diagnosis of conditions in the musculoskeletal system depends on a variety of factors, including the patient's history, the examiner's experience and skills, the validity and reliability of the assessment procedures used, and how each step in the diagnostic process supports each other step (Seffinger & Hruby, 2007). Clinical prediction rules describing patient populations with neck pain (Tseng et al., 2006; Cleland et al., 2007) and low back pain (Flynn et al., 2002; Childs et al., 2004; Fritz et al., 2005) likely to respond to joint manipulation have been developed (**Table 23.3**). It has been argued, however, that replacing specific manual diagnostic and treatment procedures with clinical guidelines undervalues the role of clinical skills, potentially posing a risk to the individual patient's safety (Grimsby & Miller, 2006).

Proposed Mechanisms of Action

Most theories for the therapeutic action of HVLA manipulation have previously focused on either the mechanical or neurophysiologic effects of manipulation. Mechanical effects from manipulation of the zygapophysial joints have been considered to be either intra- or extra-articular. The proposed intra-articular effects include releasing entrapped or ex-trapped synovial folds, plicae, or meniscoids, and disrupting intra-articular adhesions. Proposed extra-articular mechanical effects include stretching and disruption of periarticular adhesions (Evans, 2002; Maigne & Vautravers, 2003). Despite their prevalence in the literature, these theories remain unproven.

The presence of meniscoids in the cervical zygapophysial joints has been demonstrated histologically, both in cadaveric anatomic studies and using computed tomography and magnetic resonance imaging (MRI) (Adams et al., 2006; Friedrich et al., 2007). Furthermore, the presence of nociceptive fibers within these structures has been demonstrated (Inami et al., 2001). An earlier theory proposed that the entrapment of meniscoids alone was not painful, but that the traction on the zygapophysial joint capsule via the meniscoid or synovial fold could cause pain (Kos & Wolf, 1972). This theory has been refuted on the grounds that meniscoids may not be strong enough to distort the zygapophysial joint capsule (Bogduk & Jull, 1985). Alternatively, a basal tear of the meniscoid producing a subcapsular hemorrhage could be a source of pain, or the meniscoid apex might be torn from its base, producing a loose body and potentially causing an acute locked joint (Bogduk & Engel, 1984). Based on these meniscoid theories, the successful application of HVLA should separate the surfaces of the zygapophysial joints, so that the meniscoid can slip back to its normal place or position (Lewit, 1999). In the case of a subcapsular hemorrhage from a tear in the meniscoid, restoring motion to the zygapophysial joint with manual techniques may activate or enhance the function of the transsynovial pump, facilitating the formation and drainage of synovial fluid in the joint. The pump has three components, all of which are stimulated by movement: (a) a fluctuating intra-articular pressure, (b) an increased synovial blood flow, and (c) facilitated drainage into the lymphatic system, all of which help the fluxes of fluids and synovial constituents in and out of the joint cavity.

The neurophysiologic effects of joint manipulation and mobilization commonly proposed in the literature include alterations in reflex excitability (Herzog, 2006), altered sensory processing (Zhu et al., 2000; Haavik-Taylor & Murphy, 2007), altered motor excitability (Pickar, 2002), and reduced pain or hypoalgesia (Sluka &

Wright, 2001; Skyba et al., 2003; Hoeger & Sluka, 2007).

The neuromuscular effects caused by spinal manipulation have been categorized as reflex activation, reflex inhibition, and the Hoffmann (H-) reflex response associated with the technique (Herzog, 2006). In a review of the physiologic effects of spinal manipulation, Potter et al. (2005) concluded that there is some evidence to support the theory that these techniques evoke spinal stretch reflexes, and that a brief muscle contraction may be followed by a period of reduced muscle activity. Although there is little supporting evidence, reflex activation of alpha motor neurons has been proposed to lead to resetting of muscle activity and result in reduced hypertonicity (Potter et al., 2005). Apparently spinal manipulation produces multisegmental reflex responses that are associated with a variety of afferent pathways (Herzog, 2006), even to the extent of altering cortical somatosensory processing and sensomotor integration (Haavik-Taylor & Murphy, 2007).

The hypoalgesic effect, or manipulation-induced analgesia, may be a multifactorial effect resulting from beneficial influences on the chemical environment of the joint, facilitation of tissue repair processes, segmental inhibitory processes within the central nervous system, and the activation of various descending inhibitory pathways projecting from the brain to the spinal cord (Wright, 1995; Sluka et al., 2002). There is now a growing body of anatomic, physiologic, and behavioral evidence from experimental, basic science, and clinical studies suggesting that joint mobilization and manipulation activates supraspinal descending pain inhibitory systems (Zusman, 2004). It has been suggested that this hypoalgesic effect is segmentally organized and probably results from large-diameter afferent stimulation (Sluka et al., 2002).

Evidence exists that descending pain inhibitory systems may be principally responsible for the rapid hypoalgesic effect produced by manual therapy (Souvlis et al., 2004). Both animal and human studies indicate that the periaqueductal gray area of the midbrain may be a key mediator in this response involving the descending inhibitory pathways (Souvlis et al., 2004; Hoeger-Bement & Sluka, 2007). Animal studies using specific antagonists to neurotransmitters involved in endogenous opioid and nonopioid analgesia showed that the serotonergic and noradrenergic nonopioid pathways and receptors are the most likely mediators of the hypoalgesic effects (Sluka & Wright, 2001; Skyba et al., 2003). The drugs were injected into the intrathecal space in the spinal cord via catheter (Skyba et al., 2003). Spinal blockade of serotonin receptors 5-HT$_{1A}$ prevents the hypoalgesic effect of joint manipulation in acute joint inflammation. Further, spinal blockade of noradrenaline receptors partially reduced the hypoalgesic effect (Hoeger-Bement & Sluka, 2007). To differentiate between a centrally mediated neurophysiologic response and local peripheral effects from the joint mobilization, animal studies on acute and inflammatory joint pain have involved joint mobilization to the noninflamed neighboring joint (Sluka & Wright, 2001; Skyba et al., 2003). Vicenzino et al. (2000) investigated the effect of naloxone on the hypoalgesic response to cervical joint mobilization in humans, demonstrated no effect from the administered naloxone on pain relief, and concluded that the hypoalgesic effect was not opioid in nature.

Studies using a similar animal model of acute inflammatory pain and functional MRI support the observations of central changes involved in the hypoalgesic effects of manual therapy. Using functional MRI, Malisza et al. (2003a) noted areas of the dorsal horn in the rat lumbar spinal cord with increased neuronal activity following the injection of the inflammatory agent capsaicin in the hind paws of the animals, changes consistent with spinal cord physiology on pain. Further, they noted decreased activation of these areas following the application of manual therapy to the homolateral knee joint (Malisza et al., 2003a). In a second study, Malisza et al. (2003b) investigated whether there was any detectable cerebral activation due to secondary hyperalgesia from injection of capsaicin to the ankle joints and hind paws in rats. In addition, they investigated whether they could detect analgesic changes in the central nervous system response to pain as a result of the joint mobilization and noted a trend toward reduced areas of activation for animals in which joint mobilization was performed compared with those in which no mobilization was performed (Malisza et al., 2003b).

When to Administer High-Velocity, Low-Amplitude Manipulation

It is beyond the scope of this chapter to discuss all the relative and absolute contraindications to cervical joint manipulation. Numerous factors may help determine the patient's suitability to receive cervical joint manipulation. These factors depend both on the patient and the clinician. Some factors that may be associated with poor outcomes with cervical joint manipulation (Wells,

Table 23.4 Factors Associated with Poor Outcomes with Cervical Joint Manipulation

Clinician-Related Factors	Patient-Related Factors

Clinician training and experience
   Inadequate diagnostic skills
   Inadequate manipulative skills
Inadequate patient assessment
Diagnostic error
Poor choice of manipulative
   procedures
Incorrect patient positioning
   during technique
Poorly applied technique that
   uses excessive force
Excessive manipulation
Lack of interpersonal and
   communication skills
	Personal expectations of
	   patient
	Previous experiences
	   with other practitioners
	Emotional, psychological,
	   and behavioral factors
	Patient fear and
	   apprehension
	Too much pain in too
	   many directions
	Congenital abnormalities
	Multiple medical
	   comorbidities

2000; Krauss et al., 2006; Gibbons & Tehan, 2006) are listed in **Table 23.4**.

The clinical decision-making process involves excluding any contraindications (red flags), determining any psychosocial risk factors associated with chronic pain or disability (yellow flags), identifying the presence of a treatable somatic dysfunction (Table 23.1), and deciding on the appropriate manipulative intervention (Gibbons & Tehan, 2006). In determining whether joint HVLA manipulation is the appropriate intervention, some clinicians recommend assessing joint glide and end-feel at the end of the available passive range in the segment identified as dysfunctional, for detection of a firm end-feel that arrives slightly early in the passive range of motion (Krauss et al., 2006; Pettman, 2006). Use of end-feel to determine the appropriateness of a specific manipulative technique is based on the concept that the loss of motion may be caused by many factors, including myofascial shortening, periarticular capsule–ligamentous shortening, intra-articular swelling, or alteration in intra-articular mechanics (due to entrapment of meniscoid or synovial folds), all of which may influence the quality of the perceived end-feel.

There is little evidence, however, to guide the clinician with regard to the validity of assessing end-feel as an indicator for joint manipulation. Furthermore, there is little evidence of improved clinical outcomes based on factors such as the direction of the thrust or impulse in the technique (with respect to the diagnosed motion barrier) or the combination and sequencing of manipulative techniques in patients presenting with musculoskeletal pain and dysfunction (Gibbons & Tehan, 2006).

Effectiveness of High-Velocity, Low-Amplitude Manipulation for Headache and Neck Pain

The evidence for effectiveness of manipulation for headache and neck pain is growing and consists of an increasing number of clinical trials and systematic reviews of these trials. Several reviews have reported benefit from spinal manipulation for these conditions (Bronfort et al., 2001, 2004; Gross et al., 2004; Vernon et al., 2007), but, because of the poor methodologic quality of the reviewed studies and the heterogeneity of the manual techniques used, other reviews have been unable to make definitive conclusions (Astin & Ernst, 2002; Lenssinck et al., 2004; Fernández-de-las-Peñas et al., 2006).

For the treatment of different categories of headaches, the most recent Cochrane review identified potential benefit from spinal manipulation (Bronfort et al., 2004). For migraine headache, there was evidence that spinal manipulation might be an effective treatment option with a short-term effect similar to that of a commonly used, effective drug (amitriptyline). For chronic tension-type headache, spinal manipulation was superior in the short term, although less effective than this drug overall. For prophylactic treatment of cervicogenic headache, the review identified evidence that both neck exercise and spinal manipulation were effective in the short and long term when compared with no treatment, and effective in the short term when compared with massage or placebo manipulation (Bronfort et al., 2004).

For neck pain, manipulation and mobilization have been reported to demonstrate only a nonsignificant benefit in pain relief when assessed against placebo, control groups, or other treatments (Gross et al., 2004). This Cochrane review, however, did identify strong evidence of benefit favoring multimodal care, where the common elements were manipulation and/or mobilization and exercise. Vernon et al. (2007) examined and reviewed the pre- and postchange scores from clinical studies using a course of spinal manipulation or mobilization and concluded that there was moderate- to high-quality evidence that subjects with chronic neck pain show clinically important improvements.

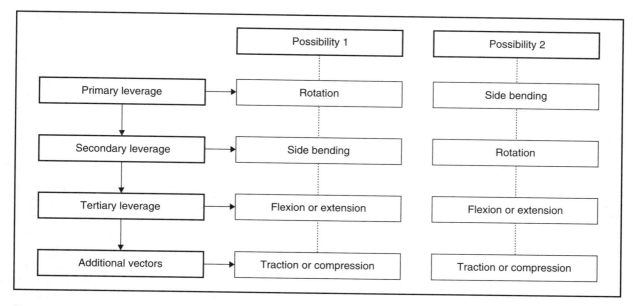

Figure 23.1 Leverages for Smooth and Easy Application of Combined Leverage and Thrust (CLT) Technique

PRINCIPLES OF TECHNIQUE APPLICATION

Leverages

Most HVLA techniques involve use of patient positioning to achieve specific leverages localized to the targeted joint. The primary purpose of using a combined leverage and thrust (CLT) technique varies according to different authors, but it may be used for localization of force to the targeted joint by relatively "locking" segments above and below, taking up the joint slack in order to minimize the amount of force required to cavitate the joint (Gibbons & Tehan, 2006; Hartman, 1997; Stoddard, 1959), or to directly engage the planes of restricted motion in the dysfunctional joint (Bourdillon et al., 1992; Greenman, 2003). The use of leverage to localize forces to targeted segments may be achieved by anatomic (facet apposition locking) or physiologic (ligamentous-tension locking) locking of adjacent joints. Additionally, some authors have proposed combinations of leverages that are claimed to minimize the overall amount of leverage required for joint tension and localization in order to improve patient comfort and safety (Gibbons & Tehan, 2006).

For smooth and easy application of CLT technique to the cervical spine, it is important to identify primary and secondary leverages. The primary leverage can be identified as the principal or executive vector of force for that particular technique. The secondary leverage is the stabilizing and enhancing vector that allows greatest efficiency in the primary leverage direction. The tertiary leverage and additional vectors are variables that are used to further localize and focus the forces to the particular segment (**Figure 23.1**). These are particularly helpful when it is necessary to "splint" the area being treated, such as in patients with very flexible or hypermobile cervical segments. The use of extension combined with end-of-range rotation is generally avoided to minimize stress on the vertebral arteries on their anatomic course through the cervical spine, especially at the level of C1 and C2.

The resultant effect of the leverage and thrust on the zygapophysial joint may theoretically promote either gliding of joint surfaces (vector of force parallel to joint surfaces) or joint separation and cavitation (vector of force perpendicular to joint surfaces). **Figure 23.2** illustrates the effect of coupled side bending and rotation leverage on joint glide and separation.

Where in the Range of Motion Is the Thrust Applied?

HVLA technique involves leverages for specificity and accurate positioning, anatomic (facet apposition locking) or physiologic (ligamentous-tension locking) locking of adjacent joints, and a high-velocity movement that is characterized more by its rapid acceleration than

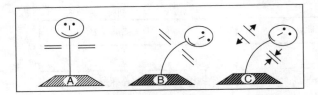

Figure 23.2 Effect of Leverage on Joint Glide and **Separation. A:** Cervical spine is in neutral position. The zygapophysial joint orientation for the right and left joints is illustrated. **B:** Side bending and rotation in the same side. This is the proposed normal physiologic coupled motion behavior, but will do little to separate the zygapophysial joint surfaces. **C:** Side bending and rotation in opposite directions will theoretically create separation of the zygapophysial joint surfaces on the side opposite the side bending.
Source: Courtesy of Christian Fossum.

its amplitude. The direction of the movement in relation to the plane of the zygapophysial joints may be:

- Parallel gliding of the joint surfaces (Possibility 1, Figure 23.1)
- Perpendicular or angular to the joint surfaces (Possibility 2, Figure 23.1).

The barrier concept is a method of describing the components of range of motion in a single plane for a given joint. Joint barriers include the anatomic barrier (limit of motion imposed by anatomic structure; the limit of passive motion), the physiologic barrier (limit of active motion), and the restrictive barrier (a functional limit, which abnormally diminishes the normal physiologic range) (Kappler & Kuchera, 2003). The neutral zone is the point or region in the range of motion where the passive osteoligamentous stability mechanisms exert little or no influence and there is very little constraint offered by the joint capsules (Panjabi, 1992).

The application of HVLA may either promote movement along the surfaces of the joint toward the restrictive barrier (gliding motion) or at right angles to the joint surface to create joint separation. **Figure 23.3** illustrates the concept of the two different directions of force in relation to the zygapophysial joint planes. In practice, it is possible that techniques aimed at promoting parallel gliding motion may also achieve separation once the capsule and ligaments are taut and prevent further gliding, which may explain why these gliding techniques frequently result in an audible pop associated with separation or cavitation.

The neutral zone is the area or the midpoint in the available range of motion where the surrounding tension in capsuloligamentous and myofascial structures is minimal and the major resistance to the separation of the two joint surfaces is the negative intra-articular pressure (Hartman, 1997, 1998; Evans & Breen, 2006).

If the aim of a technique is to achieve separation of the two joint surfaces with the joint relatively in its neutral zone, how does an operator build up the necessary joint tension in order to achieve a successful thrust? The CLT technique uses the concept of a variable barrier to motion (Hartman, 1998). This barrier is variable in that it can be under the direct control of the operator. This control is maintained by an understanding of the various vectors of motion available in an articular complex and introducing them as combined movements to limit overall amplitude. By combining several movement vectors, a barrier is formed that is at a *cumulative* end of range rather than an anatomic end of range, which implies that it is not necessary to perform thrust techniques at the end of any given range of motion (Middleton, 1971; Hartman, 1997, 1998).

This also has the effect of bringing the point of resistance or the movable barrier closer to the patient's midline neutral, rather than at the end range of any single plane of motion. This not only has clear benefits in safety and comfort, but also has the advantage that tissue stress and distortion are reduced, and position will reduce the tension on the periarticular and paravertebral structures. Additionally, the use of leverage will increase the patient's comfort and reduce the tissue resistance to the technique, and therefore less force will be required for application of a successful technique. This apparently is analogous to performing an HVLA technique from the "point of balanced ligamentous tension" (the joint's neutral zone), from which the separation of the joint surfaces is most easily achieved. This is illustrated in the following analogy attributed to A.T. Still, the founder of osteopathy:

Many say that when we have positioned a lesion for correction that we should take all the slack out of the ligaments and then thrust it a bit farther. I am very definitely opposed to this method. My father once asked Dr. Still about this point. Dr. Still said, "If you had a horse tied to a post (they still drove horses in those days) and you wanted to untie him, you wouldn't first frighten him so that he would pull back on the rope to hold it tight during the untying operation, would you?" (Fryette, 1954, pg. 62)

The Thrust or the Impulse

The thrust has three important components that require consideration: velocity, amplitude, and force. It

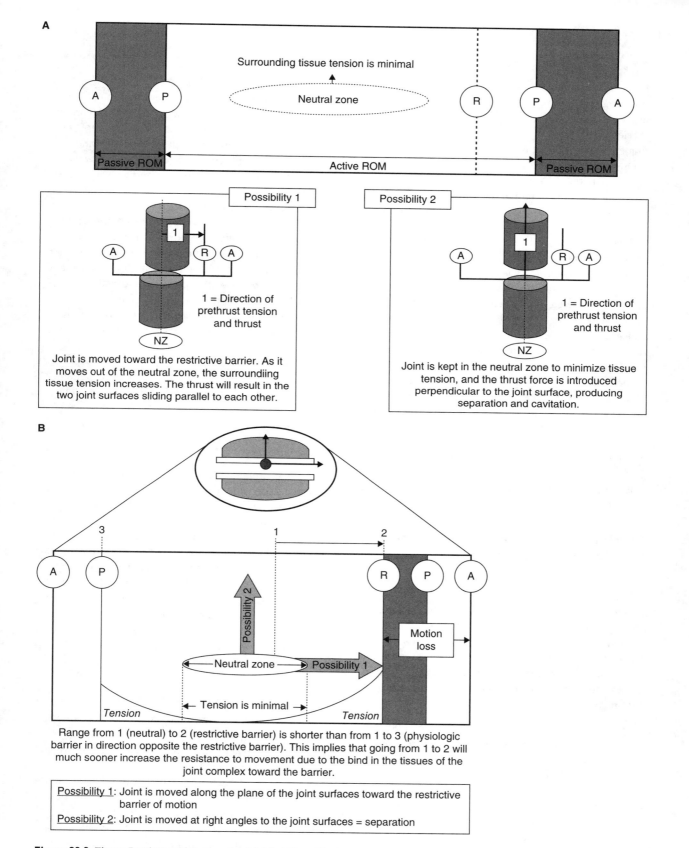

Figure 23.3 Tissue Barriers and Zygapophysial Joint Plane Motion. A, anatomic barrier; P, physiologic barrier; R, restrictive barrier; ROM, range of motion; NZ, neutral zone; from P to P, active range of motion; from P to A, passive range of motion.
Source: Courtesy of Christian Fossum.

has been argued that the term *high-velocity* may be a misnomer since the technique starts at zero velocity, and it has been referred to by several authors as a *high-acceleration* technique rather than a *high-velocity* technique (Pettman, 2006; Nicholas & Nicholas, 2007).

Operators should strive to keep the amplitude in the HVLA technique to a minimum. Keeping the amplitude low minimizes the potential risk of damage to the joint complex and its surrounding tissues. Pain and muscle spasm following an HVLA technique may be due to excessive amplitude and force in the technique, creating an inflammatory response in these tissues.

The magnitude of force is also important. If adequate localization and accumulative tension of the movable barrier is achieved, little force is required for successful technique. Replacing the word *thrust* or *impulse* with *nudge* better conveys a sense of the force that is required. The required amount of force can be greatly reduced by consideration and use of primary and secondary leverages. The direction of force used in the thrust should preferably be the same as the primary leverage, and *not* a combination of primary and secondary leverages (irrespective of how tempting that may be). If rotation was the primary leverage chosen and side bending the secondary leverage, the thrust should be a rapid increase in rotation with little or no increase of side bending, therefore allowing the facets to move with a minimum of friction (less resistance).

Considerations for Learning High-Velocity, Low-Amplitude Techniques

Mere imitation of one operator's technique by another inexperienced operator may result in awkward posture and technique and strain and sprain of the operator, because mastery of HVLA application takes practice and skill, with modifications for the individual characteristics of operator and patient. Attention to the principles of operator relaxation, balance, correct posture, and skilled motor coordination will assist novice manipulators in gaining skills in this technique.

- *Operator relaxation*. Relaxation of both operator and patient is essential for effective technique. An operator who is nervous or tense will have difficulty in localizing the leverages and successfully applying appropriate control, speed, and amplitude. Tension in the operator is easily sensed by the patient, making it difficult for the patient to fully relax, a step necessary for successful technique.

- *Operator balance*. Balance is important for adequate control of forces, generation of adequate and controlled velocity in a technique, and the unity of body motion. An unstable or uncentered operator will often overuse the shoulder and arm muscles to generate velocity, which will make amplitude and velocity more difficult to control.

- *Unity of body movement*. This principle refers to the connectedness of body movement acting in rhythmic unity for optimizing economy of movement and minimizing tension and energy wastage. This principle is difficult to explain and often comes with experience in practice. Together with the accomplishment of the previous two principles, it is analogous to the concept of "centeredness" or "maintaining the center" referred to in certain martial arts. Rhythm in technique postpones the onset of fatigue in the operator and relaxes the patient; when a technique is performed without body unity (such as performing HVLA techniques using only the arms and shoulders), control and accuracy of force become more difficult.

As an example of the importance of posture, balance, and handling in cervical techniques, to stand stooping or to sit with the arms straight when treating the supine patient would strain the operator, as well as detract from the power and sensitivity of the hands. If standing, the operator should be close enough for the lumbar spine to be straight and abdominal muscles slightly tensed, and should bend from the hips with a straight spine from a wide and steady base, or from the knees if the operator wishes to reach lower. The arms of the operator should be comfortably bent—not straight—and the part to be treated should be within the area of the operator's center of weight.

Additional Tips for the Acquisition of Technique Skills

- The operator should have a clear understanding of the following.
  - The planes of motion and leverages involved in the correction
  - The "tension sense," that is, the ability to sense when you have the necessary accumulation of tension through the leverages (the barrier)
  - How to control the rhythm, amplitude, and force involved in the correction

Table 23.5 Troubleshooting Guide for High-Velocity, Low-Amplitude Techniques

Incorrect selection of technique

Size differences between operator and patient

Inadequate diagnosis (casual use of manipulation without adequate examination)

Inexperienced with the selected technique (inadequate manipulative skills)

Inability to position the patient due to pain, discomfort, or physical limitation

Patient apprehension

Inadequate selection of technique

Incorrect application of leverages (primary and secondary)

Inability to recognize the necessary accumulative tension prior to thrust

Ineffective thrust

Loss of contact point pressure

Poor bimanual coordination

Incorrect direction of thrust

Inadequate acceleration of the thrust

Incorrect amplitude of the thrust

Incorrect force of the thrust

Loss of leverage at time of thrust

Poor operator posture

Operator not relaxed

Failure to arrest thrust and leverage adequately

Lack of practitioner confidence

Modified from Gibbons & Tehan, 2006.

- Brute strength to achieve joint cavitation is absolutely contraindicated.
- Do not grip the patient too tightly (remember to be relaxed and balanced).
- To minimize the amplitude in the HVLA technique, the operator should hold the arms as close to his or her own body or trunk as possible.
- Make your patient comfortable and then alter your own position to suit the direction of your correction.
- After any type of correction or technique, the area treated should be returned to the normal neutral position.

A number of technique, operator, and patient factors may result in technique failure. A troubleshooting guide is presented in **Table 23.5**.

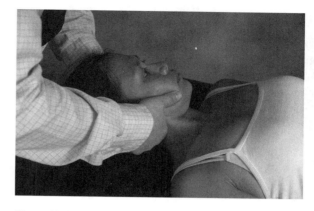

Figure 23.4 C2 to C7 Segment with Rotation as Primary Leverage (Separation of Left Zygapophysial Articular Joint)

HIGH-VELOCITY, LOW-AMPLITUDE TECHNIQUES FOR THE CERVICAL REGION

C2 to C7 Segment with Rotation as Primary Leverage (Separation of Left Zygapophysial Articular Joint) (**Figure 23.4**)

1. The operator contacts the patient's right articular pillar with the metacarpophalangeal (MCP) joint of the operator's right hand on the dysfunctional segment (for motion loss between C2 and C3, operator contacts C2).
2. The left hand supports the patient's head on the left side.
3. The cervical spine is flexed down to the dysfunctional segment.
4. Left rotation (primary leverage in thrust) is introduced until motion is felt at segment.
5. Right side-bending is introduced (this should bring the neck back into the patient's physical midline to minimize stress in cervical soft tissues).
6. When the barrier and accumulating joint tension are palpated by combining flexion, rotation, and side bending, a high-acceleration thrust (with low amplitude and little force) is executed in the direction of left rotation.

Note: Do not combine rotation and side bending in the thrusting force, because this may increase the friction of the joint surfaces and the periarticular capsuloligamentous tension, which may cause the operator to increase the force of the thrust to overcome this resistance.

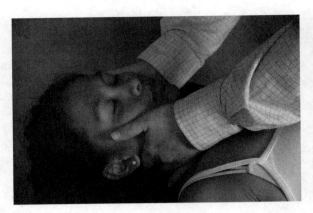

Figure 23.5 C2 to C7 Segment with Rotation as Primary Leverage (Separation of Left Zygapophysial Articular Joint): Alternative Handhold

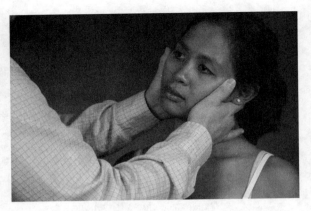

Figure 23.6 C2 to C7 Segment with Rotation as Primary Leverage (Separation of Right Zygapophysial Articular Joint): Alternative Handhold

C2 to C7 Segment with Rotation as Primary Leverage (Separation of Left Zygapophysial Articular Joint): Alternative Handhold (**Figure 23.5**)

This is a variation of the previous technique with the operator standing on the patient's left side.

1. The operator contacts the patient's right articular pillar with the proximal interphalangeal (PIP) region of the operator's left hand.
2. Operator's left hand supports the left side of the patient's head.
3. Operator introduces motion of the cervical spine in the sagittal plane until appropriate tension is felt in that plane.
4. Rotation of the cervical spine to the left is introduced until motion is felt at the point of contact with the dysfunctional segment.
5. When the barrier and accumulating joint tension are palpated using composite leverages, a high-acceleration thrust (with low amplitude and little force) is executed in the direction of left rotation.

C2 to C7 Segment with Rotation as Primary Leverage (Separation of Right Zygapophysial Articular Joint): Alternative Handhold (**Figure 23.6**)

This is a variation of the previous C2 to C7 technique with the patient seated.

1. The operator stands in front of the patient.
2. Operator contacts the left articular pillar with the PIP of the operator's right hand.

3. Operator introduces right rotation of the cervical spine until motion is palpated at the dysfunctional segment (primary leverage).
4. Left side-bending is introduced until the motion is localized to the dysfunctional segment (this should also bring the neck back into the patient's physical midline to minimize stress in cervical soft tissues).
5. A small amount of extension can be used to further localize the barrier.
6. When the barrier and accumulating joint tension are palpated using composite leverages, a high-acceleration thrust (with low amplitude and little force) is executed in the direction of right rotation.

C2 to C7 Segment Using Chin Hold with Rotation as Primary Leverage (Separation of Left Zygapophysial Articular Joint) (**Figure 23.7**)

1. The operator contacts the right articular pillar with MCP joint of right hand on the dysfunctional segment (for motion loss between C2 and C3, operator contacts C2).
2. The operator's left hand cradles the chin and supports the head.
3. The cervical spine is flexed down to the dysfunctional segment.
4. Left rotation is introduced until motion is palpated at the dysfunctional segment.
5. Right side-bending is introduced until motion is felt at the dysfunctional segment. The right side-

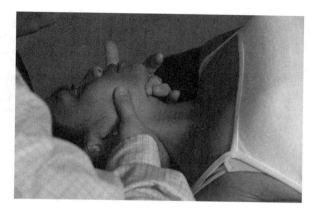

Figure 23.7 C2 to C7 Segment Using Chin Hold with Rotation as Primary Leverage (Separation of Left Zygapophysial Articular Joint)

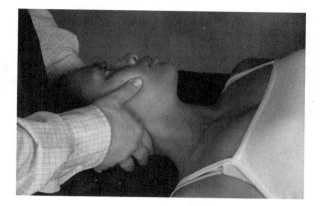

Figure 23.8 C1 Segment (Atlantoaxial Joint) Using Cradle Hold with Rotation as Primary Leverage (Separation of Left Zygapophysial Articular Joint)

bending also allows the neck of the patient to return to the patient's physical midline, thus reducing stress in cervical soft-tissue structures.

6. A small amount of extension can be used to further localize the leverages at the barrier.
7. When the barrier and accumulating joint tension are palpated using composite leverages, a high-acceleration thrust (with low amplitude and little force) is executed in the direction of left rotation.

C1 Segment (Atlantoaxial Joint) Using Cradle Hold with Rotation as Primary Leverage (Separation of Left Zygapophysial Articular Joint) (**Figure 23.8**)

1. The operator contacts and cradles the patient's head.
2. Operator contacts the right articular pillar of the dysfunctional segment with the MCP joint of the right hand.
3. The cervical spine is rotated to the left until the restrictive barrier is palpated (remember that the primary motion available in the atlantoaxial [AA] joint is rotation).
4. To further localize the barrier, a minimal amount of left side-bending is introduced (the available side bending in the AA joint is approximately 4–5°).
5. When the barrier and accumulating joint tension are palpated, a high-acceleration thrust (with low amplitude and little force) is executed in the direction of left rotation.

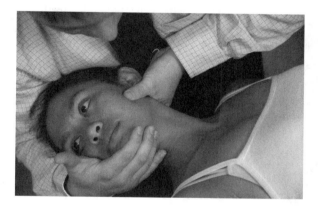

Figure 23.9 C0-C1 (Occipitoatlantal Joint) Using Chin Hold (Traction Separation of the Left Zygapophysial Articular Joint)

C0-C1 (Occipitoatlantal Joint) Using Chin Hold (Traction Separation of the Right Zygapophysial Articular Joint) (**Figure 23.9**)

1. The operator gently grasps the patient's chin and uses his or her forearm to support the patient's head.
2. The head of the patient is rotated to the right.
3. The operator contacts the area posterior to the mastoid process with the MCP joint of the left hand.
4. The operator exerts a small amount of traction with both hands to increase the sense of localization.

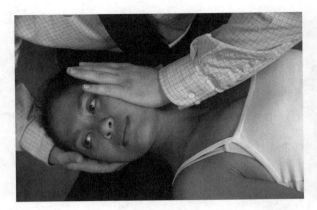

Figure 23.10 C0-C1 (Occipitoatlantal Joint) using Traction-Rotation Thrust

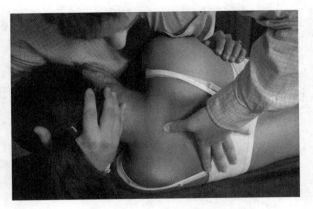

Figure 23.11 Thrust Technique for the Cervicothoracic Junction with Patient in Lateral Recumbent Position

5. When the barrier and accumulating joint tension are palpated, a high-acceleration thrust (with low amplitude and little force) is executed in the direction of the right orbit of the patient.

C0-C1 (Occipitoatlantal Joint) using Traction-Rotation Thrust Technique for the OAA (Occiput Atlas Axis) Complex on the Right Side (**Figure 23.10**)

1. The operator stands on the patient's left side.
2. With the middle and the ring finger of the right hand, the operator contacts the right mastoid process.
3. The patient's head is positioned in right rotation.
4. With the palm of the left hand, the operator contacts the patient's left jawline and cheek.
5. The fingers contacting the right mastoid process exert a moderate amount of traction; this traction is also supported and enhanced by gentle traction exerted through the operator's left hand.
6. When the barrier and accumulating joint tension are palpated, a high-acceleration thrust (with low amplitude and minimal force) is given in the direction of traction with a gentle right rotary force.

Thrust Technique for the Cervicothoracic Junction for the Left Zygapophyseal Joint with the Patient in Lateral Recumbent Position (**Figure 23.11**)

1. The patient is in a left lateral recumbent position.
2. The operator stands in front of the patient.
3. The operator's right hand and forearm support the patient's head and control the amount of leverage used in the technique.

4. The operator's left thumb contacts the right side of the spinous process of T1.
5. By controlling the head of the patient, the cervical spine is positioned into left rotation and right side-bending until leverage can be localized to C7 to T1.
6. Posterior translation is introduced (do not use extension for this technique) by the operator controlling the head of the patient.
7. The thrust is delivered as a quick downward pressure against the spinous process of T1 with the operator's left thumb, with a simultaneous low-amplitude exaggeration of cervical left rotation, right side-bending, and posterior translation with the right arm.

Note: The exaggeration of the cervical motion by the operator controlling and supporting the head of the patient can be smoothly achieved by the operator visualizing the movement as an uppercut (from boxing). The thrust should be a high-acceleration thrust with low amplitude and little force.

Thrust Technique for the Cervicothoracic Junction with Patient Seated (**Figure 23.12**)

1. The operator stands behind the patient.
2. The thumb of the operator's right hand contacts the right side of the spinous process of T1.
3. The operator contacts the head of the patient and brings the cervical spine into left rotation and right side-bending until motion is palpated and localized to the C7 to T1 segment.
4. A moderate amount of axial compression is introduced through the contact on the patient's head.

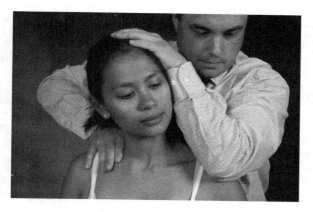

Figure 23.12 Thrust Technique for the Cervicothoracic Junction with Patient Seated

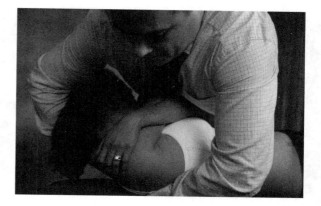

Figure 23.13 Thrust Technique for the Upper Thoracic Spine with the Patient Supine

5. When the barrier and accumulating joint tension are palpated, a thrust is given by the operator's right thumb in the direction of the patient's left axilla.
6. When delivering the thrust, the operator should avoid any use of the neck for the thrusting force.
7. The thrust should be a high-acceleration thrust with low amplitude and little force.

Thrust Technique for the Upper Thoracic Spine with the Patient Supine (**Figure 23.13**)

This is a variation of the technique that is commonly referred to as the *Kirksville crunch* (United States) or the *Dog technique* (United Kingdom).

1. The operator may stand on either side of the patient.
2. The patient's arms are crossed over the chest (the arm on the side of which the operator is standing will be the lower arm when the arms are crossed).
3. The operator's hand contacting the thoracic spine should contact both transverse processes of the inferior vertebra in the dysfunction (for a T2 dysfunction, the transverse processes of T3 are contacted).

4. The thenar eminence and the palmar MCP area are used to contact the transverse processes. (If the operator is standing on the patient's left side, the thenar eminence of the operator's left hand contacts the patient's right transverse process, and the palmar MCP the left transverse process: the operator's hand will be perpendicular to the spine.)
5. The operator may use his or her free hand and arm to adjust the patient's position to allow appropriate contact of the patient on the applicator hand.
6. The operator lifts the head of the patient and places the free hand just superior to the area being treated. This will allow the operator to exert some traction on the segment during the preloading phase.
7. The operator's arm supporting the head and the neck flexes and extends the cervical and thoracic spine until the segment is positioned in a relatively neutral position.
8. An oblique downward (toward the segment being treated) thrust is executed from the epigastric region of the operator through the elbows of the patient.

REFERENCES

Adams M, Bogduk N, Burton K, et al. *The Biomechanics of Back Pain.* 2nd ed. Edinburgh: Churchill Livingstone Elsevier; 2006.

Astin JA, Ernst E. The effectiveness of spinal manipulation for the treatment of headache disorders: a systematic review of randomized clinical trials. *Cephalalgia* 2002;22:617–623.

Barber E. *Osteopathy Complete.* Kansas City, MO: Hudson-Kimberly Publishing Company; 1898.

Bogduk N, Engel R. The menisci of the lumbar zygapophysial joints: a review of their anatomy and significance. *Spine* 1984;9:454–460.

Bogduk N, Jull G. The theoretical pathology of acute locked back: a basis for manipulative therapy. *Man Med* 1985;1:78–82.

Bolton PS, Budgell BS. Spinal manipulation and spinal mobilization influence different axial sensory beds. *Med Hypotheses* 2006;66:258–262.

Bourdillon JF, Day EA, Bookhout MR. *Spinal Manipulation*. 5th ed. Oxford: Butterworth-Heinemann; 1992.

Bronfort G, Assendelft WJ, Evans R, Haas M, Bouter L. Efficacy of spinal manipulation for chronic headache: a systematic review. *J Manipulative Physiol Ther* 2001;24:457–466.

Bronfort G, Nilsson N, Haas M, et al. Non-invasive physical treatments for chronic/recurrent headache. *Cochrane Database Syst Rev* 2004;3:CD001878.

Chaitow L. *Muscle Energy Techniques*. 3rd ed. Edinburgh: Churchill Livingstone Elsevier; 2007.

Childs JD, Fritz JM, Flynn T, et al. A clinical prediction rule to identify patients with low back pain most likely to benefit from spinal manipulation: a validation study. *Ann Intern Med* 2004;141:920–928.

Cleland JA, Glynn P, Whitman J, Eberhart SL, MacDonald C, Childs JD. Short-term response of thoracic spine thrust versus non-thrust manipulation in patients with mechanical neck pain: A randomized clinical trial. *Phys Ther* 2007;87:431–440.

Cook CE. *Orthopedic Manual Therapy: An Evidence-Based Approach*. Upper Saddle River, NJ: Pearson Prentice Hall; 2007.

Denslow JS. Patho-physiologic evidence for the osteopathic lesion: the known, unknown and controversial. *J Am Osteopath Assoc* 1975;74:415.

Educational Council on Osteopathic Principles. Glossary of Osteopathic terminology. In: Ward RC, ed. *Foundations for Osteopathic Medicine*. 2nd ed. Baltimore: Lippincott Williams & Wilkins; 2003:1229–1253.

Evans DW. Mechanisms and effects of spinal high velocity low amplitude thrust manipulation: previous theories. *J Manipulative Physiol Ther* 2002;25:251–262.

Evans DW, Breen AC. A biomechanical model for mechanically efficient cavitation production during spinal manipulation: pre-thrust position and the neutral zone. *J Manipulative Physiol Ther* 2006;29:72–82.

Fernández-de-las-Peñas C, Alonso-Blanco C, Cuadrado ML, Miangolarra JC, Barriga FJ, Pareja JA. Are manual therapies effective in reducing pain from tension-type headache? A systematic review. *Clin J Pain* 2006;22:278–285.

Flynn T, Fritz J, Whitman J, et al. A clinical prediction rule for classifying patients with low back pain who demonstrate short-term improvement with spinal manipulation. *Spine* 2002;27:2835–2843.

Friedrich KM, Trattnig S, Millington SA, et al. High-field magnetic resonance imaging of meniscoids in the zygapophysial joints of the human cervical spine. *Spine* 2007;32:244–248.

Fritz JM, Childs JD, Flynn T. Pragmatic application of a clinical prediction rule in primary care to identify patients with low back pain with a good prognosis following a brief spinal manipulation intervention. *BMC Fam Pract* 2005;6:29.

Fryer G. Somatic dysfunction: updating the concept. *Aust J Osteopathy* 1999;10:14–19.

Fryer G. Inter-vertebral dysfunction: a discussion of the manipulable spinal lesion. *J Osteopath Med* 2003;6:64–73.

Fryette HH. *Principles of Osteopathic Technique*. Carmel, CA: Academy of Applied Osteopathy; 1954.

Gatterman MI. *Foundations of Chiropractic: Subluxation*. St. Louis: Mosby Elsevier; 2005.

Gibbons P, Tehan P. *Manipulation of the Spine, Thorax and Pelvis: An Osteopathic Perspective*. Edinburgh: Churchill Livingstone; 2006.

Greenman PE. *Principles of Manual Medicine*. 3rd ed. Baltimore: Williams & Wilkins; 2003.

Grimsby O, Miller E. A critical review of Dr. Timothy Flynn's guest editorial in the April 2006 issue of JOSPT. *Sci Phys Ther* 2006;15:6–10.

Gross AR, Hoving JL, Haines TA, et al. A Cochrane review of manipulation and mobilization for mechanical neck disorders. *Spine* 2004;29:1541–1548.

Haavik-Taylor H, Murphy B. Cervical spine manipulation alters sensory-motor integration: a somatosensory evoked potential study. *Clin Neurophysiol* 2007;118:391–402.

Haldeman S. *Principles and Practice of Chiropractic*. New York: McGraw-Hill Medical; 2004.

Haldeman S, Dagenais S. Cervicogenic headaches: a critical review. *Spine J* 2001;1:31–46.

Hartman L. *Handbook of Osteopathic Technique*. 3rd ed. Cheltenham, England: Stanley Thornes; 1997.

Hartman L. An osteopathic approach to manipulation. In: Erhard R, ed. *Orthopedic Physical Therapy Clinics of North America*. Philadelphia: WB Saunders; 1998:565–580.

Herzog W. The biomechanics of spinal manipulation. In: Morris CE. *Low Back Syndromes: Integrated Clinical Management*. New York: McGraw-Hill Medical; 2006:597–610.

Hoeger Bement MK, Sluka KA. Pain: perception and mechanisms. In: Magee DJ, Zachazewski JE, Quillen WS, eds. *Scientific Foundations and Principles and Practice in Musculoskeletal Rehabilitation*. St. Louis, MO: Saunders Elsevier; 2007:217–237.

Howell JN, Willard FH. Nociception: new understandings and their possible relation to somatic dysfunction and its treatment. *Ohio Research and Clinical Review*; Spring 2005.

Huijbregts P. Clinical prediction rules: time to scarify the holy cow of specificity? *J Manual Manipulative Therapy* 2007;15:5–8.

Inami S, Shiga T, Tsujino A, et al. Immunohistochemical demonstration of nerve fibers in the synovial fold of the human cervical facet joint. *J Orthop Res* 2001;19:593–596.

Isaac ER, Bookhout MR. *Bourdillon's Spinal Manipulation*. 6th ed. London: Butterworth-Heinemann; 2006.

Kappler R, Kuchera WA. Diagnosis and plan for manual treatment: a description. In: Ward RC, ed. *Foundations for Osteopathic Medicine*. 2nd ed. Baltimore: Lippincott Williams & Wilkins; 2003:574–579.

King W, Lau P, Lees R, Bogduk N. The validity of manual examination in assessing patients with neck pain. *Spine J* 2007;7:22–26.

Korr IM. The emerging concept of the osteopathic lesion. *J Am Osteopath Assoc* 1948;48:127–138.

Korr IM. Proprioceptors, and somatic dysfunction. *J Am Osteopath Assoc* 1975;74:638.

Kos J, Wolf J. Die "menisci" der Zwischenwirbelgelenke und ihre mogliche Rolle bei Wirbelblockierungen. *Man Med* 1972;10:105–114.

Krauss JR, Evjenth O, Creighton D. *Translatoric Spinal Manipulation*. Minneapolis, MN: Lakeview Media; 2006.

Kuchera ML. Somatic dysfunction. In: Hutson M, Ellis R. *Textbook of Musculoskeletal Disorders*. Oxford: Oxford University Press; 2006:27–46.

Lederman E. *The Science and Practice of Manual Therapy*. 2nd ed. Edinburgh: Elsevier Churchill Livingstone; 2005.

Lenssinck ML, Damen L, Verhagen AP, Berger MY, Passchier J, Koes BW. The effectiveness of physiotherapy and manipulation in patients with tension-type headache: a systematic review. *Pain* 2004;112:381–388.

Lewit K. *Manipulative Therapy in Rehabilitation of the Locomotor System*. 3rd ed. Oxford: Butterworth-Heinemann; 1999.

Lewit K. Managing syndromes and finding the key link. In: Liebenson C, ed. *Rehabilitation of the Spine: A Practitioner's Manual*. 2nd ed. Baltimore: Lippincott Williams & Wilkins; 2007:776–797.

Lewit K, Kolar P. Chain reactions related to the cervical spine. In: Murphy DR, ed. *Conservative Management of Cervical Spine Syndromes*. New York: McGraw-Hill; 2000:515–530.

Liebenson C, ed. *Rehabilitation of the Spine: A Practitioner's Manual*. 2nd ed. Baltimore: Lippincott Williams & Wilkins; 2007.

Maigne R. *Diagnosis and Treatment of Pain of Vertebral Origin: A Manual Medicine Approach*. Baltimore: Williams & Wilkins; 1996.

Maigne JY, Vautravers P. Mechanisms of action of spinal manipulative therapy. *Joint Bone Spine* 2003;70:336–341.

Malisza KL, Stroman PW, Turner A, et al. Functional MRI of the rat lumbar spinal cord involving painful stimulation and the effect of peripheral joint mobilization. *J Magn Reson Imaging* 2003a;18:152–159.

Malisza KL, Gregorash L, Turner A, et al. Functional MRI involving painful stimulation of the ankle and the effect of physiotherapy joint mobilization. *Magn Reson Imaging* 2003b;21:489–496.

Mennell JM. *Back Pain: Diagnosis and Treatment Using Manipulative Techniques*. Boston: Little Brown; 1960.

Mennell JM. *The Musculoskeletal System: Differential Diagnosis from Symptoms and Physical Signs*. Gaithersburg, MD: Aspen Press; 1992.

Middleton HC. Osteopathic technique: fines in high velocity thrust techniques. *Br Osteopath J* 1971;5:9–15.

Mitchell FL Jr. Towards a definition of somatic dysfunction. *Osteopath Ann* 1979;7:12–25.

Murphy DR, ed. *Conservative Management of Cervical Spine Syndromes*. New York: McGraw-Hill; 2000.

Murphy DR, Morris C. Manual examination of the patient. In: Haldeman S, ed. *Principles and Practice of Chiropractic*. 3rd ed. New York: McGraw-Hill; 2004:593–610.

Nicholas AS, Nicholas EA. *Atlas of Osteopathic Techniques*. Philadelphia: Lippincott Williams & Wilkins; 2007.

Panjabi M. The stabilizing system of the spine. Part II: neutral zone and stability hypothesis. *J Spinal Disorders* 1992;5:390–397.

Parsons J, Marcer N. *Osteopathy: Models for Diagnosis, Treatment and Practice*. Edinburgh: Churchill Livingstone Elsevier; 2006.

Pettman E. *Manipulative Thrust Techniques: An Evidence-Based Approach*. Abbotsford, Canada: Aphema Publishing; 2006.

Pickar JG. Neurophysiological effects of spinal manipulation. *Spine J* 2002;2:357–371.

Potter L, McCarthy C, Oldham J. Physiological effects of spinal manipulation: a review of proposed theories. *Phys Ther Rev* 2005;10:163–170.

Rome PL. Usage of chiropractic terminology in the literature: 296 ways to say "subluxation." *Chiropractic Technique* 1996;8:49–60.

Sammut E, Searle-Barnes P. *Osteopathic Diagnosis*. Cheltenham, England: Stanley Thornes; 1998.

Seffinger MA, Hruby RJ. *Evidence-Based Manual Medicine: A Problem-Oriented Approach*. Philadelphia: Saunders Elsevier; 2007.

Seffinger MA, Najm WI, Mishra SL, et al. Reliability of spinal palpation for diagnosis of back and neck pain: a systematic review of the literature. *Spine* 2004;29:E413–E425.

Skyba DA, Rhadakrishnan R, Rohlwing JJ, et al. Joint manipulation reduces hyperalgesia by activation of monoamine receptors but not opioid or GABA receptors in the spinal cord. *Pain* 2003;106:159–168.

Sluka K, Wright A. Knee joint mobilization reduces secondary mechanical hyperalgesia induced by capsaicin injection into the ankle joint. *Eur J Pain* 2001;5:81–87.

Sluka KA, Hoeger MK, Skyba DA. Basic science mechanism of non-pharmacological treatments of pain. In: Giamberaridino MA, ed. *Pain. An Updated Review: Refresher Course*. Seattle: IASP Press; 2002.

Souvlis T, Vicenzino B, Wright A. Neurophysiological effects of spinal manual therapy. In: Boyling JD, Jull GA, eds. *Grieves Modern Manual Therapy*. Edinburgh: Churchill Livingstone; 2004:367–380.

Stochkendahl MJ, Christensen HW, Hartvigsen J, et al. Manual examination of the spine: a systematic critical literature review of reproducibility. *J Manipulative Physiol Ther* 2006;29:475–485.

Stoddard A. *Manual of Osteopathic Technique*. London: Hutchinson Medical Publications; 1959.

Stoddard A. *Manual of Osteopathic Practice*. London: Harper Row; 1969.

Triano JJ. The mechanics of spinal manipulation. In: Herzog W, ed. *Clinical Biomechanics of Spinal Manipulation*. New York: Churchill Livingstone; 2000:92–190.

Triano JJ. Biomechanics of spinal manipulative therapy. *Spine J* 2001;1:121–130.

Triano JJ. Manipulation. In: Cole AJ, Herring S, eds. *Low Back Pain Handbook: A Guide for the Practicing Clinician*. 2nd ed. Philadelphia: Hanley & Belfus; 2003:169–178.

Tseng YL, Wang WT, Chen WY, et al. Predictors for the immediate responders to cervical manipulation in patients with neck pain. *Man Ther* 2006;11:306–315.

Van Buskirk RL. Nociceptive reflexes and the somatic dysfunction: a model. *J Am Osteopath Assoc* 1990;90:792.

Van Buskirk RL. *The Still Technique Manual*. 2nd ed. Indianapolis, IN: American Academy of Osteopathy; 2007:24–34.

Van Trijffel E, Anderegg O, Bossuyt PM, Lucas C. Inter-examiner reliability of passive assessment of intervertebral motion in the cervical and lumbar spine: a systematic review. *Man Ther* 2005;10:256–269.

Vernon H, Humphreys K, Hagino C. Chronic mechanical neck pain in adults treated by manual therapy: a systematic review of change scores in randomized clinical trials. *J Manipulative Physiol Ther* 2007;30:215–227.

Vicenzino B, O'Callaghan J, Felicity K, Wright A. No influence of naloxone on the initial hypoalgesic effects of spinal manual therapy. Presented at the Ninth World Congress on Pain; Vienna, Austria; 2000.

Wells K. *A Model for Teaching and Assessing Skills in High Velocity Low Amplitude Thrust Techniques*. Victoria, Australia: Keri Moore; 2000.

Woolf AD, Pfleger B. Burden of major musculoskeletal conditions. *Bull World Health Org* 2003;81:646–656.

Wright A. Hypoalgesia post-manipulative therapy: a review of potential neuro-physiological mechanism. *Man Ther* 1995;1:11–16.

Wright A, Sluka K. Non-pharmacological treatments for musculoskeletal pain. *Clin J Pain* 2001;17:33–46.

Zhu Y, Haldeman S, Hsieh CY, et al. Do cerebral potentials to magnetic stimulation of paraspinal muscles reflect changes in palpable muscle spasm, low back pain, and activity scores? *J Manipulative Physiol Ther* 2000;23:458–464.

Zusman M. Mechanisms of musculoskeletal physiotherapy. *Phys Ther Rev* 2004;9:39–49.

Thoracic Spine Interventions for the Management of Patients with Headache

Paul Glynn, PT, DPT, OCS, FAAOMPT, Bill Egan, PT, DPT, OCS, FAAOMPT, and Josh Cleland, PT, DPT, PhD, OCS, FAAOMPT

The concept of addressing impairments in areas remote to the patient's primary zone of pain symptoms has been termed *regional interdependence*, and the effectiveness of treating these distant regions has been well documented (Vicenzino et al., 1996; Cleland et al., 2004b; Boyle, 1999; Bergman et al., 2004; Bang & Deyle, 2000; Struijs et al., 2003; Cibulka et al., 1986; Suter et al., 1999, 2000; Deyle et al., 2000, 2005; Whitman et al., 2005, 2006; Cliborne et al., 2004; Currier et al., 2007; Sutlive et al., in press). More specifically related to the cervicocranial region, studies have demonstrated the favorable benefit of addressing thoracic spine impairments in individuals with mechanical neck pain (Cleland et al., 2005a, 2007a, 2007b; Flynn et al., 2001), whiplash-associated disorders (Fernández-de-las-Peñas et al., 2004), cervical radiculopathy (Cleland et al., 2005b; Piva et al., 2000), and low-grade cervical myelopathy (Browder et al., 2004).

In a randomized controlled trial, Cleland et al. (2005a) demonstrated that patients with mechanical neck pain who receive thoracic spine thrust manipulation experienced immediate and significant (P <0.001) improvements in pain, as measured by the Visual Analogue Scale, compared with patients receiving a placebo manipulation. The improvement in pain in the group receiving thoracic spine thrust manipulation was 15.5 mm (SD 7.7) (95% CI: 11.8, 19.2), compared with a 4.2 mm (SD 4.6) (95% CI: 1.9, 6.6) change in the group receiving placebo manipulation. Thoracic spine manipulation has also been compared with nonthrust manipulation in individuals with mechanical neck pain (Cleland et al., 2007b). Results at a 48-hour follow-up indicated significant improvement in both disability and pain (P <0.001) for those receiving thrust manipulation. Disability as measured by the Neck Disability Index (NDI) was reduced by 15.5% in those receiving thrust manipulation, compared with a 5.5% reduction in those receiving nonthrust manipulation. Pain as measured by the Numerical Pain Rating Scale (NPRS) was reduced by 2.6 points in those receiving thrust manipulation and 0.5 points in those receiving nonthrust manipulation. Despite the growing evidence for the application of thoracic spine thrust manipulation in individuals with mechanical neck pain, until recently clinicians did not have a means of identifying those who would most benefit from these techniques. This subgroup of patients has recently been identified through the derivation of a clinical prediction rule (Cleland et al., 2007a).

Clinical prediction rules are designed to assist in the decision-making process. They improve diagnostic accuracy or prediction of outcomes based on a subset of possible predictor variables identified during the historical or physical examination (Childs & Cleland, 2006). In Cleland's clinical prediction rule, a parsimonious set of six variables was retained in the logistic regression analysis as maximizing the accuracy of predicting patients with neck pain likely to respond to thoracic spine thrust manipulation. Variables included symptom duration of less than 30 days, no symptoms distal to the shoulder, patient reports that looking up does not aggravate symptoms, Fear Avoidance Belief Questionnaire–Physical Activity Subscale (FABQPA) less than 12, decreased upper thoracic spine kyphosis (T3-T5), and cervical extension less than 30°. If four of the six criteria were met, a positive likelihood ratio (+LR) of 12 was noted, producing a large and conclusive shift in post-test probability that those individuals would benefit from the techniques. As mentioned by the authors, wide confidence intervals were found with four of six variables (95% CI: 2.28, 70.8). Therefore, clinicians may demonstrate greater accuracy by using three of six criteria as the treatment threshold to implement thoracic thrust manipulation (+ LR of 5.5; 95% CI: 2.72, 12.0).

Fernández-de-las-Peñas et al. (2004) conducted a randomized controlled trial comparing the effects of a physical therapy package consisting of electrical modalities, stretching, active exercise, and nonthrust manipulation to a group who also received two thoracic thrust manipulations in individuals suffering from whiplash-associated disorders. Those receiving thoracic spine thrust manipulation experienced a significantly greater (P <0.003) reduction in pain than those who did not receive the thrust procedure.

In a prospective case series involving 11 individuals with cervical radiculopathy, a physical therapy package consisting of manual therapy, cervical traction, and strengthening produced clinically meaningful gains (Cleland et al., 2005b). The manual therapy component included cervical lateral glides performed with the involved upper extremity in the dynamic neural tension position of shoulder abduction, external rotation, elbow extension, and wrist/finger extension. Additionally, thrust manipulations were applied to the upper and middle thoracic spine. The mean number of treatment sessions was 7.1, with 91% of patients experiencing a clinically meaningful improvement in pain and functioning (Cleland et al., 2005b).

In a prospective case series involving seven patients with grade 1 cervical compressive myelopathy, Browder et al. (2004) utilized thrust manipulation aimed at the upper and middle thoracic spine in combination with cervical traction over an average of nine treatment sessions. A clinically meaningful decrease in pain of 5 points was found on the NPRS. The functional rating index improved by a mean of 26%, and dizziness was eliminated in three of four patients. There were three patients with headache complaints, and full resolution occurred in two of three by the end of treatment. Despite a lack of full headache resolution, the remaining patient exhibited a reduction in headache frequency and intensity, thus presenting preliminary evidence for the benefit of treating the thoracic spine in this patient population.

Despite this growing body of scientific literature, evidence supporting treatment of the thoracic spine in individuals with tension-type or cervicogenic headache has just begun to emerge. Therefore, although many of the techniques described in this chapter have been shown to be beneficial in the management of patients with several cervical conditions, further research is necessary to determine whether a cause and effect relationship exists between manual therapy directed at the thoracic spine and improved outcomes in patients with headaches.

One rationale to include thoracic spine interventions in the treatment of patients with cervicogenic and tension-type headache results from the theory that disturbances in joint mobility in the thoracic spine may be an underlying contributor to musculoskeletal disorders in the neck (Greenman et al., 1996; Johansson & Sojka, 1991; Knutson, 2001). Although the biomechanical link between the thoracic and cervical spine appears intuitive, this theory has only recently been investigated (Norlander et al., 1996, 1997; Norlander & Nordgren, 1998). Norlander et al. investigated whether mobility in the cervicothoracic motion segment was associated with musculoskeletal neck/shoulder pain symptoms. They reported a significant association between decreased mobility in the thoracic spine and the presence of subjective complaints associated with neck pain. Although the exact mechanism by which thoracic spine thrust manipulation decreases pain and spasm and increases mobility is not clear, researchers have reported changes in muscle electrical activity (Shambaugh, 1995), reduced reflex muscle spasm (Johansson & Sojka, 1991), and increased intersegmental joint play

subsequent to a spinal manipulation (Cassidy et al., 1992; Norlander et al., 1997; Norlander & Nordgren, 1998). Preliminary evidence exists suggesting that thoracic spine manipulation reduces pain and disability in patients with neck pain (Cleland et al., 2005a, 2007a, 2007b; Flynn et al., 2001; Fernández-de-las-Peñas et al., 2007a). Norlander and Nordgren (1998) also noted that reduced upper thoracic mobility was a significant predictor of headaches, with 50% of individuals demonstrating headache symptoms over a 12-month time frame. Because of this emerging evidence, assessment and subsequent treatment of the thoracic spine should be considered in individuals with headaches.

Another theoretical link between the thoracic spine and headaches is derived from the potential influence of posture on both the articular and muscular structures in the area. Forward head posture (FHP) has been found in individuals with both cervicogenic and tension-type headaches as compared with controls (Fernández-de-las-Peñas et al., 2006a, 2006b, 2007a, 2007b; Watson & Trott, 1993). In three separate studies, Fernández-de-las-Peñas et al. (2006a, 2006b, 2007a) demonstrated a significantly reduced craniovertebral angle—that is, increased FHP—in patients with chronic tension-type headache as compared with controls ($P <0.01$). Watson and Trott (1993) also documented an increased FHP in patients with cervicogenic headache and migraine as compared with a nonheadache population ($P <0.001$). Postural deviations, including FHP, have also been linked to higher headache frequency and longer headache duration (Fernández-de-las-Peñas et al., 2006a). Because of the evolving connection between FHP and headaches and the potential influence of the thoracic spine on both soft-tissue and articular structures of the cervical spine, the authors recommend examination and subsequent treatment of identified impairments.

Preliminary evidence has begun to suggest that an interdependent link may exist between the thoracic spine and cervical spine because the combined treatment of these regions has resulted in excellent outcomes in patients presenting with cervicogenic and tension-type headaches. For example, research has indicated that a multimodal approach utilizing postural reeducation and endurance training of the scapular stabilizing muscles in addition to cervical interventions produced decreased headache frequency and intensity and neck pain ($P <0.05$) in a population of 200 subjects with cervicogenic headaches (Jull et al., 2002). Van Duijn et al. (2007) treated an individual with cervicogenic headaches with a combination of thrust and nonthrust manipulations applied to the cervical spine, thoracic spine, and ribs, as well as stretching and strengthening of the cervicothoracic musculature. A significant reduction in both neck disability and head pain was produced over 16 visits. Hammill et al. (1996) found a significant reduction in tension-type headache (P <0.001), produced over 6 visits, with the use of postural reeducation, strengthening, massage, and cervicothoracic muscle stretching. The obtained benefits continued at a 12-month follow-up. In a single case report, Issa and Huijbregts (2006) have demonstrated a regionally applied multimodal approach to the treatment of an individual with chronic tension-type headache and migraine that included orthopaedic manual therapy, exercise, patient education, and myofascial trigger point work. Both the cervical and thoracic regions were incorporated into treatment producing clinically meaningful changes in disability and headache symptoms. Petersen (2003) noted that the combination of manual therapy applied to the cervical spine, as well as muscle reeducation of the neck flexor and scapula stabilizers, decreased headache frequency and intensity after 8 treatment sessions in a single-subject study of a patient with cervicogenic headache. McDonnell et al. (2005) addressed the impairments of the cervical, thoracic, and lumbar regions in a patient with cervicogenic headache. Headache frequency and intensity decreased, and clinically meaningful change was produced in the patient's level of neck disability.

The interventions of this chapter focus on manual therapy techniques used in the clinical literature as well as techniques commonly used in the management of cervicogenic and tension-type headache in the clinic by the authors. The techniques include both thrust and nonthrust manipulation directed at the cervicothoracic junction and thoracic spine. Thrust manipulation has been defined as a high-velocity, low-amplitude therapeutic movement applied near the end range of motion, whereas nonthrust manipulations include therapeutic passive movements that do not involve thrust (American Physical Therapy Association, 2004). These are the accepted terms of the American Academy of Orthopedic Manual Physical Therapists (AAOMPT), and in keeping with the goal of the AAOMPT to standardize nomenclature, we use these terms throughout the chapter.

THORACIC SPINE SOFT-TISSUE INTERVENTIONS

Forward head posture has been associated with compensatory changes throughout the musculoskeletal system (Donatelli & Wooden, 2001). Because of the upper thoracic flexion, the scapula may assume a position of protraction and downward rotation (Donatelli & Wooden, 2001). This may lead to a loss of proper postural functioning of the middle and lower trapezius muscles as well as the serratus anterior (Donatelli & Wooden, 2001; Jull, 1997). Conversely, the pectoralis major and minor, levator scapula, scalene, sternocleidomastoid (SCM), and upper trapezius muscles may be placed in a shortened position (Jull, 1997). Because of the above adaptive changes and their potential to perpetuate FHP, which has been linked to headaches, it is recommended that these soft-tissue impairments be addressed through the use of self- and manual stretching (Jull, 1997).

Stretching of the Cervicothoracic Musculature

The benefit of incorporating cervicothoracic muscle stretching into a multimodal treatment program for the headache patient is well documented (Jull, 1997; Jull et al., 2002; Hammill et al., 1996; Issa & Huijbregts, 2006; Van Duijn et al., 2007; McDonnell et al., 2005). The decision to initiate stretching may be based on the identification of impairments through a side-to-side comparison during the physical examination.

Stretching the Left Anterior and Middle Scalene

The patient lies supine with the head off the end of the plinth, supported by the therapist's right hand (**Figure 24.1**). Apply gentle downward pressure with your right shoulder onto the patient's forehead, creating and maintaining upper cervical flexion throughout the remainder of the stretch. Depress the clavicle and first rib with your left hand. Extend the middle/lower cervical spine by translating the head-neck in an anterior-to-posterior direction. Side-bend the head and neck toward the right side until a stretch is felt. Initiate left rotation if further refinement is needed.

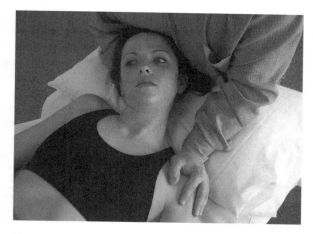

Figure 24.1 Scalene (Anterior and Middle) Stretch

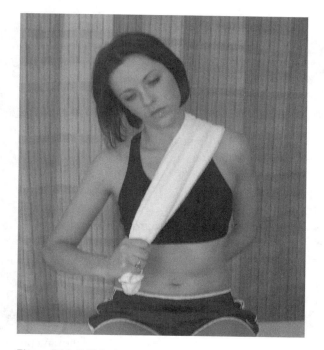

Figure 24.2 Self Scalene Stretch

Self-Stretch of the Left Anterior and Middle Scalene

In the upright sitting position, the patient places a towel over the left medial shoulder and pulls down through the towel to depress the first rib (**Figure 24.2**). Chin-tuck and then side-bend to the right until a stretch is felt in the lateral cervical spine area. Add gentle left cervical rotation as needed to refine the stretch.

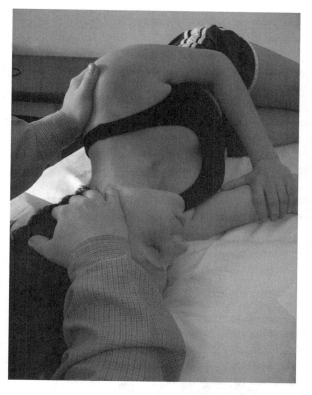

Figure 24.3 Levator Scapula, Splenius Cervicis, and Posterior Scalene Stretch

Stretching the Left Levator Scapulae, Splenius Cervicis, and Posterior Scalene

With the patient lying on his or her right side, position the supported head and neck in flexion, right side-bending, and right rotation (**Figure 24.3**). Use your right hand to stabilize this position through the lateral aspect of the middle/upper cervical area. The left hand grasps the anteromedial aspect of the left scapula. Depress, upwardly rotate, and posteriorly tilt the scapula until a stretch is felt.

Self-Stretch of the Left Levator Scapulae, Splenius Cervicis, and Posterior Scalene

In the sitting position, have the patient place his or her left hand on the upper back to create scapular upward rotation (**Figure 24.4**). Flex, right side-bend, and right rotate the cervical spine until a stretch is noted in the posterolateral cervicothoracic area. To refine the stretch, the patient can further abduct and extend the arm at the end of inhalation followed by gentle manual

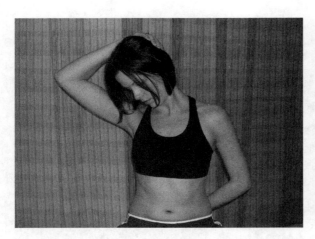

Figure 24.4 Self Levator Scapula, Splenius Cervicis, and Posterior Scale Stretch

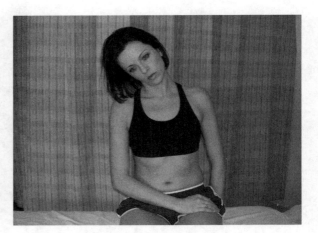

Figure 24.6 Self Upper Trapezius Stretch

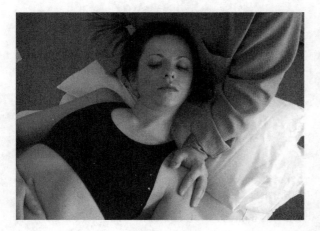

Figure 24.5 Upper Trapezius Stretch

pressure of the cervical spine into flexion, side bending, and rotation while he or she exhales.

Stretching the Left Upper Trapezius and Sternocleidomastoid

With the patient supine, the therapist uses his or her left hand to press caudad through the lateral shoulder and clavicle (**Figure 24.5**). With the right hand, flex, right side-bend, and left rotate the patient's head and neck until a stretch is noted. Final adjustments can be made by adding further downward left shoulder pressure.

Self-Stretch of the Left Upper Trapezius and Sternocleidomastoid

In the upright sitting position, the patient places his or her left hand under the buttocks to maintain shoulder depression during the motion (**Figure 24.6**). The cervical spine is flexed, right side-bent, and left rotated until a stretch is felt in the left upper trapezius. To further refine the motion, the patient may add a chin tuck. To increase emphasis on the left sternocleidomastoid, the cervical spine is extended slightly, right side-bent, and left rotated until the stretch is felt.

Stretching the Left Pectoralis Major

With the patient in prone position, apply downward stabilizing pressure through the left scapula with your right hand (**Figure 24.7**). Externally rotate the humerus and then raise the patient's left arm into varying degrees of flexion and abduction to emphasize the sternal and clavicular portions of the muscle. Ensure that the stretch is felt though the chest and not the anterior shoulder.

Self-Stretch of the Pectoralis Major

The patient faces inward into a corner with the feet approximately 12 inches away. The arms are placed in a W position to emphasize the clavicular portion of the muscle (**Figure 24.8**) or an overhead Y position to emphasize the sternal head of the muscle. The patient leans forward until a stretch is felt in the pectoralis muscle.

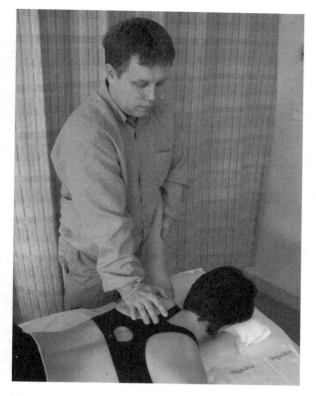

Figure 24.7 Pectoralis Major Stretch

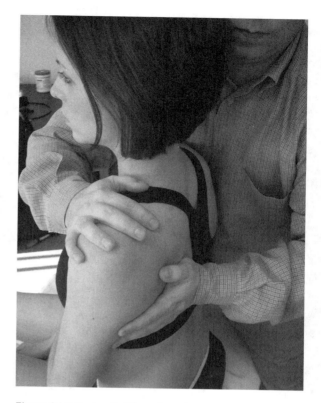

Figure 24.9 Pectoralis Minor Stretch

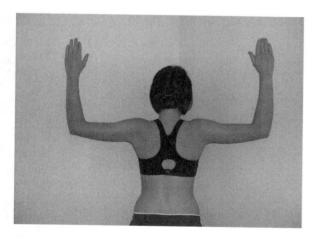

Figure 24.8 Self Pectoralis Major Stretch

Stretching the Left Pectoralis Minor

With the patient in the seated position, place your right hand over the patient's left coracoid process (**Figure 24.9**). Use the soft area between the thenar and hypothenar eminences because the process is often very tender to pressure. Place your left hand over the inferior angle of the scapula. Ask the patient to take a deep breath in, and at the end of inhalation apply anterior-to-posterior pressure over the coracoid process and posterior-to-anterior pressure through the inferior angle of scapula. This will create a posterior tilt of the scapula. Hold the position as the patient exhales. Confirm a stretch in the area of the pectoralis minor.

Self-Stretch of the Left Pectoralis Minor

With the patient in the supine position, have him or her take a deep breath in (**Figure 24.10**). At the end of inhalation, the patient depresses, adducts, and posteriorly tips the scapula. This position is held during exhalation.

Strengthening of the Scapular Muscles

Muscular endurance training of the scapular muscles in individuals with headache disorders has been studied

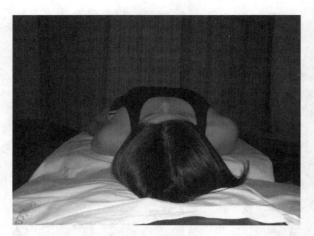

Figure 24.10 Self Pectoralis Minor Stretch

by Jull et al. (2002). In a large randomized controlled trial, patients with cervicogenic headache were randomized to receive cervical mobilization/manipulation, endurance training of the scapular stabilizers and deep neck flexor muscles, or both manual therapy and exercise, or to act as a control group. Results demonstrated a significant reduction in headache frequency and intensity lasting 1 year for all treatment groups versus the control group (P <0.05 for all). At the 7-week follow-up, the combination of endurance training exercise and manual therapy demonstrated a 10% higher percentage of good to excellent outcomes as compared with the other groups. Additionally, numerous less robust evidence has indicated the benefit of including scapular muscle strengthening in a physical therapy package for patients with both cervicogenic and tension-type headache (McDonnell et al., 2005; Hammill et al., 1996; Petersen, 2003; van Duijn et al., 2007). The decision to initiate strengthening may be based on the identification of weakness through manual muscle testing during the physical examination.

Middle Trapezius Strengthening

With the patient in the prone position, the arms are actively elevated to approximately 90° of abduction (**Figure 24.11**). The arms are externally rotated until the thumb is pointing toward the ceiling. The patient then adducts the scapula while horizontally abducting the arm. This position has demonstrated significant middle trapezius activity during surface electromyographic testing (Ekstrom et al., 2003).

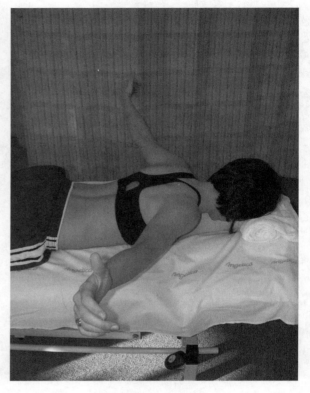

Figure 24.11 Middle Trapezius Strengthening

Lower Trapezius Strengthening

With the patient in the prone position, the arms are elevated to approximately 120° of abduction (**Figure 24.12**). The arms are then externally rotated until the thumbs are pointing toward the ceiling. The patient adducts and depresses the scapula while flexing the arm overhead. Ekstrom et al. (2003) demonstrated that this technique significantly increased lower trapezius contraction as compared with other conventional exercises. If patients are unable to assume the prone position or tolerate this approach, they can begin by performing the motion as described previously, but in the standing position.

Serratus Anterior Strengthening

Research has described the push-up with a plus position as the most effective means of contracting the serratus anterior (Ludewig et al., 2004; Decker et al., 1999). With the patient in the push-up or modified push-up position, he or she is instructed to arch the upper back while keeping the elbows straight (**Figure 24.13**).

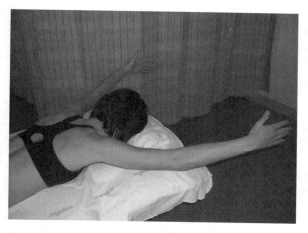

Figure 24.12 Lower Trapezius Strengthening

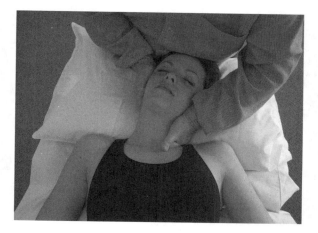

Figure 24.14 Supine First Rib Thrust Manipulation

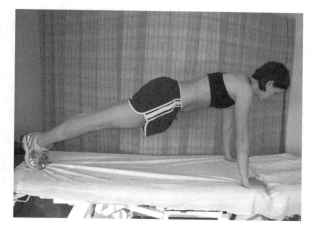

Figure 24.13 Serratus Anterior Strengthening

Emphasis should be placed on protracting the scapula. If these positions are uncomfortable for the patient, an alternative may be the wall push-up position.

FIRST RIB THRUST AND NONTHRUST MANIPULATIONS

The anterior and middle scalenes have attachment on the first rib and run superiorly until their attachment in the subcranial area. Theoretically, an elevated first rib may allow for scalene shortening and subcranial compression, which may create cervicogenic headache. Because of its potential influence, this area should be treated if it is found to be hypomobile and painful during examination. The cervical rotation lateral flexion test (CRLF) described in Chapter 15 may further assist in identifying mobility limitations in this area (Lindgren et al., 1992).

Left First Rib Inferior-Medial Thrust and Nonthrust Manipulations

Left Rib Management with the Patient Supine

The patient is supine with the head resting on the plinth. The therapist side-bends the head and neck toward the involved left side of the patient. Use your left hand to push the upper trapezius from an anterior to posterior direction. Follow this with gentle caudal pressure until you feel the first rib. Using the palmar surface of your second metacarpophalangeal joint, apply further inferomedial pressure until the end-feel is noted. The therapist can then apply a thrust or nonthrust manipulation (**Figure 24.14**).

Left Rib Management with the Patient Seated

If the patient is unable to assume the supine position, a seated technique may also be applied. The therapist places the patient's lower extremity on the side opposite to the hypomobile first rib, onto the table (in this case the right lower extremity). The knee is flexed, allowing the leg to support the patient's trunk. The patient's right arm is placed on the therapist's right lower extremity. The therapist uses his or her body to introduce thoracic extension and right lateral translation to the patient's thoracic spine. The patient's head is

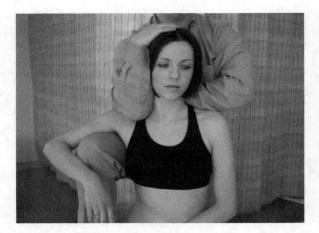

Figure 24.15 Sitting First Rib Thrust Manipulation

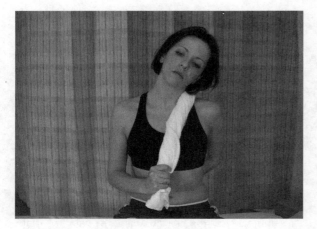

Figure 24.16 Self First Rib Nonthrust Manipulation

side-bent to the left and rotated right down to the cervicothoracic junction. Place your left hypothenar eminence on the first rib, just lateral to the transverse process. Apply inferomedial pressure until the end-feel is noted and follow this with either a thrust or nonthrust manipulation (**Figure 24.15**).

Self Nonthrust Manipulation of the Left First Rib

Sitting with upright posture, the patient places a towel over the left first rib (**Figure 24.16**). The cervical spine is side-bent to the left to relax the scalene muscles. The patient pulls in an inferomedial direction through the towel to impart an inferior nonthrust manipulation.

THORACIC THRUST AND NONTHRUST MANIPULATIONS

The thrust techniques in this section may be indicated when physical examination reveals hypomobility as detected through passive mobility assessment of the cervicothoracic junction, as well as decreased upper thoracic motion noted during active movement of the cervical spine. Various versions of the following techniques have been utilized in the care of patients with mechanical neck pain (Cleland et al., 2005a, 2007a, 2007b; Flynn et al., 2001; Fernández-de-las-Peñas et al., 2007a), cervical radiculopathy (Cleland et al., 2005b; Piva et al., 2000), whiplash-associated disorder (Fernández-de-las-Peñas et al., 2004), and grade 1 cervical myelopathy (Browder et al., 2004). Currently three case reports exist indicating the positive effect of thoracic spine thrust and nonthrust manipulations in individuals with headaches (Viti & Paris, 2000; Issa & Huijgbregts, 2006; van Duijn et al., 2007). In all instances manual therapy was utilized in conjunction with exercise, which agrees with the current recommendations of systematic reviews for patients with mechanical neck pain both with and without headaches (Gross et al., 2004). Despite the lack of high-quality evidence indicating the benefit of thoracic manipulative techniques, both biomechanical and anatomic associations have been outlined by Norlander et al. (1996, 1997; Norlander & Nordgren, 1998).

Upper Thoracic Extension Thrust Manipulation

With the patient in the supine position, have the patient clasp his or her hands at the base of the neck (**Figure 24.17**). Roll the patient toward you and place your hand, which is in the pistol-grip position (**Figure 24.18**), over the central upper thoracic region. The spinous processes of the thoracic vertebrae should sit between the flexed fingers and the thenar and hypothenar eminences. Your manipulative hand stabilizes the inferior vertebrae of the hypomobile motion segment. Roll the patient back onto your hand and apply downward pressure through the elbows until you feel the superior vertebrae of the motion segment begin to move. Pull your manipulative hand caudally to impart final minor extension adjustments. If further refinement is necessary, have the patient bridge upward until increased pressure is noted on the inferior vertebrae. Using your body weight, push downward through the patient's arms,

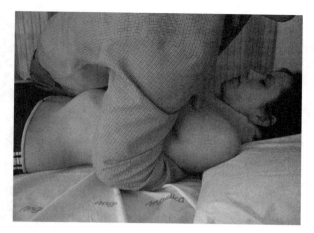

Figure 24.17 Upper Thoracic Extension Thrust Manipulation

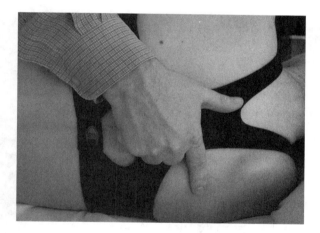

Figure 24.18 Pistol-Grip Hand Position

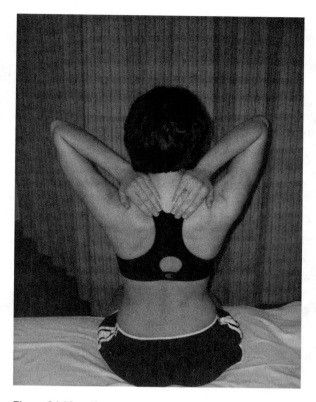

Figure 24.19 Self Upper Thoracic Extension Nonthrust Manipulation

A chair may also be used to create the extension fulcrum if the patient's hands are unable to create an acceptable level of posteroanterior pressure (**Figure 24.20**).

Upper Thoracic Flexion Thrust Manipulation

With the patient supine and hands clasped behind the neck, roll the patient toward you and place your pistol-grip hand at the level of the dysfunction (**Figure 24.21**). Roll the patient back onto your hand and flex the patient's cervical spine up until you feel the superior vertebrae of the motion segment begin to move. Place downward pressure through the patient's elbows and impart a thrust manipulation.

If the patient is unable to assume the supine position, an alternative technique can be used in a sitting position (**Figure 24.22**). Have the patient place his or her hands with interlaced fingers at the superior vertebrae of the motion segment. Standing behind the patient, loop your hands through the patient's arms.

taking up the soft-tissue slack, and apply a thrust manipulation at the restrictive barrier.

Self Upper Thoracic Nonthrust Extension Manipulation

While sitting, the patient places his or her fingertips on both sides of the vertebrae at the upper level of the motion segment (**Figure 24.19**). The patient should be cued to sit up tall and then add further posteroanterior pressure at the level of the facet joints. Shoulder horizontal abduction and scapula retraction may further emphasize the extension moment. To avoid overextension of the cervical spine, the patient should be asked to maintain a chin tuck throughout the motion.

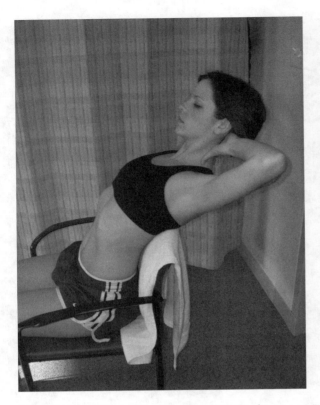

Figure 24.20 Self Upper Thoracic Extension Nonthrust Manipulation with Chair

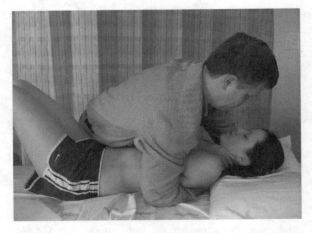

Figure 24.21 Upper Thoracic Flexion Thrust Manipulation

Gently push forward through your hands and chest until motion is localized to the target area. Using your legs and trunk as the primary force, lift quickly upward, creating a distraction manipulation at the cervicothoracic junction.

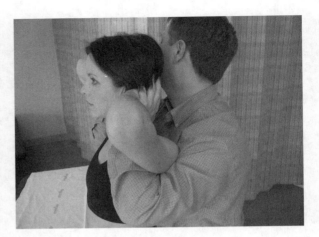

Figure 24.22 Self Upper Thoracic Flexion Nonthrust Manipulation

Self Upper Thoracic Flexion Nonthrust Manipulation

While sitting, the patient places his or her fingertips on both sides of the vertebrae at the upper level of the motion segment (**Figure 24.23**). Thoracic flexion is introduced by allowing the upper back to round. Overpressure is added to the segment of interest by placing the elbows in by their side and pulling forward and downward through the motion segment. Verbal cues should be given to avoid strain on the neck.

Supine Thoracic Distraction Thrust Manipulation

This technique may be used when a patient demonstrates hypomobility or pain provocation or both in the middle thoracic area. In the author's opinion, this approach may be more comfortable for patients who have noted discomfort with attempts to flex or extend the middle thoracic spine, because the thrust is directed cranially, creating distraction. Place your pistol-grip hand over the inferior vertebrae of the motion segment and roll the patient back into the supine position (**Figure 24.24**). Cross the patient's arms in front over his or her chest with the opposite arm on top. A towel roll placed between the arms and chest can be utilized if further comfort is required. Pivot your hips and body so that they are facing toward the patient's head. With the uninvolved arm, reach around the upper trunk and introduce slight flexion to

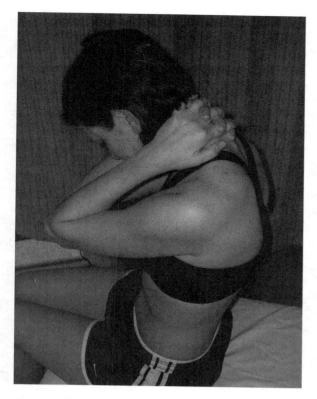

Figure 24.23 Sitting Cervicothoracic Junction Thrust Manipulation

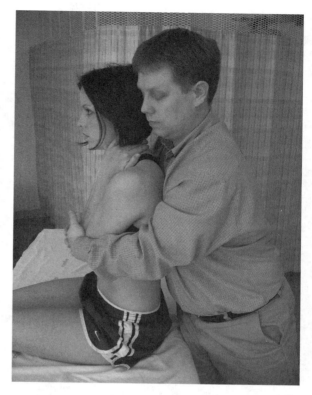

Figure 24.25 Sitting Thoracic Distraction Thrust Manipulation

Seated Thoracic Distraction Thrust Manipulation

If the patient is unable to assume the supine position, an alternative technique may be utilized. Position the patient in a sitting position with his or her hands behind the base of the neck (**Figure 24.25**). Stand behind the patient and place your chest at the level of the thoracic spine to be manipulated. Reach around the patient and grasp his or her elbows, pulling the patient in tightly against your sternum. A towel roll placed between the patient's arms and sternum may be used for patient or therapist comfort. Localize the force by performing fine motor adjustments until you feel the area has been identified and all soft-tissue slack has been removed. Perform the manipulation by pulling the patient's elbows toward you and thrusting in a cranial direction.

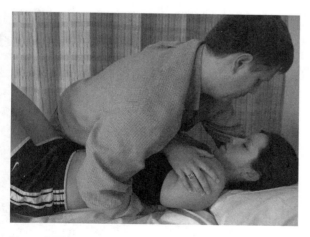

Figure 24.24 Supine Thoracic Distraction Thrust Manipulation

Supine Thoracic Flexion Thrust Manipulation

Place your pistol-grip hand over the lower vertebrae of the motion segment (**Figure 24.26**). Roll the patient onto

lift the trunk off the plinth. Press your body weight through the patient's arms to take up the slack and then thrust manipulate upward toward the head of the table.

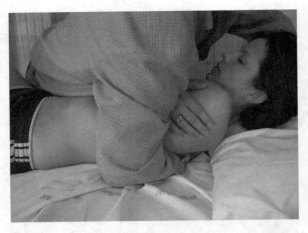

Figure 24.26 Supine Thoracic Flexion Thrust Manipulation

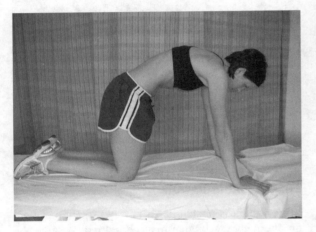

Figure 24.27 Self Thoracic Flexion Nonthrust Manipulation in Quadruped Position

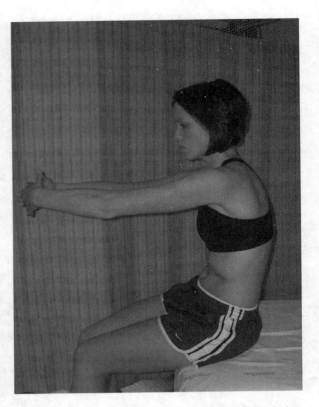

Figure 24.28 Self Thoracic Flexion Nonthrust Manipulation in Sitting Position

If the patient is unable to assume the quadruped position, an alternative stretch can be performed while sitting. The patient interlaces the hands and protracts the scapula as if to hug a barrel. Next have the patient flex forward through the thoracic spine until a stretch is noted (**Figure 24.28**).

Supine Thoracic Extension Thrust Manipulation

Locate your pistol-grip hand over the inferior vertebrae of the motion segment (**Figure 24.29**). Roll the patient back onto your hand and have the patient cross his or her arms over the chest. Pull your hand caudally as you push cranially through the crossed arms, introducing a thoracic extension moment. Place your forearm over the patient's forearms and apply downward pressure with your body. Once the tissue slack is taken up, perform a thrust manipulation. Cleland et al. (2004a) found an immediate, statistically significant improvement in lower trapezius strength ($P < 0.025$) after the application of this technique to vertebral levels T6 to T12. As

your hand in the supine position. Cross the patient's arms over the chest, with the opposite arm on top. Reach around the patient's upper trunk and flex them upward until you feel the upper vertebrae of the motion segment begin to move. Push your body weight downward through the patient's arms onto your hand. Once the slack is taken up, perform a thrust manipulation.

Self Thoracic Flexion Nonthrust Manipulation

In the quadruped position, the patient arches the thoracic spine upward, introducing flexion until a stretch is felt (**Figure 24.27**). Cervical flexion may be added to further emphasize the flexion moment.

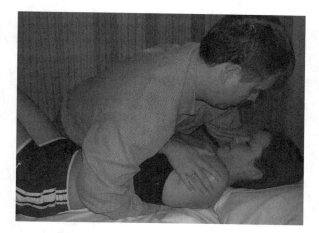

Figure 24.29 Supine Thoracic Extension Thrust Manipulation

noted previously, lower trapezius weakness is often associated with postural deviations, which may place stress on the cervical spine.

Prone Thoracic Extension Thrust Manipulation

An alternative position for the previous intervention has the patient in the prone position (**Figure 24.30**). Standing on the patient's left side, place your left hand on the left transverse process of the vertebrae to be extended. Place your right hand on the right transverse process of the same vertebrae. Introduce an anterior force through your right hand and an inferior force through your left hand until the soft-tissue slack is removed. Apply a thrust or nonthrust manipulation. Liebler et al. (2001) studied the effects of prone, grade IV posterior-anterior mobilizations to T6-T12 on lower trapezius strength. A statistically significant improvement in lower trapezius strength was noted ($P < 0.05$) immediately after the mobilizations.

Self Thoracic Extension Nonthrust Manipulation

A home exercise to reinforce the extension motion may include use of a towel roll. The patient lies supine, and the towel roll is placed horizontally over the inferior vertebra. The patient crosses his or her arms over the chest and applies a gentle rocking moment, creating a fulcrum over the towel into extension. Alternatively, a

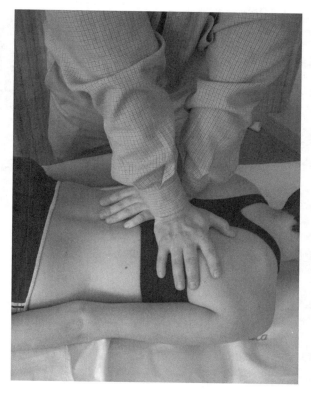

Figure 24.30 Prone Thoracic Extension Thrust Manipulation

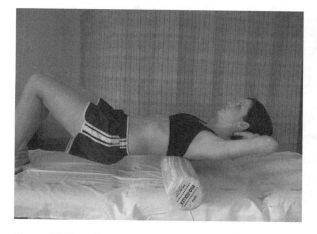

Figure 24.31 Self Thoracic Extension Nonthrust Manipulation with Foam Roller

foam roller may also be placed horizontally under the patient's thoracic spine (**Figure 24.31**). The patient supports the head and neck by interlacing the hands behind the head. While allowing the body to relax into extension, the patient bridges upward, placing further

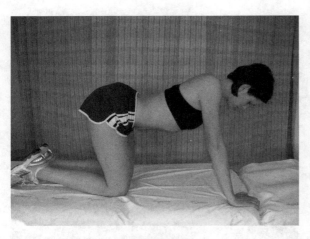

Figure 24.32 Self Thoracic Extension Nonthrust Manipulation in Quadruped Position

weight onto the thoracic spine. Using the legs, the patient rolls the trunk up and down the thoracic spine.

In quadruped position, the patient may also impart an extension moment at the thoracic spine by allowing the trunk to slump forward while retracting the scapula (**Figure 24.32**).

CONCLUSION

The concept of regional interdependence is well exemplified through the use of thoracic spine interventions for patients with various conditions of the cervical spine. Research has supported the use of exercise and manual therapy aimed at the thoracic spine for such conditions as mechanical neck pain (Cleland et al., 2005a, 2007a, 2007b; Flynn et al., 2001; Fernández-de-las-Peñas et al., 2007a), whiplash-associated disorders (Fernández-de-las-Peñas et al., 2004), cervical radiculopathy (Cleland et al., 2005b; Piva et al., 2000), and low-grade cervical myelopathy (Browder et al., 2004). Research has only recently begun to acknowledge the potential link between the thoracic spine and headaches of cervicogenic or tension-type origin.

The current best available evidence shows that a multimodal approach to the headache patient produces decreased headache intensity, frequency, and duration (Jull et al., 2002; Hammill et al., 1996; Petersen, 2003; Issa & Huijbregts, 2006; McDonnell et al., 2005; Viti & Paris, 2000; van Duijn et al., 2007). Various manual physical therapy interventions aimed at addressing cervicothoracic impairments have been utilized throughout the available research. Interventions include both thrust and nonthrust manipulations applied to the thoracic spine (Jull et al., 2002; Viti & Paris, 2000; Issa & Huijbregts, 2006; van Duijn et al., 2007), cervicothoracic musculature stretching (Issa & Huijbregts, 2006; McDonnell et al., 2005; van Duijn et al., 2007), and scapula stabilization strengthening (Peterson, 2003; Jull et al., 2002; McDonnell et al., 2005; van Duijn et al., 2007). The available studies to date linking thoracic spine interventions to subjects with cervicogenic and tension-type headache fall low in the hierarchy of evidence, because the majority are case reports. High-quality randomized controlled trials comparing the effect of evidence-based multimodal treatment plans with and without thoracic spine interventions currently do not exist, indicating the need for future research in this area.

The purpose of this chapter has been to update the reader on the current state of evidence for thoracic spine interventions in the headache patient. Theoretical links explaining the regional interdependence have been suggested, and the evidence for each theory has been noted. The interventions included are those that have been used in the literature as well as those that are commonly used by the listed authors.

REFERENCES

American Physical Therapy Association. *Manipulation Education Manual: For Physical Therapist Professional Degree Programs*. Alexandria, VA: APTA; 2004:1–51.

Bang MD, Deyle GD. Comparison of supervised exercise with and without manual physical therapy for patients with shoulder impingement syndrome. *J Orthop Sports Phys Ther* 2000;30:126–137.

Bergman GJ, Winters JC, Klaas HG, et al. Manipulative therapy in addition to usual medical care for patients with shoulder dysfunction and pain. *Ann Intern Med* 2004;141:432–439.

Boyle JW. Is the pain and dysfunction of shoulder impingement lesion really second rib syndrome in disguise? Two case reports. *Man Ther* 1999;4:44–48.

Browder DA, Erhard RE, Piva SR. Intermittent cervical traction and thoracic manipulation for management of mild cervical compressive myelopathy attributed to cervical herniated disc: a case series. *J Orthop Sports Phys Ther* 2004;34:701–712.

Cassidy JD, Lopes AA, Yong-Hing K. The immediate effect of manipulation versus mobilization on pain and range of motion in the cervical spine: a randomized controlled trial. *J Manipulative Physiol Ther* 1992;15:570–575.

Childs JD, Cleland JA. Development and application of clinical prediction rules to improve decision making in physical therapy practice. *Phys Ther* 2006;86:122–131.

Cibulka MT, Rose SJ, Delitto A, et al. Hamstring muscle strain treated by mobilizing the sacroiliac joint. *Phys Ther* 1986;66:1220–1223.

Cleland JA, Selleck B, Stowell T, et al. Short-term effects of thoracic manipulation of lower trapezius strength. *J Manual Manipulative Ther* 2004a;12:82–90.

Cleland JA, Whitman JA, Fritz JM. Effectiveness of manual physical therapy to the cervical spine in the management of lateral epicondylalgia: a retrospective analysis. *J Orthop Sports Phys Ther* 2004b;34:713–724.

Cleland JA, Childs JD, McRae M, et al. Immediate effects of thoracic manipulation in patients with neck pain: a randomized trial. *Man Ther* 2005a;10:127–135.

Cleland JA, Whitman JM, Fritz JM, et al. Manual physical therapy, cervical traction, and strengthening exercises in patients with cervical radiculopathy: a case series. *J Orthop Sports Phys Ther* 2005b;35:802–811.

Cleland JA, Childs JD, Fritz JM, et al. Development of a clinical prediction rule for guiding treatment of a subgroup of patients with neck pain: use of thoracic spine manipulation, exercise and patient education. *Phys Ther* 2007a;87:9–23.

Cleland JA, Glynn PE, Whitman JM, et al. The short-term effects of thrust versus non-thrust mobilization/manipulation directed at the thoracic spine in patients with neck pain: a randomized clinical trial. *Phys Ther* 2007b;87:431–440.

Cliborne AV, Wainner RS, Rhon DI, et al. Clinical hip tests and a functional squat test in patients with knee osteo-arthritis: reliability, prevalence of positive test findings, and short-term response to hip mobilizations. *J Orthop Sports Phys Ther* 2004;34:676–685.

Currier L, Froehlieh R, Carow S, et al. Development of a clinical prediction rule to identify patients with knee osteo-arthritis who demonstrate a favorable short-term response to hip mobilizations. *Phys Ther* 2007;87:1106–1119.

Decker MJ, Hintermeister RA, Faber KJ, et al. Serratus anterior muscle activity during selected rehabilitation exercises. *Am J Sports Med* 1999;27:784–791.

Deyle GD, Henderson NE, Matekel RL, et al. Effectiveness of manual physical therapy and exercise in osteo-arthritis of the knee. *Ann Intern Med* 2000;132:173–181.

Deyle GD, Allison SC, Matekel RL, et al. Physical therapy treatment effectiveness for osteo-arthritis of the knee: a randomized comparison of supervised clinical exercise and manual therapy procedures versus a home exercise program. *Phys Ther* 2005;85:1301–1317.

Donatelli RA, Wooden MJ. *Orthopaedic Physical Therapy.* 3rd ed. Philadelphia: Churchill Livingstone; 2001:46–61.

Ekstrom RA, Donatelli RA, Soderberg GL. Surface electromyographic analysis of exercises for the trapezius and serratus anterior muscles. *J Orthop Sports Phys Ther* 2003;33:247–258.

Fernández-de-las-Peñas C, Fernández-Carnero J, Plaza-Fernández A, et al. Dorsal manipulation in whiplash injury treatment: a randomized controlled trial. *J Whiplash Rel Disord* 2004;3:55–72.

Fernández-de-las-Peñas C, Alonso-Blanco C, Cuadrado ML, et al. Forward head posture and neck mobility in chronic tension-type headache: a blinded, controlled study. *Cephalgia* 2006a;26:314–319.

Fernández-de-las-Peñas C, Alonso-Blanco C, Cuadrado ML, Gerwin RD, Pareja JA. Trigger points in the suboccipital muscles and forward head posture in tension-type headache. *Headache* 2006b;46:454–460.

Fernández-de-las-Peñas C, Palomeque-del-Cerro L, Rodríguez C, et al. Changes in neck pain and active range of motion after a single thoracic spine manipulation in patients with mechanical neck pain: a case series. *J Manipulative Physiol Ther* 2007a;330:312–320.

Fernández-de-las-Peñas C, Pérez-de-Heredia M, Molero A, et al. Performance of the cranio-cervical flexion test, forward head posture, and headache clinical parameters in patients with chronic tension-type headache: a pilot study. *J Orthop Sports Phys Ther* 2007b;37:33–39.

Flynn T, Wainner R, Whitman J. Immediate effects of thoracic spine manipulation on cervical spine range of motion and pain. *J Manual Manipulative Ther* 2001;9:165–166.

Greenman P. *Principles of Manual Medicine.* 2nd ed. Philadelphia, PA: Lippincott Williams & Wilkins; 1996.

Gross AR, Hoving JL, Haines TA, et al. A Cochrane review of mobilization and manipulation for mechanical neck disorders. *Spine* 2004;29:1541–1548.

Hammill JM, Cook TM, Rosecrance JC. Effectiveness of a physical therapy regimen in the treatment of tension-type headache. *Headache* 1996;36:149–153.

Issa TS, Huijbregts PA. Physical therapy diagnosis and management of a patient with chronic daily headache: a case report. *J Manual Manipulative Ther* 2006;14: E88–E123.

Johansson H, Sojka P. Patho-physiological mechanisms involved in genesis and spread of muscular tension in occupational muscle pain and in chronic musculoskeletal pain syndromes: a hypothesis. *Med Hypotheses* 1991;35:196–203.

Jull G. Management of cervical headache. *Man Ther* 1997;2: 144–149.

Jull G, Trott P, Potter H, et al. A randomized controlled trial of exercise and manipulative therapy for cervicogenic headache. *Spine* 2002;27:1835–1843.

Knutson GA. Significant changes in systolic blood pressure post vectored upper cervical adjustment vs. resting control groups: a possible effect of the cervico-sympathetic and/or pressor reflex. *J Manipulative Physiol Ther* 2001;24:101–109.

Liebler EJ, Tufano-Coors L, Douris P, et al. The effects of thoracic spine mobilization on lower trapezius strength testing. *J Manual Manipulative Ther* 2001;9:207–212.

Lindgren K-A, Leino E, Manninen H. Cervical rotation lateral flexion test in brachialgia. *Arch Phys Med Rehabil* 1992;73:735–737.

Ludewig PM, Hoff MS, Osowski EE, et al. Relative balance of serratus anterior and upper trapezius muscle activity during push-up exercises. *Am J Sports Med* 2004;32:484–493.

McDonnell MK, Sahrmann SA, Van Dillen L. A specific exercise program and modification of postural alignment treatment of cervicogenic headache: a case report. *J Orthop Sports Phys Ther* 2005;35:3–15.

Norlander S, Nordgren B. Clinical symptoms related to musculoskeletal neck-shoulder pain and mobility in the cervico-thoracic spine. *Scand J Rehabil Med* 1998;30: 243–251.

Norlander S, Aste-Norlander U, Nordgren B, Sahlstedt B. Mobility in the cervico-thoracic motion segment: an indicative factor of musculo-skeletal neck-shoulder pain. *Scand J Rehabil Med* 1996;28:183–192.

Norlander S, Gustavsson BA, Lindell J, Nordgren B. Reduced mobility in the cervico-thoracic motion segment—a risk factor for musculoskeletal neck-shoulder pain: a two-year prospective follow-up study. *Scand J Rehabil Med* 1997;29:167–174.

Petersen SM. Articular and muscular impairments in cervicogenic headache: a case report. *J Orthop Sports Phys Ther* 2003;33:21–30.

Piva SR, Erhard RE, Al-Higail M. Cervical radiculopathy: a case problem using a decision-making algorithm. *J Orthop Sports Phys Ther* 2000;30:745–754.

Shambaugh GE Jr. Manipulating medicine. *Lancet* 1995;345: 1574.

Struijs PA, Damen PJ, Bakker EW, et al. Manipulation of the wrist for management of lateral epicondylitis: a randomized pilot study. *Phys Ther* 2003;83:608–616.

Suter E, McMorland G, Herzog W, et al. Decrease in quadriceps inhibition after sacroiliac joint manipulation in patients with anterior knee pain. *J Manipulative Physiol Ther* 1999;22:149–153.

Suter E, McMorland G, Herzog W, et al. Conservative lower back treatment reduces inhibition in knee-extensor muscles: a randomized controlled trial. *J Manipulative Physiol Ther* 2000;23:76–80.

Sutlive T, Moore J, Garber M, et al. A clinical prediction rule for classifying patients with patello-femoral pain who respond successfully to lumbo-pelvic manipulation. In press.

Van Duijn J, Van Duijn AJ, Nitsch W. Orthopaedic manual physical therapy including thrust manipulation and exercise in the management of a patient with cervicogenic headache: a case report. *J Manual Manipulative Ther* 2007;15:10–24.

Vicenzino B, Collins D, Wright A. The initial effects of a cervical spine manipulative physiotherapy treatment on the pain and dysfunction of lateral epicondylalgia. *Pain* 1996;68:69–74.

Viti JA, Paris SV. The use of upper thoracic manipulation is a patient with headache. *J Manual Manipulative Ther* 2000;8:25–28.

Watson DH, Trott PH. Cervical headache: an investigation of natural head posture and upper cervical flexor muscle performance. *Cephalalgia* 1993;13:272–284.

Whitman JM, Childs JD, Walker V. The use of manipulation in a patient with an ankle sprain injury not responding to conventional management: a case report. *Man Ther* 2005;10:224–231.

Whitman JM, Flynn TW, Childs JD, et al. A comparison between two physical therapy treatment programs for patients with lumbar spinal stenosis: a randomized clinical trial. *Spine* 2006;31:2541–2549.

Muscle Energy Techniques

Gary Fryer, PhD, BSc (Osteopathy), ND, and Christian Fossum, DO

Muscle energy technique (MET) is a manual procedure that was developed and systemized by osteopathic physicians Fred Mitchell Sr. and Jr. MET has continued to evolve with contributions from many individuals, and is now practiced by clinicians from many different manual therapy disciplines. MET can be applied to address dysfunctions involving myofascial tissues, or to primary spinal or peripheral joint dysfunctions. MET has been claimed to be effective for lengthening a shortened muscle, mobilizing an articulation with restricted mobility, strengthening a physiologically weakened muscle, and reducing localized edema and passive congestion (Mitchell et al., 1979; Bourdillon et al., 1992; Mitchell & Mitchell, 1995; Goodridge & Kuchera, 1997; Chaitow, 2006).

Although there are different approaches for the application of MET, postisometric relaxation (or "contract-relax") is the most commonly advocated technique. This involves the accurate localization of forces to the joint or muscle barrier (with the shortened tissue placed on stretch position), an isometric contraction (3–7 seconds) of the lengthened muscle against an unyielding counterforce supplied by the clinician, followed by patient relaxation and careful engagement of the new barrier to take up the slack. Three to five repetitions of the procedure are usually recommended (Mitchell et al., 1979; Bourdillon et al., 1992; Mitchell & Mitchell, 1995; Goodridge & Kuchera, 1997; Chaitow, 2006).

There are similarities between MET and other forms of postisometric stretching, at least when applied to facilitate the lengthening of a muscle. The most common forms of postisometric stretching referred to in the research scientific literature are variations of proprioceptive neuromuscular facilitation (PNF) techniques, and include contract-relax (CR) (Wallin et al., 1985; Handel et al., 1997; Spernoga et al., 2001), where the muscle being stretched is contracted and then relaxed and further stretched; agonist contract-relax (ACR) (Osternig et al., 1990; Ferber et al., 2002), where contraction of the agonist (rather than the muscle being stretched) actively moves the joint through the restrictive barrier for increased range of motion (ROM); and contract-relax agonist-contract (CRAC) (Etnyre & Abraham, 1986; Godges et al., 2003), a combination of these two methods. Other than when applied to increase muscle length, the two treatment procedures, MET and PNF, have different approaches and goals. MET was developed to address pelvic, intervertebral, or peripheral joint dysfunction according to biomechanical principles, whereas PNF emphasizes the need to improve rotational trunk stability and generally uses stronger contraction forces (Chaitow, 2006).

PRINCIPLES OF TREATMENT APPLICATION

The principles of MET application differ depending on whether MET is applied primarily to muscle or segmental joint dysfunctions. In essence, the aim of applying MET to a muscle is to lengthen the muscle (by elongating the sarcomeres and promoting viscoelastic and plastic change to the connective tissue elements), to normalize tissue tone, and to deactivate muscle trigger points (TrPs). When applied to spinal joint dysfunctions, the chief goals of MET are to produce a change in the range and quality of joint motion, to reduce pain or tenderness, and to improve the palpable tone of the surrounding soft tissues.

The physiologic mechanisms by which these therapeutic changes are achieved are still largely speculative, but it appears likely that manual techniques may act by both neurologic and biomechanical mechanisms. Traditionally, MET has been proposed to produce reflex muscle relaxation via Golgi tendon organ and muscle spindle reflexes (Kuchera & Kuchera, 1992; Mitchell & Mitchell, 1995), but this seems unlikely given that studies have generally reported an increase—not a decrease—in electromyographic activity following postisometric stretching procedures (Osternig et al., 1987, 1990), and it appears that motor activity does not play a significant role in limiting stretch of a muscle (Magnusson et al., 1996a, 1996b). It is more plausible that MET activates descending inhibitory pain pathways

and possibly improves proprioception and motor control, as well as a biomechanical action to promote tissue fluid drainage and structural change to the viscoelastic connective tissues (see Chapter 19).

The force and duration of isometric contraction during MET can be varied, as can the force and the duration of stretch, depending on the tissues targeted. In general, a gentle force of contraction is recommended for MET directed at spinal segments and for TrPs in order to selectively recruit the local segmental muscles or the irritable TrP fibers. More moderate stretching and contraction forces are recommended for increasing the extensibility of shortened, painless, or fibrotic muscles, in order to maximize the postcontraction hypoalgesia and create substantial tension on the connective tissue elements for plastic change (Mitchell & Mitchell, 1995; Fryer, 2006).

Some authors have recommended different durations of isometric contraction for cervical MET, from 2 to 3 seconds (Mitchell & Mitchell, 1995), 3 to 5 seconds (Greenman, 2003; DiGiovanna et al., 2005), to 5 to 7 seconds (Chaitow, 2006). The research literature provides little guidance regarding the most effective application; in the only study found that examined contraction duration of MET applied to the cervical spine, there were no benefits in using a 20-second contraction compared with a 5-second contraction (Fryer & Ruszkowski, 2004). The authors of this chapter recommend a 3- to 5-second contraction when applied to spinal joints, whereas a 5- to 7-second contraction is recommended when applied to larger muscles, because a longer contraction may promote more viscoelastic changes in these structures.

This chapter describes the application of MET to the cervical spine and related musculature. It should be clearly understood, however, that treatment of patients with headaches should not be limited to treatment of the neck and shoulders or even to the use of MET. In the context of a holistic approach, muscle energy procedures would seldom be the only treatment applied to a patient with a musculoskeletal cause of headaches, and should be integrated with other interventions, such as soft-tissue manipulation, joint mobilization or manipulation, postural reeducation, and exercise prescription. This chapter outlines techniques for the head and upper body region, but consideration of the patient with headaches should also include assessment of global posture, the thoracic spine and rib cage, lumbar spine and pelvis, and sometimes the lower extremities. Any of these regions may have postural or functional consequences that may affect the neck and induce or maintain headache, so these regions should be assessed and, if necessary, treated. Readers are advised to consult other texts for specific MET approaches for these regions (Mitchell et al., 1979; Bourdillon et al., 1992; Mitchell & Mitchell, 1995; Goodridge & Kuchera, 1997; Greenman, 2003; Chaitow, 2006).

CAUTIONS AND CONTRAINDICATIONS

MET is a safe technique, and there are no reports of serious adverse reactions in the literature. The cautions and contraindications for MET are common to those of other soft-tissue techniques, and involve caution with use of stretching force when dealing with acute pain conditions and caution with forces and leverages in the presence of weakened bone. With MET, very light to moderate applications of stretch or isometric contraction are normally performed, and thus MET is perceived to be a safe technique with little risk of serious injury. When applied to previously injured, healing tissues, forces of contraction or stretch should be matched to the stage of healing and repair to avoid further tissue damage and promote optimal healing (Lederman, 2005).

Cerebrovascular accidents following high-velocity manipulation to the cervical spine have been reported as unpredictable rare complications (Di Fabio, 1999; Haldeman et al., 2001), and, although no such incidents have been reported for MET, care and caution should be taken when treating the cervical spine. Fortunately, the leverages advocated for MET applied to the cervical spine are generally subtle and minimal, and the avoidance of end-range rotation and extension leverages may reduce the risks posed by MET.

EVIDENCE OF EFFICACY FOR MUSCLE ENERGY TECHNIQUES
Application to Cervical Musculature

There has been almost no research investigating the effect of MET on the muscles of the cervical region. Inferences may be drawn, however, from the considerable research into related postisometric stretching techniques for increasing the extensibility of other muscles, primarily the hamstring muscle group. MET and PNF stretching methods have been shown to bring about greater improvements in joint range of motion and muscle extensibility compared with passive, static

stretching, both in the short and long term (Sady et al., 1982; Wallin et al., 1985; Osternig et al., 1990; Magnusson et al., 1996c; Feland et al., 2001; Ferber et al., 2002; Ballantyne et al., 2003). Researchers have reported immediate hamstring length and ROM increases from 3° (Ballantyne et al., 2003) to 33° (Magnusson et al., 1996c) following the application of MET or similar postisometric stretching methods. Because of differences in the study designs and measurement methodology, it is difficult to determine the most efficacious elements of the various treatment protocols, but it appears that ACR and CRAC methods are more effective for increasing ROM than CR when applied to the hamstring muscles.

Caution must be exercised when attempting to generalize the results to treatment of the cervical musculature, because the neck and shoulder muscles are smaller, less fibrous, and more painful in subjects with neck and head pain than the hamstring muscles in subjects from these studies. This is an area that deserves considerable investigation, and researchers should look to establish reliable methods of measuring neck and shoulder muscle length, the effect of MET on muscle extensibility and motor recruitment, and the effect of MET on clinical outcomes for patients with neck pain and headache.

Application to Cervical Spinal Dysfunction

Few researchers have investigated the effects of MET applied to the spine, despite the fact that many authors in the field of MET have emphasized its application for spinal dysfunction (Mitchell et al., 1979; Bourdillon et al., 1992; Mitchell & Mitchell, 1995; Goodridge & Kuchera, 1997; Greenman, 2003; DiGiovanna et al., 2005). A small number of studies have reported that MET produces increased ROM in the cervical, thoracic, and lumbar spine. Schenk et al. (1994) investigated the effect of MET treatment over a 4-week period on cervical ROM. Eighteen asymptomatic subjects with limitations (10° or more) of active motion in one or more planes (rotation, side bending, flexion, or extension) were randomly assigned to either the treatment or control group. Those subjects in the MET group achieved significant gains in rotation (approximately 8°), whereas the control group showed little change. Fryer and Ruszkowski (2004) examined the effect of a single application of MET directed at the rotational restriction of the atlantoaxial (AA) articulation in 52 volunteers who displayed at least 4° of asymmetry in active AA rotation. Subjects received a single application of MET using a light isometric contraction (5 or 20 seconds) or a sham treatment. Fryer and Ruszkowski (2004) found that MET using a 5-second contraction phase produced a significantly greater increase in the restricted direction than the control group. The increase in ROM was not made at the expense of the unrestricted direction, which also made small mean increases. The 20-second isometric contraction phase MET also induced increased ROM, but appeared to be less effective than the 5-second contractions. Similarly, Burns and Wells (2006) found an immediate increase in active rotation, lateral bending, and overall range of cervical motion (approximately 4°) following the application of MET, compared with a control sham procedure, in an asymptomatic group with multiplanar motion restrictions.

In the only randomized clinical trial that examined the application of MET as a sole treatment, Wilson et al. (2003) treated 19 patients with acute low back pain who were diagnosed with a segmental lumbar dysfunction. Patients assigned to the MET group received a specific MET for their diagnosed dysfunction and were given a home exercise program that included a MET self-treatment component, abdominal "drawing in," and progressive strengthening exercises, whereas those patients assigned to the control group received a sham treatment and the home exercise program. Those patients treated with MET showed a significantly higher change in Oswestry Disability Index scores than the control patients (mean change of 83% vs. 65%), and every patient treated with MET had a greater improvement than those in the control group.

Similarly, Brodin (1982) claimed that MET treatment of 41 low back pain patients over 3 weeks produced a reduction in pain, but no details of the techniques used in the MET sessions were reported and the author did not offer statistical analysis to support this conclusion. MET is rarely used as a standalone technique, but as part of a treatment program. Fryer et al. (2005) treated 17 patients with chronic or subacute neck pain using a semistandardized osteopathic treatment approach that included MET of the cervical and shoulder muscles, as well as to other regions as required. Self-reported pain and disability were significantly reduced over the course of treatment.

These studies support the use of MET to increase spinal ROM and improve clinical indicators of pain and disability, but further investigation of the duration of these effects and the clinical benefit to symptomatic individuals is needed.

MUSCLE ENERGY TECHNIQUES APPLIED TO THE CERVICAL MUSCLES

Muscle energy techniques can be applied to the muscles and soft tissues of the cervical region to stretch and lengthen these tissues, to deactivate muscle TrPs, and to improve lymphatic drainage. The main principles for application of MET to myofascial structures are as follows.

1. *Stretch the involved muscle to its barrier* (sense of palpated resistance or end range).
   - Light stretching force to the initial or first barrier if the muscle is acutely painful
   - Moderate stretching force (to a comfortable sensation of stretch experienced by the patient) if the muscle is only mildly painful or not painful
2. *Isometric contraction.* Request the patient to gently contract the targeted muscle (push away from the barrier) against your controlled, unyielding resistance for 5 to 7 seconds. A light contraction force should be used if the muscle is painful or contains active TrPs. If it is relatively pain free, a moderate contraction force is permitted.
3. *Muscle relaxation.* The patient should fully relax for several seconds, with the stretch maintained. A deep inhalation or exhalation may assist relaxation. Chaitow (2006) recommends maintaining this stretch for up to 60 seconds in the case of chronically shortened muscles (and then removing the muscle from stretch for a rest period), but this long period of stretch may not be appropriate for small cervical muscles. A stretch maintained for approximately 10 seconds is generally recommended for neck and shoulder muscles that are judged to be shortened, fibrotic, and are not provoked by stretching, whereas a few seconds is appropriate for symptomatic muscles.
4. *Reengage barrier.* The slack that has developed in the tissues following the contraction and relaxation phases is taken up, and usually the muscle can be lengthened to a new barrier without using increased force. This process is repeated two to four times, or until a change in length and tissue texture is noted.

The following section describes techniques for muscles commonly identified as developing TrPs (Simons et al., 1999) or those susceptible to becoming shortened (Greenman, 2003; Chaitow, 2006; Liebenson, 2007). Not all cervical muscles that are claimed to refer pain to the head are covered (see Chapter 6), because some of the smaller muscles are difficult to stretch and are more amenable to other therapeutic techniques, such as direct manual pressure release (Chapter 26). Additionally, the pectoral muscles are included in this section because shortness in these muscles may profoundly affect cervical posture and produce strain and irritation of headache-producing structures.

For optimal localization or effectiveness, many of the following stretches require subtle fine-tuning for each individual patient. Clinicians are encouraged to experiment with small amounts of additional leverage—flexion, rotation, side bending, and traction—using palpation of tissue stretch and patient feedback to maximize the localization of the techniques.

Caution: The following stretching techniques should be applied slowly, carefully, and with a request for patient feedback. If the patient experiences discomfort, or any sensation other than a pleasant stretching sensation, cease the procedure immediately and reassess the patient. Additionally, if any of the following signs of vertebrobasilar insufficiency appear (Gibbons & Tehan, 2006), the technique should be stopped and the patient reassessed: vertigo, visual disturbances, dysphagia, dysarthria, hoarseness, facial numbness, paresthesias, confusion, or syncope (drop attacks).

Upper Trapezius Muscle and Levator Scapulae Muscles

The upper trapezius muscle is reported to be frequently beset by TrPs and is a commonly overlooked source of temporal headaches (Simons et al., 1999; Fernández-de-las-Peñas et al., 2007). The levator scapulae muscle, which is reported to produce local pain in the ipsilateral neck, will also be stretched during the treatment of the trapezius.

Procedure

1. Patient is supine, with arms resting by side. Stand at the head of the table.
2. Stabilize the shoulder of the treated side with one hand, and contact the occiput, mastoid region, and upper neck with the other hand (**Figure 25.1**). If the weight of the patient's head is heavy, support and stabilize your hand using the support of your abdomen or chest (**Figure 25.2**). Alternatively, use a crossed-arm position, in which your hands contact and stabilize both of

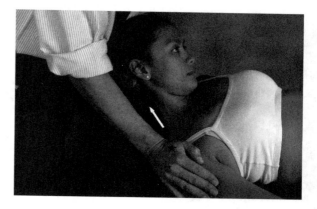

Figure 25.1 Muscle Energy Techniques Applied to the Upper Trapezius and Levator Scapulae Muscles. Note that the prime leverages are cervical flexion and lateral flexion away from the treated side; however, subtle rotation may be introduced to localize particular fibers of the trapezius or levator scapulae muscles. The patient is instructed to gently push the head back against the resistance provided by the practitioner, or to elevate the shoulder.

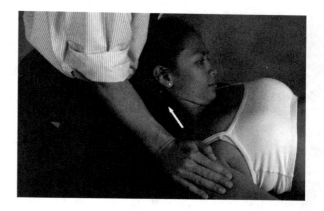

Figure 25.2 Muscle Energy Techniques Applied to the Upper Trapezius and Levator Scapulae Muscles: Use of the Abdomen to Support the Clinician's Hand and Patient's Head

the patient's shoulders and your crossed arms support the upper neck and head (**Figure 25.3**).
3. Fully flex and side bend the neck away from the involved side until a sense of tissue resistance is palpated and the patient reports a pleasant stretching sensation (Figure 25.1).
4. Addition of cervical rotation may selectively stretch particular fibers. There are different views as to the amount and direction of rotation needed to select specific parts of the muscle. Liebenson (2007) advocates contralateral rotation

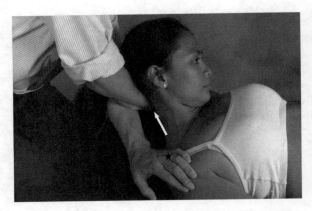

Figure 25.3 Muscule Energy Techniques Applied to the Upper Trapezius and Levator Scapulae Muscles with Crossed-Hands Position

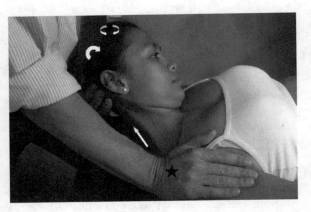

Figure 25.4 Muscle Energy Techniques Applied to the Posterior Cervical Muscles. The neck should be flexed and laterally flexed away from the treated side. In this position, subtle occipital traction and flexion should be introduced to localize the stretch to the suboccipital muscles. Further modification using occipital rotation and side bending can be based on palpatory and patient feedback to optimize localization of the stretch. The patient is requested to look up at the ceiling or to gently press the head back against the resistance provided by the practitioner.

for stretch of the upper trapezius, and ipsilateral rotation for the levator scapulae. Chaitow (2006) suggests full contralateral rotation for the posterior fibers of the trapezius, half rotation for the middle fibers, and slight ipsilateral rotation for the anterior fibers. Subtle fine-tuning of rotation using palpatory and patient feedback to determine the most effective position for each individual is recommended.

5. Request the patient to gently push the head and neck back against your controlled, unyielding resistance for 5 to 7 seconds. The direction of patient force can either be in extension or side bending; however, rotation is not recommended because it is more difficult to control and stabilize. Alternatively, shoulder elevation can be requested and resisted.
6. Allow the patient to relax for a few seconds (or more), maintaining the stretch.
7. Reengage the new barrier by taking up any slack that has developed since the contraction-relaxation phases (the muscle is further lengthened), using shoulder depression.
8. Repeat the procedure two to four times.
9. Reassess after treatment.

Suboccipital and Posterior Cervical Muscles

The deep suboccipital muscles—rectus capitis posterior major and minor, inferior and superior oblique—are reported to be a common source of headache (Fernández-de-las-Peñas et al., 2006a), particularly head pain that is

deep, poorly localized, and refers from the occiput to the orbit (Simons et al., 1999). The posterior cervical muscles, including the cervical multifidus, semispinalis capitis, longissimus capitis, and the more superficial splenius capitis and cervicis, have all been reported to produce referred pain to the head (Simons et al., 1999). The following stretches should be modified using subtle additions of leverage (flexion, rotation, or side bending) according to changes in palpated resistance and reports of sensation of stretching from the patient in order to localize the stretch to the most involved fibers.

Procedure

1. Patient is supine, arms resting by side. Stand at the head of the table.
2. Stabilize the shoulder of the treated side with one hand, and contact the occiput and mastoid region (not the neck) with the other hand (**Figure 25.4**). If the weight of the patient's head is heavy, support and stabilize the hand using the support of your abdomen or chest.
3. Fully flex the patient's neck and then side bend away from the treated side until a sense of resistance is palpated.
4. Introduce subtle occipital flexion and traction until a sense of resistance is palpated and the patient reports a pleasant stretching sensation in

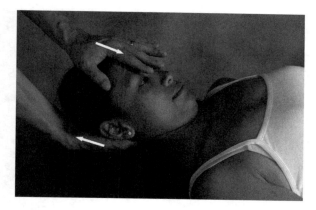

Figure 25.5 Muscle Energy Techniques Applied to the Suboccipital Muscles. The neck is in neutral and the practitioner introduces occipital traction and head flexion until a sense of resistance is palpated. The patient is instructed to nod the head upward against the resistance provided by the practitioner.

the suboccipital region. Subtle addition of rotation and side bending can be made according to changes in palpated resistance and sensation of stretching from the patient in order to localize the stretch to the most involved fibers.

5. Request the patient to gently look up to the ceiling and push the head back against the resistance of the practitioner for 5 to 7 seconds.
6. Allow the patient to relax for a few seconds.
7. Reengage the new barrier by taking up any slack that has developed since the contraction and relaxation phases (the muscle is further lengthened).
8. Repeat the procedure two to four times.
9. Reassess after treatment.

A variation on this technique that may be more specific to the suboccipital muscles is as follows:

1. Patient is supine, arms resting by side. Stand at the head of the table.
2. Contact the occiput with the first finger and medial hand, and rest the other hand over the frontal region of the patient's head.
3. Flex the head on the neutral neck using a combination of cephalic traction with the lower hand and caudal pressure with the upper until a pleasant stretch is perceived (**Figure 25.5**). Subtle addition of rotation and side bending can be made as required.
4. Request the patient to nod the head upward against the offered resistance for 5 to 7 seconds.

5. Allow the patient to relax for a few seconds.
6. Reengage the new barrier by taking up any slack that has developed since the contraction and relaxation phases (the muscle is further lengthened).
7. Repeat the procedure two to four times.
8. Reassess after treatment.

Sternocleidomastoid Muscle

This muscle has been cited as a frequent cause of atypical facial neuralgia and tension headache (Simons et al., 1999; Fernández-de-las-Peñas et al., 2006b). Referred muscle pain from the sternal division may extend to the vertex, cheek, eye, and throat, whereas referred pain from the clavicular division typically produces frontal headache or earache. The sternocleidomastoid (SCM) muscle requires careful positioning when treated with MET, because of the potential for strain of related structures—particularly the upper cervical spine—when positioning the patient for an effective stretch. The clavicular division is more amenable to MET stretching than the sternal division, but care is needed to avoid excessive cervical extension and patient discomfort. In the techniques described here, the anterior neck fascia and muscles such as the digastric and anterior scalene may be lengthened, which may contribute to the effectiveness of the techniques.

Caution: Upper cervical extension should be avoided or minimized because it can be uncomfortable for the patient and potentially irritate the cervical zygapophysial joints and compress the vertebral artery. The cervical extension required for this technique is minimal, should always be comfortable for the patient, and should be discontinued in the event of any discomfort or signs of vertebrobasilar insufficiency (see earlier).

The SCM muscle can be treated with MET with the patient either sitting or prone.

Procedure (sitting)

1. Patient is seated on a low bench or stool. Stand behind patient.
2. Place your forearm on or under the patient's clavicle on the involved side. It is important that you anchor your hand or forearm into the region by applying a compressive and downward force to take up tissue slack. Inadequate locking of the tissues will result in the need for more cervical leverage to achieve a stretch.

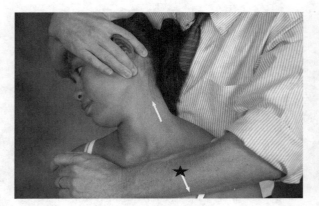

Figure 25.6 Muscle Energy Techniques Applied to the Sternocleidomastoid Muscle (Clavicular Head). The clavicular head and the anterior fascia of the neck can be stretched with the patient in seated position by firmly anchoring the fascia around the clavicle and applying the leverages of cervical side bending, slight rotation, and slight extension. The patient is asked to gently push the head forward against the resistance of the practitioner.

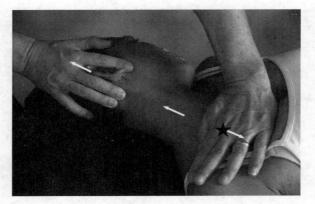

Figure 25.7 Muscle Energy Techniques Applied to the Sternocleidomastoid Muscle (Clavicular Head) in Supine Position. The clavicular head and the anterior fascia of the neck can be stretched with the patient supine by firmly anchoring the fascia around the clavicle and applying the leverages of cervical side bending, slight rotation, and slight extension. The patient is asked to gently lift the head from the table against the resistance provided by the practitioner.

3. Contact both the mastoid process and anterior ear region with the fingers of one hand, and introduce a small amount of neck rotation and side bending away from the treated side, with *slight* neck extension (avoid upper neck extension, which will produce a stretching sensation in the suprahyoid region). The anchoring of the clavicular tissues should be maintained during this movement. The patient should report a pleasant stretching sensation over the region of the SCM (**Figure 25.6**).
4. Request the patient to push the head forward against your resistance for 5 to 7 seconds.
5. Allow the patient to relax for a few seconds.
6. Reengage the new barrier by taking up any slack that has developed since the contraction and relaxation phases (the muscle is further lengthened) by traction on the mastoid, side bending, or slight extension.
7. Repeat the procedure two to four times.
8. Reassess after treatment.

Procedure (supine)

1. Patient is supine, without pillow, arms resting by side. A small folded towel can be placed under the thoracic region (not the shoulders) to accentuate slight cervical extension. Stand at the head of the table.

2. Place your hand on or under the patient's clavicle on the involved side (a small folded towel under the hand may improve patient comfort). It is important that a compressive and downward force be applied to take up tissue slack.
3. Contact the mastoid process and anterior ear region with the fingers, and introduce a small amount of neck rotation and side bending away from the treated side (**Figure 25.7**). Keep the head in neutral or slight flexion, but avoid head extension. The anchoring of the clavicular tissues should be maintained during this movement. The patient should report a pleasant stretching sensation over the region of the SCM.
4. Request the patient to lift the head forward against your resistance for 5 to 7 seconds.
5. Allow the patient to relax for a few seconds.
6. Reengage the new barrier by taking up any slack that has developed since the contraction and relaxation phases (the muscle is further lengthened).
7. Repeat the procedure two to four times.
8. Reassess after treatment.

The sternal division of the SCM is more difficult to stretch than the clavicular division, and direct massage and myofascial release techniques are often more suitable. Although a stretch using ipsilateral rotation would seem logical according to the action of this muscle, such leverages are rarely effective.

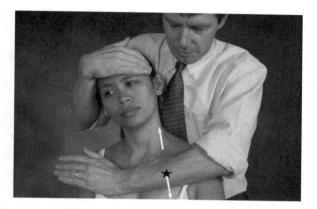

Figure 25.8 Muscle Energy Techniques Applied to the Sternocleidomastoid Muscle (Sternal Head). The sternal head can be stretched by anchoring the tissues around the medial clavicle and sternum and introducing cervical rotation away from the treated side, followed by side bending to the same side and slight extension. The patient is requested to gently push the head forward against the resistance of the practitioner.

Procedure (sternal division)

1. Patient is seated on a low bench or stool. Stand behind the patient.
2. Place your forearm on or under the patient's clavicle on the involved side. It is important that you anchor your forearm by applying a compressive and downward force to take up tissue slack. Inadequate locking of the tissues will result in the need for more cervical leverage to achieve a stretch.
3. Contact the mastoid process and anterior ear region with the fingers of your hand, and introduce a small amount of neck rotation to the side of the treated muscle. Following this, introduce posterior translation of the chin and head (avoid upper cervical extension), followed by lateral flexion to the *opposite side* (**Figure 25.8**). Anchoring of the clavicular tissues should be maintained during this movement. The patient should report a pleasant stretching sensation over the region of the sternal head of the SCM.
4. Request the patient to push the head forward against your resistance for 5 to 7 seconds.
5. Allow the patient to relax for a few seconds.
6. Reengage the new barrier by taking up any slack that has developed since the contraction and relaxation phases (the muscle is further lengthened).
7. Repeat the procedure two to four times.
8. Reassess after treatment.

Scalene Muscles

The scalene muscles (anterior, middle, and posterior) are reported to be a commonly overlooked source of back, shoulder, and arm pain, and TrPs in these muscles are claimed to frequently contribute to symptoms in patients with cervicogenic headache (Simons et al., 1999). Opinions differ on the degree and direction of rotation required for the stretch of the scalene muscles. Chaitow (2006) recommended slight rotation to the opposite side to localize the anterior scalene, 45% of rotation for the middle scalene, and full rotation for the posterior scalene. Gerwin (2005) advocated ipsilateral rotation, whereas Liebenson (2007) recommended rotation to the involved side for the anterior fibers, no rotation for the middle fibers, and rotation to the opposite direction for the posterior. Experimentation using palpatory and patient feedback is recommended.

Procedure

1. Patient is supine, arms resting by side. Stand at the head of the table.
2. Contact the mastoid, lateral occiput, and upper cervical pillars to stabilize the neck and prevent excessive upper cervical lateral flexion. Place your other hand over the patient's shoulder and lateral clavicle region for stabilization. Alternatively, your hand can be placed over the patient's hand and thenar eminence, which is placed below the medial clavicle to stabilize the first and second ribs.
3. Place the patient's neck in slight extension (remove pillow), laterally flex the neck away from the treated side, and introduce slight rotation (**Figure 25.9**). Experiment with varying degrees of rotation for the most effective stretch.
4. Request the patient to gently laterally flex the head against your resistance for 5 to 7 seconds.
5. Allow the patient to relax for a few seconds. A deep inhalation and exhalation may assist relaxation of the scalene muscles.
6. Reengage the new barrier by taking up any slack that has developed since the contraction and relaxation phases (the muscle is further lengthened).
7. Repeat the procedure two to four times.
8. Reassess after treatment.

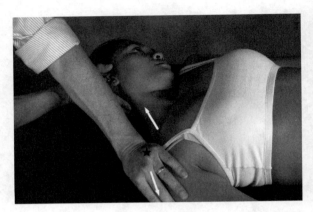

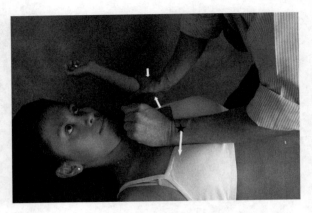

Figure 25.9 Muscle Energy Techniques Applied to the Scalene Muscles. The scalene muscles can be stretched using slight cervical extension (no pillow, hand fixing on first or second ribs), contralateral lateral flexion, and varying amounts of rotation. The patient is instructed to gently laterally flex the head and neck against the resistance of the practitioner. Cervical rotation may be varied in order to stretch different fibers.

Figure 25.10 Muscle Energy Techniques Applied to the Pectoralis Major Muscle. The pectoralis major muscle is stretched by anchoring the fascia around the chest and sternum and slowly introducing shoulder horizontal extension with traction. The patient is instructed to gently push the arm toward the ceiling against the resistance of the practitioner.

Pectoralis Major Muscle

Although TrPs in the pectoralis major typically refer pain to the chest and arm (Simons et al., 1999), shortened muscles can produce a round-shouldered, head-forward posture that may lead to ongoing strain to the cervical tissues and further contribute to cervicogenic headaches.

Caution: This technique is not suitable for any patient with an unstable shoulder joint, previous shoulder injury, or limited shoulder movement due to pain. Do not use external rotation as the primary leverage, because this will frequently cause pain and discomfort, even in the healthy shoulder joint.

Procedure

1. Patient is supine, arms resting by side. Stand at the side of the table, on the side to be treated.
2. Abduct the patient's shoulder to 90°, and place in comfortable external rotation. The amount of arm abduction can be varied to select particular fibers, with decreased abduction (below 90°) tending to localize the clavicular fibers and increased abduction (above 90°) localizing the sternal fibers.
3. Anchor the tissues by placing your hand or forearm over the patient's sternum (close to the border with the rib cage), using a light compressive and lateral force away from the

treated side. Pre-tension of the fascia will help minimize the amount of leverage necessary on the shoulder.
4. Grasp the patient's arm close to the elbow.
5. Gently apply horizontal extension and traction (down the length of the humerus) to the shoulder, while maintaining the anchoring pressure near the sternum. The patient should experience a pleasant stretching sensation through the pectoral region (**Figure 25.10**).
   Note: The addition of traction frequently produces a much more effective stretch, and will minimize the amount of leverage required on the shoulder.
6. Request the patient to gently push the arm toward the ceiling for 5 to 7 seconds, against your resistance. Ensure you are positioned so your applicator arm is straight and the isometric force is easily resisted against your body weight.
7. Allow the patient to relax for a few seconds.
8. Reengage the new barrier by taking up any slack that has developed since the contraction and relaxation phases (the muscle is further lengthened) by gently increasing the horizontal extension.
9. Repeat the procedure two to four times.
10. Reassess after treatment.

Pectoralis Minor Muscle

The pectoralis minor muscle may refer pain to the anterior deltoid region or the ulnar side of the arm, hand, and fingers, and may entrap the axillary artery and brachial plexus to mimic cervical radiculopathy (Simons et al., 1999). Like the pectoralis major, shortened pectoralis minor muscle may affect posture to produce round shoulders and a head-forward posture, which may contribute to the production of cervicogenic headaches. There are several variations for the application of MET to shortened pectoralis minor muscles.

Procedure 1

1. Patient is supine, close to the edge of the bench so that the involved shoulder slightly overhangs the bench. The involved arm is left to hang comfortably over the edge. Stand at the side of the table on the involved side.
2. Rest your hand or forearm on either the sternum or upper chest, and apply a compressive and lateral force to take up tissue slack in the direction away from the involved muscle.
3. Cup your hand over the patient's anterior shoulder and slowly apply a force in a posterior and lateral direction with a straight arm (the bench should be low), while maintaining a firm anchor on the pectoral tissues. A small towel can be folded and placed on the patient's anterior shoulder to cushion the practitioner's hand if the patient experiences discomfort from the pressure. The patient should perceive a pleasant stretching sensation in the pectoral region (**Figure 25.11**).
4. The patient is requested to gently push the shoulder in an anterior direction "toward the ceiling" for 5 to 7 seconds.
5. Allow the patient to relax for a few seconds.
6. Reengage the new barrier by taking up any slack that has developed since the contraction and relaxation phases (the muscle is further lengthened) by gently increasing the posterior and lateral pressure on the shoulder.
7. Repeat the procedure two to four times.
8. Reassess after treatment.

An alternative application for the pectoralis minor muscle that incorporates a modified myofascial release technique is as follows.

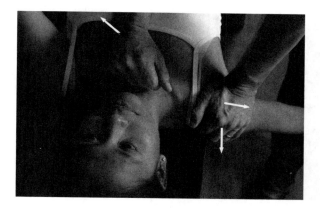

Figure 25.11 Muscle Energy Techniques Applied to the Pectoralis Minor Muscle: Procedure 1. The chest and pectoral tissues are anchored by the hand or forearm, a posterior and lateral pressure is introduced to the shoulder (arrows), and the patient is instructed to push the shoulder toward the ceiling against the practitioner's resistance.

Procedure 2

1. Patient is supine, with elbows bent and hands resting on abdomen (or under the small of the back if the arm tends to move during the treatment). Stand at the side of the table, on the side to be treated. The patient should be warned that the technique may cause discomfort and will be discontinued if the discomfort becomes substantial.
2. Slide one hand, with the fingertips together and extended, under the patient's anterior axillary fold. Slowly move medially and superiorly toward the direction of the sternal notch (under the pectoralis major and lateral edge of pectoralis minor) until tissue resistance is palpated.
3. Using your other hand, cup the anterior shoulder and exert a posterior and lateral force (a small folded towel may be placed under the hand), while maintaining the pressure under the axillary fold. The table should be low enough to allow your arm to be straight and resist the contraction force using your body weight (**Figure 25.12**).
4. Request the patient to gently push the shoulder in an anterior direction "toward the ceiling" against the resistance of your hand for 5 to 7 seconds.
5. Allow the patient to relax for a few seconds.
6. Reengage the new barrier by taking up any slack that has developed since the contraction and relaxation phases (the muscle is further

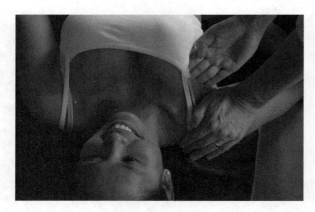

Figure 25.12 Muscle Energy Techniques Applied to the Pectoralis Minor Muscle: Procedure 2. The hand and extended fingertips are introduced under the anterior axillary fold and directed medially and superiorly until tissue resistance is palpated. A posterior and lateral pressure is introduced to the shoulder, and the patient is instructed to push the shoulder toward the ceiling against the practitioner's resistance.

lengthened) by gently increasing the posterior and lateral pressure on the shoulder.

7. Repeat the procedure two to four times.
8. Reassess after treatment.

MUSCLE ENERGY TECHNIQUES APPLIED TO THE CERVICAL JOINTS

Although MET can be directed primarily to myofascial structures, the vast majority of technique descriptions in MET texts relate to intervertebral and pelvic dysfunction, reflecting that MET is a manipulative procedure as much as a soft-tissue technique. MET is offered as a gentle alternative to high-velocity, low-amplitude thrust techniques, and procedures have been described to address specific biomechanical dysfunctions of the spine and pelvis (Mitchell, 1979; Bourdillon et al., 1992; Mitchell & Mitchell, 1995; Goodridge & Kuchera, 1997; Greenman, 2003; DiGiovanna et al., 2005).

The traditional paradigm for the application of MET to the spine is a mechanical one: precise ranges of joint motion loss are determined, and subtle leverages are applied to precisely engage each restrictive barrier in order to increase the joint motion in all the restricted planes (Bourdillon et al., 1992; Mitchell & Mitchell, 1995; Goodridge & Kuchera, 1997; Greenman, 2003; DiGiovanna et al., 2005). This biomechanical paradigm is likely to be oversimplistic, and alternative explana-

tions for the therapeutic effect are offered in Chapter 19 of the present textbook. Deficiencies in explanations of therapeutic mechanisms or biomechanical models (see below) associated with MET, however, should not discourage practitioners from using this safe and gentle technique and adapting it to the unique requirements of individuals in clinical practice.

Spinal Coupled Motion

The MET approach for segmental somatic dysfunction has traditionally been based on the biomechanical principles of spinal coupled motion proposed by Fryette (1954) and the pelvic biomechanical model developed by Mitchell (1958). Coupled motion is the involuntary segmental coupling of one plane of motion with another, which has been attributed to a combination of anatomic joint plane, ligamentous tension, and intervertebral disc mechanics. Fryette's model described neutral (type 1) coupled motion, in which lateral flexion in one direction is accompanied by rotation to the opposite direction, and nonneutral coupled motion (type 2, named because the motion occurred if the segment was hyperflexed or hyperextended), in which lateral flexion and rotation are coupled to the same side. According to this model, only three combinations of multiple-plane motion restrictions are possible: neutral type 1 dysfunctions (restriction of lateral flexion and rotation to opposite sides), and two nonneutral type 2 dysfunctions: ERS dysfunction (*extended*, being a motion restriction of flexion, rotation and to the same side) or FRS dysfunction (*flexed*, being a motion restriction of extension, rotation side bending to the opposite side). Type 2 spinal dysfunctions are proposed to be indicative of zygapophysial joint dysfunction ("open" facet, where the joint fails to glide downward and back into extension, or a "closed" facet, where it fails to glide upward and forward into flexion) and are considered more clinically significant than the compensatory type 1 dysfunctions. Further, this model has been used as a predictive diagnostic model, in which restricted coupled motions are predicted based on apparent neutral or nonneutral spinal posture or involvement of flexion or extension restriction, and clinical decisions (specific techniques) are based on these predictions.

The model, when used as a diagnostic tool, has been criticized for its prescriptive diagnostic labeling and for making invalid inferences from static positional assessment (Gibbons & Tehan, 1998; Fryer, 2000). According to the Fryette model, motion restrictions will either be coupled in a type 1 (not involving flexion or extension) or type 2 (involving either flexion or extension) pattern, with no possibility of other combinations (for example, type 1 with extension), and therefore no descriptions of techniques for these combinations are found in MET texts. Authors of MET texts commonly advocate the assessment of positional landmark asymmetry (spinal transverse process or sacral base) with the spine in different postures (neutral, flexion, and extension). Based on these findings, inferences are made concerning specific motion restriction combinations, and specific MET applications are advocated. Assessment of segmental static asymmetry has not proved to be reliable (Spring et al., 2001), and spinal coupled motion appears to be inconsistent, with variability between spinal levels and between individuals (Gibbons & Tehan, 1998; Legaspi & Edmond, 2007). In a review of lumbar coupled motion studies, Legaspi and Edmond (2007) found little agreement on the existence or type of coupled motion and concluded that physical therapists should not rely on presumed coupling for evaluation or treatment. Similarly, a review of thoracic spinal coupling studies did not find evidence of consistent patterns of motion coupling, but concluded that more quality studies are required to confirm spinal coupling patterns in flexed and extended postures (Sizer et al., 2007).

Cervical spinal kinematics is complex; in addition to coupled rotation and lateral flexion, coupled motions also include flexion, extension, and translation. Coupled motion in the typical cervical spine (C2 to C7) is claimed to occur only as type 2 motion in MET texts. Consistent ipsilateral side bending and rotation has been observed in some studies (Cook et al., 2006; Ishii et al., 2006), whereas others have suggested there may be variability in the amount and direction of these movements, influenced by gender, age, and cervical posture (Edmondston et al., 2005; Malmstrom et al., 2006). In the upper cervical region, coupled motion appears to be consistent, with opposite side bending and rotation occurring at the occipitoatlantal (OA) and AA joints, and coupled extension observed to consistently occur with rotation (Ishii et al., 2004).

Because of the variability and complexity of coupled motions in the cervical spine, practitioners are advised to be guided by the motion restrictions that present on palpation (despite the issues of reliability of motion palpation), rather than by an expectation of what "should be" according to any biomechanical model. In addition, regardless of whether spinal segmental coupling is consistent or variable between individuals, when the primary motion is introduced by the practitioner performing MET, spinal coupling (in whatever direction is normal for that individual) will occur automatically— because of the very nature of conjunct motion—and without the need to be consciously introduced by the practitioner. The pragmatic approach is therefore to address the key range(s) of motion restriction, and coupled motions will look after themselves.

Principles of Application of Muscle Energy Techniques to Cervical Intersegmental Joints

The application of MET to the intervertebral joints of the spine differs from the application to large muscles in terms of the need for localization, control, and force (Mitchell & Mitchell, 1995; Greenman, 2003). The basic principles of application to intervertebral segments include the following.

1. *Localization.* Careful attention is required to accurately engage the restricted barrier to the initial sense of increasing resistance to motion ("first" or "feather edge" of barrier) (Mitchell & Mitchell, 1995) *at the involved level.* The primary plane of motion restriction should be engaged first, and then fine-tuning performed using secondary planes of motion restriction (if detected) or translation, or both. It is essential that the patient be relaxed, so that active muscle contraction does not help or hinder the engagement of the restrictive barrier.

2. *Contraction and control.* The patient is instructed to actively push—using a *very gentle* force—away from the restrictive barrier, against the clinician's controlled, unyielding counterforce, for 3 to 5 seconds. Too strong a contraction will recruit larger, multisegmental muscles and create difficulty in maintaining accurate localization. The practitioner should give clear instructions to the patient and be relaxed and well balanced in order to facilitate patient relaxation.

3. *Relaxation.* The patient should be allowed to relax fully for several seconds.

4. *Reengage the barrier.* Usually the restrictive barrier is perceived to diminish, and the practitioner should take up the slack to reengage this barrier.

5. *Repetition.* The procedure is typically performed three to five times.

6. *Reexamination.* Segmental motion should be reassessed.

Application for Segmental Cervical Dysfunction

Middle and Lower Cervical Spine (C2 to C7)

Lateral translation is commonly advocated as the initial diagnostic procedure to identify motion restriction in the cervical spine and is most analogous to the primary motion of lateral flexion. Side bending activation force is easily controlled by the practitioner. Many authors recommend introducing either cervical flexion or extension first, and then localizing the lateral flexion (depending on whether lateral translation is most restricted in either of these positions during assessment); this order of motion introduction is easily controlled and localized. Although MET texts traditionally describe only type 2 multiplanar restrictions (ERS and FRS dysfunctions), procedures may be adapted and applied for restrictions in either a single plane (side bending, rotation, flexion, or extension) or multiple planes, depending on the individual clinical findings.

Procedure 1: restriction of flexion, side bending, and rotation (**Figure 25.13**)

1. Patient is supine. Stand or sit at head of table.
2. Place the fingertips (first to third) of both hands on the right and left articular pillars of the upper segment (e.g., C3 pillars for a C3/4 dysfunction).

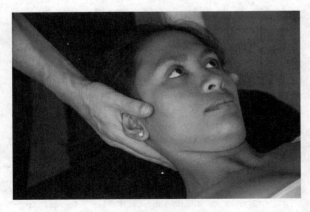

Figure 25.13 Treatment of C2 to C7 Dysfunction (Involving Restriction of Flexion, Side Bending, and Rotation). The operator carefully engages each restricted plane, and the patient is instructed to gently push back (side bending or extension) against the operator's resistance.

3. Flex the neck to the level of dysfunction. Introduce side bending and/or lateral translation until the first barrier at that segment is engaged. Fine-tune with very subtle additional leverage (rotation, more or less flexion or extension) as required.
4. Request the patient to gently push the head towards the midline (side-bending away from the restrictive barrier) *or* extend against your resistance for 3 to 5 seconds.
5. Allow the patient to relax for a few seconds.
6. Reengage the new barrier by taking up any slack in side bending or extension that has developed since the contraction and relaxation phases.
7. Repeat two to four times.
8. Reassess.

Procedure 2: primary restriction of extension, side bending, and rotation

1. Patient is supine. Stand or sit at head of table.
2. Two alternative hand positions are suitable for introducing segmental extension:
   a. Place the fingertips (first to third) of both hands on the right and left articular pillars of the upper segment (e.g., C3 pillars for a C3/4 dysfunction).
   b. Place the index and middle finger on one articular pillar and the thumb on the opposite pillar (right and left pillars of the lower segment). The other hand contacts the patient's head. This pincer hold is useful for introducing highly localized extension (without the need to extend the neck) and lateral translation, as well as creating a local fulcrum for lateral flexion (**Figures 25.14 and 25.15**).
3. Extend the segment by lifting the fingertips on the pillars until the extension barrier is palpated. Introduce side bending (using the cephalic hand to introduce motion and either the fingers or thumb of the pincer hand acting as a fulcrum) and/or lateral translation (using the pincer contact) of the segment until the barrier is engaged. Fine-tune with very subtle additional leverage (rotation, more or less flexion or extension) as required (Figure 25.15).
4. Request the patient to gently push the head toward the midline (side bending away from the restrictive barrier) *or* flex against your resistance for 3 to 5 seconds.

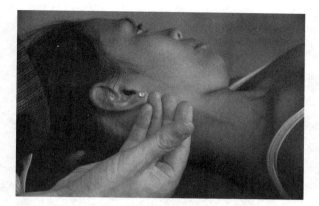

Figure 25.14 **Manual Contact for Treatment of C2 to C7 Dysfunction Involving Restriction of Extension, Side Bending, and Rotation.** Pincer hold is used for contact on articular pillars to introduce localized segmental extension and translation.

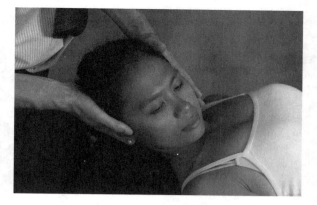

Figure 25.16 **Treatment of the Atlantoaxial Joint.** The operator flexes the patient's neck to minimize rotation below C1, and rotates the C1 segment to the restrictive barrier. The patient is instructed to gently rotate toward the midline against the operator's resistance.

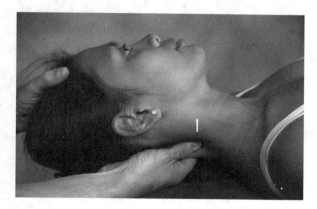

Figure 25.15 **Treatment of C2 to C7 Dysfunction Involving Restriction of Extension, Side Bending, and Rotation.** The operator carefully engages each restricted plane, and the patient is instructed to gently push back (side bending or flexion) against the operator's resistance.

perience of the authors of this chapter the engagement of AA rotation as the primary plane is highly effective. The neck is placed in flexion that relatively locks the lower cervical joint segments and localizes the rotation to the AA segment (Ogince et al., 2007).

Procedure (**Figure 25.16**)

1. Patient is supine; practitioner stands or sits at head of table.
2. The fingertips of both hands are placed on the articular pillars of the upper segment, with palms cradling the head. The chest or abdomen can also be used to support your hands.
3. Flex the patient's neck fully (until a sense of resistance) in order to relatively lock the middle and lower cervical spine. Maintain the flexion and rotate the neck until the barrier of restricted rotation is engaged. Fine-tune with additional leverages (side bending, flexion, extension), as determined with palpation.
4. Request the patient to gently rotate the head toward the midline (rotate away from the restrictive barrier) against your unyielding resistance for 3 to 5 seconds.
5. Allow the patient to relax for a few seconds.
6. Reengage the new barrier by taking up any slack in rotation that has developed since the contraction and relaxation phases.
7. Repeat three to five times.
8. Reassess.

5. Allow the patient to relax for a few seconds.
6. Reengage the new barrier by taking up any slack in side bending (or extension) that has developed since the contraction and relaxation phases.
7. Repeat two to four times.
8. Retest.

Atlantoaxial Joint

The primary movement at the AA segment is rotation, and, although some authors have advocated addressing additional planes (Mitchell & Mitchell, 1995), in the ex-

Occipitoatlantal Joint

The primary movement at the OA joint is flexion and extension, but examination and treatment of the restricted side bending and rotation components appear also to be clinically rewarding. Techniques can be used to address a single plane (usually either flexion or extension) or multiple planes (contralateral side bending and rotation, with flexion or extension).

Procedure for single-plane restricted flexion (or extension)

1. Patient is supine; practitioner stands or sits at head of table.
2. Place one hand under the occiput with the fingertips palpating the suboccipital tissues close to the OA joint line, and the other hand resting on the patient's forehead.
3. Gently flex (or extend) the head without engaging movement in the cervical spine until the initial sense of barrier at the OA is palpated (**Figure 25.17**).
4. Request the patient to gently extend (or flex) the head, using the instruction to "nod the head upward" or "look upward" (or downward) against your unyielding resistance for 3 to 5 seconds.
5. Allow the patient to relax for several seconds.
6. Reengage the new barrier by taking up any slack in flexion (or extension) that has developed since the contraction and relaxation phases.
7. Repeat two to four times.
8. Reassess.

Procedure for multiple-plane restriction: flexion (or extension), contralateral side bending and rotation (**Figure 25.18**)

1. Patient is supine. Stand or sit at head of table.
2. Cradle the occiput and head using both hands, with the fingertips palpating the suboccipital muscles near the OA joint line.
3. Gently flex (or extend) the head until the initial sense of barrier is palpated.
4. Introduce side bending by a combination of gentle side bending and lateral translation of the head on the neck until the barrier is engaged. Fine-tune with subtle contralateral rotation, if required.
5. Request the patient to gently push the head toward the midline (side bending away from the

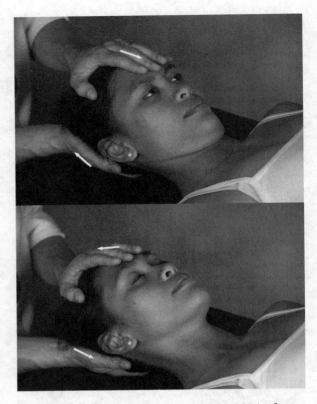

Figure 25.17 Treatment of the Occipitoatlantal Joint for Single-Plane Restriction. Top: Single-plane restriction, flexion. The operator carefully flexes the head to the barrier, and the patient is requested to gently extend the head against the operator's resistance. **Bottom:** Single-plane restriction, extension. The operator carefully extends the head to the barrier, and the patient is requested to gently flex the head against the operator's resistance.

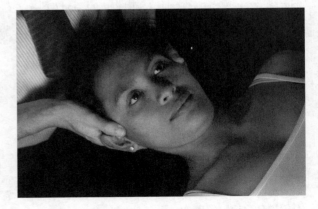

Figure 25.18 Treatment of the Occipitoatlantal Joint for Multiple-Plane Restriction Involving Side Bending. The operator carefully flexes (or extends) the head to the barrier, and then introduces side bending, lateral translation, and/or rotation.

restrictive barrier) against your unyielding resistance for 3 to 5 seconds. Alternatively, a flexion (or extension) activating force can be used.

6. Allow the patient to relax for several seconds.
7. Reengage the new barrier by taking up any slack in flexion (or extension) or side bending that has developed since the contraction and relaxation phases.

8. Repeat two to four times.
9. Reassess.

Acknowledgment

The authors express gratitude to Rolena Stephenson for her contribution as model.

REFERENCES

Ballantyne F, Fryer G, McLaughlin P. The effect of muscle energy technique on hamstring extensibility: the mechanism of altered flexibility. *J Osteopath Med* 2003;6: 59–63.

Bourdillon JF, Day EA, Bookhout MR. *Spinal Manipulation*. 5th ed. Oxford: Butterworth-Heinemann; 1992.

Brodin H. Lumbar treatment using the muscle energy technique. *Osteopath Ann* 1982;10:23–24.

Burns DK, Wells MR. Gross range of motion in the cervical spine: the effects of osteopathic muscle energy technique in asymptomatic subjects. *JAOA* 2006;106:137–142.

Chaitow L. *Muscle Energy Techniques*. 3rd ed. Edinburgh: Churchill Livingston; 2006.

Cook C, Hegedus E, Showalter C, Sizer PS Jr. Coupling behavior of the cervical spine: a systematic review of the literature. *J Manipulative Physiol Ther* 2006;29:570–575.

Di Fabio RP. Manipulation of the cervical spine: risks and benefits. *Phys Ther* 1999;79:50–65.

DiGiovanna EL, Schiowitz S, Dowling DJ. *An Osteopathic Approach to Diagnosis and Treatment*. 3rd ed. Philadelphia: Lippincott Williams & Wilkins; 2005.

Edmondston SJ, Henne SE, Loh W, Ostvold E. Influence of cranio-cervical posture on three-dimensional motion of the cervical spine. *Man Ther* 2005;10:44–51.

Etnyre BR, Abraham LD. Gains in range of ankle dorsi-flexion using three popular stretching techniques. *Am J Phys Med* 1986;65:189–196.

Feland JB, Myrer JW, Schulthies SS, Fellingham GW, Measom GW. The effect of duration of stretching of the hamstring muscle group for increasing range of motion in people aged 65 years or older. *Phys Ther* 2001;81:1100–1117.

Ferber R, Osternig LR, Gravelle DC. Effect of PNF stretch techniques on knee flexor muscle EMG activity in older adults. *J Electromyogr Kinesiol* 2002;12:391–397.

Fernández-de-las-Peñas C, Alonso-Blanco C, Cuadrado ML, Gerwin RD, Pareja JA. Trigger points in the suboccipital muscles and forward head posture in tension type headache. *Headache* 2006a;46:454–460.

Fernández-de-las-Peñas C, Alonso-Blanco C, Cuadrado ML, Gerwin RD, Pareja JA. Myofascial trigger points and their relationship to headache clinical parameters in chronic tension type headache. *Headache* 2006b;46: 1264–1272.

Fernández-de-las-Peñas C, Ge HY, Arendt-Nielsen L, Cuadrado ML, Pareja JA. Referred pain from trapezius muscle trigger point shares similar characteristics with chronic tension type headache. *Eur J Pain* 2007;11:475–482.

Fryer G. Muscle energy concepts: a need for change. *J Osteopath Med* 2000;3:54–59.

Fryer G. Muscle energy technique: research and efficacy. In: Chaitow L, ed. *Muscle Energy Techniques*. 3rd ed. Edinburgh: Churchill Livingston; 2006:109–132.

Fryer G, Ruszkowski W. The influence of contraction duration in muscle energy technique applied to the atlanto-axial joint. *J Osteopath Med* 2004;7:79–84.

Fryer G, Alivizatos J, Lamaro J. The effect of osteopathic treatment on people with chronic and sub-chronic neck pain: a pilot study. *Int J Osteopath Med* 2005;8:41–48.

Fryette H. *Principles of Osteopathic Technique*. Carmel, CA: Academy of Applied Osteopathy; 1954.

Gerwin R. Headache. In: Ferguson LW, Gerwin R, eds. *Clinical Mastery in the Treatment of Myofascial Pain*. Baltimore: Lippincott Williams & Wilkins; 2005:1–29.

Gibbons P, Tehan P. Muscle energy concepts and coupled motion of the spine. *Man Ther* 1998;3:95–101.

Gibbons P, Tehan P. *Manipulation of the Spine, Thorax and Pelvis: An Osteopathic Perspective*. 2nd ed. London: Churchill Livingston; 2006.

Godges JJ, Mattson-Bell M, Thorpe D, Shah D. The immediate effects of soft tissue mobilization with proprioceptive neuromuscular facilitation on gleno-humeral external rotation and overhead reach. *J Orthop Sports Phys Ther* 2003;33:713–718.

Goodridge JP, Kuchera ML. Muscle energy treatment techniques for specific areas. In: Ward RC, ed. *Foundations for Osteopathic Medicine*. Baltimore: Williams & Wilkins; 1997:696–761.

Greenman PE. *Principles of Manual Medicine*. 3rd ed. Philadelphia: Lippincott Williams & Wilkins; 2003.

Haldeman S, Kohlbeck FJ, McGregor M. Unpredictability of cerebro-vascular ischemia associated with cervical spine manipulation therapy: a review of sixty-four cases after cervical spine manipulation. *Spine* 2001;27:49–55.

Handel M, Horstmann T, Dickhuth HH, Gulch RW. Effects of contract-relax stretching training on muscle performance in athletes. *Eur J Appl Physiol* 1997;76:400–408.

Ishii T, Mukai Y, Hosono N, Sakaura H, Nakajima Y, Sato Y, et al. Kinematics of the upper cervical spine in rotation: in vivo three-dimensional analysis. *Spine* 2004;29: E139–E144.

Ishii T, Mukai Y, Hosono N, Sakaura H, Fujii R, Nakajima Y, et al. Kinematics of the cervical spine in lateral bending: in vivo three-dimensional analysis. *Spine* 2006;31:155–160.

Kuchera WA, Kuchera ML. *Osteopathic Principles in Practice.* Missouri: Kirksville College of Osteopathic Medicine Press; 1992.

Lederman E. *The Science and Practice of Manual Therapy.* 2nd ed. Edinburgh: Elsevier Churchill Livingston; 2005.

Legaspi O, Edmond SL. Does the evidence support the existence of lumbar spine coupled motion? A critical review of the literature. *J Orthop Sports Phys Ther* 2007;37: 169–178.

Liebenson C. *Rehabilitation of the Spine: A Practitioner's Manual.* 2nd ed. Baltimore: Lippincott Williams & Wilkins; 2007.

Liebenson C, Tunnell P, Murphy DR, Gluck-Bergman N. Manual resistance techniques. In: Liebenson C, ed. *Rehabilitation of the Spine: A Practitioner's Manual.* 2nd ed. Baltimore: Lippincott Williams & Wilkins; 2007:407–459.

Magnusson M, Simonsen EB, Aagaard P, Sorensen H, Kjaer M. A mechanism for altered flexibility in human skeletal muscle. *J Physiol* 1996a;497(pt 1):293–298.

Magnusson M, Simonsen EB, Dyhre-Poulsen P, Aagaard P, Mohr T, Kjaer M. Visco-elastic stress relaxation during static stretch in human skeletal muscle in the absence of EMG activity. *Scand J Med Sci Sport* 1996b;6:323–328.

Magnusson SP, Simonsen EB, Aagaard P, Dyhre-Poulsen P, McHugh MP, Kjaer M. Mechanical and physiological responses to stretching with and without pre-isometric contraction in human skeletal muscle. *Arch Phys Med Rehabil* 1996c;77:373–377.

Malmstrom E, Karlberg M, Fransson PA, Melander A, Magnusson M. Primary and coupled cervical movements. The effect of age, gender, and body mass index. A 3-dimensional movement analysis of a population without symptoms of neck disorders. *Spine* 2006;31:E44–E50.

Mitchell FL Sr. Structural pelvic function. In: Barnes MW, ed. *Year Book 1958: Selected Osteopathic Papers.* Carmel, CA: Academy of Applied Osteopathy; 1958:71–90.

Mitchell FL Jr, Mitchell PKG. *The Muscle Energy Manual.* Vol. 1. East Lansing, MI: MET Press; 1995.

Mitchell FL Jr, Moran PS, Pruzzo NA. *An Evaluation and Treatment Manual of Osteopathic Muscle Energy Procedures.* Valley Park, MO: Mitchell, Moran and Pruzzo; 1979.

Ogince M, Hall T, Robinson K, Blackmore AM. The diagnostic validity of the cervical flexion-rotation test in C1/2-related cervicogenic headache. *Man Ther* 2007;12:256–262.

Osternig LR, Robertson RN, Troxel RK, Hansen P. Muscle activation during proprioceptive neuromuscular facilitation (PNF) stretching techniques. *Am J Phys Med* 1987;66: 298–307.

Osternig LR, Robertson RN, Troxel RK, Hansen P. Differential responses to proprioceptive neuromuscular facilitation (PNF) stretch techniques. *Med Sci Sports Exerc* 1990;22: 106–111.

Sady SP, Wortman M, Blanke D. Flexibility training: ballistic, static or proprioceptive neuromuscular facilitation? *Arch Phys Med Rehabil* 1982;63:261–263.

Schenk RJ, Adelman K, Rousselle J. The effects of muscle energy technique on cervical range of motion. *J Manual Manipulative Ther* 1994;2:149–155.

Simons DG, Travell JG, Simons LS. *Myofascial Pain and Dysfunction: The Trigger Point Manual.* Vol. 1. 2nd ed. Baltimore: Williams & Wilkins; 1999.

Sizer PS Jr, Brismee JM, Cook C. Coupling behavior of the thoracic spine: a systematic review of the literature. *J Manipulative Physiol Ther* 2007;30:390–399.

Spernoga SG, Uhl TL, Arnold BL, Gansneder BM. Duration of maintained hamstring flexibility after a one-time, modified hold-relax stretching protocol. *J Athletic Training* 2001;36: 44–48.

Spring F, Gibbons P, Tehan P. Intra-examiner and inter-examiner reliability of a positional diagnostic screen for the lumbar spine. *J Osteopath Med* 2001;4:47–55.

Wallin D, Ekblam B, Grahn R, Nordenborg T. Improvement of muscle flexibility. A comparison between two techniques. *Am J Sports Med* 1985;13:263–268.

Wilson E, Payton O, Donegan-Shoaf L, Dec K. Muscle energy technique in patients with acute low back pain: a pilot clinical trial. *J Orthop Sports Phys Ther* 2003;33:502–512.

Neuromuscular Approaches

Luis Palomeque del Cerro, PT, DO, and
César Fernández-de-las-Peñas, PT, DO, PhD

Neuromuscular techniques (NMT) refers to the manual application of specialized digital pressure or strokes, most commonly applied through finger, thumb, or elbow contact. These digital contacts can have either a diagnostic (assessment) or therapeutic objective, and the degree of pressure employed varies considerably among therapists and modes of application.

NMT attempts to identify altered states of soft tissues of the human body, since they affect patients' health, and sometimes offers therapeutic intervention that reduces the load or assists the self-regulatory functions of the body (homeostasis). These techniques may be used in all areas of the human body to reduce the structural distress that often accompanies injury or pain conditions. For instance, when a patient suffers from an ankle sprain, compensatory gait changes, as well as crutch usage and redistribution of weight, may stress the lower back, hip joint, or even cervical spine. The application of NMT to these regions may help reduce structural adaptations and decrease the overall effects of the injury. Further, neuromuscular approaches also seek to correct dysfunctional postural patterns by releasing stressful tension in muscular and fascial tissues.

Boris Chaitow, DC (personal communication, 1983) wrote:

To apply NMT successfully it is necessary to develop the art of manual palpation and sensitivity of fingers by constantly feeling the appropriate regions and assessing any abnormality in tissue structure for tensions, contractions, adhesions, or spasms. It is very important to acquire with practice an appreciation of the "feel" of normal tissue so that one is better able to recognize abnormal tissue. Once some level of diagnostic sensitivity with fingers has been achieved, subsequent application of the technique will be much easier to develop. The whole secret is to be able to recognize the "abnormalities" in the feel of tissue structures. Having become accustomed to understanding the texture and character of "normal" tissue, the pressure applied by the thumb in general, especially in the spinal structures, should always be firm but never hurtful or bruising. To this end the pressure should be applied with a "variable" pressure, i.e. with an appreciation of the texture and character of the tissue structures and according to the feel that sensitive fingers should have developed.

The level of the pressure applied should not be consistent because the character and texture of tissue is always variable. The pressure should therefore be so applied that the thumb is moved along its path of direction in a way which corresponds to the feel of the tissues. This variable factor in finger pressure constitutes probably the most important quality a practitioner of NMT can learn, enabling him to maintain more effective control of pressure, develop a greater sense of diagnostic feel, and be far less likely to bruise the tissue.

THERAPEUTIC EFFECTS OF NEUROMUSCULAR APPROACHES

Modern pain research has demonstrated that a feature of the etiology of chronic pain is the presence of areas of soft-tissue dysfunction that promote pain and distress in soft-tissue structures (Lewit, 1999; Simons et al., 1999; Mense et al., 2000). Manual modalities are often able to encourage optimal regeneration and repair, particularly during the remodeling phase of tissue recovery.

Therapeutically, NMT aims to induce modifications in dysfunctional soft tissue, encouraging a restoration of functional normality, with a particular focus of deactivating focal points of reflexogenic activity (Chaitow, 2001). An alternative focus of NMT focuses on normalizing imbalances in hypertonic or fibrotic tissues. NMT can be used as the sole technique during a treatment or prior to joint mobilization or manipulation interventions. Mechanical elongation of shortened, stiff, or fibrotically soft tissues can be modified, and sometimes normalized, by means of a variety of manual modalities, such as massage, mobilization, muscle energy techniques, oscillatory methods, and NMT.

The therapeutic effects of NMT arise from two distinct approaches: one that reduces adaptive load (improved posture, ergonomics, breathing function, etc.) and one that encourages soft tissues to have a greater ability to adapt by improving flexibility, stability, stamina, and function.

Fluid Movement

This physiologic effect is related to injuries, including inflammation, ischemia, and wherever there is an impediment to normal blood or lymph flow. NMT and other manual techniques may assist in fluid movement by the following mechanisms:

- Enhancing local circulation and drainage
- Reducing swelling and improving washout of inflammatory chemicals
- assisting in normalization of trigger point pain
- modifying neural irritation caused by local edema

Mechanical Stimulus

Possibly the most distinctive therapeutic effect of NMT is related to the mechanical stimulus exerted by manual compression. The range of physiologic effects resulting from sustained or intermittent compression includes several aspects.

- Simons (2002) proposed that local pressure may equalize the length of sarcomeres in the involved soft-tissue trigger point and consequently decrease the pain.
- Hou et al. (2002) suggested that pain relief from pressure treatment may result from reactive hyperemia, or a spinal reflex mechanism for the relief of muscle spasm.
- Cantu and Grodin (1992) believe that NMT induces a degree of mechanical stretching, which

occurs when creep of connective tissue commences.

- Hong et al. (1993) suggested that deep pressure can offer effective stretching and mobilization of muscle taut bands.
- Barnes (1997) suggested that soft-tissue interventions induce piezoelectric effects, which modify the gel state of tissues to a more solute state (as in myofascial induction approaches, Chapter 27).
- Melzack and Wall (1988) established the pain-gate theory; hence, NMT may induce rapid mechanoreceptor impulses (stimulation of Aδ fibers), which interfere with slower pain messages (inhibition of C fibers).
- Other authors (Jones, 1981; Chaitow, 2001) suggested that some manual interventions (e.g., strain/counterstrain) achieve their benefits by means of an automatic resetting of muscle spindles that would help dictate the length and tone into the affected tissues.

Whether the therapeutic goal is to focus on pain relief, motor system rehabilitation, enhanced proprioception, or other neurologically mediated processes, manual modalities inevitably rely on, or influence, the nervous system—generally, locally, significantly, or peripherally. There is also most likely the impact of neuromuscular modalities on what can be termed the psychophysiologic aspect. This might involve mechanisms modulating sympathetic nerve function, reducing arousal, stimulating parasympathetic functions, or assisting in reintegration of the mind-body complex (as in psychodynamic bodywork or somatic experiencing work).

SCIENTIFIC EVIDENCE FOR NEUROMUSCULAR APPROACHES

There is limited research into the use of NMT, although it is included in some studies investigating treatment of muscle or post-traumatic pain in which some techniques, particularly muscle energy, have been combined with NMT (Fernández-de-las-Peñas et al., 2005).

Patel (2002) compared the effects on cervical range of motion of either NMT or muscle energy technique applied bilaterally to both scalene muscles in a cohort of 40 asymptomatic female subjects. Participants were randomly divided into two groups: group 1 received NMT on week 1, followed by a rest period on week 2,

followed by NMT on week 3; whereas group 2 received muscle energy technique on week 1, followed by a rest period on week 2, followed by NMT on week 3. This study found that either NMT or muscle energy technique significantly increased cervical range of motion in all planes of movement ($P < 0.05$), with muscle energy application being more effective than NMT.

Palmer (2002) investigated the effectiveness of both NMT and muscle energy techniques on quadriceps muscle strength in a cohort of 30 asymptomatic subjects (20 females and 10 males). The participants were randomly allocated to two groups: group 1, which received a muscle energy intervention during the first week and NMT during the second week; and group 2, which received NMT first and the muscle energy intervention the second week. Quadriceps strength of the dominant leg was assessed before and after the intervention by means of a digital myograph (Myo-tech, model DM 2000). This study showed that both NMT and muscle energy techniques applied separately produced a significant change in muscle strength of the quadriceps muscle ($P < 0.05$).

Tomlinson (2002) investigated whether the inclusion of NMT or muscle energy technique in a clinical approach was effective in increasing restricted ankle dorsiflexion in 21 subjects (12 females and 9 males) who were treated on three separate visits over 5 weeks. NMT or muscle energy technique was applied to the plantar flexors in two separate treatments on two separate occasions, with a week of no treatment dividing the two. The final treatment included both techniques. The results found a significant increase in passive ankle dorsiflexion range of motion ($P < 0.05$) for both techniques used alone, as well as for both interventions when combined, with no significant difference between the effectiveness of the two techniques used alone. In addition, the combination of both interventions was more effective than the application of each intervention ($P < 0.05$).

Rice (2002) investigated the effects of the application of NMT to the diaphragm on cervical mobility in a cohort of 24 healthy subjects (13 females and 11 males). A within-subject repeated measures design was used in which each subject was exposed first to the control procedure and then received the intervention. The results demonstrated an increased range of motion following the application of NMT to the diaphragm muscle ($P > 0.05$), with no significant differences between males and females.

Ibáñez-García et al. (2008) compared the immediate effects on pressure pain sensitivity and active mouth opening following the application of either NMT or strain/counterstrain technique applied over trigger points in the masseter muscle. Seventy-one subjects (34 men and 37 women) were divided randomly into three groups: group A, which was treated with an NMT intervention; group B, treated with the strain/counterstrain technique; and group C, which was the control group. Each treatment group received a weekly treatment session during 3 consecutive weeks. Outcomes measures were pressure pain thresholds (PPT), mouth opening, and local pain (Visual Analogue Scale) elicited by the application of 2.5 kg/cm^2 of pressure over the trigger point. The results found a significant group versus time interaction ($F = 25.3$; $P <0.001$) for changes in PPT, changes in active mouth opening ($F = 10.5$; $P <0.001$), and local pain evoked by 2.5 kg/cm^2 of pressure ($F = 10.1$; $P <0.001$). Both interventions were effective for reducing pressure pain sensitivity and increasing mouth opening compared with the control procedure ($P <0.001$), but without differences between NMT or strain/counterstrain techniques.

Finally, there are some studies that have investigated different pressure application of neuromuscular approaches, such as ischemic compression (Hong et al., 1993; Fryer & Hodgson, 2005; Fernández-de-las-Peñas et al., 2006) or muscle energy techniques (Rodriguez-Blanco et al., 2006).

Although the sort of evidence summarized above shows that NMT can be clinically effective, almost all studies were conducted on healthy subjects who are not typical of the population presenting to manual therapists for treatment. Until more rigorous studies evaluate NMT in some patient populations, the effectiveness of this technique remains hypothetical.

CLINICAL CONSIDERATIONS FOR THE USE OF NEUROMUSCULAR APPROACHES

When Should Neuromuscular Techniques Be Applied?

If an injury has occurred within 72 hours of therapy, great care must be taken to protect the tissues and modulate blood flow and swelling. The body will, in most cases, naturally splint the area and often produces swelling as part of the recovery process (Cailliet, 1996). The normal response after injury involves inflammation, vasodilation, swelling, relative ischemia (and the pain this induces), an influx of white blood cells that, together with macrophages, remove damaged cells and

debris, and the arrival of fibroblasts that proliferate to form connective tissue and that subsequently turn into myofibroblasts that have the ability to contract to help consolidate the damaged area (MacIntosh et al., 2006). As the remodeling phase of the healing process progresses, collagen fibers are laid down in line with tension forces. This is the stage at which appropriate exercise, movement, and careful manual therapy may usefully assist the intrinsic repair process. However, neuromuscular interventions should not be applied directly to the injured tissues within the first 72 hours following the injury, because this would tend to encourage increased blood flow to the already congested tissues and reduce the natural splinting that is needed in this phase of recovery. After 72 hours, NMT may be carefully applied to the injured tissues and to the supporting structures and muscles involved in possible compensating patterns.

In addition, caution should be taken with the following situations: acute arthritis or other inflammatory conditions (NMT is contraindicated during acute stages), aneurysm, bone fractures, acute soft-tissue injury, hemophilia, osteoporosis, leukemia, malignancy with metastasis involving bone, patients on cortisone or with high fever, phlebitis, recent scar tissue, syphilitic articular or periarticular lesions, or uncontrolled diabetic neuropathy.

Clinical Guideline for the Use of Neuromuscular Interventions

Based on the clinical experiences, it is suggested that the following be used as a general guideline when addressing soft-tissue problems.

- Knowledge of the anatomy of each muscle, including innervation, fiber arrangement, nearby neurovascular structures, and overlying and underlying muscles, will greatly assist the practitioner in quickly locating the appropriate affected tissue.
- The most superficial tissue should usually be treated before the deeper layers.
- The proximal portions of an extremity should be treated before the distal portions so that proximal restrictions of lymph flow are removed before distal lymph movement is increased.
- In a two-jointed muscle, both joints should be assessed, whereas in multijointed muscles, all

involved joints are treated. For instance, if biceps muscle is examined, both glenohumeral and elbow joints should be assessed.

- Where multiple areas of pain are present, a general rule of thumb, based on clinical experience, can be suggested: treat the most proximal, most medial, and most painful tissue first, avoiding overtreating the patient as a whole (including the assignment of homework) as well as the individual tissues.

Use of Lubricant During Neuromuscular Interventions

In general, soft-tissue treatment techniques often involve the use of a lubricant to prevent skin irritation and facilitate smooth movement. The use of a lubricant during a neuromuscular application facilitates the smooth passage of the thumb, finger, or elbow. A suitable balance between lubrication and adherence can be found by mixing two parts of almond oil to one part limewater. It is important to avoid excessive oiliness, because the essential aspect of slight traction from the contact digit will be lost. In addition, NMT often involves dry-skin techniques prior to lubrication. If the skin or muscles need to be lifted following lubrication, this can be accomplished through a cover sheet or a piece of cloth, paper towel, or tissue placed on the skin. Finally, the lubricant may be removed using an appropriate alcohol-based medium.

Discomfort or Unpleasant Responses from the Patient

NMT, although extremely effective, can be uncomfortable for the patient because one of the main objectives is to locate and then to introduce an appropriate degree of pressure into areas of dysfunctional soft tissues. Temporary discomfort may be produced, which may require the technique to be adjusted in order to avoid excessive painful responses during the intervention. The patient is instructed to report, when requested or when he or she wants, if the level of perceived discomfort increases or decreases.

GLIDING OR SLIDING TECHNIQUES

Neuromuscular applications involve different manual techniques, such as compression, stretching, transverse friction massage, and so on. Nevertheless, the most important maneuver is the gliding or sliding technique. These longitudinal strokes are ideal for exploring the tissue for ischemic bands or muscle trigger points and may also be followed by other interventions, such as compression or stretching techniques. Gliding or sliding techniques also help the clinician to become familiar with the quality, muscle tension, and degree of tenderness in the tissues being assessed or treated. The degree of pressure applied over the tissue is determined by a constantly fluctuating stream of information regarding the status of the patient's tissue. As the thumb, fingers, or elbow move from normal tissue to tense or fibrotic tissue, the amount of pressure will need to be modified. Some regions will feel hard or tense, and pressure should be slightly lightened but not increased. After assessment of the extent of tissue involvement (i.e., the size of area involved, a sense of depth of tissue involvement, and degree of tenderness), pressure can be increased if appropriate. Some areas will feel doughy, although they may be extremely tender (tender points), whereas others may feel stringy or ropy. Indurations may be felt as the thumb or index finger glides transversely across taut bands (muscle trigger points). Manual palpation can then be altered to include flat or pincer palpation, depending on the tissue's availability to be grasped (see Chapter 16).

Finally, if trigger points are found, other modalities can be applied, including trigger point pressure release, transverse friction massage (Fernández-de-las-Peñas et al., 2006), stretching, vibration, and so on, which will encourage the release of the taut fibers housing the muscle trigger point (Simons et al., 1999). Clinical experience indicates that the best result usually comes from gliding on the tissues repetitively (six to eight times).

Clinical Application of Gliding or Sliding Techniques

Gliding strokes are usually effective in lengthening shortened connective tissue. It is especially useful to apply strokes using one or both thumbs. Nevertheless, some clinicians prefer the index finger or the elbow. These gliding strokes may be started at the center of the fibers and stroked toward one attachment and then repeated toward the other attachment or by using both fingers and gliding from the center to both muscle ends simultaneously. The treatment is usually the same each time. The pattern suggests a framework and useful starting and ending points, but the degree of therapeutic response offered to the various areas of dysfunction encountered varies depending on individual considerations.

The positioning of the clinician's body in relation to the area being treated is very important to achieve economy of effort and comfort. The optimum height *vis-à-vis* the couch and the most effective angle of approach to the body areas being addressed should be considered. Because the angle of pressure to the skin surface is usually between 40° and 50°, the clinician should carefully consider his or her position.

To glide most effectively on the tissues, the practitioner's fingers are spread slightly and lead the thumbs. The fingers support the weight of the hands and arms, which relieves the thumbs of that responsibility. As a result, the pressure exerted by the thumb is more easily controlled and can be changed as varying tensions are matched in the tissues. The fingers stabilize the hands, while the thumbs are the actual treatment tools in most cases, although sometimes the elbow can serve to deliver the treatment. The wrist needs to remain stable so that the hands move as a unit, with little or no motion occurring in the wrist or the thumb joints. When two-handed glides are employed, the lateral aspects of the thumbs are placed side by side or one slightly ahead of the other with the tips of both pointing in the same direction, that being the direction of the glide. In addition, a two-handed knuckles contact can also be used. Pressure is applied through the wrist and longitudinally through the thumb (elbow, index finger, knuckle) joints (osteoarticular column), not against the medial aspects of the thumbs. A stroke or glide of 2 to 3 inches (5–8 cm) will usually take 4 to 5 seconds, seldom more unless a particularly obstructive indurate area is involved.

Speed of Gliding Movements

Unless the tissue being treated is excessively tender, the gliding stroke should cover 3 to 4 inches (8–10 cm) per second. However, if the tissue is sensitive, a slower pace and reduced pressure is suggested. It is important to develop a moderate gliding speed in order to feel what is present in the tissue. Movement that is too rapid may skim over congestion or other tissue abnormality, or cause excessive pain or discomfort in the patient, whereas movement that is too slow may make identification of individual muscles difficult. A moderate speed will allow for numerous repetitions

that will significantly increase blood flow and soften fascia for further manipulation. Nevertheless, the speed should be adapted to each patient on each session of treatment.

NEUROMUSCULAR INTERVENTIONS FOR HEADACHE PATIENTS

Neuromuscular Techniques Applied to the Sacrum and Iliac Bones

The technique starts with the treatment of the sacrum and both iliac bones. The clinician contacts over the center of the base of the sacrum bone with the thumbs. From this point, the thumbs slide laterally over the base of the sacrum, reaching the superior border. The sliding continues along the lateral aspects of the sacrum to the lower point (**Figure 26.1**). Second, the therapist also performs different strokes over the superior border of the iliac bone (**Figure 26.2**).

Neuromuscular Techniques Applied to the Paraspinal Extensor Muscles

The first contact is applied over the posterior-superior spine of the iliac bone of one side. From this point, the clinician slides cranially along the lumbar extensor muscles (**Figure 26.3**) and the thoracic and cervical muscles until the thumb reaches the external occipital protuberance (**Figure 26.4**). The other hand of the therapist rests on the upper thoracic or shoulder area as a stabilizing contact. Unless serious underlying dysfunction is found, it is usually necessary to repeat three superimposed strokes at each level of the extensor muscles. If underlying fibrotic tissue is felt under the thumb of the clinician, a fourth stroke can be applied. A second series of strokes may also be applied in the lateral border of the extensor muscles (**Figure 26.5**). Finally, an alternative contact can be applied with the elbow (**Figure 26.6**).

Neuromuscular Techniques Applied to the Lower Trapezius Muscle

The thumb is placed on the right lateral aspect of the twelve dorsal vertebrae, and different strokes are performed cranial and laterally (i.e., diagonally) toward the inferior border of the spine of the scapula (**Figure 26.7**).

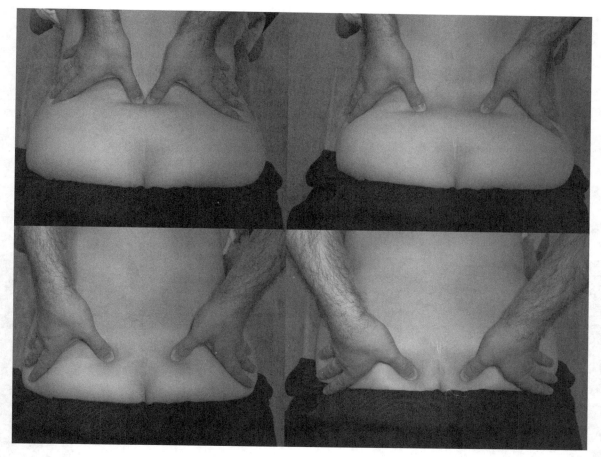

Figure 26.1 Neuromuscular Techniques Applied to the Sacrum Bone

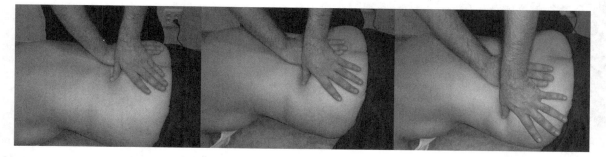

Figure 26.2 Neuromuscular Techniques Applied to the Iliac Bone

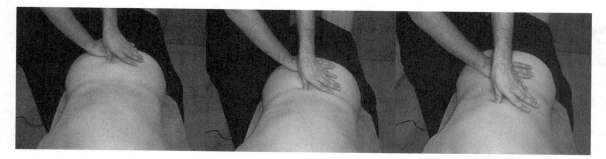

Figure 26.3 Neuromuscular Techniques Applied to the Lumbar Extensor Muscles

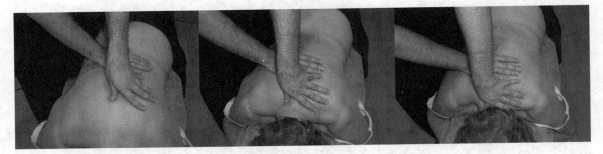

Figure 26.4 Neuromuscular Techniques Applied to the Cervical Extensor Muscles

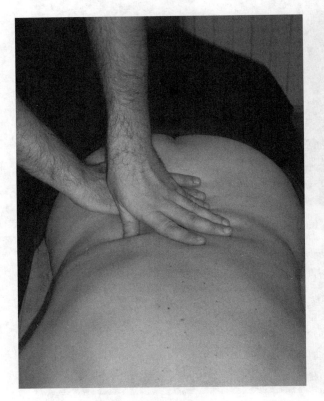

Figure 26.5 Neuromuscular Techniques Applied to the Thoracic Extensor Muscles

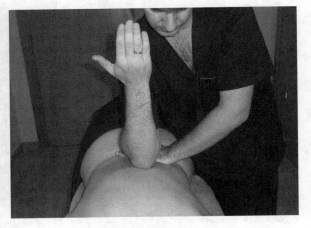

Figure 26.6 Neuromuscular Techniques Applied to the Extensor Muscles with an Elbow Contact

(atlas), and a series of strokes is performed caudad toward the superior border of the scapula (**Figure 26.9**).

Neuromuscular Techniques Applied to the Occipital Bone

The clinician places both thumbs over the middle of the external occipital protuberance, and a series of strokes is performed laterally toward the mastoid process (**Figure 26.10**). This technique releases the insertion of all the cervical muscles.

Neuromuscular Techniques Applied to the Sternocleidomastoid Muscle

With the patient in supine position, the therapist uses the thumb and the index fingers to contact the center region of the sternocleidomastoid muscle. From this contact point, the therapist applies a series of strokes toward both insertions of the muscle (**Figure 26.11**).

Neuromuscular Techniques Applied to the Upper Trapezius and Levator Scapulae Muscles

For the upper trapezius muscle, the thumb is placed over the external occipital protuberance, and the stroke is performed caudad and laterally (i.e., diagonally) toward the spine of the scapula (**Figure 26.8**).

For the levator scapulae muscle, the thumb is placed over the transverse process of the first cervical vertebra

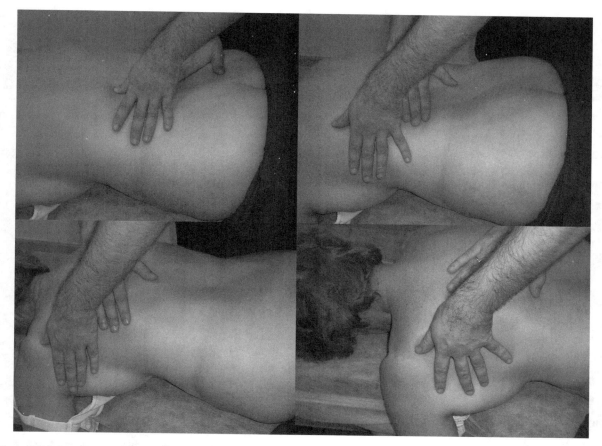

Figure 26.7 Neuromuscular Techniques Applied to the Lower Trapezius Muscle

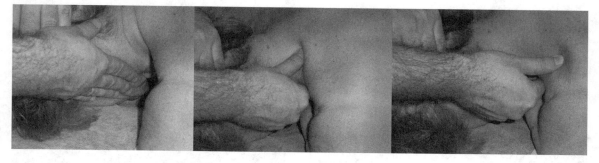

Figure 26.8 Neuromuscular Techniques Applied to the Upper Trapezius Muscle

Neuromuscular Techniques Applied to the Digastric Muscle

The therapist makes contact under the mandible bone, using the middle finger of both hands. From this position, the fingertips of the therapist cranially slide to the angle of the mandible (**Figure 26.12**).

Neuromuscular Techniques Applied to the Masseter Muscle

The therapist places the thumb under the zygomatic insertion of the masseter muscle. A series of strokes are caudally performed toward the superior border of the mandible bone (**Figure 26.13**).

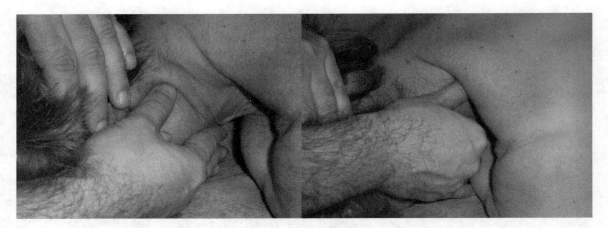

Figure 26.9 Neuromuscular Techniques Applied to the Levator Scapulae

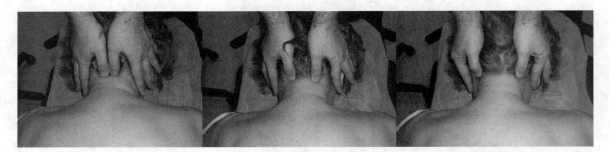

Figure 26.10 Neuromuscular Techniques Applied to the Occipital Bone

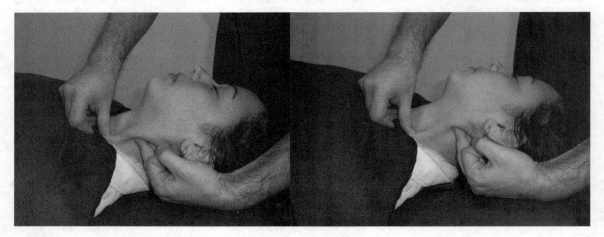

Figure 26.11 Neuromuscular Techniques Applied to the Sternocleidomastoid Muscle

Neuromuscular Techniques Applied to the Mandible Muscle

The therapist contacts with both thumbs over the chin of the patient. A series of strokes is performed laterally toward the inferior border of the mandible bone (**Figure 26.14**).

Neuromuscular Techniques Applied to the Frontalis Muscle

The therapist uses the palms of both hands to contact the forehead of the patient. A series of strokes is laterally performed toward the sphenoid bone (**Figure 26.15**). This technique is usually conducted unilaterally.

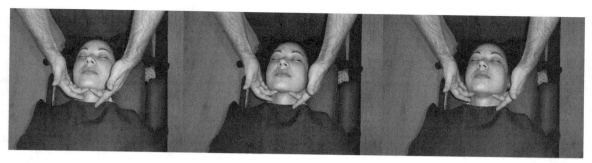

Figure 26.12 Neuromuscular Techniques Applied to the Digastric Muscle

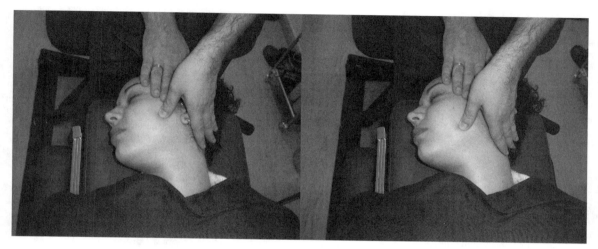

Figure 26.13 Neuromuscular Techniques Applied to the Masseter Muscle

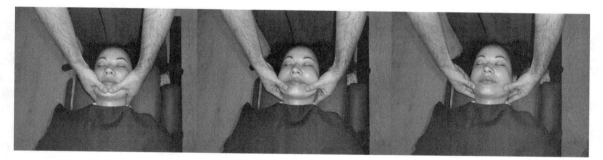

Figure 26.14 Neuromuscular Techniques Applied to the Mandible Muscle

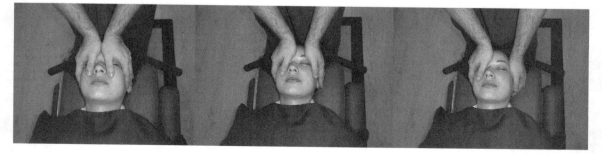

Figure 26.15 Neuromuscular Techniques Applied to the Frontalis Muscle

REFERENCES

Barnes M. The basic science of myofascial release. *J Bodywork Movement Ther* 1997;1:231–238.

Cailliet R. *Soft Tissue Pain and Disability*. 3rd ed. Philadelphia; FA Davis; 1996.

Cantu R, Grodin A. *Myofascial Manipulation*. Gaithersburg, MD: Aspen Publications; 1992.

Chaitow L. *Muscle Energy*. Edinburgh: Churchill Livingstone; 2001.

Fernández-de-las-Peñas C, Sohrbeck-Campo M, Fernández-Carnero J, Miangolarra-Page JC. Manual therapies in the myofascial trigger point treatment: a systematic review. *J Bodywork Movement Ther* 2005;9:27–34.

Fernández-de-las-Peñas C, Alonso-Blanco C, Fernández-Carnero J, Miangolarra-Page JC. The immediate effect of ischemic compression technique and transverse friction massage on tenderness of active and latent myofascial trigger points: a pilot study. *J Bodywork Movement Ther* 2006;10:3–9.

Fryer G, Hodgson L. The effect of manual pressure release on myofascial trigger points in the upper trapezius muscle. *J Bodywork Movement Ther* 2005;9:248–255.

Hong CZ, Chen YC, Pon CH, Yu J. Immediate effects of various physical medicine modalities on pain threshold of an active myofascial trigger point. *J Musculoskeletal Pain* 1993;1:37–53.

Hou CR, Tsai LC, Cheng KF, Chung KC, Hong CZ. Immediate effects of various physical therapeutic modalities on cervical myofascial pain and trigger-point sensitivity. *Arch Phys Med Rehabil* 2002;82:1406–1414.

Ibáñez-García J, Alburquerque-Sendín F, Rodríguez-Blanco C, Girao D, Atienza-Meseguer A, Planella-Abella S, Fernández-de-las-Peñas C. Changes in masseter muscle trigger points following strain-counterstrain or neuro-muscular technique. *J Bodywork Movement Ther* 2008 (in press).

Jones LN. *Strain and Counter-strain*. Newark, OH: American Academy of Osteopathy; 1981.

Lewit K. *Manipulative Therapy in Rehabilitation of the Locomotor System*. 3rd ed. Oxford: Butterworth Heinemann; 1999.

MacIntosh B, Gardiner P, McComas A. *Skeletal Muscle Form and Function*. Champaign, IL: Human Kinetics; 2006.

Melzack R, Wall P. *The Challenge of Pain*. 2nd ed. Middlesex, UK: Penguin Harmondsworth; 1988.

Mense S, Simons DG, Russell IJ. *Muscle Pain: Understanding Its Nature, Diagnosis and Treatment*. Philadelphia: Lippincott Williams & Wilkins; 2000.

Palmer D. Comparison of a muscle energy technique and neuro-muscular technique on quadriceps muscle strength. 2002. Available at: http://www.osteopathic-research.com/.

Patel P. Comparison of neuromuscular technique and a muscle energy technique on cervical range of motion. British College of Osteopathic Medicine; 2002. Available at: http://www.osteopathic-research.com/cgi-bin/or/Search1.p?show_one=30175.

Rice G. The effect of a NMT to the diaphragm on cervical range of motion. 2002. Available at: http://www.osteopathic-research.com/.

Rodríguez-Blanco C, Fernández-de-las-Peñas C, Hernández-Xumet JE, Peña-Algaba G, Fernández-Rabadán M, Lillo MC. Changes in active mouth opening following a single treatment of latent myofascial trigger points in the masseter muscle involving post-isometric relaxation or strain/counter-strain. *J Bodywork Movement Ther* 2006;10:197–205.

Simons DG. Understanding effective treatments of myofascial trigger points. *J Bodywork Movement Ther* 2002;6:81–88.

Simons DG, Travell J, Simons L. *Myofascial Pain and Dysfunction: The Trigger Point Manual*. Vol. 1. 2nd ed. Baltimore: Williams & Wilkins; 1999.

Tomlinson K. Comparison of neuromuscular technique and muscle energy technique on dorsi-flexion range of motion. 2002. Available at: http://www.osteopathic-research.com/.

ETIOLOGY AND PATHOGENESIS OF CERVICAL HEADACHE

Currently, clinicians specializing in headache management focus their approach on circulatory impairments; however, mechanical factors related to the cervical spine are misleading. The term *cervicogenic headache* (CeH) was introduced by Sjaastad in 1983 (Sjaastad & Bovim, 1991). This concept was based on previous studies by Bogduk related to the greater occipital nerve (GON) and the C2 nerve (Bogduk, 1981). An essential criterion for diagnosis according to Sjaastad is mechanical unleashing pain. From a theoretical viewpoint, impairments in either cervical structure or biomechanically related segments can be a nociceptive source responsible for CeH symptoms. Therefore, the genesis of CeH may differ between patients.

Different opinions about the role of cervical musculoskeletal impairments in headache disorders induce divisions between clinicians. For instance, neurologists believe that only 2% of headaches have their origin in the cervical spine (Admeads, 1998). This is opposite to the opinion held by clinicians specializing in musculoskeletal disorders, who believe that 80% of headaches can be attributed to cervical disorders (Vautravers & Maigne, 2003). In addition, the fact that there is no anatomic evidence of any structural lesion detectable with magnetic resonance imaging or computed tomography increases these disagreements among clinicians.

There are several current concepts related to the etiologic factors for CeH. For instance, some authors support the relevance of muscle and aponeurotic factors as the origin of cervical headache (Travell & Simons, 1983). This idea agrees with the clinical reasoning previously published by Cyriax and Cyriax (1989) about referred pain and explores the idea of a global mechanical or pathomechanical response of the cervical spine. In this conceptual model, we should recognize that CeH may represent a complex, dynamic, and fluctuating process, with a multifactorial pathogenesis. Recent studies support this clinical reasoning, focusing the attention on a global anatomic communication network established by the fascial tissue located at the cervical region.

FASCIAL TISSUE

Fascia represents a dense (regular and irregular) connective tissue that forms, in different ways (aponeurosis, tendons, ligaments, joint capsules, and nerve

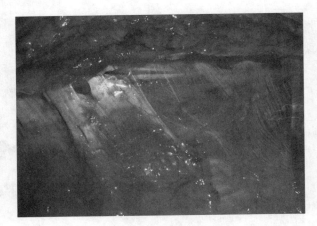

Figure 27.1 Different Forms of Fascial Tissue Representing Regular and Irregular Connective Tissue

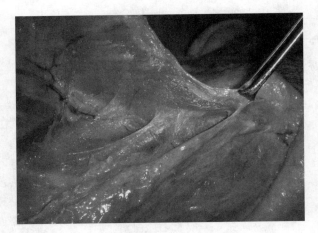

Figure 27.2 Multiple Levels of Connective Tissue Establishing a Network Between the Musculoskeletal Systems

sheets) (**Figure 27.1**) a continuous network between the musculoskeletal system components (**Figure 27.2**). Fascia is also the loose connective tissue that fills the human body's intermedium spaces, linking all the anatomic body structures (veins, arteries, viscera, nerves). These are not only anatomic links, but also meet extensive functional tasks (Pilat, 2003).

From this point of view, it seems that the fascia plays a relevant role in body posture (Langevin, 2006). Studies performed on fresh cadavers (Pilat, 2003; Meyers, 2001) and also some observations during surgical procedures (Guimbertenau et al., 2005) demonstrate that the fascia not only envelops muscle structures (epimysium) but also infiltrates muscles and fatty tissue

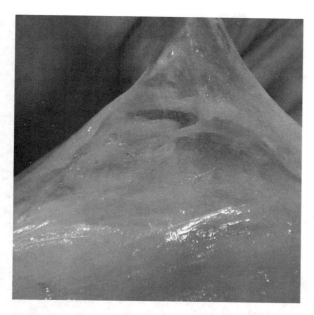

Figure 27.3 Fatty Nodules Infiltrated in the Superficial Fascia of the Cervical Region

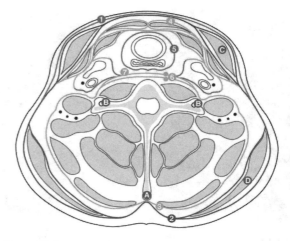

Figure 27.4 **System of Concentric Tubes of the Cervical Fascial System (Transversal Slide at C5 Level).** 1, superficial fascia (subcutaneous fascia); 2, superficial lamina of the deep fascia; 3, prevertebral fascia; 4, infrahyoid lamina; 5, visceral lamina; 6, prevertebral lamina; 7, alar lamina; A, spinous process; B, transverse process; C, sternocleidomastoid muscle; D, trapezius muscle.

Source: Modified from Khrustcheva et al., 2003.

in a very individual manner (**Figure 27.3**). In that way, fascia creates a tridimensional network on macro- and microstructure levels penetrating within the deepest levels of its structure (Swartz et al., 2001; Guimbertenau et al., 2005). These networks may also reach cellular and intracellular levels (Chiquet, 1999).

The extracellular matrix of the connective tissue is the medium of the complex process of mechanotransduction, through which the cellulae dynamically respond, detecting and interpreting the mechanical inputs (Ghosh & Ingber, 2007; Parker & Ingber, 2007; Ingber, 1998, 2005, 2006; Pilat, 2003, 2005). Therefore, it is logical to think about the possibility of the influence of this multidimensional network on the biomechanical or biochemical processes related to the pathogenesis of headaches.

ANATOMY OF THE CERVICAL FASCIA

Geometry of the Cervical Fascial System

The fascial system of the cervical region represents a dynamic connection between the head and the thorax. In this region, there is no clear division between muscle, nerve, and vascular structures. None of them is related to one particular segment. The fascial system establishes several spaces with a longitudinal orientation (Upledger, 1987; Bienfait, 1987; Bochenek & Reicher,

1997; Pilat, 2003), which divide, envelop, support, and connect the muscles, bones, viscera, vascular vessels, and peripheral nerves; this can be compared to a system of tubes concentrically placed inside one another, all interconnected at different levels and in several forms (Pilat, 2003) (**Figure 27.4**). These interconnections unfolded between the muscles establish mechanical links, which determine the direction and the amplitude of the movement (Bochenek & Reicher, 1997). The lubrication of these compartments, due to a greater amount of fatty tissue or loose connective tissue, permits great liberty of movements (particularly sliding) to the fascial system. For instance, this lubrication permits the movement of the hyoid bone during some daily activities such as talking, swallowing, and coughing. The fascial system is responsible for the transmission of the dynamic (active) forces between the cranium, mandible, hyoid, sternum, clavicles, scapula, and the first two ribs. The fascial system deeply connects the endocranium with the endothorax, influencing not only the mechanics of the cervical region, the shoulder complex, and the temporomandibular joint but also the mechanics of the respiratory system and the suitability of the vascular input to the cephalic region.

The route and the connection between the different fascial layers are individual for each person. This is

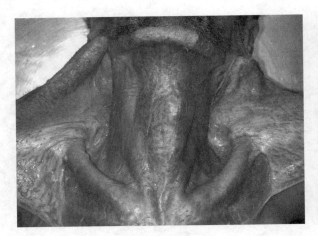

Figure 27.5 Superficial Fascia of the Cervical Cutaneous Muscle

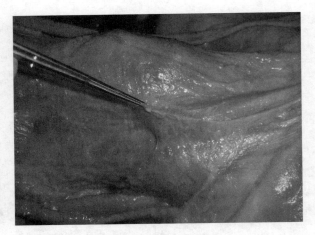

Figure 27.6 Superficial Fascia. Note the great elasticity.

why it is difficult to classify its exact anatomy in regard to the trajectory and interrelations. Nevertheless, most anatomists agree with the following classification and distribution of the fascial system:

Superficial fascia
Deep fascia
   Superficial lamina
   Pretracheal lamina
     Infrahyoid fascia
     Visceral lamina
   Prevertebral lamina
   Alar lamina

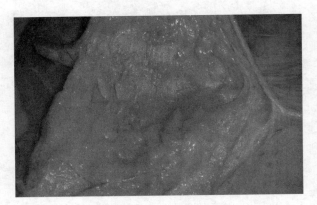

Figure 27.7 Superficial Lamina of the Deep Cervical Fascia with a Higher Amount of Fatty Nodules

Superficial Cervical Fascia (Subcutaneous Fascia)

The most superficial part of the cervical fascial system is formed by a thin lamina called superficial fascia or subcutaneous fascia (**Figure 27.5**). This fascia is located between the skin and the deep fascia. It contains a platysma muscle, cutaneous nerves, capillaries, and lymphatic vessels and is an elastic structure (**Figure 27.6**). The superficial fascia controls the quantity, form, and size of the fatty nodules (**Figure 27.7**). Therefore, the superficial fascia also participates in the distribution of the total fat accumulation.

The dynamic activity of the superficial fascia is related to the platysma muscle, which expands superficially over the anterolateral neck region. On the upper side, the superficial fascia along the platysma muscle envelops the mandible and continues to the superficial

face muscles (depressor anguli, depressor labii inferioris, and the orbicularis oris). On its lower side, the superficial fascia extends beyond the level of the clavicle and inserts to the second and third ribs; on the lateral side it continues to the platysma insertions (**Figure 27.8**).

Deep Cervical Fascia

The second part of the fascial system is formed by the deep fascia, previously called the *fascia colli*. It is a complex system that forms control compartments of the muscular dynamics of the cervical region. As has been previously mentioned, the deep cervical fascia is divided into a series of concentric tubes, all interconnected, at different levels and of several forms that are individual to each person (Pilat, 2003). The following

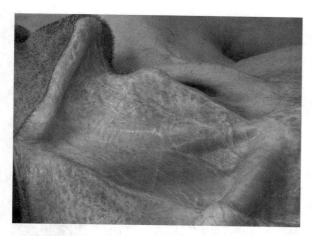

Figure 27.8 Cervical Cutaneous Muscle. Note its expansion under the clavicle level.

levels can be distinguished within the deep fascial system of the cervical region (**Figure 27.9**):

Superficial lamina
Pretracheal lamina
  Infrahyoid fascia
  Visceral lamina
Prevertebral lamina
Alar lamina

Superficial Lamina of the Deep Cervical Fascia

The superficial lamina of the deep fascia (**Figure 27.10**) permits a continuous mechanical action between the cranium and the face bones. It is located under the skin, the superficial fascia, and the platysma muscle. As a thin lamina, it envelops, like a collar, the neck region (**Figure 27.11**). Its insertions involve several structures acting as a distribution network of the cervical region and linking different functional levels. The superficial lamina of the cervical fascia has the following insertions (Gallaudet, 1931; Bochenek & Reicher, 1997):

- *Anterior insertions (this part is also called cervical fascia):* Inserts on the inferior border of the mandible and on the hyoid bone, creating a fold for the stylomandibular ligament.
- *Posterior insertions (this part is also called nuchal fascia):* Inserts on the spinous processes of the cervical vertebrae (continuum to their bone periostium), on the nuchal and supraspinous ligaments.

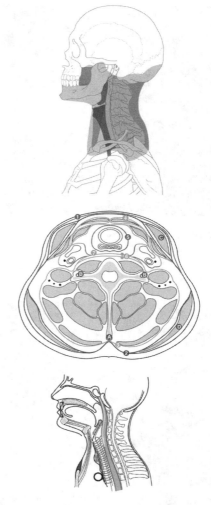

Figure 27.9 Scheme of the Fascial Anatomy of the Cervical Region
Source: Modified from Khrustcheva et al., 2003.

- *Superior insertions:* Inserts on the periostium of the occipital external protuberance, mastoid process of the temporalis bones, the external acoustic meatus, inferior border of the zygomatic arch, and the masseter fascia.
- *Inferior insertions:* Inserts on the spine of the scapulae, acromium, and clavicle. At this level, this lamina assembles with the superficial lamina of the pectoral fascia and with the sternal manubrium, forming the suprasternal space (Upledger, 1987; Bochenek & Reicher, 1997). The connection of this lamina with the sternum is very interesting because the fascial system ends

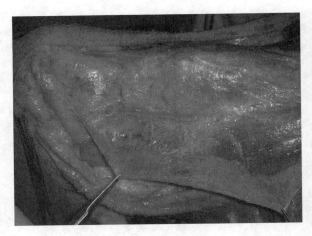

Figure 27.10 Superficial Lamina of the Deep Cervical Fascia

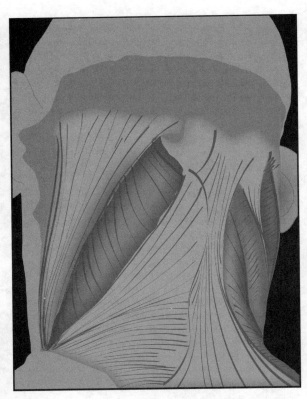

Figure 27.12 Posterior Compartment of the Superficial Lamina of the Deep Cervical Fascia. Note that the sternocleidomastoid and trapezius muscles are located at the same fascial level.

at the manubrium but does not continue over the sternal surface. On the lateral and inferior point, the superficial lamina of the deep fascia changes to the deltoid fascia, whereas under the spine of the scapulae, the superficial lamina of the deep fascia changes to the infraspinatus muscle fascia.

From its posterior insertions, the superficial lamina of the deep cervical fascia is bilaterally divided into two compartments, enveloping first the upper trapezius (**Figure 27.12**) and then the sternocleidomastoid muscle (**Figure 27.13**). At the anterior border of the trapezius muscle, the fascia expands into a fibrotic lamina that communicates with the fascia of the scalene muscles. The sternocleidomastoid fascial envelope is asymmetric, and in its deep trajectory is thin and low-load resistant. The superficial layer is thicker and stronger, particularly at the superior part of the muscle belly. At the superior border the cervical fascia of the sternocleidomastoid muscle forms several fibrotic trabecules and, crossing the subcutaneous tissue, joins the dermis (**Figure 27.14**).

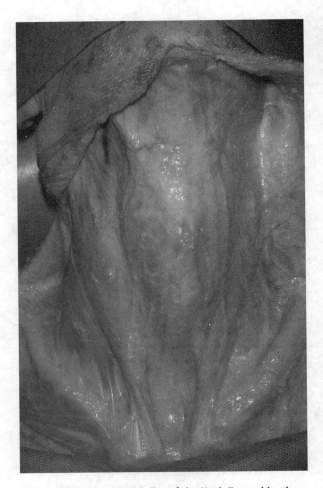

Figure 27.11 Protective Collar of the Neck Formed by the Superficial Lamina of the Deep Cervical Fascia

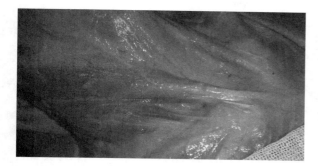

Figure 27.13 Sternocleidomastoid Muscle Enveloped in the External Lamina of the Deep Cervical Fascia

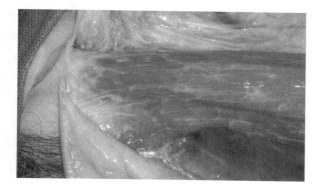

Figure 27.14 Superior Insertions of the Sternocleidomastoid Muscle

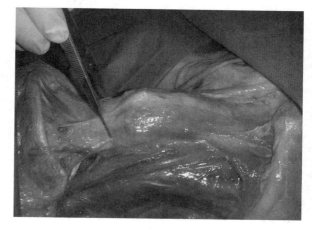

Figure 27.15 Infrahyoid Fascia. Note the hyoid bone positioning.

Pretracheal Lamina

The pretracheal fascia forms the intermediate lamina of the deep cervical fascia, divided into two clearly differentiated structures: the infrahyoid fascia and the visceral lamina.

Infrahyoid Fascia

The infrahyoid fascia comes from the superficial lamina and is divided into two parts: the superficial fascia enveloping the omohyoid and sternohyoid muscles; and the deep fascia that, wrapping and surrounding the thyroid and sternothyroid muscles, joins with the superficial lamina.

The infrahyoid fascia assembles with the superficial fascia at the level of the deep lamina of the sternocleidomastoid muscle. Its trajectory is only anterior (Gallaudet, 1931; Bochenek & Reicher, 1997) (Figure 27.9). At its lateral border, the infrahyoid fascia extends to the omohyoid muscles, whereas posteriorly it continues with the anterior lamina of the upper trapezius muscle. The infrahyoid fascia represents a resistant aponeurotic lamina.

The infrahyoid fascia forms a narrowing space, creating the fibrotic insertion of the digastric muscle that facilitates the hyoid bone suspension (**Figures 27.15, 27.16**). Its extension is smaller than others because it is located only under the hyoid bone. The infrahyoid fascia has the following insertions (Gallaudet, 1931; Bochenek & Reicher, 1997):

- *Anterior insertions:* Located between both omohyoid muscles and in front of the trachea

Another relevant connection is a bandolier structure that goes to the mandibular angle, which originates at the anterior border of the fascial layer and inserts at the proximity of the inferior border of the mandible bone. It has been suggested that this fascial structure plays a relevant role in the dynamic mechanics of the temporomandibular joint.

The sternocleidomastoid and upper trapezius muscles envelop, like a collar, all of the borders of the neck region, establishing several free spaces, which permit access to the deepest lamina of the cervical fascial system. Furthermore, if we look at the cranial and clavicle insertions of both muscles, it seems that they appear as only one muscle with some segments divided in between. This can be related to the fact that both muscles come from the same embryonic lamina, or to the fact that they are innervated by the same cranial nerve (XI). Finally, other structures mechanically controlled by the superficial lamina of the deep cervical fascia are the submandible glandule and the fibrotic capsule of the parotid glandule.

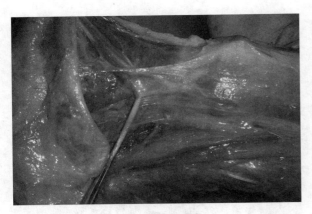

Figure 27.16 Relationship of the Digastric Muscle with the Fibrotic Ansa. Note its continuity to the cervical fascia.

- *Superior insertions:* At the hyoid bone
- *Inferior insertions:* At the inferior border jugular point and around the sternal portion of both clavicle bones

Visceral Lamina of the Pretracheal Fascia

The visceral lamina of the pretracheal fascia is very thin and is located at the deep level of the infrahyoid muscles. This fascia covers the thyroid, the trachea, the esophagus, and the pharynx (Figure 27.9) and joins the prevertebral fascia through the lateral septum. The visceral lamina of the pretracheal fascia has the following insertions (Gallaudet, 1931; Bochenek & Reicher, 1997; Rouviere & Delmas, 2005; Khrustcheva & Zemnick, 2007):

- *Anterior insertions:* Joins the muscular infrahyoid lamina
- *Posterior insertions:* It continues to the prevertebral fascia, particularly at the thyroid level
- *Superior insertions:* Cricoid cartilage, thyroid cartilage, and hyoid bone
- *Inferior insertions:* Together with the infrahyoid muscles go to the sternum bone

In addition, the visceral lamina of the pretracheal fascia has the following expansions:

- *Lateral expansions:* The fascia creates a fold for the carotid lamina and continues with the fascial structures of the heart.
- *Posterior expansions:* The fascia extends from the buccopharyngeal fascia to the sphenoid bone.

- *Inferior expansions:* The fascia continues to the pericardium and mediastinum.

Therefore, this fascial system constitutes a connective network between the endocranium and the endothorax.

Prevertebral Fascia

The prevertebral fascia is the deepest level of the cervical fascial system that envelops all the cervical muscles except the sternocleidomastoid, upper trapezius, and the infrahyoid muscles (Figure 27.9). The trajectory of the prevertebral fascia is similar to the tubular system that surrounds the cervical spine and the related muscles. The reason this fascial system is called *prevertebral* is that its origin is in the vertebral longitudinal anterior ligament. The prevertebral fascia has the following insertions:

- *Anterior insertions:* Vertebral longitudinal anterior ligament
- *Posterior insertions:* The prevertebral fascia continues in its inferior end with the superficial lamina of the thoracolumbar fascia
- *Superior insertions:* Base of the skull
- *Inferior insertions:* At the third thoracic vertebrae the prevertebral fascia joins the thoracolumbar fascia and continues up to the lumbar region

In its lateral trajectory the prevertebral fascia goes bilaterally to the axillar fascia and, at its anterior-inferior border, continues toward the vertebral longitudinal anterior ligament and the posterior border of the mediastinum. Laterally it covers the three scalenes, anteriorly the longus collis and longus cervicis muscles. It rests over the transverse processes of the cervical vertebrae. Finally, on its anterior trajectory, the prevertebral fascia creates a division between the anterior (visceral) and posterior (muscle) regions of the neck (Gallaudet, 1931; Bochenek & Reicher, 1997). In this prevertebral fascial compartment are the following 13 muscles relevant for the dynamic action of the head and neck: longus capitis, longus collis, anterior scalene, middle scalene, posterior scalene, levator scapulae, splenius cervicis, thoracic iliocostalis, cervical and capitis longissimus, semispinalis capitis and cervicis, and the multifidus muscles.

Alar Lamina

The alar lamina constitutes a separate subdivision of the prevertebral fascia on its anterior trajectory and is located posteriorly to the esophagus (Gallaudet, 1931; Bochenek & Reicher, 1997), forming bridges between the transverse processes. Longitudinally it extends from the base of the skull to the mediastinum.

Clinical Considerations of the Cervical Fascia Anatomy

The anatomy of the cervical fascia has several clinical implications (Pilat, 2003).

- The mastoid process is the prominent bone subjected to a constant traction force induced by muscles inserted on it. From the most superficial to the deep level, they are the sternocleidomastoid, the splenius capitis, and the longus colli muscles. All of them are long muscles capable of developing a strong traction force.
- The splenius capitis muscle, when acting bilaterally, exerts an important extension movement to the head and the neck. Nevertheless, this muscle is not important for the maintenance of the upright posture of the head.
- Both longus capitis and cervicis muscles are extremely important for the maintenance of this upright position of the head in the sagittal plane. These muscles are powerful flexors and are responsible for counteracting the extensor force created by the posterior cervical extensor muscles.
- The scalene muscles place the lower cervical spine in flexion, whereas the suboccipital muscles position the upper cervical spine in extension, contributing to a forward head posture (Chapter 8). The scalene muscles stabilize the first rib, but they can also exert a caudal and anterior force to the lower cervical vertebrae. It is important to remember that during the application of any deep fascial technique to this cervical region, the clinician should avoid applying compression to the brachial plexus. If the patient reports pins and needles or a tingling sensation in the limb, the clinician should move his or her fingers away from the brachial plexus.

Conclusions

The introduction to this chapter mentioned the continuity of the fascial structure between all the body's me-

chanical levels. The cervical region represents one of the best anatomic examples of this fascial continuity, evidencing the relationship that the fascial system induces over the structures. The fascial tissue organizes and divides, permits the protection and autonomy of each muscle and viscera, and joins all the components of the cervical region into several functional units. In this way, fascial tissue establishes spatial relationships between these functional units, creating a continuous network. In addition, the fascia permits the expansion of nerve and lymphatic vessels. This fascial property connects this tissue with the metabolic changes of the water and the nutrition function related to blood and lymph. Thus, the fascia is converted into a sophisticated transport medium between and within all the systems.

THEORETICAL ASPECTS FOR THE MANAGEMENT OF FASCIAL DYSFUNCTION SYNDROME

Principles of Fascial Dysfunction

The proper quality and mobility of the fascial tissue is essential for the optimal functioning of all the corporeal systems. Fascial tissue is also related to the proper interchange of fluids. A decrease of fascial mobility will alter the blood circulation, causing it to become slower and heavier, and, in some extreme cases, could induce an ischemia and a deterioration of the muscle fibers' quality.

One possible reason for a restriction of the fascial tissue may be an excess stimulation of collagen, which will induce fibrosis in the fascial system, resulting in loss of its quality and the creation of entrapment areas. These entrapment areas may alter physiologic movements in relation to amplitude, velocity, resistance, and coordination. In that situation, the human body will adopt alternative and compensatory motor control strategies. If this fascial restriction is prolonged, the body becomes overloaded and creates dysfunctional consequences (Pilat, 2003). These changes first affect the loose connective tissue structures and then reorganize the specialized tissue (regular or irregular dense connective tissue, for example, tendons, ligaments, or capsules), creating an excessive density and reorientation. Fascial restrictions of shorter durations will affect the local function of the tissue, whereas restrictions of long duration will induce a global dysfunction.

Mechanisms of the Myofascial Release Approach

The result of the myofascial induction approach is the mechanical stimulation of the connective tissue. The following three mechanisms have been proposed as the liberation and reorganization phenomena of the fascial tissue: viscoelastic, neurophysiologic, and piezoelectric reactions.

These responses will appear with the correct application of a mechanical stimulus in regard to proper force, velocity, and time. Each of these proposed mechanisms occurs at different levels of body movement (micro or macro) and at different timescales. In addition, each of these mechanisms has the potential of influencing the behavior of the others (Langevin, 2006). In spite of the fascial tissue response during the treatment, all signals (mechanisms) can interact (Pilat, 2003). Therefore, as a result of the therapy, we can obtain (a) a more efficient circulation of antibodies in the ground substance, (b) an increase in the blood supply (release of histamine) toward the region of restriction, (c) a correct orientation in the fibroblast mechanics, (d) greater blood supply toward the nervous system, and (e) increases in the metabolite flow to and from the tissue, facilitating the recovery process (Evans, 1980; Barlow & Willoughby, 1992; Barnes, 1990; Hamwee, 1999; Pilat, 2003).

Mechanical Response of the Fascia Tissue: Viscoelasticity

Viscoelasticity is one of the most important fascial mechanical responses and is defined as the behavior of the material with respect to time. When a mechanical force is applied to a viscoelastic material, a deformation occurs. The deformation will increase in time with the application of the same force.

The viscoelastic properties of the fascial tissue were investigated in several studies related to the specific analysis of certain fascial body structures: thoracolumbar fascia (Yahia et al., 1993), fascia latae (Wright & Rennels, 1964), and subcutaneous fascia in rats (Latridies et al., 2003). Other studies were related to global concepts of practical applications (Rolf, 1977; Threlkeld, 1992; Barnes, 1990; Cantu & Grodin, 2001; Pilat, 2003; Schleip et al., 2005).

Viscoelasticity is linked to the remodeling process of the extracellular matrix related to the density changes and to the proper orientation of the collagen fibers. Studies conducted with the fascia latae, plantar fascia,

and nasal septum (Chaudhry, 2007) supported the viscoelastic properties of these structures and provided important data about the viscoelasticity mechanism and its utility in the therapeutic process:

- The viscoelastic response appears after 60 seconds' application of a continuous force of traction or compression.
- To avoid the fascial tissue block, the therapist should not progressively increase the applied force; it must be constant.
- Different fascial structures demand different levels of the applied force; nevertheless, the time required for the fascial movement response remains the same.

The viscoelastic response originated in the fascial tissue during application of the myofascial induction approach is perceived by the therapist's hand as a movement. This movement can appear on different fascial construction levels (macro- or microscopic). This movement can be visible or only perceived by the subtle perception of therapist's hand. The possibility for manual perception of the fascial movement, without the simultaneous visible response of this phenomenon, can be explained as follows:

- Observations made during surgical procedures and analyzed with 25× microscopy of extension and a videocamera suggest the presence of a continuous network of "multimicrovacuolar collagenous absorbing systems." This is defined as a "chaotic matrix" that maintains its form by the action of physical forces that connect it to a hierarchical complex related to time and space (Guimberteau et al., 2005).
- Ingber's studies related to cellular dynamics and the cytoskeleton's active response (while receiving the mechanical force action emitted from the extracellular matrix) demonstrate the relevance of tissue reorganization at both cellular and subcellular levels (Ingber, 1998, 2004, 2006; Stamenovic et al., 2007; Parker & Ingber, 2007). Ingber's theory focuses on an interconnected system based on the *Tensegrity* principles (Ingber, 1998; Chen & Ingber, 1999). This system of shared tensions in the distribution of the mechanical forces along several levels of the body's construction also explains the fascial system when the system receives an appropriate mechanical impulse during the therapeutic process.

Neurophysiologic Mechanism of Myofascial Induction

Because the muscle is a contractile tissue permitting the human body to perform different kinds of movements, we should also consider the fascia as intramuscular connective tissue. The muscle fibers and the fascia form a functional unit, since each muscle contraction will mobilize the fascial system, and a fascial system restriction will affect the proper functioning of the muscle system (Pilat, 2003). Analysis of the fascial microstructure suggests the hypothesis of an inherent fascial movement induced by the contraction of the myofibroblasts (Staubesand & Li, 1997; Schleip et al., 2006).

The fascial system is richly innervated by an extraordinary network of mechanoreceptors (e.g., Golgi receptors) similar to other structures such as ligaments, joint capsules, or musculotendinous junctions. Fascial mechanoreceptors were described by Schleip (2003a, 2003b). The infrafascial receptors can be divided into three groups:

1. *Paccini corpuscles:* These receptors respond to both rapid mechanical and vibrational inputs. Because these receptors have an extremely rapid response, they react to thrust and vibratory techniques.
2. *Ruffini organs:* These receptors respond to slower impulses and to constant-pressure application. Therefore, they respond to the sustained and deep pressure applied over the soft tissues and with the application of tangential forces in a transverse direction.
3. *Type III receptors (myelin receptors) or type IV receptors (nonmyelin receptors):* These are the sensitive receptors that are most abundant in the human body, which transmit the information from the fascia to the central nervous system.

The application of a stimulus of sustained pressure activates some mechanoreceptors, such as Ruffini corpuscles, which have been described by López (1987) as encapsulated endings where the thick myelin fibers (alpha fibers) arrive. These nerve endings are arranged on concentric layers, creating different compartments with liquid accumulation. This system controls mechanical effects depending on pressure changes. As a result, only high-intensity stimuli can be transmitted. The myofascial induction techniques with constant-pressure application will send inputs to the central nervous system through the anterior spinocerebellar tract.

Snell (2006) described this situation as follows: "The receptor is located in the free nerve endings, or mechanoreceptors (Ruffini corpuscles, tendons, Golgi organs). The axons enter to the spinal cord from the second order neurons ganglion, specifically on the dorsal nucleus on the posterior gray horn base. Most of the axons of second order neurons are crossed toward the opposed tract, ascend through it to the bulb as part of the anterior spinocerebellous tract. They ascend along the peduncular protuberance, penetrating the paleocerebellum through the superior cerebellous stem, and moving to the cerebellous cortex."

It seems that myofascial induction reduces the neural tone via this route since the cerebellum is responsible for its regulation by inhibitory or facilitatory effects. These effects originate in the anterior spinocerebellar tract, particularly when the anterior lobe of the paleocerebellum is stimulated. It appears that the afferent cerebellum tract is the fastigial nucleus that impulses influence over the vestibular nucleus and the alpha motor neurons. In that way, this afferent route permits muscle tone inhibition, facilitating an optimal application of the manual technique.

Piezoelectric Reaction

Piezoelectricity (from the Greek word *piezein*, which means "squeeze" or "pull") is a phenomenon present in certain crystals. This property establishes that when the crystal is subjected to a mechanical tension, it acquires a polarization on its mass; that is, potential differences and electrical load appear on its surface. The crystal deforms under the application of internal forces when an electric field is applied (Pilat, 2003).

The crystals in our body are liquid crystals (Bouligard, 1978; Szent-Gyorgi, 1941). When a mechanical action is performed—for example, the stretching of a muscle tendon—the fascial system is activated and a tiny electrical pulsation is produced. This pulsation, which will represent consecutive mechanical actions, is usually harmonic and oscillatory. The information is electrically transmitted, crossing the fundamental substance of the connective tissue (Oschman, 2003). Since collagen is a semiconductive structure (Cope, 1975), we can conclude that the fascia has the property of forming an integrated electronic network permitting the intercommunication of all the elements of the connective tissue. Therefore, the basic properties of the fascial system (elasticity, flexibility, elongation, and resistance) will depend on the ability to maintain the continuous flow of this information.

MYOFASCIAL INDUCTION TECHNIQUES

There are many different approaches for the management of the fascial system (Barnes 1990; Rolf, 1977; Manheim, 1998; Cantu & Grodin, 2001; Chaitow & Delany, 2002; Pilat, 2003). Most of the approaches are based on a biomechanical analysis and clinical experiences. Currently, enough data from basic research exist to demonstrate that both mechanical and pathomechanical phenomena exist relative to therapeutic approaches involving the fascial tissue. Nevertheless, there currently exists no consensus as to the most beneficial clinical approach (Remvig, 2007).

The techniques described in this chapter focus on a clinical approach and are based on previously described anatomic principles (Pilat, 2003). These techniques focus on the treatment of the three relevant fascial structures related to the cervical region: the superficial lamina of the deep fascia, the prevertebral fascia, and the pretracheal fascia.

Techniques Aimed at the Superficial Lamina of the Deep Fascia

Those changes or restrictions located in the superficial lamina of the deep fascia can be related to a forward head posture (Chapter 8), shortening of suboccipital muscles, dysfunctional respiratory patterns, or impairments in the scapulae region.

Myofascial Induction of the Sternocleidomastoid Muscle

The aim of this technique is to release fascial restrictions of the sternocleidomastoid muscle (**Figure 27.17**) (Pilat, 2003). The patient is in supine position and the therapist is seated at the head of the table. The therapist contacts bilaterally (with a pincer palpation between the thumb and the index finger) the muscle belly of both sternocleidomastoid muscles. With this contact the therapist feels for the restricted side (**Figure 27.18**). Next, the patient's head is rotated to the contralateral side, and again the therapist palpates for the side with the most restriction (**Figure 27.19**). The head of the patient may be brought into slight extension; the hand of the therapist should slide over the region of the restriction. It is important to note that the most restricted region of

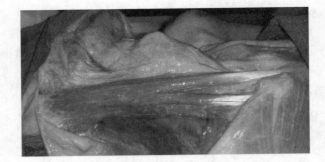

Figure 27.17 Sternocleidomastoid Muscle in a Human Cadaver

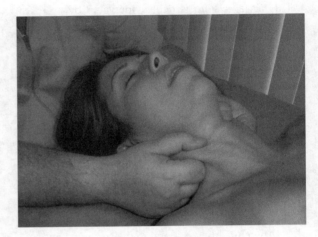

Figure 27.18 Bilateral Pincer Palpation of the Sternocleidomastoid Muscle

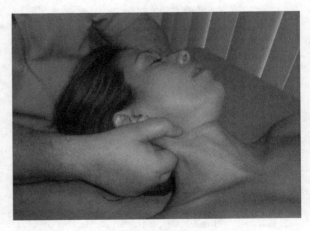

Figure 27.19 Unilateral Pincer Palpation of the Sternocleidomastoid Muscle

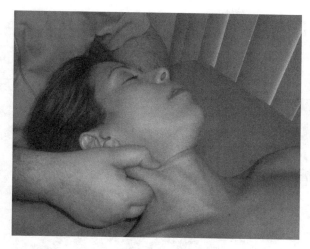

Figure 27.20 Unilateral Pincer Palpation of the Sternocleidomastoid Muscle with Contralateral Cervical Rotation

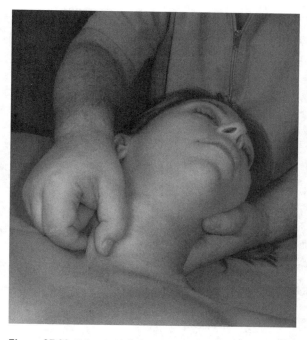

Figure 27.22 Palpation of the Sternocleidomastoid Muscle with the Fingertips

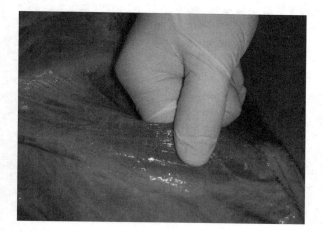

Figure 27.21 Unilateral Pincer Palpation of the Sternocleidomastoid Muscle in a Human Cadaver

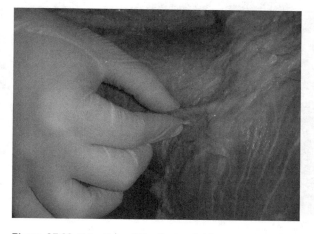

Figure 27.23 Palpation of the Sternocleidomastoid Muscle with the Fingertips in a Human Cadaver

this muscle may be different among patients. Therefore, the pincer palpation should be adapted to the region of the muscle. For instance, if the fascial restriction is located in the muscle belly, the palpation should be conducted with the thumb and the index fingers (**Figures 27.20, 27.21**). On the contrary, if the restriction is located in the tendon of the muscle, the palpation should be done with the fingertips (**Figures 27.22, 27.23**). In either application, the therapist should conduct 7 to 15 sliding passes.

The sliding can be applied in different regions of the muscle belly or the tendon, depending on the location of

the fascial restriction. This technique can be applied unilaterally or bilaterally. If the therapist decides to treat both muscles in the same session, the most restricted side should be treated first. After the treatment, it is recommended that the clinician perform bilateral slides with the aim of checking the symmetry of the elasticity of both sternocleidomastoid muscles (**Figure 27.24**).

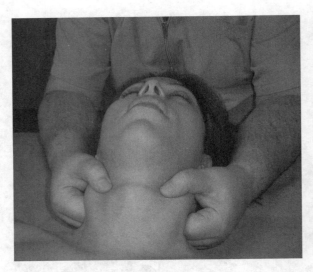

Figure 27.24 Bilateral Pincer Palpation of the Sternocleidomastoid Muscle

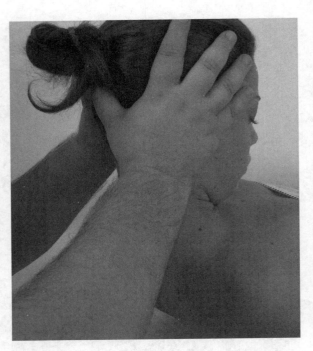

Figure 27.26 Lifting the Patient's Head for the Stroke of the Cervical Extensors

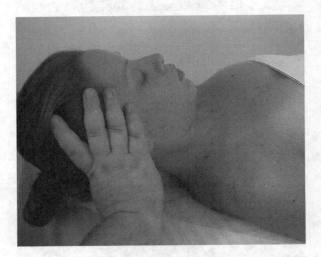

Figure 27.25 Manual Contact for the Stroke of the Cervical Extensor Muscles

Stroke Technique for the Cervical Extensors and the Upper Trapezius Muscle

The aim of this technique is to stretch the fascial structures of the posterior cervical extensor region (Pilat, 2003). The patient is in a supine position and the therapist is seated at the head of the table. The therapist holds the patient's head with both hands (**Figure 27.25**). Next, the patient's head is raised toward the ceiling (**Figure 27.26**). In this position, the therapist

changes the manual contact and with his or her non-dominant hand supports the patient's head from the occipital bone (**Figure 27.27**). The elbow of the therapist is supported on the table. With the other hand, the therapist contacts the cervical extensor muscles. The contact point is placed between the knuckles of the thumb and the index fingers (**Figure 27.28**). The technique consists of longitudinal slides in a caudal direction (**Figure 27.29**). This procedure can be repeated three to seven times. It should be slowly and progressively performed; that is, the movement should be retained for approximately 7 seconds (maintaining the same force) and not continued until the release happens.

This technique can also be performed with the patient in prone position (**Figure 27.30**). The therapist follows the same procedures as previously described. **Figure 27.31** shows the technique conducted on a fresh human cadaver.

Techniques Aimed at the Prevertebral Fascia

The changes located in the prevertebral fascial level can be associated with a forward head posture (Chapter 8) or cervicobrachial symptoms.

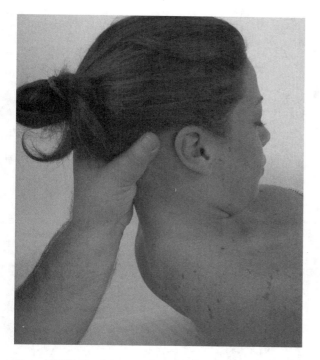

Figure 27.27 Head Contact for the Stroke of the Cervical Extensor Muscles

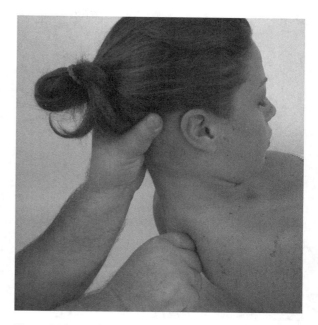

Figure 27.29 Stroke of the Cervicothoracic Extensor Muscles

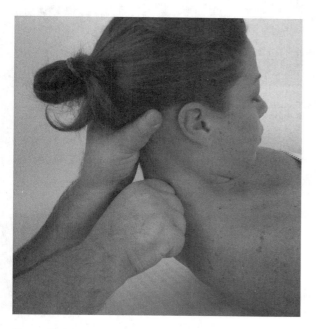

Figure 27.28 Stroke of the Cervical Extensor and Upper Trapezius Muscles

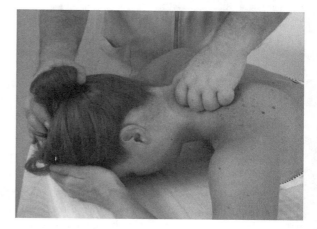

Figure 27.30 Stroke of the Cervical Extensor and Upper Trapezius Muscles in Prone Position

Myofascial Induction of the Levator Scapulae Muscle

The aim of this technique is to release fascial restrictions located in the levator scapulae muscle (Pilat, 2003). The patient is in a supine position and the therapist is seated at the head of the table.

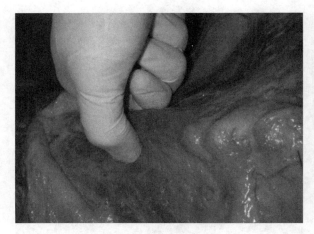

Figure 27.31 Stroke of the Cervical Extensors in a Human Cadaver

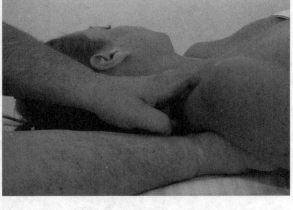

Figure 27.33 Myofascial Induction of the Levator Scapulae Muscle

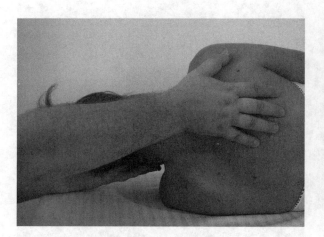

Figure 27.32 Manual Contact over the Scapula's Inferior Angle

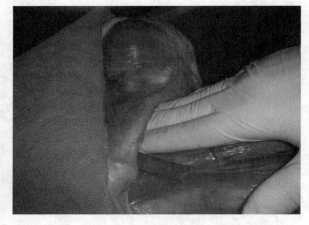

Figure 27.34 Manual Contact over the Scalene Muscle Region in a Human Cadaver

The therapist places one hand below the scapula bone, with the fingertips located in the scapula's inferior angle (**Figure 27.32**). In this position the therapist pulls from the scapula in a cranial direction, which will release the superior angle of the scapula. The other hand contacts the origin of the levator scapulae muscle, located in front of the upper trapezius muscle (**Figure 27.33**). The therapist pulls the scapula in a cranial direction with one hand, and introduces the fingers of his or her other hand in a caudal direction into the origin of the levator scapulae muscle. Once tension is placed on the fascial system, the therapist can follow with a slight movement.

Myofascial Induction of the Scalene Muscles

The aim of this technique is to release fascial restrictions located in the scalene muscles (Pilat, 2007). Patients with a thoracic breathing pattern or those presenting with a forward head posture may have increased tension in the scalene muscles (Pilat, 2003). The release of the fascial tissue of the scalene muscle is extremely relevant for the restoration of the dynamic equilibrium between the anterior, lateral, and posterior parts of the cervical spine. The patient is supine and the therapist is seated at the head of the table.

The therapist makes contact with his or her caudal hand, with the fingers in extension, within the space located under the clavicle bone (**Figure 27.34**). The

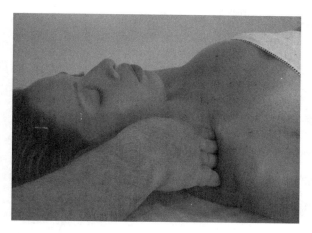

Figure 27.35 Location of the Therapist's Hand for the Scalene Technique

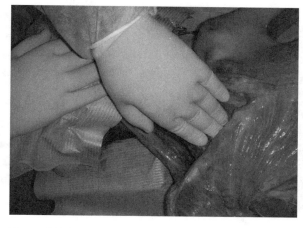

Figure 27.37 Myofascial Induction of the Scalene Muscles with Cross-Hand Contact (Cadaver View)

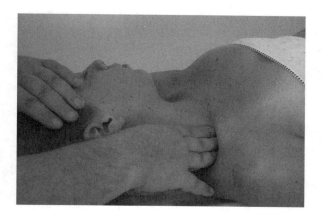

Figure 27.36 Myofascial Induction of the Scalene Muscles with Cervical Rotation

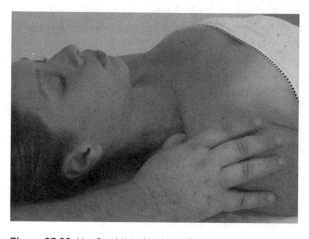

Figure 27.38 Myofascial Induction of the Scalene Muscles with Thumb Contact

anterior scalene muscle is located under the clavicle muscle belly of the sternocleidomastoid (**Figure 27.35**). The therapist can focus the tension on the scalene muscle by positioning the cervical region, for example, by contralateral rotation (**Figure 27.36**). For the middle scalene, the contact is very similar. Because this technique sometimes needs a long time for its application, a cross-hand contact is also recommended (**Figure 27.37**). Finally, for the posterior scalene, thumb contact is more useful (**Figure 27.38**).

In each approach, the fascial tissue is positioned to the barrier tissue, and the therapist waits for the viscoelastic response of the fascial tissue. This response usually appears within approximately 60 seconds of be-

ginning the technique. Again, for this technique, the therapist should treat the restricted barrier three to six consecutive times.

Note: For the myofascial release of the scalene muscles, it is important to control the force applied to avoid painful responses, to avoid pressing the carotid artery, and to control the presence of paresthesia in the upper extremity.

Myofascial Induction of the Longus Collis and Cervicis Muscles

The aim of this technique is to release fascial restrictions located in the longus collis and cervicis muscles (Pilat, 2003). Fascial restrictions of these muscles can

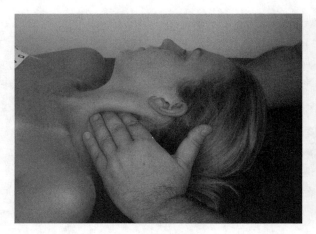

Figure 27.39 Myofascial Induction of the Longus Collis and Cervicis Muscles

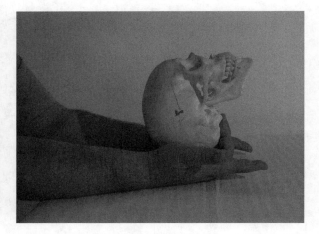

Figure 27.41 Occipital Bone Contact for the Suboccipital Induction Technique

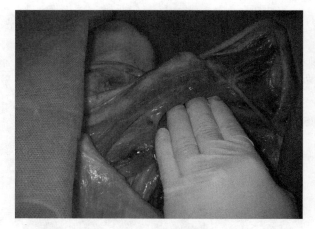

Figure 27.40 Myofascial Induction of the Longus Collis and Cervicis Muscles in a Human Cadaver

The therapist should wait 60 to 90 seconds for the viscoelastic response of the fascial tissue. The therapist should treat the restricted barrier three to six consecutive times, which usually requires 5 to 10 minutes of treatment.

Note: It is important that the clinician apply only slight pressure to avoid painful or antalgic responses from the fascia.

Myofascial Induction of the Connective Tissue Bridge at the Suboccipital Region

The aim of this technique is to release restrictions located in the connective tissue bridge between the rectus capitis posterior minor muscle and the dura mater (Hack et al., 1995; Pilat, 2003) (Chapter 7). The patient is supine and the therapist is seated at the head of the table with forearms firmly over its surface.

The therapist puts his or her fingers under the patient's head in such a way that the fingertips of the index and middle fingers are placed at the C5–C6 level. From this position, the fingers are flexed in a cranial direction until they reach the occipital bone (**Figure 27.41**). Next, the therapist's contact point should be adjusted until the space between the occipital bone and C1–C2 vertebrae is reached. Once the therapist has located this point, the metacarpophalangeal joints are flexed 90° and the interphalangeal joints are extended (**Figures 27.42, 27.43**). This maneuver will raise the patient's head slightly. The therapist should make contact with the tips of the index and middle fingers. The remaining fingers should be moved away from the patient's head (**Figure 27.44**). This position

overload the superficial neck flexors, particularly the sternocleidomastoid muscle. In addition, fascial restriction in these muscles will make it more difficult to perform cervical flexion, and hence compensatory movements during daily activities could be evident (Jull, 1998; von Piekartz, 2001; Pilat, 2003). The patient is supine and the therapist is seated at the head of the table. The therapist rotates the head of the patient to the contralateral side. The therapist's contact point should be located below the sternocleidomastoid muscle, over the scalene muscles, and over the transverse processes of the middle-lower cervical vertebrae (**Figures 27.39, 27.40**). The fingertips of the therapist should be placed over the longitudinal canal formed by the cervical vertebrae. It is very important to avoid compression of the carotid artery or the trachea.

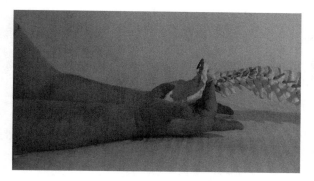

Figure 27.42 Position of the Therapist's Fingers at the C1–C2 Level (Skeleton View)

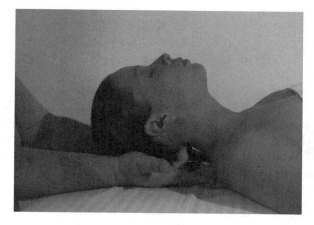

Figure 27.43 Position of the Therapist's Fingers at the C1–C2 Level (Patient View)

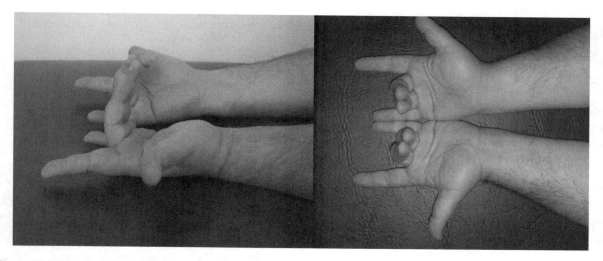

Figure 27.44 Detail of the Contact over the Atlantoaxial Region (Lateral and Upper View)

will induce a constant pressure over the connective tissue bridge between the rectus capitis posterior minor muscle and the dura mater. The pressure should be painless and be maintained for minutes until the fascia is released.

Myofascial Induction of the Suboccipital Triangle

The aim of this technique is to release fascial restrictions located in the craniocervical junction, particularly the suboccipital muscles: rectus capitis posterior minor, rectus capitis posterior major, and superior and inferior oblique muscles. The patient is supine and the therapist is seated at the head of the table.

The therapist places his or her cranial hand under the occipital bone of the patient, with the fingers directed in a caudal direction. The other hand is transversely placed in the cervical region at the C1 vertebra level (**Figures 27.45, 27.46**). The therapist applies a slight cranial traction to the occipital bone, and the opposite hand stabilizes the upper cervical region. The therapist waits for the facilitated movement elicited by the fascial tissue, probably smoothly inducing movements of the patient's head. This procedure takes a few minutes according to the principles of the deep technique application.

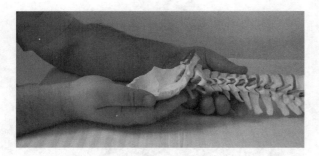

Figure 27.45 Manual Contact for Myofascial Induction of the Suboccipital Triangle (Skeleton View)

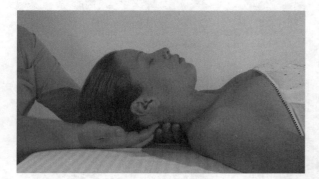

Figure 27.46 Myofascial Induction of the Suboccipital Triangle (Patient View)

Techniques Aimed at the Hyoid Region and Pretracheal Fascia

The hyoid bone is located in the anterior part of the neck region, between the mandible and the clavicle bone (**Figures 27.47, 27.48**). The anatomic relationship is unique because the hyoid bone is not joined with any other bones. Nevertheless, the hyoid plays an important role in the biomechanical equilibrium of the fascial system of the cervical and orofacial (temporomandibular joint) region. There are 14 pairs of muscles and other connective structures related to the hyoid, which is sometime referred to as the "little mandible" (Pilat, 2003). From a functional viewpoint, this bone assists with several daily activities, such as swallowing, speaking, chewing, and blowing. The anatomic position of the hyoid bone is controlled by the action of three muscle groups (Gallaudet, 1931; Bochenek & Reicher, 1997):

- *Infrahyoid muscles:* Serve to move the hyoid bone in a caudal direction
- *Suprahyoid muscles:* Serve to move the hyoid bone in a cranial direction

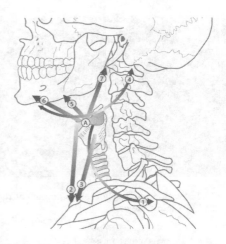

Figure 27.47 Dynamic Equilibrium of the Hyoid Region. The hyoid bone is the "sensor" of the tension of the anterior region of the neck. The figure shows the fascial relationships between the bones. A, hyoid bone; 1, omohyoid muscle; 2, sternohyoid muscle; 3, sternothyroid muscle; 4, digastric muscle; 5, mylohyoid muscle; 6, geniohyoid muscle; 7, stilohyoid muscle.

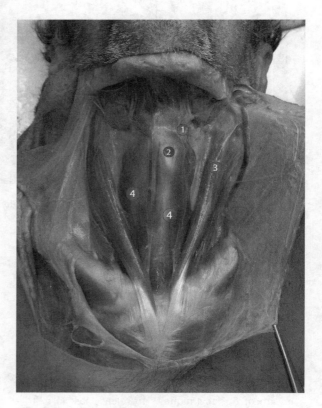

Figure 27.48 Location of the Hyoid Bone and Its Relationship with the Adjacent Structures. 1, hyoid bone; 2, thyroid cartilage; 3, sternocleidomastoid muscle; 4, infrahyoid muscles.

- *Retrohyoid muscles:* Serve to move the hyoid bone in a dorsal direction

The hyoid bone supports the following tongue muscles: genioglossus, hyoglossus, and chondroglossus. They control the tongue's movements through reciprocal contraction. In addition, the hyoid bone is fixed to both the prevertebral and superficial fascia. Therefore, a fascial restriction of these regions could influence the functioning of the hyoid. For this reason, the supra-, infra-, and retrohyoid muscles play a key role in head and neck posture. For instance, a forward head posture (Chapter 8), which implies an extension of the occipital bone, induces an excessive fascial tension over the hyoid bone. If this tension is prolonged, it will translate the mandible to a posterior and lower anatomic position, increasing the tension in the masseter and temporalis muscles. This functional change will induce fascial restrictions and overload of the orofacial system (Pilat, 2003).

The treatments of the hyoid region are focused on the restoration of the functional equilibrium of all the above-mentioned structures. Clinical applications start with the fascial release of the anterior-posterior structures, which facilitates the approach of the hyoid region.

Transversal Induction of the Clavicle Level

The aim of this technique is to release fascial restriction of the clavicle region (Pilat, 2003). This region is very important because the fascial structures originated in the cervical region extend below the clavicle (e.g., the cervical cutaneous muscle in the surface or the infrahyoid muscles in the depth). Further, the infrahyoid fascia also extends below the sternum bone, whereas the visceral lamina of the cervical fascia continues with the mediastinum. In addition, other fascial structures can insert in the clavicle region, so any restriction in this level could potentially contribute to the development of headaches.

The patient is supine and the therapist seated on a chair at the side of the treatment table. The therapist makes contact with his or her nondominant hand on the interscapular region of the patient, and the dominant hand makes contact over the superior point of the sternum bone and below the clavicle bone (**Figure 27.49**).

The technique consists of performing a slight and smooth anterior-to-posterior pressure over the clavicle region (the therapist's superior hand is placed over the sternum and the other on the interscapular region). The

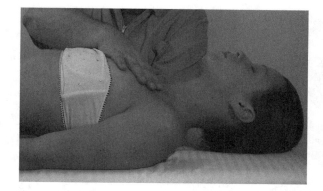

Figure 27.49 Transversal Induction of the Clavicle Level

therapist waits 60 to 90 seconds until the first response is elicited by the tissue. The pressure should be constant during the entire technique. At the end of the technique, the therapist should first very slowly remove the dominant hand (sternum) and then the nondominant hand 10 seconds afterward.

Note: It is important that the application of pressure be slight to avoid painful or antalgic responses from the fascia.

Transversal Induction of the Hyoid Level

The aim of this technique is to release fascial restriction of the hyoid region (Pilat, 2007). The patient is supine and the therapist is seated at one side of the table. The therapist makes contact with his or her nondominant hand on the cervical region. The dorsum of the hand contacts the table. If necessary, the therapist can use a pillow between the dorsum of the hand and the table. The therapist's dominant hand embraces, using the index and thumb fingers, the hyoid bone. The nondominant hand is used as support, and the dominant hand applies a slight and smooth anterior-posterior pressure (**Figure 27.50**). The therapist waits 60 to 90 seconds until the first response is elicited from the fascial tissue. The therapist should treat the barrier three to six consecutive times, which usually requires 5 to 10 minutes of treatment.

Note: It is important that the application of pressure be slight to avoid painful or antalgic responses from the fascia.

Transversal Myofascial Induction of the Hyoid: The Rocking Chair Technique

The aim of this technique is to release fascial restriction of the hyoid region (Pilat, 2003). The patient is supine

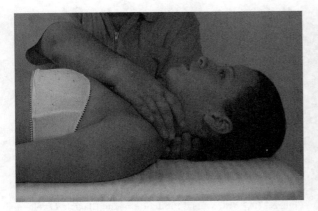

Figure 27.50 Transversal Induction of the Hyoid Level

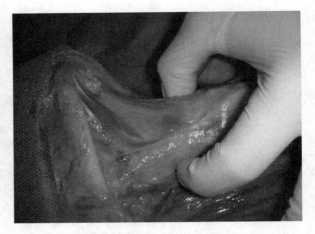

Figure 27.52 Rocking Chair Technique over the Hyoid Bone in Human Cadaver

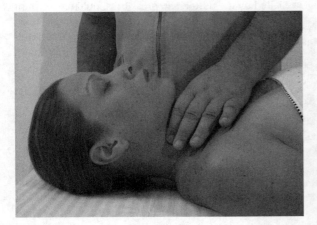

Figure 27.51 The Rocking Chair Technique over the Hyoid Bone

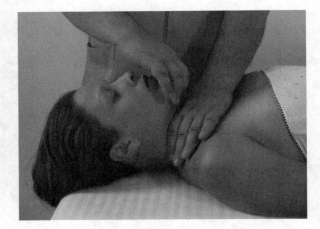

Figure 27.53 Myofascial Induction of the Suprahyoid Region

and the therapist seated or standing at one side of the table. The dominant hand of the therapist embraces, with the index and thumb fingers, the hyoid bone (**Figure 27.51**). With this manual contact, the therapist moves the hyoid bone laterally (**Figure 27.52**). The therapist repeats a slight and smooth movement 7 to 15 times, until the barrier tissue is perceived and maintained.

Myofascial Induction of the Suprahyoid and Infrahyoid Fascia

The aim of this technique is to release fascial restrictions of the suprahyoid and infrahyoid region (Pilat, 2003). The patient is supine and the therapist stands at one side of the table at the patient's shoulder level.

1. *Myofascial induction of the suprahyoid region:* The caudal hand of the therapist embraces, with the index and thumb fingers, the hyoid bone. The fingertips of the index, middle, and ring fingers contact under the mandible bone at the chin level (**Figure 27.53**). In that position, the lower hand applies a caudal traction, and the top hand applies a cranial traction (**Figure 27.54**).
2. *Induction of the infrahyoid region:* The therapist applies a cross-hand position contact as follows: the cranial hand embraces the hyoid bone, whereas the caudal hand is placed in the space between the clavicles and the hyoid bone (**Figure 27.55**). In this position, the sternal

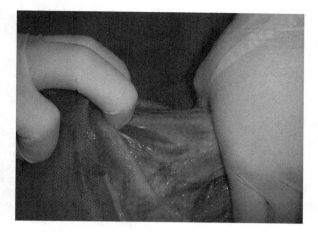

Figure 27.54 Myofascial Induction of the Suprahyoid Region in Human Cadaver

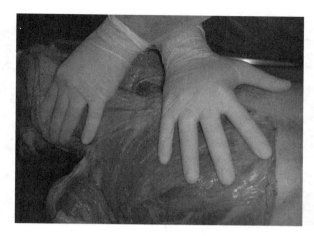

Figure 27.56 Myofascial Induction of the Infrahyoid Region in Human Cadaver

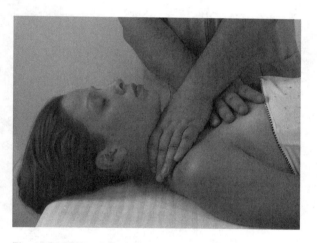

Figure 27.55 Myofascial Induction of the Infrahyoid Region

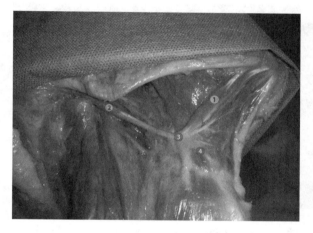

Figure 27.57 Digastric Muscle and Its Fascial Relations. 1, anterior belly of the digastric muscle; 2, posterior belly of the digastric muscle; 3, intermedium tendon of the digastric muscle and the fibrotic expansion of the external lamina of the deep cervical fascia; 4, superficial cervical fascia.

hand applies a caudal traction, whereas the hyoid hand applies a cranial traction (**Figure 27.56**).

In both techniques, pressure must be smooth and the therapist should wait 60 to 90 seconds until the first response from the tissue before continuing the facilitated movement. The therapist treats the fascial barrier three to six consecutive times, which usually requires 3 to 5 minutes of treatment.

Note: It is important that pressure be carefully applied to avoid painful or antalgic responses from the fascia.

Myofascial Induction of the Digastric Muscle

The aim of this technique is to release fascial restriction of the suprahyoid region, particularly the superior digastric muscle belly (**Figure 27.57**) (Pilat, 2003). The patient is supine and the therapist is seated at the head of the table.

The therapist makes contact under the mandible bone, using the middle and ring fingers of both hands (**Figure 27.58**). From this position, the fingertips of the therapist cranially move to the angle of the mandible,

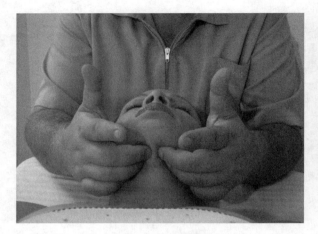

Figure 27.58 Manual Contact over the Digastric Muscle

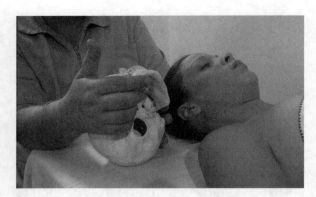

Figure 27.60 Contact for the Myofascial Induction of the Digastric Muscle

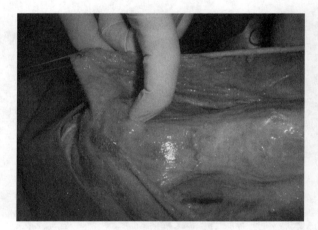

Figure 27.59 Manual Contact over the Digastric Muscle in Human Cadaver

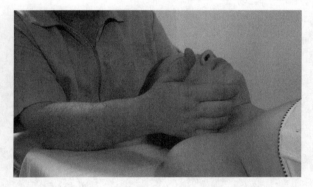

Figure 27.61 Myofascial Induction of the Digastric Muscle

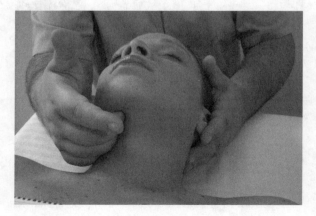

Figure 27.62 Unilateral Myofascial Induction of the Digastric Muscle

keeping contact with the lower border of the mandible bone (**Figure 27.59**). These slides are repeated seven times. If a restricted point is felt by the therapist, a slight and smooth pressure should be applied for 7 seconds to release the fascial restriction. This technique can be applied either unilaterally or bilaterally.

If the technique is performed unilaterally, one hand repeats the same procedure and the other hand stabilizes the head of the patient (**Figures 27.60, 27.61**). If the fascial restriction is deep, the therapist should use the hand placed on the head of the patient to follow the involuntary movement of the head (**Figure 27.62**).

Note: It is very important to avoid the application of pressure over the submandible glands.

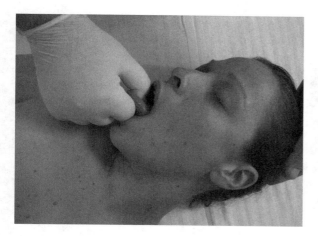

Figure 27.63 Myofascial Induction of the Muscles of the Tongue

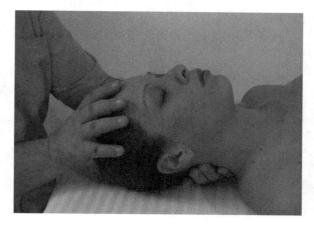

Figure 27.64 Assisted Induction of the Cervical Fascia

Myofascial Induction of the Muscles of the Tongue

The aim of this technique is to release the fascial restriction of the muscle complex of the tongue (Pilat, 2003). This technique is relevant because of the relationship between the extrinsic muscles of the tongue and the hyoid bone: genioglossus, hyoglossus, or chondroglossus muscles. The patient is supine, with the head slightly rotated to one side, and the therapist is seated or stands at the head of the table.

The therapist stabilizes the slightly rotated patient's head with one hand, whereas the other hand embraces the tongue between the index and thumb fingers (**Figure 27.63**). It is recommended that the therapist use a latex or vinyl glove and a piece of gauze to avoid sliding the tongue. Finally, it is recommended that the therapist wait an adequate time to obtain a deep fascial release.

Global Myofascial Induction Techniques

These techniques are used to coordinate the movement between all the fascial layers of the cervical region. The therapist should follow only the facilitated movement, avoiding any arbitrary movement. These techniques are usually performed for 5 to 20 minutes.

Assisted Induction of the Cervical Fascia

The aim of this technique is to release fascial restrictions of the cervicothoracic region. It can be employed as

a preparatory method before the application of any other specific technique. The patient is supine and the therapist is seated at the head of the table.

The therapist puts one of his or her hands on the neck of the patient with a smooth contact. The other hand is placed over the frontoparietal region (**Figure 27.64**). This position is maintained for 60 to 90 seconds until the therapist feels a spontaneous movement of the patient's head, which is usually a neck rotation. The therapist should continue with the facilitated movement of the tissue, but never increase it. The therapist should avoid any extreme joint movement. This spontaneous movement is usually asymmetric. This technique usually requires 5 to 15 minutes of treatment.

Myofascial Induction of the Anterior Thoracic Wall

The aim of this technique is to release fascial restrictions of the anterior part of the thoracic region (Pilat, 2003). It can be employed as a preparatory method before the application of any other specific technique. The patient is supine, with his or her arms relaxed along the body, and the therapist is seated at the head of the table.

The therapist makes contact with his or her dominant hand over the sternum and with the nondominant hand over the forehead (**Figure 27.65**). The therapist applies a smooth pressure over the forehead of the patient; the dominant hand of the therapist applies a posterior and caudal pressure over the sternum bone. With this contact, the therapist waits for the facilitated movement elicited by the fascial tissue. It is important to remember that

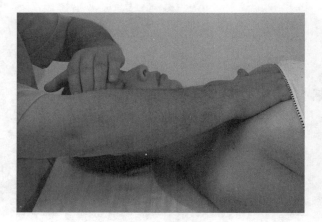

Figure 27.65 Myofascial Induction of the Anterior Thoracic Wall

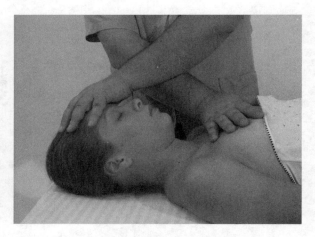

Figure 27.66 Myofascial Induction of the Anterior Thoracic Wall with Cross-Hand Contact

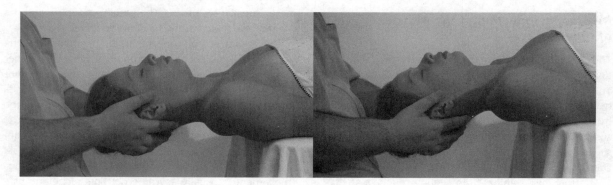

Figure 27.67 Cervical Traction of the Global Myofascial Release of the Cervical Fascia

the fascial barrier should be smoothly reached to avoid any painful reaction from the tissue. The pressure applied over the forehead of the patient should be less than the weight of the therapist's hand. The therapist should avoid any extreme passive movement. This spontaneous movement is generally asymmetric. This technique usually requires 5 to 15 minutes.

An alternative application can be done with a cross-hand contact, with one hand over the frontal region and the other over the sternum (**Figure 27.66**).

Global Myofascial Release of the Cervical Fascia

The aim of this technique (adapted from Barnes, 1990) is to release fascial restrictions of both the anterior and posterior regions of the cervical segments. The patient is

supine with the head off the table (up to the T4 level), and the therapist is seated at the head of the table.

1. *Cervical traction (beginning of the extension movement)*: The therapist holds the patient's head with both hands and induces a slight and smooth extension along with axial traction (**Figure 27.67**).
2. *Three-dimensional thoracic release*: The therapist makes contact with one hand over the sternal region, which will apply a caudal pressure. The other hand contacts the head of the patient, increasing the extension motion. It is important this movement be conducted three-dimensionally (**Figure 27.68**).
3. *Oblique myofascial release*: At this stage, it is expected that the tissue of the patient will induce

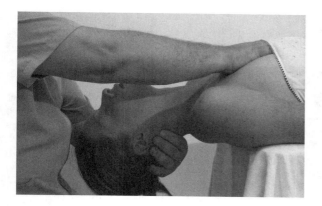

Figure 27.68 Three-Dimensional Thoracic Release of the Global Myofascial Release of the Cervical Fascia

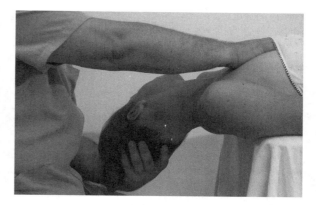

Figure 27.70 Oblique Myofascial Release to the Left of the Global Myofascial Release of the Cervical Fascia

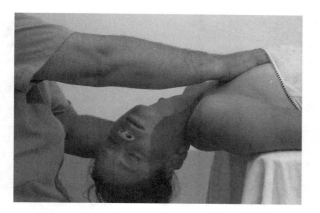

Figure 27.69 Oblique Myofascial Release to the Right of the Global Myofascial Release of the Cervical Fascia

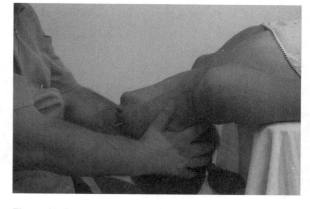

Figure 27.71 Final Point of the Global Myofascial Release of the Cervical Fascia

a facilitated movement until the release occurs. The therapist should guide and follow this motion without increasing the force or the velocity (**Figures 27.69, 27.70**). Hence the movement increases gradually until a complete individual extension occurs (**Figure 27.71**). This process is usually slow and requires at least 10 minutes.

Note: This technique is complex and requires extensive skill on the part of the therapist. The therapist should only follow the facilitated movement during the application, avoiding any arbitrary passive movement. In addition, any cervical movement in the sagittal plane is usually contraindicated, since motion should be tridimensional. Finally, it is recommended to perform a vertebral artery evaluation (extension-rotation test) before beginning this technique.

REFERENCES

Admeads J. The cervical spine and headache. *Neurology* 1998;38:1875–1878.

Barlow Y, Willoughby S. Patho-physiology of soft tissue repair. *Br Med Bull* 1992;48:698–711.

Barnes J. *Myofascial Release.* Paoli, PA: MFR Seminars; 1990.

Bienfait M. *Estudio e tratamento do esqueleto fibroso: Fascias e pompages.* São Paulo: Summus Editorial; 1987.

Bochenek A, Reicher M. *Anatomia czlowieka.* Warsaw: PZWL; 1997.

Bogduk N. The anatomy of occipital neuralgia. *Clin Exp Neurol* 1981;17:167–184.

Bouligard Y. Liquid crystals and their analogues in biological systems. *Solid State Physics* 1978;14:259–294.

Cantu TI, Grodin AJ. *Myofascial Manipulation: Theory and Clinical Application.* Gaithersburg, MD: Aspen; 2001.

Chaitow L, Delany J. *Clinical Application of Neuromuscular Techniques.* Vol. 2. *The Lower Body.* London: Churchill Livingstone; 2002.

Chaudhry H. Visco-elastic behaviour of human fasciae under extension in manual therapy. *J Bodywork Movement Ther* 2007;11:159–167.

Chen CS, Ingber DE. Tensegrity and mechano-regulation: from skeleton to cytoskeleton. *Osteoarthritis Cartilage* 1999;7:81–94.

Chiquet M. Regulation of extra-cellular matrix gene expression by mechanical stress. *Matrix Biol* 1999;18:417–426.

Cope FW. A review of the applications of solid state physics concepts to biological systems. *J Biol Phys* 1975;3:1–41.

Cyriax JH, Cyriax PJ. *Illustrated Manual of Orthopaedic Medicine.* 2nd ed. London: Butterworth; 1989.

Evans P. The healing process at cellular level: a review. *Physiotherapy* 1980;66:256–259.

Gallaudet BB. *A Description of the Planes of Fascia of the Human Body.* New York: Columbia University Press; 1931.

Ghosh K, Ingber DE. Micromechanical control of cell and tissue development: implications for tissue engineering. *Adv Drug Deliv Rev* 2007;59:1306–1308.

Guimbertau JC, Sentucq-Rigall J, Panconi B. Introduction to the knowledge of subcutaneous sliding system in humans. *Ann Chir Plast Esthet* 2005;50:19–34.

Hack C, Koritzer R, Robinson W, Hallgren R, Greeman P. Anatomic relation between the rectus capitis posterior minor muscle and the dura mater. *Spine* 1995;20:2484–2486.

Hamwee J. *Zero Balancing: Touching the Energy of Bone.* Berkeley, CA: North Atlantic Books; 1999.

Ingber D. The architecture of life. *Scientific American* 1998;278:48–57.

Ingber D. Mechanochemical basis of cell and tissue regulation. *NAE Bridge* 2004;34(3):4–10.

Ingber DE. Tissue adaptation to mechanical forces in healthy, injured and aging tissues. *Scand J Med Sci Sports* 2005;15:199–200.

Ingber DE. Cellular mechano-transduction: putting all the pieces together again. *FASEB J* 2006;20:811–827.

Jull G. Physiotherapy management of neck pain of mechanical origin. In: Giles LGF, Singer KP, eds. *Clinical Anatomy and Management of Cervical Spine Pain.* Oxford: Butterworth-Heinemann; 1998:168–191.

Khrustcheva N, Zemnick C. Department of Gross Anatomy at Tufts University. Available at: http://iris3.med.tufts.edu/medgross/medgross2008.html.

Langevin HM. Connective tissue: a body-wide signaling network? *Med Hypotheses* 2006;66:1074–1077.

Latridies J, Wu J, Yandow J, Langevin H. Subcutaneous tissue mechanical behavior is linear and visco-elastic under uni-axial tension. *Connective Tissue Res* 2003;44:208–217.

López A. *Anatomía funcional del sistema nervioso.* Mexico: Lamersa; 1987.

Manheim C. *The Myofascial Release Manual.* 2nd ed. Thorofare, NJ: Slack; 1998.

Meyers T. *Anatomy Trains: Myofascial Meridians for Manual and Movement Therapists.* Edinburgh: Churchill Livingstone; 2001.

Oschman J. *Readings on the Scientific Basis of Bodywork.* Dover, NH: Natures' Own Research Association; 1993.

Oschman J. *Energy Medicine in Therapeutics and Human Performance.* Dover, NH: Natures' Own Research Association; 2003.

Parker KK, Ingber D. Extra-cellular matrix, mechano-transduction and structural hierarchies in heart tissue engineering. *Philos Trans R Soc Lond B Biol Sci* 2007;362:1267–1279.

Pilat A. *Inducción miofascial.* Madrid: McGraw-Hill; 2003.

Pilat A. El peligro de moverse y el peligro de no moverse. Interpretación del dolor desde la práctica fisioterapéutica. Libro de Ponencias XV Jornadas de Fisioterapia de la Escuela de Fisioterapia de la ONCE, Universidad Autónoma de Madrid; 2005.

Pilat A. *Inducción miofascial técnicas globales. Manual del seminario.* Madrid: Escuela de Terapias Miofasciales; 2007.

Remvig L. *Fascia Research. Myofascial Release: An Evidence Based Treatment Concept.* London: Elsevier, Urban & Fischer; 2007.

Rolf I. *Structural Integration.* Boulder, CO: The Rolf Institute; 1963.

Rolf I. *La integración de las estructuras del cuerpo humano.* Barcelona: Ediciones Urano; 1977.

Rouviere H, Delmas A. *Anatomía humana.* Barcelona: Masson; 2005.

Schleip R. Facial plasticity: a new neurobiological explanation. Part I. *J Bodywork Movement Ther* 2003a;7:11–19.

Schleip R. Facial plasticity: a new neurobiological explanation. Part II. *J Bodywork Movement Ther* 2003b;7:104–116.

Schleip R, Klingler W, Lehmann-Horn F. Active fascial contractility: fascia may be able to contract in a smooth muscle-like manner and thereby influence musculoskeletal dynamics. *Med Hypotheses* 2005;65:273–277.

Schleip R, Naylor IL, Ursu D, et al. Passive muscle stiffness may be influenced by active contractility of intramuscular connective tissue. *Med Hypotheses* 2006;66:66–71.

Sjaastad O, Bovim G. Cervicogenic headache: the differentiation from common migraine. An overview. *Funct Neurol* 1991;6:93–100.

Snell R. *Clinical Neuroanatomy.* Philadelphia: Lippincott Williams & Wilkins; 2006.

Stamenovic D, Rosenblatt N, Montoya-Zavala M, et al. Rheological behavior of living cells is timescale dependent. *Biophys J* 2007;93:39–41.

Staubesand J, Li Y. Begriff und Substrat der Faziensklerose bei chronisch-venöser Insuffizienz. *Phlebologie* 1997;26:72–77.

Swartz MA, Tschumperlin DJ, Kamm R, Drazen JM. Mechanical stress is communicated between different cell types to elicit matrix remodeling. *Proc Natl Acad Sci U S A* 2001;98:6180–6185.

Szent-Gyorgyi A. The study of energy-levels in biochemistry. *Nature* 1941;148:157–159.

Threlkeld AJ. The effects of manual therapy on connective tissues. *Phys Ther* 1992;72:893–902.

Travell J, Simons D. *Myofascial Pain and Dysfunction: The Trigger Point Manual.* Baltimore: Williams & Wilkins; 1983.

Upledger J. *Craniosacral Therapy II.* Seattle, WA: Eastland Press; 1987.

Vautravers P, Maigne JY. Manipulations du rachis cervical: risques-bénéfices-précautions. *Rev Neurol (Paris)* 2003;159:1064–1066.

Von Piekartz H, Bryden L. *Craniofacial Dysfunction and Pain: Manual Therapy, Assessment and Management.* Oxford: Butterworth-Heinemann; 2001.

Wright DG, Rennels DC. A study of the elastic properties of plantar fascia. *J Bone Joint Surg (Am)* 1964;46:482–492.

Yahia LH, Pigeon P, DesRosiers EA. Visco-elastic properties of the human lumbo-dorsal fascia. *J Biomed Eng* 1993;15:425–429.

Physical Therapy Interventions for the Orofacial Region

Anton de Wijer, RPT, SCS, MT, PhD, and Michel H. Steenks, DDS, PhD

Temporomandibular disorders (TMD) is a collective term embracing a number of clinical problems that involve the masticatory musculature, the temporomandibular joint (TMJ), and associated structures (Okeson, 1996). Most patients with TMD typically show signs of pain or discomfort in the muscles of mastication or the neck; limitations of jaw movement, especially mouth opening; pain and TMJ sounds; or a combination of these.

The American Academy of Orofacial Pain (AAOP) and the European Academy of Craniomandibular Disorders (EACD) cite physical therapy as one relevant treatment. Physiotherapy in this chapter is defined according to the World Confederation for Physical Therapy ([WCPT], 1995), namely, as "a health profession concerned with the assessment, diagnosis and treatment of disease and disability through physical means. It is based on principles of medical sciences, and is generally held to be within the sphere of conventional medicine and [to] be evidence based." Evidence-based practice (EBP) is part of the decision-making process described by

Sackett et al. (1998) as "the integration of the best research evidence with clinical expertise and patient values." Physiotherapy applications for TMD include a wide variety of techniques and treatment modalities that have been commonly used to inform and advise the patient and to alleviate pain, reverse the dysfunction, and restore optimal muscle and joint function, including oral activities such as mouth opening, chewing, laughing, and talking. Exercises normally include education, joint mobilization, biofeedback, relaxation, postural correction for the basic activities of daily life and ergonomic instructions, and, when necessary, strengthening and mobilization or stretching exercises to make a postural correction possible.

THEORETICAL MODELS: GENERAL CONSIDERATIONS

The physiotherapeutic approach is tailored to the individual patient, based on the principles of a self-supportive strategy and the knowledge that most nonspecific TMD problems are benign and that a conservative (reversible) therapy is the intervention of first choice. In complex cases, there is a special need for cooperation between the dental profession or medical specialist(s) and an orofacial physical therapist. As discussed in Chapter 17, we adopt the clinical guidelines of the AAOP (Okeson, 1996) for the clinical examination of the orofacial region. This means that the physiotherapeutic approach is based on a biopsychosocial model and that both diagnostic and therapeutic procedures cover biomedical and psychosocial issues. To analyze the patient's problems, the physiotherapist can use the rehabilitation problem-solving form, which allows the clinician to focus on specific targets and to relate the symptoms to disabilities and modifiable variables. The RPS Form is based on the International Classification of Functioning, Disability and Health (ICF) (Steiner et al., 2002).

In daily practice, it is possible to implement diagnostic and therapeutic strategies related to different theoretical constructs or rationales. Diagnosis and therapy should always proceed from a theoretical construct. This construct dictates the choice of how to diagnose or what kinds of interventions will be followed, but can also dictate the choice of outcome measurement for research evaluation.

In the beginning of the treatment process, at the end of the consultation phase, it is necessary to change patients' unrealistic beliefs and counsel them that their problem is a benign and self-limited condition. Patients are informed that chronic pain may follow if they stop normal activities, stop work, fail to enter into an active exercise program, develop poor posture, allow stress, pay too much attention to their condition and worry, or rely on medications rather than activity.

The traditional biomedical paradigm has its roots in the Cartesian division between mind and body and considers disease primarily as a failure within the soma, resulting from injury, infection, inheritance, and the like. This model has been extraordinarily productive for medicine but prevents accounting for all relevant medical aspects of health and illness. Therapies that are appropriate for acute disease are not often useful in the care of those with chronic conditions. Therefore, treatment as care focuses on pathophysiology, whereas management seeks to reduce the impact of the condition without necessarily curing it. In an acute condition, treatments are usually discrete and simple, with short-term goals. Chronic conditions generally involve a mixture of therapies to manage the condition.

Hansson et al. (1980) introduced the theoretical model or construct of James Cyriax (1975) in dentistry. He introduced the functional examination of the masticatory system based on the Cyriax approach in order to make a more precise diagnosis. The clinician working in this biomedical model examines the locomotor system with functional tests in order to find the body structure that causes the pain. The intervention that follows then focuses on that specific structure (e.g., muscle, ligament, capsule, or other joint structure). It is a disease-centered approach for the locomotor system.

In recent years, the so-called biopsychosocial model has found broad acceptance in some academic and institutional domains. It is now generally accepted that, in contrast to the disease model, illness and health are the result of an interaction between biological, psychological, and sociocultural factors. Engel proposed this model in 1977. This model presumes that it is important to handle the two (biological and psychosocial) aspects together because they are interlinked. Therefore, clinicians who are working with this model should collect data on both axes. This has consequences for outcome studies in research as well. The biopsychosocial model in physiotherapy and rehabilitation is implemented in the disablement process and was acknowledged in 1994. This model proposes a pathway that links pathology with impairments, functional limitation, and perceived disability. There is a bidirectional relation between all these entities. Extraindividual and intraindividual factors, and comorbidity as a special case of an intraindividual factor, may act upon this pathway and modify the course of the disease and the extent to which an individual is affected. Many studies have attempted to determine the relative contributions of diseases to the total perceived disability of patients. Di Fabio (1998) showed that clinical change can occur in these areas in patients with TMD.

In rehabilitation and allied health care such as physiotherapy, there is a need to describe the functioning of the patient in daily life—in other words, the consequences of disease for the patient. This is in addition to the medical diagnosis. The ICF, the current framework, was approved by the World Health Organization. It is in use in more than 200 countries and fits the ideas of the disablement process and the biopsychosocial model. Steiner et al. (2002) discussed the concept that one disease can have different consequences for patients and that they can be explained using the ICF model. Swinkels (2005) showed that the outcome measurements in most research studies on physiotherapy in patients with rheumatoid arthritis are limited to one of the categories, namely, body functions and structures. He emphasizes the need to put effort into designing instruments that will cover the other areas of the ICF in research settings.

PHYSICAL THERAPY INTERVENTIONS FOR THE OROFACIAL REGION

Scientific Evidence for Physical Therapy in Temporomandibular Disorders

Based on information from several databases, meta-analyses, and Cochrane reviews, the overall conclusion regarding physical therapy is that effectiveness is especially well proven for exercise therapy in all domains, that is, musculoskeletal, neurologic, and cardiopulmonary. The results for physical therapy modalities and massage therapy are still inconclusive at this moment because of a lack of high-quality studies. For manual therapy, clinically relevant results exist for spinal disorders and for shoulder and hip disorders.

A frequently cited article in the scientific literature focused on physiotherapy and TMD is that written by Feine and Lund (1997). They published a review article on physical therapy and modalities for the control of chronic musculoskeletal pain as a follow-up to their report for the National Institutes of Health (NIH) Technology Assessment Conference on Management of Temporomandibular Disorders in 1996. The general conclusion was that although some forms of therapy appeared promising, no definite conclusions could be drawn because of the overall low quality of the trial designs. The studies included were from the period 1980 to 1995. Using the methodologic standard of that period, they showed that treatment was almost always better than no intervention (15 of 16 clinical studies). Systematic reviews and discussions regarding clinical relevance have improved during the last two decades. Early single-center studies did little to clarify the clinical relevance of physiotherapy, due to fragmentary description of the therapy involved, vague criteria for the patients included and the symptom relief obtained, and insufficient controls and blinding procedures. In an editorial, Furlan (2007) supports the latest techniques in meta-analysis to assess the robustness of conclusions by conducting sensitivity analysis and metaregression techniques to determine why studies included in an analysis reach different conclusions. These modern techniques make it possible to show the consequences of underpowered studies, in this case showing electrical nerve stimulation for chronic musculoskeletal pain to be effective, in contrast with earlier systematic reviews. Because of the methodologic shortcomings of earlier studies, the results should be interpreted with caution. The fact that there is no external support in the databases yet does not mean that the intervention does not work. We do know that therapy in most musculoskeletal cases is better than no treatment at all, with the same results for totally different interventions frequently shown in databases. We therefore would like to know whether a specific physiotherapy intervention works better (and on which outcome measures) than no intervention, placebo, or another intervention. The therapist's clinical experiences and the patient's values and preferences are also important factors in the clinical reasoning process and need to be evaluated.

In a systematic review conducted by McNeely et al. (2006) on the effectiveness of physical therapy for TMD, the same methodologic shortcomings were found as earlier. In their search, McNeely et al. (2006) included 36 potentially relevant articles of the 1,138 first selected; in the end 14 articles, representing 12 studies, were analyzed. There was considerable heterogeneity among the studies in the type of TMD, the treatment modality, comparison groups, and the frequency or duration of the interventions. They used the Jadad scale and a critical appraisal especially relevant for daily practice (e.g., clinically relevant variables; Vet de et al., 1997). Their review gives a good overview of the available studies, but no extra analyses (pooled data, sensitivity analyses) were conducted. Significant improvements in active mouth opening were found in the studies using muscular awareness relaxation therapy, biofeedback training, and low-level laser therapy.

McNeely et al. (2006) also analyzed exercise therapy as part of the physiotherapy program. They included single-center studies by Komiyama et al. (1999) and Wright et al. (2000). Both trials investigated the effect of posture training as additional therapy for myogenous TMD and found a significant improvement in pain and active mouth opening. Within the patient group for which posture correction was added to the cognitive behavioral program, the opening value increased markedly within 1 month, from 35.0 to 43.1 mm, and there were significant and clinical relevant decreases in pain intensity (Komiyama et al., 1999). Other studies in this review also discussed aspects of posture training. For example, Carmeli et al. (2001) and Schiffman et al. (2007) added posture training to TMD self-management instructions for patients with arthrogenous TMD (anterior displaced disc). They found clinically relevant effects in the combination group and an improvement in symptom severity in patients with neck pain and TMD. In conclusion, McNeely et al. (2006) supported the use of active and passive oral movement exercises and of exercises to improve posture as effective interventions to reduce symptoms associated with TMD.

Medlicott and Harris (2006) analyzed studies examining the following physical therapy interventions: manual therapy, electrotherapy, relaxation training, and biofeedback. Their recommendations should also be viewed cautiously because of the methodologic problems they encountered. None of the studies they reviewed could be judged as studies with strong scientific rigor. In the 30 studies reviewed, more than 75 different outcome measures, using different tools or methods, were utilized. After studying the 30 articles that met the inclusion criteria, they recommended both active and passive exercises, postural training in combination with other interventions, relaxation techniques, and biofeedback as forms of reversible physiotherapy interventions.

Physical Modalities
Electrical Nerve Stimulation

A meta-analysis by Johnson and Martinson (2007) regarding the efficacy of electrical nerve stimulation (ENS) for chronic musculoskeletal pain in any anatomic location showed a significant decrease in pain at rest with ENS therapy as compared with placebo. The working mechanism is based on the gate control theory of Melzack and Wall (1965) and stimulation-induced release of endogenous endorphins (Sjolund & Eriksson, 1976). ENS is generally believed to be an effective, safe, and relatively noninvasive intervention that can be used to alleviate many different sorts of pain. In their analyses, these authors concluded that the mixed results of the majority of the existing studies were a result of low statistical power. The standard deviations were typically large relative to the scale on which pain was measured, which necessitates large sample sizes. In their review, the pain relief provided by ENS was, on average, three times greater than the pain relief provided by placebo. Further, from the 38 studies included in the analysis, 35 favored ENS therapy with respect to placebo, with 24 studies showing a significant benefit of ENS therapy versus placebo. This review showed that answers regarding the efficacy of the various frequencies, modalities, and durations of ENS therapy can only be obtained by studies with sufficient power. Other benefits of ENS therapy were a decreased use of other therapies, including medication, and less pain interference at home and work (Fisbain et al., 1996).

Low-Level Laser Therapy

Low-level laser therapy (LLLT) reduces inflammation through reduction of prostaglandin E2 levels and inhibition of cyclooxygenase-2 in cell cultures. We currently lack data on what biological effects lasers cause in the human body. In a review, Bjordal et al. (2003) included 11 trials with 565 patients with an average Physiotherapy Evidence Database (PEDro) score of 6.9 of 10 points. The results showed a mean weighted difference in change of pain on the Visual Analogue Scale (VAS) of 29.8 mm (95% CI: 18.9–40.7) in favor of the active LLLT groups. Global health status improved for more patients in the active groups (relative risk, 0.52; 95% CI: 0.36–0.76). In this review, two studies were related to TMD (Gray et al., 1994; Conti, 1997). Conti (1997) used a dose outside the suggested range that Bjordal et al. (2003) assumed as therapeutic (doses of 0.4–19 J and power density of 5–21 mW/cm^2). Bjordal et al. (2003) could not find a significant effect compared with placebo treatment, whereas Gray (1997) found a significant pain reduction. Finally, Kulekcioglu et al. (2003) investigated the effectiveness of LLLT in a placebo-controlled study in both myogenous and arthrogenous subgroups of TMD patients. They found significant improvement in the active treatment group in both subjective parameters (e.g., pain and number of tender points) as well as in objective functional parameters (e.g., mouth opening or lateral motions).

Exercise Therapy

Two pragmatic randomized controlled trials (Van der Glas et al., 2000; Michelotti et al., 2004), which included the myogenous type of TMD patients, compared the effectiveness of physiotherapy and dental treatments such as an appliance and education and found clinically relevant effects. Van der Glas et al. (2000) included 71 myogenous TMD patients without occlusal interference and contrasted physiotherapy and splint therapy. Splint therapy aims to effect pain reduction and restore function by a change in TMJ position, muscle length, and occlusal relationship with changes in oral behavior (e.g.,

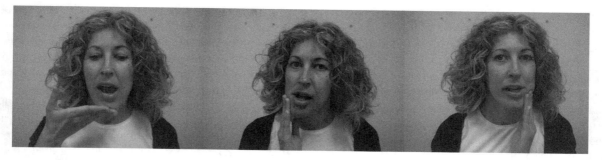

Figure 28.1 Exercise Therapy for Temporomandibular Joint

clenching, grinding, or nail biting). Physiotherapy in this study was a self-supportive program based on the principles of the biopsychosocial model, with emphasis on patient education, oral instruction including the rest position of the tongue, postural (head and neck) alignment, relaxation techniques, automassage techniques, habit reversal procedures, and muscle strength exercises (**Figure 28.1**). Regardless of the treatment choice, a single intervention was successful in the short term for two-thirds of the patients, with a similar reduction of pain for facial as well as nonfacial areas. In the long term, the chance of treatment success varied between 50% and 66%. The authors argue that physiotherapy might be preferred as a starting option with respect to splint therapy because of the lower costs, similar efficacy, and shorter treatment duration. Other factors may modify the choice as well (such as tooth grinding or attrition).

In this study by Michelotti et al. (2004), the summed VAS score (24 areas in the upper quarter of the body; 0–10 cm) was used (Grootel et al., 2005). The successful treatment group had an outcome at the start of the study of 332.4 of 2,400 mm (SEM 36.8; $n = 63$); the nonsuccessful treatment group scored 494.5 of 2,400 mm (SEM 62.2; $n = 44$). Predicting factors for success of treatment were pain severity and the duration of preceding TMD symptoms. Next to a pain reduction (>55%) in facial areas (87%), the authors found a reduction in pain in the nonfacial areas, such as neck and shoulders (84%), as well. This study found an average pain reduction of 27% after the first consultation, which only provided a diagnosis and no treatment. Myogenous pain in TMD patients could be characterized in two daily pain patterns: 79% had maximal pain after lunchtime or late in the day (PM group) and 21% had pain early in the day (AM group). The PM subgroup (pain intensity, 29.1 mm; frequency, 69% of the scoring times; duration, 5.5 hours a day) frequently had a more widespread pain condition that had consequences for the therapy. The incidence of pain-free days was 12%. The mean VAS score averaged across AM and PM group patients was 29 mm (SD 18.8). During the day there was a continuous increase in mean VAS scores for the PM group and a decrease for the AM group. Forty-four percent of all patients did not use pain medication.

Türp et al. (2004) conducted a systematic review on the efficacy of stabilization splints for the management of patients with masticatory muscle pain. These authors identified 13 publications, including 9 controlled clinical trials. Their conclusion was that a stabilization splint does not appear to yield a better clinical outcome than a soft splint or physical therapy. Schiffman et al. (2007) did a pragmatic follow-up study comparing four treatment strategies (medical management, rehabilitation, arthroscopy with postoperative rehabilitation, and arthroplasty with postoperative rehabilitation) for chronic and nonchronic TMJ closed lock. Their rehabilitation program included the participation of a dentist, physical therapist, and health psychologist. Physical therapy involved joint mobilization modalities and a home exercise program. They were unable to detect any net benefit associated with surgery over that of medical management or rehabilitation at any follow-up period (3–60 months). Their study showed that the short-term improvement with regard to pain and function, as measured at 3 months, was similar for all four treatment strategies. This result did not change during a 5-year follow-up period. In their view the primary treatment for patients with a closed lock consists of medical management (education, a 6-day regimen of oral methylprednisolone followed by NSAIDs for 3 to 6 weeks, and a self-help program) or rehabilitation (medical management, splinting, physical therapy, and cognitive behavioral therapy).

Regarding behavioral therapy in general, there is agreement that behavioral and educational programs are useful and effective in the management of many chronic pain conditions. Spending extra time in physiotherapy programs to educate patients seems to be effective, because adequate information in simple terms assists in making choices and overcoming unhelpful beliefs. Further, when it is necessary, it helps patients to modify their behavior. In addition, management of myogenous TMD may also benefit from behavioral interventions. Behavioral programs have focused on information about the disorder and skills training in self-control strategies to modify pain perception, such as relaxation training or cognitive restructuring techniques by psychologists to alter dysfunctional belief systems. The label *biobehavioral treatment* encompasses a large collection of modalities, the most commonly studied of which are biofeedback, relaxation, education, and cognitive-behavioral methods. The common aims of these methods are self-management and the acquisition of self-control over pain symptoms as well as the cognitive attributions or meanings given to those symptoms.

In more complex patients, a multidisciplinary approach is usually recommended. Dentists, physiotherapists, and psychologists work together to improve function and decrease the need for active treatment in order to let the patient be self-supportive as much as possible. Conclusions related to research data in the field of orofacial pain for such a multidisciplinary approach are scarce.

IMPLEMENTATION OF PHYSICAL THERAPY IN THE MYOGENOUS OR ARTHROGENOUS TYPE OF TEMPOROMANDIBULAR DISORDER

Physiotherapy is frequently chosen for the treatment of TMD and is especially focused on the main target regarding the patient's demand. The physiotherapist normally explains the natural course of the pain condition and discusses the relation between load and tolerance and the relation between the complaints and the correlated variables (ICF, problem-solving form: impairments, level of activity, and participation and psychosocial context). Next to general information, more specific information about the diagnosed condition is provided. It is important to have visual information to explain what is going on, and therefore there is a need for proper instruction material. The main goals of the treatment depend on whether the disorder can be categorized as caused by movement disorders, biomechanical patterns, segmental disturbances, or personal or psychosocial factors. Promoting an adequate way of coping seems to be as useful as relieving the muscle tone with massage techniques.

The physical therapy program is usually part of a self-management approach and demands the active participation of the patient. Normally the home exercise program will include several procedures, such as counseling, patient education that includes habit reversal techniques, (auto) massage, and proper use of the jaw (Laat de et al., 2003; Michelotti et al., 2005). Exercise therapy normally is the cornerstone of the therapy, and there is strong evidence that it is effective for a wide spectrum of musculoskeletal disorders, including TMD. The most useful techniques for muscle rehabilitation include muscle stretching, mobilization of the joint (**Figure 28.2**), proprioception, posture training, breathing exercises or other relaxation training, and exercises to improve relevant functions such as muscle tone, mobility, strength, and stability (kinetic and ergonomic parameters). When indicated (VAS score above 6/10, impact of the pain on the patient's functioning and activities high, or an abnormal course), medication such as the pain medication cyclobenzaprine (Flexeril) or tricyclic antidepressants (amitriptyline) can be effective. Occlusal splints can be the dental treatment of choice. The number needed to treat (NNT) calculated from the study conducted by Ekberg et al. (1998) was 2.3 (95% CI: 1.7–4.5), indicating that almost two in three patients with myogenous TMD pain will have to be treated before one of them experiences at least 50% pain reduction.

The role of occlusal factors has changed during the last decade. The consequence is that irreversible (occlusal adjustment) and extensive occlusal therapy take a minor position in the treatment of the majority of patients. A surgical approach could be indicated if conservative interventions fail and the condition negatively affects daily activities such as speech, chewing, singing, and yawning.

Therefore, in most simple, nonspecific conditions, the physiotherapist can play a role in treatment of these painful conditions; in more chronic or complex conditions, the physical therapist is part of the management team that includes a dental specialist and psychologist. Sometimes a consultant medical specialist (e.g., anesthesiologist) is also needed within the treatment team.

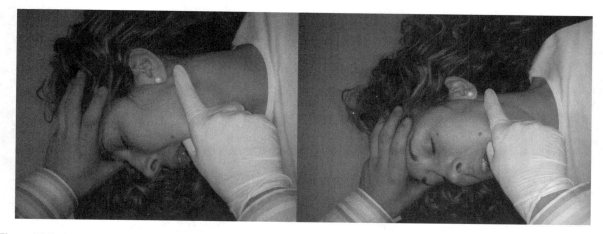

Figure 28.2 Manual Joint Mobilization of the Temporomandibular Joint

CONCLUSION

The quality of the randomized controlled trials conducted should be improved. Concealed allocation, blinding of the assessor, increasing the sample size and follow-up time, intention-to-treat analyses, and standardization of the outcome measurements will help improve studies and stimulate discussion on the clinical relevance of their results. The outcome assessment must be placed in a broader perspective and related to the ICF domains. It will also be of interest to avoid chronicity in acute and subacute conditions; therefore, studies must start in this time frame as well. Instead of pragmatic studies, we need to do more placebo-controlled studies.

The clinical expertise and the information in the literature give the impression that physiotherapy, especially exercise therapy, is an adequate treatment option for TMD. Physical therapy modalities (e.g., ultrasound, shortwave diathermy, iontophoreses) can be discouraged until the moment that we have better studies with clinically relevant results. ENS and laser treatment in different settings and populations call for special mention. Thermotherapy and massage therapy and other soft-tissue techniques, in spite of the lack of external evidence, are frequently used in treatment protocols of patients with orofacial pain or TMD. The outcome for patients and therapists are positive, whereby the results of the massage treatment are believed to be a stimulation of parasympathetic activity, engaging a relaxation response, and a reduction of stress and anxiety. These techniques alleviate musculoskeletal pain conditions involving muscle trigger points, pain points, hypertonus, and stiffness.

The approach for the acute TMD condition with a normal course should be counseling, including general information, and, when indicated, a tailored exercise program depending on the type of the disorder (AAOP or RDC-TMD criteria) and other conditions, such as those related to the ICF domains or to local factors such as attrition.

When there is a deviating course in an acute or subacute condition, it is essential to avoid chronicity; effort must be placed into influencing the risk factors, including pain intensity, depression, anxiety, and self-esteem (Steenks et al., 2007; Dworkin et al., 2002; Brister et al., 2006). In chronic pain and more complex conditions, an exercise program that uses behavior-oriented principles in relation to functioning, activity-related goal setting, and pacing of activity can play a key role in rehabilitation. The approach can be time contingent, that is, a step-by-step advancement of activities on the basis of a previously determined period of time, rather than on the basis of pain, which is meant to focus the attention of the patient on activities rather than on pain.

REFERENCES

Bjordal JM, Couppe C, Chow RT, Tunér J, Ljunggren EA. A systematic review of low level laser therapy with location-specific doses for pain from chronic joint disorders. *Aust J Physiother* 2003;49:107–116.

Brister H, Turner JA, Aaron LA, Mancl L. Self-efficacy is associated with pain, functioning, and coping in patients with chronic TMD. *J Orofacial Pain* 2006,20:115–124.

Carmeli E, Sheklow SL, Bloomenfeld I. Comparative study of repositioning splint therapy and passive manual range of motion techniques for anterior displaced temporomandibular discs with unstable excursive reduction. *Physiotherapy* 2001;87:26–36.

Conti PC. Low level laser therapy in the treatment of temporomandibular disorders (TMD): a double blind pilot study. *Cranio Clin Int* 1997;15:144–149.

Cyriax J. *Textbook of Orthopaedic Medicine: Diagnosis of Soft Tissue Lesions*. Vol. 1. 7th ed. London: Ballière Tindall; 1975.

Di Fabio RP. Physical therapy for patients with TMD: a descriptive study of treatment, disability, and health status. *J Orofacial Pain* 1998;12:124–135.

Dworkin SF, Huggins KH, Wilson L, et al. Randomized clinical trial using research diagnostic criteria for temporomandibular disorders-Axis II to target clinical cases for a tailored self-care TMD treatment program. *J Orofacial Pain* 2002;16:48–63.

Ekberg EC, Vallon D, Nilner M. Occlusal appliance therapy in patients with temporomandibular disorders. A double blind controlled study in a short-term perspective. *Acta Odont Scand* 1998;56:12–18.

Engel GL. The need for a new medical model: a challenge for biomedicine. *Science* 1977;196:129–136.

Feine S, Lund JP. An assessment of the efficacy of physical therapy and physical modalities for the control of chronic musculoskeletal pain. *Pain* 1997;71:5–23.

Fisbain DA, Chabal C, Abbott A, Wipperman Heine L, Cutler R. Transcutaneous electrical nerve stimulation (TENS) treatment outcome in long-term users. *Clin J Pain* 1996;12: 201–214.

Furlan AD. Igniting the spark? *Pain* 2007;130:1–3.

Gray RJM, Qualle AA, Hall CA, Schofield MA. Physiotherapy in the treatment of temporomandibular disorders: a comparative study of four treatment methods. *Br Dental J* 1994;176:257–261.

Grootel RJ, Glas van der HW, Buchner R, Leeuw de RJ, Passchier J. Patterns of pain variation related to myogenous temporomandibular disorders. *Clin J Pain* 2005;21:154–165.

Hansson TL, Wessman CH, Oberg T. Sakräre diagnoser med ny teknik. Förslag till funktionsbedömning av käkleder och tuggmuskler. *Tandläkartidningen* 1980;72:1372.

Johnson M, Martinson M. Efficacy of electrical nerve stimulation for chronic musculoskeletal pain: a meta-analysis of randomized controlled trials. *Pain* 2007;130:157–165.

Komiyama O, Kawara M, Arai M, Asano T, Kobayashi K. Posture correction as part of behavioural therapy in treatment of myofascial pain with limited opening. *J Oral Rehabil* 1999;26:428–435.

Kulekcioglu S, Sivrioglu K, Ozcan O, Parlak M. Effectiveness of low-level laser therapy in temporomandibular disorder. *Scand J Rheumatol* 2003;32:114–118.

Laat de A, Stappaerts K, Papy S. Counselling and physical therapy as treatment for myofascial pain of the masticatory system. *J Orofacial Pain* 2003;17:42–49.

McNeely ML, Olivo SA, Magee DJ. A systematic review of the effectiveness of physical therapy interventions for temporomandibular disorders. *Phys Ther* 2006;86: 710–725.

Medlicott MS, Harris SR. A systematic review of the effectiveness of exercise, manual therapy, electrotherapy, relaxation training, and biofeedback in the management of temporomandibular disorder. *Phys Ther* 2006;86: 955–973.

Melzack R, Wall P. Pain mechanisms: a new theory. *Science* 1965;150:971–979.

Michelotti A, Steenks M, Farella M, et al. The additional value of a home physical therapy regimen versus patient education only for the treatment of myofascial pain of the jaw muscles: short-term results of a randomized clinical trial. *J Orofacial Pain* 2004;18:114–125.

Michelotti A, Wijer de A, Steenks M, Farella M. Home exercise regimes for the management of non-specific temporomandibular disorders. *J Oral Rehabil* 2005;32: 779–785.

Okeson JP, ed. *Orofacial Pain: Guidelines for Assessment, Diagnosis and Management*. Chicago: Quintessence Publishing Company; 1996.

Sackett DL, Scott Richardson W, Rosenberg W, Haynes RB. *Evidence-Based Medicine*. Edinburgh: Churchill Livingstone; 1998.

Schiffman EL, Look JO, Hodges JS, et al. Randomized effectiveness study of four therapeutic strategies for TMJ closed lock. *J Dent Res* 2007;86:58–63.

Sjolund B, Eriksson M. Electro-acupuncture and endogenous morphines. *Lancet* 1976:1085.

Steenks MH, Hugger A, Wijer de A. Painful arthrogenous temporomandibular disorders. In: Türp JC, Sommer C, Hugger A, eds. *The Puzzle of Orofacial Pain. Integrating Research into Clinical Management*. Basel: Karger; 2007: 124–152.

Steiner WA, Ryser L, Huber E, Uebelhart D, Aeschlimann A, Stucki G. Use of the ICF model as a clinical problem-solving tool in physical therapy and rehabilitation medicine. *Phys Ther* 2002;82:1098–1107.

Swinkels RAHM. *Measurement Instruments for Patients with Rheumatic Disorders: A Clinimetric Appraisal*. Amsterdam: Vrije Universiteit; 2005.

Türp JC, Komine F, Hugger A. Efficacy of stabilization splints for the management of patients with masticatory muscle pain: a qualitative systematic review. *Clin Oral Invest* 2004;8:179–195.

Van der Glas HW, Buchner R, Grootel van RJ. Vergelijking tussen behandelings-vormen bij myogene temporomandibulaire dysfucntie. *Ned Tijdschr Tandheelkd* 2000;107:505–512.

Vet de HCW, Verhagen AP, Ostelo RWJG. Literature search: aims and design of systematic reviews. *Aust J Physiother* 2005;51:125–129.

World Confederation for Physical Therapy. *Declarations of Principle and Position Statements*. London: World Confederation for Physical Therapy, 1995.

World Health Organization. *International Classification of Functioning, Disability, and Health (ICF): ICF Full Version*. Geneva: World Health Organization; 2001.

Wijer de A. *Temporomandibular and Cervical Spine Disorders* [PhD dissertation]. The Netherlands: Universiteit Utrecht; 1995.

Wijer de A, Leeuw de JRJ, Steenks MH, Bosman F. Temporomandibular and cervical spine disorders: self-reported signs and symptoms. *Spine* 1996;21:1638–1646.

Wright EF, Domenech MA, Fischer JR. Usefulness of posture training for patients with temporomandibular disorders. *JADA* 2000;131:202–211.

Therapeutic Exercise of the Cervical Spine for Patients with Headache

César Fernández-de-las-Peñas, PT, DO, PhD, and
Peter A. Huijbregts, PT, MSc, MHSc, DPT, OCS, MTC, FAAOMPT, FCAMT

MUSCLE IMPAIRMENTS OF THE CERVICAL SPINE IN HEADACHE

It is now known that patients with tension-type or cervicogenic headache present with an array of neuromuscular changes that are not substantially different from those observed in patients with mechanical neck pain. Studies have reported that patients with cervicogenic headache showed deficits in the strength and endurance of cervical flexor and extensor muscles (Watson & Trott, 1993; Dumas et al., 2001; Jull et al., 2007a). Other studies have demonstrated an altered motor strategy when patients with cervicogenic headache perform the clinical craniocervical flexion test (Zito et al., 2006; Jull et al., 2007a). The craniocervical flexion test (Jull et al., 1999) is designed to provide a clinical indicator of impaired activation of the deep cervical flexor muscles. When patients with cervicogenic headache perform the craniocervical flexion test, greater activation of the sternocleidomastoid muscle has been observed (Zito et al., 2006; Jull et al., 2007a).

Fernández-de-las-Peñas et al. (2007a) found in a pilot study that patients with chronic tension-type headache showed reduced holding capacity of the deep neck flexor muscles as assessed with the craniocervical flexion test when compared with healthy subjects; however, greater activation of the sternocleidomastoid muscle has not been reported (Zito et al., 2006; Jull et al., 2007a). In a recent study, women with chronic tension-type headache displayed greater coactivation of cervical antagonist muscles (i.e., greater activation of sternocleidomastoid muscle during cervical extension motion) during isometric cervical extension and flexion contractions when compared with healthy women (Fernández-de-las-Peñas et al., 2008). When flexors were tested, this study found unilateral antagonist coactivation; that is, there was a greater coactivation of the left splenius capitis muscle (Fernández-de-las-Peñas et al., 2008).

Finally, some studies have reported reduced cross-sectional area of various cervical muscles in both headache disorders. Jull et al. (2007a) found that patients with cervicogenic headache showed atrophy of the semispinalis capitis muscle assessed at the level of the C2 vertebrae on the symptomatic side. No such atrophy was found in patients with migraine or tension-type headache. Fernández-de-las-Peñas et al. (2007b) demonstrated that women with chronic tension-type headache had a reduced cross-sectional area of both the rectus capitis posterior minor and major muscles compared with healthy women. In contrast, cross-sectional areas of the semispinalis capitis and splenius capitis muscles were not significantly different between patients and controls. Readers are referred to Chapter 12 of this textbook for a more in-depth analysis of motor control impairments in cervicogenic headache.

Therefore, low-load therapeutic exercises emphasizing motor control rather than muscle strength are advocated for an effective management of patients presenting with cervicogenic (Jull et al., 2004) and tension-type headache (Fernández-de-las-Peñas, 2008). This chapter focuses on clinical application of therapeutic exercise targeting the cervical musculature impaired in either cervicogenic or tension-type headache. In addition, clinicians should consider that the proposed exercises be included in a multimodal conservative physical therapy approach, since a reduction in pain alone may be insufficient to induce changes in the motor control strategy (Falla et al., 2008).

SCIENTIFIC EVIDENCE FOR THERAPEUTIC EXERCISE PROGRAMS FOR HEADACHE

Several therapeutic approaches have been proposed for the management of headache disorders (cognitive therapy, exercise, manual therapy, and biofeedback), with physical therapy being one of the most commonly utilized treatments (Eisenberg et al., 1998). The findings of published systematic reviews investigating the benefit of physical therapy or exercise in chronic headache are inconclusive (Lenssinck et al., 2004; Fernández-de-las-Peñas et al., 2006a), probably because of the small sample sizes and the lack of adequate control groups (Fernández-de-las-Peñas et al., 2006b). This section summarizes the most relevant research in which an exercise program was included as part of the therapeutic intervention.

Hamill et al. (1996) evaluated the effectiveness of a treatment program that included ergonomic and posture education, strengthening exercises for the cervical musculature, massage, and stretching in patients with tension-type headache. The authors included a program that consisted of chin retraction exercise to improve head position and prone isotonic exercise to strengthen the posterior cervical muscles. The results showed a reduction in headache frequency (P <0.01) 6 weeks postdischarge (Hamill et al., 1996).

Marcus et al. (1998) investigated the effectiveness of a physical therapy program that included correction of head posture, cervical range of motion exercises, isometric neck strengthening exercises, active cervical self-mobilization exercises, and a general body stretching and reconditioning program in patients with migraine. A headache diary was used for assessing migraine parameters. The results supported the use of this physical therapy program for reducing symptoms in patients with migraine immediately after the application of the program. Physical therapy proved to be a useful adjunctive treatment for those women who had failed to achieve significant headache relief after biofeedback. Therefore, physical therapy may be recommended as a second-line treatment for those migraineurs who fail to achieve adequate improvement with other therapies (Marcus et al., 1998).

Jull et al. (2002) analyzed, in a high-quality randomized trial, the effectiveness of joint mobilizations and low-load exercises for cervicogenic headache when used alone and in combination. The therapeutic exercise program included low-load endurance exercises to train muscle control of the cervicoscapular region (Jull,

1997). The first stage consisted of specific exercises to address the impairment in neck flexor synergy (Jull, 1997). Craniocervical flexion exercises were intended to target the deep neck flexors (the longus capitis and colli muscles), which have an important supporting function for the cervical region (Mayoux-Benhamou et al., 1994). At 12-month follow-up assessment, both mobilization therapy and specific exercise resulted in significantly reduced headache frequency and intensity. The combination of both interventions was not significantly superior to either therapy alone, but 10% more patients gained relief with the combination (Jull et al., 2002).

Lemstra et al. (2002) tested the effectiveness of a multidisciplinary management program including physical therapy, submaximal aerobic exercise, stretching, and light resistive exercise in patients with migraine. The results revealed that the program was effective for reducing headache pain frequency, intensity, and duration (P <0.001 for all measures). In addition, the application of the multidisciplinary program increased the functional status and quality of life of the patients (P <0.001).

Torelli et al. (2004) evaluated the therapeutic effect of a physical therapy program in patients with either episodic or chronic tension-type headache. The physiotherapy program consisted of 4 weeks of twice-weekly physical therapy sessions and 4 weeks of physical exercise. They found a reduction in headache frequency (P <0.001) but not in intensity or duration as collected on the headache diary. The program was more effective in chronic tension-type headache than in the episodic form (P <0.002). No differences were found between patients with or without pericranial tenderness (Torelli et al., 2004).

Söderberg et al. (2006) compared acupuncture, relaxation training, and physical exercise training in the management of patients with chronic tension-type headache. The patients performed two 45-minute training sessions a week for 5 weeks and then a home-training program three times a week for 5 weeks (a total of 25 training sessions) or one training session and a home training program once or twice a week for 10 weeks (a total of 25 training sessions). Each training session consisted of five exercises repeated 35 times and three sets of each (105 times). The patient rested for 1 to 2 minutes between each exercise. The exercises focused on the neck and shoulder muscles. Both relaxation training and physical training resulted in a long-lasting reduction in headache intensity, more headache-free

days, and more headache-free periods than the application of acupuncture in chronic tension-type headache.

Van Ettekoven and Lucas (2006) evaluated, in a randomized controlled trial, the short- and long-term effects of physical therapy that included a craniocervical flexor training program versus physical therapy alone. Both groups received a standard physical therapy program: massage techniques, cervical posterior-anterior joint mobilizations, and posture correction (active correction of the forward head posture through craniocervical flexion, cervicothoracic extension, retraction of the shoulders, extension of the thoracic spine, and normalization of lumbar lordosis). The craniocervical program was based on low-load endurance exercises to train or to regain muscle control of the cervicoscapular and craniocervical regions (Jull, 1997). Patients were instructed to perform a slow and controlled craniocervical flexion over various ranges of motion, resulting in various resistances, and to read with various speeds using isometric contractions in various positions. At the 6-month follow-up, the craniocervical training group showed significantly reduced headache frequency, intensity, and duration (P <0.001). Furthermore, effect sizes were large and clinically relevant (Van Ettekoven & Lucas, 2006).

These studies support the inclusion of therapeutic exercise of the cervical spine in patients with cervicogenic or tension-type headache. Nevertheless, clinicians know that not all patients will benefit in the same degree from different interventions. Therefore, future studies investigating clinical features of those patients who will benefit most from these interventions, culminating in the development of validated clinical prediction rules, are recommended (Jull & Stanton, 2005).

NEUROPHYSIOLOGIC EFFECTS OF EXERCISE

Physical therapy, particularly exercise, has multiple neurophysiologic effects. However, there are two main mechanisms that may account for the relief of pain in headache disorders: reduction of peripheral nociceptive inputs and activation of central antinociceptive processes. Review of these mechanisms is beyond the scope of this chapter, so it briefly summarizes the results of those studies directly related to the proposed therapeutic exercises and those studies related to headache disorders.

Studies suggest that segmental exercises induce local effects, whereas global aerobic exercises have more general effects. O'Leary et al. (2007a) investigated the immediate pain-modulating properties (to mechanical and thermal stimuli) of specific therapeutic exercise involving the neck, at sites both local and remote to the cervical spine in patients with chronic neck pain. They compared the effects of a craniocervical flexion coordination exercise (Jull et al., 2004) with that of a conventional cervical flexion endurance exercise protocol that used the resistance provided by the weight of the head. This study suggested that specific muscle training of the cervical spine might have immediate localized hypoalgesic effects; however, these effects were dependent on the type of exercise intervention. For instance, the craniocervical flexion exercise produced the most significant immediate localized hypoalgesic effect (improvement of 14–21% on pressure pain thresholds as opposed to a 3–7% change for the cervical flexion exercise). Therefore, a craniocervical flexion exercise is likely to provide immediate mechanical hypoalgesic effects with translation into perceived pain relief during movement in patients with chronic neck pain (O'Leary et al., 2007a). These authors hypothesized that the craniocervical flexion exercise may directly influence pain-sensitive structures of the upper cervical region more than does the cervical flexion exercise (O'Leary et al., 2007a).

Immediate hypoalgesia to noxious stimuli after exercise has been shown in response to aerobic (Hoffman et al., 2004, 2005), dynamic resistance (Koltyn & Arbogast, 1998), and isometric exercise programs (Koltyn et al., 2001). Furthermore, exercise is known to increase plasma β-endorphin levels in healthy subjects (Pierce et al., 1993). Köseoglu et al. (2003) evaluated immediate changes in β-endorphin levels after the application of exercise in patients with migraine. Patients exercised on the treadmill at submaximal capacity (i.e., 80% of maximal heart rate). This submaximal exercise level was attained gradually and was continued for 3 minutes and thereafter gradually decreased. At the end of the in-total 10-minute period, the exercise was gradually stopped. The study found that exercise induced an increase in β-endorphin levels in patients with migraine. Further, the beneficial effect of exercise was greater in those patients with lower β-endorphin base levels; changes in β-endorphin levels were not correlated with changes in headache parameters (Köseoglu et al., 2003). Narin et al. (2003) evaluated the exercise-related changes in blood nitric oxide levels and the impact of such changes on migraine episodes. Patients received a moderate aerobic training program plus their medical treatment. The program involved 1 hour of exercise per day three times weekly. The results showed that regular long-term aerobic exercise reduced the severity, frequency, and duration of migraine attacks, possibly due to increased nitric oxide production.

In summary, evidence supports the hypothesis that global aerobic exercise appears to have systemic pain-modulating properties dissimilar from those found or hypothesized for the segmental (cervical) exercise protocols, reflecting differences in the neurophysiologic mechanisms of these different exercise forms.

THERAPEUTIC EXERCISES OF THE CERVICAL SPINE FOR PATIENTS WITH HEADACHE

It would seem that improvement in cervical muscle function following training is task specific and directly related to the exercise protocol (Jull et al., 2005; Falla et al., 2006). Therefore, this section discusses different exercises for the cervical flexor and extensor muscles.

Craniocervical Flexion Coordination Exercise

The low-load craniocervical flexion exercise emphasizes motor control rather than muscle strength. The craniocervical flexion test is clinically used to investigate the anatomic action of the deep cervical flexors, particularly the longus colli and longus capitis muscles (Jull et al., 2004), by specifically targeting flexion motion of the upper cervical motion segments (O'Leary et al., 2007b). This exercise has been shown to improve the temporal control of the deep cervical flexor muscles (Jull et al., 2005) and the proprioception of the neck (Jull et al., 2007b), as well as leading to changes in pain and disability in cervicogenic headache patients (Jull et al., 2002). Further, patients with neck pain who received a craniocervical flexion exercise program demonstrated an improved ability to maintain a neutral cervical posture during prolonged sitting (Falla et al., 2007a). However, the craniocervical flexion exercise does not have an effect on restoring normal muscle activity during untrained functional upper limb tasks (Falla et al., 2008).

The craniocervical flexion exercise aims to improve the activation of the deep flexors of the upper cervical region while minimizing activation of the superficial neck flexors, particularly the sternocleidomastoid and anterior scalene muscles, which flex the neck but not the head. Therefore, the craniocervical flexion exercise is a more ideal strategy to reduce activity of the sternocleidomastoid muscle in those patients in whom mechanical overload of this musculature could be related to their symptoms (Fernández-de-las-Peñas et al., 2006c).

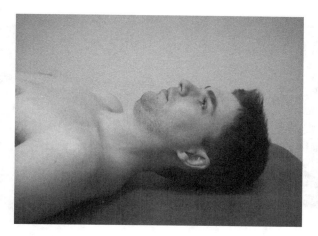

Figure 29.1 Position of the Patient's Head for the Beginning of the Standard Craniocervical Flexion Exercise

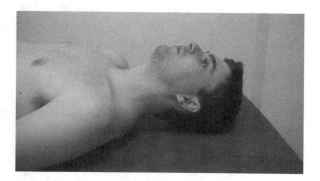

Figure 29.2 Forward Head Position in Supine Position

Standard Craniocervical Flexion Exercise

The standard exercise is usually conducted with the patient in a supine position. This task involves flexion of the head on the neck while making sure that the back of the head remains in contact with the table in an effort to facilitate activation of the deep craniocervical flexors with minimal activity of the superficial neck flexors. The correct posture of the patient's head for the beginning of the exercise is a craniocervical region midrange neutral position (**Figure 29.1**). In some patients, clinicians should correct the presence of a forward head posture before beginning the exercise (**Figure 29.2**).

A pressure biofeedback sensor (Stabilizer; Chattanooga South Pacific, USA) that monitors and grades the flattening effect of the cervical lordosis can be used for helping the patient (**Figure 29.3**). The sensor is placed behind the neck and inflated to 20 mm Hg, which is sufficient to fill the space between the table and the neck without pushing the neck into lordosis.

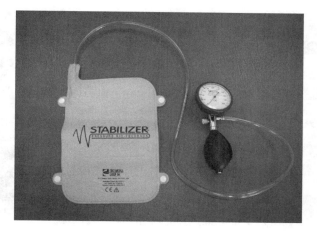

Figure 29.3 Pressure Biofeedback Sensor (Stabilizer; Chattanooga Pacific, USA)

The sensor will monitor the slight flattening of the cervical lordosis that occurs with the contraction of the deep neck flexor muscles (Mayoux-Benhamou et al., 1997). Any unwanted head lift or general cervical flexion results in a decrease in pressure.

The patient is taught the action of a slow and gentle head flexion as though nodding to indicate "yes" and to hold the end position (**Figure 29.4**). A clinician should observe and correct any substitution movement to ensure that all subjects can perform the exercise correctly. Signs of incorrect performance, such as jerking the chin down with a fast movement or performing a chin retraction action to push the neck onto the sensor, should be corrected. Patients can learn how to monitor their sternocleidomastoid muscle activity by palpating this muscle with their own fingers (**Figure 29.5**).

Clinical use of the craniocervical flexion test suggests that an ideal contraction of the deep cervical flexors can increase the pressure of the sensor to 30 mm Hg and hold this pressure for 10 seconds without any compensation strategy (Jull et al., 2004). The inflatable pressure sensor can be used to guide the patient through five pressure-progressive stages (from 20 mm Hg to 30 mm Hg). During subsequent training sessions, patients should maintain the contraction for 10 repetitions of 10-second duration, with a 10-second rest interval between each contraction.

Craniocervical Flexion Exercise in Inclined Position

In patients with forward head posture or those with a higher impairment of the cervical neck flexors, the

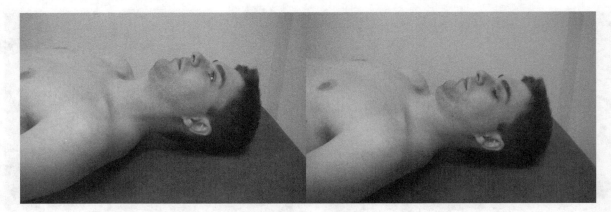

Figure 29.4 Slow and Gentle Head Flexion (as Though Nodding to Indicate "Yes")

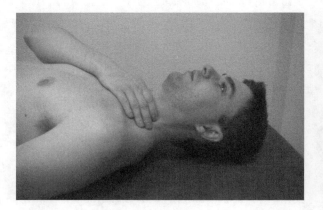

Figure 29.5 Patient Monitoring of the Sternocleidomastoid Muscle Activity

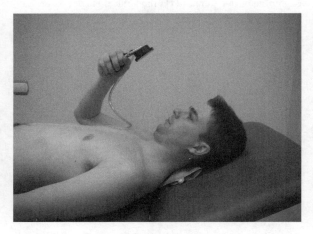

Figure 29.6 Craniocervical Flexion Exercise in Inclined Position with Sensor

craniocervical flexion exercise can be started with the table in an inclined position. In this position, gravity assists with the contraction of the deep cervical flexors. At the beginning of the exercise program, an inflatable pressure sensor can be used (**Figure 29.6**). With progressive control of the exercise, the sensor should be removed (**Figure 29.7**).

Craniocervical Flexion Exercise in Supine Position

A rational progression of the exercise would be the craniocervical flexion exercise in supine position. In this position, gravity does not assist with the contraction of the deep cervical flexors. Again, at the beginning of the exercise program, the sensor can be used to provide feedback to the patient (**Figure 29.8**). With progressive

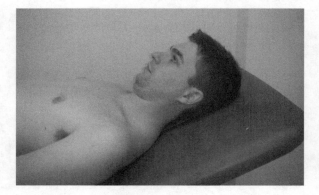

Figure 29.7 Craniocervical Flexion Exercise in Inclined Position Without Sensor

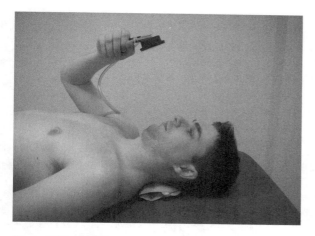

Figure 29.8 Craniocervical Flexion Exercise in Supine Position with Sensor

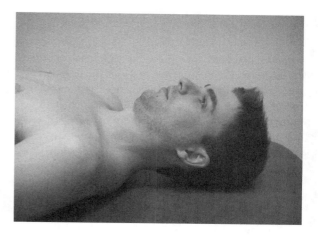

Figure 29.9 Craniocervical Flexion Exercise in Supine Position Without Sensor

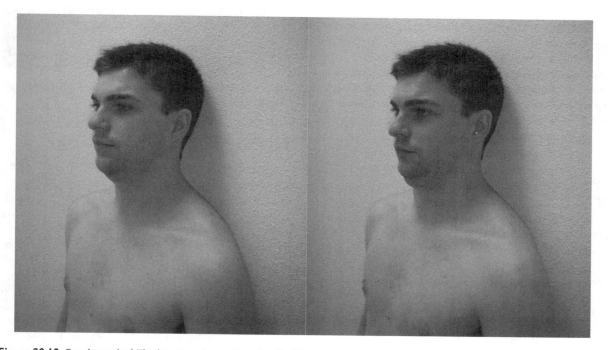

Figure 29.10 Craniocervical Flexion Exercise in Standing Position

control of the exercise, the sensor should be removed (**Figure 29.9**).

Craniocervical Flexion Exercise in Standing Position

From a clinical point of view, it is important that rehabilitation programs include exercises with the action of the gravity, that is, in a more functional position. When the patient reaches good control of the craniocervical flexion exercise in supine position and can maintain a controlled contraction of the deep cervical flexors for 10 repetitions of 10-second duration, the next step should be conducting the exercise in standing position. For that purpose, the patient should be positioned with his or her back against a wall (similar to a table), and the exercise should be conducted following the same principles as described previously (**Figure 29.10**).

Craniocervical Flexion Exercise and Breathing Patterns

Cagnie et al. (2008) investigated the influence of breathing pattern, expiration, and cervical posture on the performance of the craniocervical flexion exercise in a cohort of healthy subjects. They reported that during normal inspiration, higher activity of both sternocleidomastoid muscles was observed in subjects with an upper costal breathing pattern compared with those subjects with a costodiaphragmatic breathing pattern. A significantly lower activity of both sternocleidomastoid muscles was observed when the craniocervical flexion exercise was done during slow expiration. Therefore, performing the craniocervical flexion exercise during slow expiration is one way to diminish the activity of the superficial neck flexors.

Based on these results, the craniocervical flexion exercise should be conducted during expiration. For instance, patients with a predominantly upper costal breathing pattern should be taught to perform the craniocervical flexion exercise during slow expiration after a deep inspiration. However, clinicians should take into account that expiration requires good coordination, which makes the test complex and perhaps less feasible for some patients.

Posture Correction Exercise in Seated Position

Finally, activation of deep cervical flexors should be achieved during functional tasks. Falla et al. (2007b) analyzed the activation of cervical (deep cervical flexors), thoracic (thoracic erector), and lumbar (multifidus) segmental muscles during facilitated postural correction in a seated position in patients with chronic neck pain. This study demonstrated that activation of the deep cervical flexors and lumbar multifidus muscles (P <0.05) was significantly greater when the therapist facilitated (verbal and manual) postural correction compared with independent sitting correction.

Therefore, the patient can be instructed by the therapist with regard to adopting a proper erect sitting position. At the beginning, the back of the patient can be positioned against a wall to establish a good reference starting point (**Figure 29.11**). When the patient adopts a proper and relaxed erect position against the wall, the exercise should be done without feedback (**Figure 29.12**). It is extremely important that the therapist guide the patient with manual and verbal corrections.

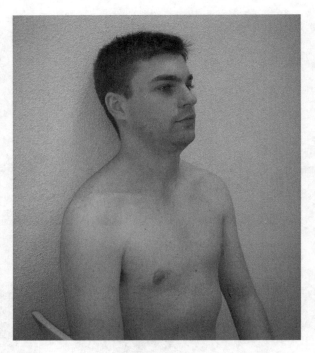

Figure 29.11 Posture Correction Exercise in Sitting Position Against a Wall

Cervical Flexion Endurance Exercise

The emphasis of the cervical flexion exercise is on flexion motion at the lower cervical motion segments and training the endurance of the entire cervical flexor muscle group (O'Leary et al., 2007b). This exercise promotes activation of all muscles that contribute to a head lift, including the sternocleidomastoid, scalenes, longus capitis and longus colli, and hyoid muscles (O'Leary et al., 2007b). The cervical flexion exercise has been shown to increase endurance of the cervical flexor muscles and improve pain and disability in people with neck pain (Falla et al., 2006). This exercise should be only introduced once the imbalance between the deep and superficial neck synergists has been addressed (Falla, 2004).

For the cervical flexion exercise, the patient is in a supine position. The exercise is conducted with the upper cervical spine in a neutral position (see Figure 29.1) while the head is lifted approximately 2 cm above the table (**Figure 29.13**). Patients are to slowly move the head and neck through as full a range of cervical flexion motion as possible without causing discomfort or reproduction of their symptoms. An emphasis on movement precision and control is essential.

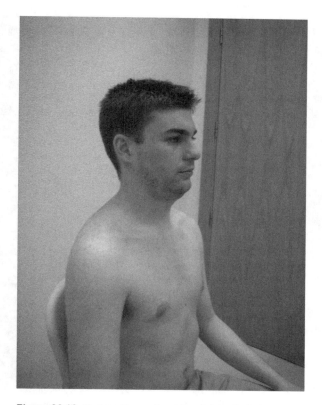

Figure 29.12 Posture Correction Exercise in Sitting Position Without Wall

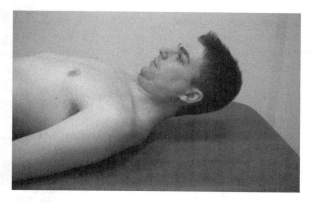

Figure 29.13 Cervical Flexion Endurance Exercise in Supine Position

Progression in the cervical flexion test is achieved by increasing the weight that the patient lifts. At the beginning of the program, patients should reach around 12 to 15 pain-free repetitions without weight. If the patient can perform all the repetitions and reports fatigue at the completion of the repetitions but not pain, the patient

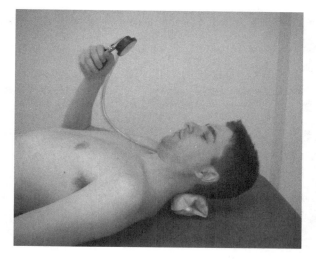

Figure 29.14 Cervical Flexion Endurance Exercise in Supine Position with Sensor

should continue on this level. During subsequent sessions, patients should perform three sets of 10 repetitions at the predetermined intensity level. If three sets of 12 to 15 repetitions are easily performed with only the weight of the head as resistance, half-kilogram weight increments can be added to the forehead.

On the other hand, if the patient is unable to perform 12 repetitions with his or her head weight, or if pain is present, a pressure biofeedback device can be used to assist the movement. The inflatable pressure sensor is placed under the occiput, inflated to 40 mm Hg, and the patient can be instructed to lift the head until the pressure is reduced by 10 mm Hg (**Figure 29.14**).

Cervical Extension Exercises

The emphasis on the neck flexor synergy does not imply a lack of importance attributed to the neck extensor synergy or neck flexor-extensor synergy (Jull et al., 2004). Therefore, it is also important to conduct an exercise program targeting both deep and superficial neck extensors.

Cervical Extension Contraction During the Craniocervical Flexion Exercise (Neck Flexor-Extensor Synergy)

O'Leary et al. (2005) demonstrated that healthy subjects and patients with neck pain performing the craniocervical flexion exercise exert a similar dorsal head

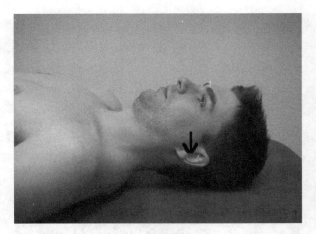

Figure 29.15 Cervical Extension Contraction in Supine Position

contact force during testing. Therefore, clinicians can include the contraction of neck extensor muscles at the end position of the craniocervical flexion exercise. For that purpose, when the patient reaches a desired target level on the craniocervical flexion exercise, he or she applies a posteriorly directed force with the head, which will induce a contraction of the cervical extensor muscles (**Figure 29.15**).

Cervical Extension Contraction in Standing Position (Neck Flexor-Extensor Synergy)

When the patient reaches proper control of flexion and extension exercises, the next step should be the inclusion of this flexor-extensor synergy in a standing position. For that purpose, the back of the patient is positioned against a wall (similar to the supine or inclined position on a treatment table) and the exercise conducted following the same principles as described earlier (**Figure 29.16**).

Dynamic Cervical Retraction Exercise

Van Ettekoven and Lucas (2006) demonstrated that the inclusion of this exercise in a physical therapy program was effective for decreasing parameters related to tension-type headache. The exercise is conducted in a sitting position with a natural lumbar lordosis, while maintaining slight scapular retraction-adduction and minimal elongation of the cervical spine. Patients are instructed to perform a slow and controlled cervical retraction exercise. Cervical retraction implies moving the head backwards from a forward head position in a linear motion in the horizontal plane. Retraction involves a

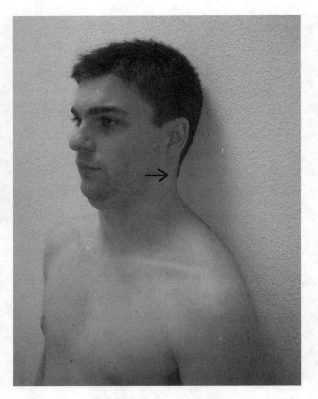

Figure 29.16 Cervical Extension Contraction in Standing Position

simultaneous combination of cranio-cervical flexion and lower and mid-cervical extension. The exercise is started without resistance (**Figure 29.17**). During subsequent sessions, the resistance or speed can be increased.

Eccentric Cervical Extension Exercise

Fernández-de-las-Peñas et al. (2007b) found muscle atrophy in both the rectus capitis posterior minor and major muscles in patients with chronic tension-type headache. Because these are the deepest muscles of the posterior neck region, their contraction is sometimes difficult to achieve. In our clinical practice, an effective method employed to recruit all the cervical extensors is conducting an eccentric cervical extension exercise with the patient supine. The therapist's hands are placed behind the occiput of the patient (**Figure 29.18**). The exercise can be divided into three stages. First, the patient actively places the craniocervical region in a flexed position. Second, the patient applies a posterior force with the head suspended over the table (in a similar way to that described in the first neck flexor-extensor

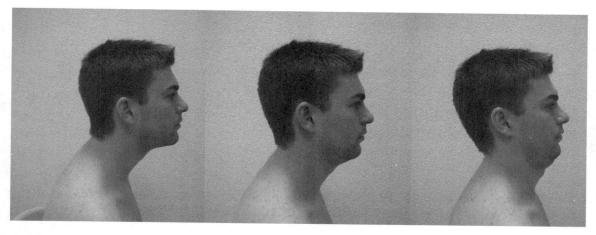

Figure 29.17 Dynamic Cervical Retraction Exercise

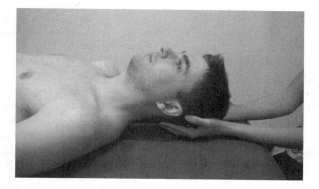

Figure 29.18 Contact over the Occiput Bone for the Eccentric Cervical Extension Exercise

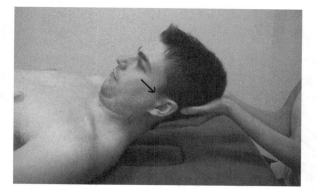

Figure 29.19 Eccentric Cervical Extension Exercise

synergy exercise discussed previously). Third, the therapist flexes the neck and head of the patient, while the patient maintains the posterior extensor force (**Figure 29.19**). This procedure induces an eccentric contraction of the cervical extensor muscles.

Cervical Flexor-Extensor Synergy

Because patients with chronic tension-type headache display a greater coactivation of cervical flexors (antagonist muscle) during cervical extension motion (Fernández-de-las-Peñas et al., 2008), it is necessary to reestablish the normal cervical flexor-extensor synergy. In our clinical practice, we alternate either flexion or extension exercises of the neck for training this synergy. For instance, the patient can start with the craniocervical flexion exercise. Afterward, the patient can follow with a neck flexion exercise and then finish with a cervical extension (**Figure 29.20**). Other combinations may

consist of the patient starting with the craniocervical flexion exercise, followed by the cervical extension exercise in supine position, and then finishing with the neck flexion exercise.

CONCLUSION

Therapists who treat patients with tension-type or cervicogenic headache should include some therapeutic exercise for the cervical flexor and extensor muscles in their clinical management approach. The exercise program should be progressive and pain free for the patient. Future studies are required to investigate which exercise protocol provides superior results and how to best combine such a protocol with other conservative modalities. Obviously, other exercises for cervical flexors and extensors exist. The current chapter summarized the exercises most commonly used in our own clinical practice.

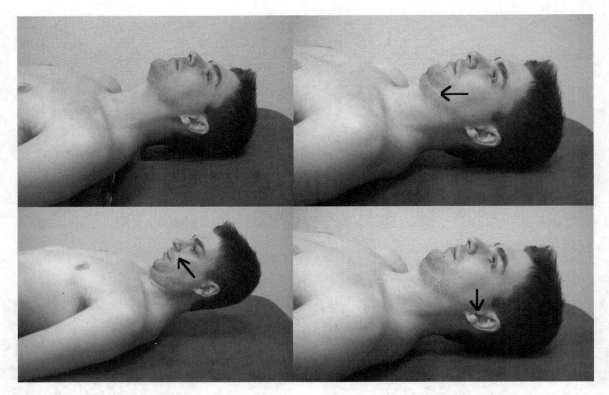

Figure 29.20 Cervical Flexor-Extensor Synergy. The patient starts with the craniocervical flexion exercise, then follows with a neck flexion exercise, and finishes with a cervical extension contraction.

REFERENCES

Cagnie B, Danneels L, Cools A, Dick N, Cambier D. The influence of breathing type, expiration and cervical posture on the performance of the cranio-cervical flexion test in healthy subjects. *Man Ther* 2008;13:232–238.

Dumas JP, Arsenault A, Boudreau G, et al. Physical impairments in cervicogenic headache: traumatic vs. non-traumatic onset. *Cephalalgia* 2001;21:884–893.

Eisenberg DM, Davis RB, Ettner SL, et al. Trends in alternative medicine use in the United States, 1990–97: results of a follow-up national survey. *JAMA* 1998;280:1569–1575.

Falla D. Unravelling the complexity of muscle impairment in chronic neck pain. *Man Ther* 2004;9:125–133.

Falla D, Jull G, Hodges P, Vicenzino B. An endurance strength training regime is effective in reducing myoelectric manifestations of cervical flexor muscle fatigue in females with chronic neck pain. *Clin Neurophysiol* 2006;117:828–837.

Falla D, Jull G, Russell T, Vicenzino B, Hodges P. Effect of neck exercise on sitting posture in patients with chronic neck pain. *Phys Ther* 2007a;87:408–417.

Falla D, O'Leary S, Fagan A, Jull G. Recruitment of the deep cervical flexor muscles during a postural-correction exercise performed in sitting. *Man Ther* 2007b;12:139–143.

Falla D, Jull G, Hodges P. Training the cervical muscles with prescribed motor tasks does not change muscle activation during a functional activity. *Man Ther* 2008;13:507–512.

Fernández-de-las-Peñas C. Physical therapy and exercise in headache. *Cephalalgia* 2008;28(suppl 1):36–38.

Fernández-de-las-Peñas C, Alonso-Blanco C, Cuadrado ML, Miangolarra JC, Barriga FJ, Pareja JA. Are manual therapies effective in reducing pain from tension-type headache? A systematic review. *Clin J Pain* 2006a;22:278–285.

Fernández-de-las-Peñas C, Alonso-Blanco C, San-Román J, Miangolarra JC. Methodological quality of randomized controlled trials of spinal manipulation and mobilization in tension type headache, migraine and cervicogenic headache. *J Orthop Sports Phys Ther* 2006b;36:160–169.

Fernández-de-las-Peñas C, Alonso-Blanco C, Cuadrado ML, Gerwin R, Pareja JA. Myofascial trigger points and their relationship to headache clinical parameters in chronic tension type headache. *Headache* 2006c;46:1264–1272.

Fernández-de-las-Peñas C, Pérez-de-Heredia M, Molero A, Miangolarra-Page JC. Performance of the cranio-cervical flexion test, forward head posture, and headache clinical parameters in patients with chronic tension type headache: a pilot study. *J Orthop Sports Phys Ther* 2007a;37:33–39.

Fernández-de-las-Peñas C, Bueno A, Ferrando J, Elliott JM, Cuadrado ML, Pareja JA. Magnetic resonance imaging of the morphometry of cervical extensor muscles in chronic tension type headache. *Cephalalgia* 2007b;27:355–362.

Fernández-de-las-Peñas C, Falla D, Arendt-Nielsen L, Farina D. Cervical muscle co-activation in isometric contractions is enhanced in chronic tension type headache. *Cephalalgia* 2008;28:744–751.

Hammill JM, Cook TM, Rosecrance JC. Effectiveness of a physical therapy regimen in the treatment of tension type headache. *Headache* 1996;36:149–153.

Hoffman MD, Shepanski MA, Ruble SB, Valic Z, Buckwalter JB, Clifford PS. Intensity and duration threshold for aerobic exercise-induced analgesia to pressure pain. *Arch Phys Med Rehabil* 2004;85:1183–1187.

Hoffman MD, Shepanski MA, Mackenzie SP, Clifford PS. Experimentally induced pain perception is acutely reduced by aerobic exercise in people with chronic low back pain. *J Rehabil Res Dev* 2005;42:183–190.

Jull G. The management of cervicogenic headache. *Man Ther* 1997;2:182–189.

Jull G, Stanton WR. Predictors of responsiveness to physiotherapy management of cervicogenic headache. *Cephalalgia* 2005;25:101–108.

Jull G, Barrett C, Magee R, Ho P. Further clinical clarification of the muscle dysfunction in cervical headache. *Cephalalgia* 1999;19:179–185.

Jull G, Trott P, Potter H, et al. A randomized controlled trial of exercise and manipulative therapy for cervicogenic headache. *Spine* 2002;27:1835–1843.

Jull G, Falla D, Treleaven J, Sterling M, O'Leary S. A therapeutic exercise approach for cervical disorders In: *Grieves' Modern Manual Therapy: The Vertebral Column.* 3rd ed. Edinburgh: Churchill Livingstone; 2004.

Jull G, Falla D, Hodges P, Vicenzino B. Cervical flexor muscle retraining: physiological mechanisms of efficacy. Presented at the 2nd International Conference on Movement Dysfunction; Edinburgh, Scotland; 2005.

Jull G, Amiri M, Bullock-Saxton J, Darnell R, Lander C. Cervical musculo-skeletal impairment in frequent intermittent headache. Part 1: subjects with single headaches. *Cephalalgia* 2007a;27:793–802.

Jull G, Falla D, Treleaven J, Hodges P, Vicenzino B. Retraining cervical joint position sense: the effect of two exercise regimes. *J Orthop Res* 2007b;25:404–412.

Koltyn KF, Arbogast RW. Perception of pain after resistance exercise. *Br J Sports Med* 1998;32:20–24.

Koltyn KF, Trine MR, Stegner AJ, Tobar DA. Effect of isometric exercise on pain perception and blood pressure in men and women. *Med Sci Sports Exerc* 2001;33:282–290.

Köseoglu E, Akboyraz A, Soyuer A, Ersoy AÖ. Aerobic exercise and plasma beta endorphin levels in patients with migrainous headache without aura. *Cephalalgia* 2003;23:972–976.

Lenssinck M, Damen L, Verhagen A, Berger M, Passchier J, Koes B. The effectiveness of physiotherapy and manipulation in patients with tension-type headache: a systematic review. *Pain* 2004;112:381–388.

Lemstra M, Stewart B, Olszynski WP. Effectiveness of multidisciplinary intervention in the treatment of migraine: a randomized clinical trial. *Headache* 2002;42:845–854.

Marcus DA, Scharffl L, Merce S, Turk DC. Non-pharmacological treatment for migraine: incremental utility of physical therapy with relaxation and thermal biofeedback. *Cephalalgia* 1998;18:266–272.

Mayoux-Benhamou MA, Revel M, Vallee C, et al. Longus colli has a postural function on cervical curvature. *Surg Radiol Anat* 1994;16:367–371.

Mayoux-Benhamou MA, Revel M, Vallee C. Selective electromyography of dorsal neck muscles in humans. *Exp Brain Res* 1997;113:353–360.

Narin SO, Pinar L, Erbas D, Oztürk V, Idiman F. The effects of exercise and exercise-related changes in blood nitric oxide level on migraine headache. *Clin Rehabil* 2003;17:624–630.

O'Leary S, Jull G, Vicenzino B. Do dorsal head contact forces have the potential to identify impairment during graded cranio-cervical flexor muscle contractions? *Arch Phys Med Rehabil* 2005;86:1763–1766.

O'Leary S, Falla D, Hodges PW, Jull G, Vicenzino B. Specific therapeutic exercise of the neck induces immediate local hypoalgesia. *J Pain* 2007a;8:832–839.

O'Leary S, Falla D, Jull G, Vicenzino B. Muscle specificity in tests of cervical flexor muscle performance. *J Electromyogr Kinesiol* 2007b;17:35–40.

Pierce EF, Eastman NW, Tripathi HL, Olson KG, Dewey WI. Beta-endorphin response to endurance exercise: relationship to exercise dependence. *Percept Mot Skills* 1993;77:767–770.

Söderberg E, Carlsson J, Stener-Victorin E. Chronic tension-type headache treated with acupuncture, physical training and relaxation training: between group differences. *Cephalalgia* 2006;26:1320–1329.

Torelli P, Jensen R, Olesen J. Physiotherapy for tension type headache: a controlled study. *Cephalalgia* 2004;24:29–36.

Van Ettekoven H, Lucas C. Efficacy of physiotherapy including a cranio-cervical training programme for tension-type headache: a randomized clinical trial. *Cephalalgia* 2006;26:983–991.

Watson DH, Trott PH. Cervical headache: an investigation of natural head posture and upper cervical flexor muscle performance. *Cephalalgia* 1993;13:272–284.

Zito G, Jull G, Stoty I. Clinical tests of musculoskeletal dysfunction in the diagnosis of cervicogenic headache. *Man Ther* 2006;11:118–129.

Neurodynamic Interventions for the Management of Patients with Headache

Emilio "Louie" Puentedura, PT, DPT, GDMT, CSMT, OCS, FAAOMPT,
Adriaan Louw, PT, MAppSc, CSMT,
and Paul Mintken, PT, DPT, OCS, FAAOMPT

The goal of this chapter is to define and describe the neurodynamic approach to patients with cervicogenic and tension-type headache (TTH). The biological plausibility of a neurodynamic mechanism in patients with headache has been discussed in Chapter 20. This chapter expands upon the normal movement properties of the neural structures of the head and neck. It then describes the various neurodynamic test procedures and how they can be modified and used in the management of patients with cervicogenic and TTH. Finally, it presents a case study as an example of how neurodynamic interventions may be used effectively in this patient population.

NEURODYNAMICS DEFINED

Neurodynamics is defined as the study of the mechanics and physiology of the nervous system and how they relate to each other (Shacklock, 1995a). Two key principles central to this definition are that the nervous system is capable of withstanding movement, stretch, and compression, and that there is a normal response (as well as abnormal) by the nervous system to movement, stretch, and compression. Both Butler (2000) and Shacklock (2005) propose the use of the term *neurodynamic* as opposed to *neural tension* because it places less emphasis on stretching and takes into account the other mechanisms taking part in the production of symptoms and physical signs during neurodynamic testing. These other mechanisms include changes to intraneural blood flow (Ogata & Naito, 1986), neural inflammation (Zochodne & Ho, 1991), mechanosensitivity (Calvin et al., 1982; Nordin et al., 1984), and muscle responses (Hall, 1995; van der Heide et al., 2001).

Neurodynamic dysfunction is now being conceptualized as any specific physical dysfunction found on testing that is presumed to physically challenge the nervous system. It can arise from mechanical or sensitivity changes in the system, and it is usually associated with changes in other tissues (e.g., musculoskeletal). Therefore, in neurodynamic dysfunctions, neural tissues may have a tension impairment (a problem handling the mechanical loads imparted to them), be hypersensitive (a problem of pathophysiologic changes within them), or a combination of both (Shacklock, 1995b). Additionally, the primary mechanical fault within the nervous system may be one of reduced sliding (neural sliding dysfunction) or could be a compression problem that relates to the tissues that form a mechanical interface with the nervous system, or both.

As noted in Chapter 20, Butler (2000) considers electrochemical communication to be one of the main roles of the nervous system. The nervous system needs to perform complex signaling processes while dealing with pressure and pinching from surrounding tissues as it passes through the various anatomic tunnels and compartments to reach its target tissue (Breig, 1960, 1978; Breig & Marions, 1963; Breig & El-Nadi, 1966; Breig & Troup, 1979; Butler, 1991, 2000; Shacklock, 2005). It must also deal with demands that it move (lengthen and/or slide) in response to limb and trunk motions (Coppieters & Butler, 2008). Finally, the nervous system must function as the effects of this pressure and movement create blood flow changes (increased or decreased blood flow) (Breig, 1978; Butler, 1991, 2000; Shacklock, 2005).

The nervous system is beautifully designed to handle the forces of compression and movement while maintaining adequate blood supply. In fact, it could be argued that its health and normal functioning might actually be enhanced by the various physical forces it encounters throughout normal human movement. As with any other human tissue, there is an optimal loading range that maintains its physical health and function, and it can suffer injury if loads are too high (Ginn et al.,

2007; Omar et al., 2007) or undergo neuroplasticity changes if loads are too low (deloading) (Richardson, 2004). From the anatomic and physiologic perspective, the nervous system is optimally loaded when it has enough space, is given enough freedom to allow unimpeded movement, and receives uninterrupted and adequate blood supply (Butler, 1991, 2000). If any or all of these three requirements (space, movement, or blood supply) are compromised, clinical signs and symptoms may develop. For greater detail on the nervous system's responses to challenges to its space, movement, and blood supply, refer to Chapter 20.

CLINICAL NEUROBIOMECHANICS IN HEADACHE

Neurobiomechanics is the study of the normal and pathologic range of motion of the nervous system. Most of what is known has been based on somewhat limited research using animals and cadavers (Breig, 1978; Elvey, 1979; Selvaratnam et al., 1988); however, there have been some significant advances in the field thanks to new studies that have utilized real-time ultrasound imaging. There is no doubt that this is an area in need of further research, and the current level of interest and effort is certainly helping to expand our knowledge base. For recent work, see Coppieters and Butler (2008), Kleinrensink et al. (1995, 2000), Wright et al. (2001), and Dilley et al. (2003).

A key concept in the understanding of neurobiomechanics is the idea that the nervous system is a continuous tissue tract (**Figure 30.1**). The system is continuous mechanically via its connective tissue interface, electrically via conducted impulses, and chemically via its common neurotransmitters. Considering the nervous system as a mechanical continuum is most relevant to the study of neurodynamic impairment because it implies transmission of movement (sliding/gliding) and development of tension (stretching) within and along the system. That is, trunk flexion, as in slump sitting, stretches and moves the spinal cord and dura within the vertebral canal. Bilateral straight leg rising would add a further caudad pull, whereas cervical flexion would cause a pull in the opposite (cephalad) direction. This has been demonstrated in cadaveric studies (Breig & Marions, 1963; Breig & El-Nadi, 1966; Breig, 1978), where the dura and nerve roots are marked with paper markers or pins. When the cervical spine is flexed, the cervical cord and nerve roots unfold or straighten out so that, in a sense, they are pulled upward toward the base

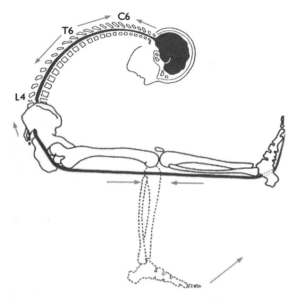

Figure 30.1 Postulated Neurobiomechanics from Spinal Extension to Spinal Flexion. The approximate points C6, T6, and L4 are where the neuraxis and meninges do not move in relation to the movements of the spinal canal.

Source: Modified from Butler, 1991, *Mobilization of the Nervous System*, Churchill Livingstone, Edinburgh, with permission.

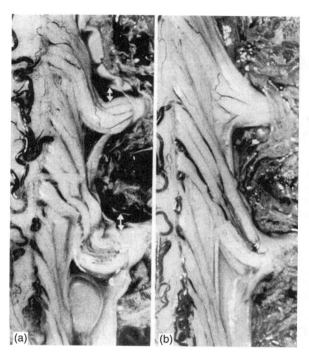

Figure 30.2 Movement, Tension, and Strain in the Cervical Spinal Cord and Nerve Roots During Spinal Flexion. **A**: Cervical spine in extension, showing loose tissue and separation between the neural tissues and the intervertebral foramen (white arrows). **B**: Elongation of the neural and vascular tissues, along with sliding and contact of the neural tissues against the structures of the intervertebral foramen.

Source: Reprinted from Shacklock, 2008, *Biomechanics of the Nervous System: Breig Revisited*, Neurodynamic Solutions, Adelaide, with kind permission.

of the skull (**Figure 30.2**). This is basically the slump test, as it was described by Maitland (1979).

Another key concept to consider in neurodynamic dysfunction is that of the mechanical interface between the nervous system and its surrounding tissues, and the role this can play in abnormal biomechanics. The mechanical interface is defined as "that tissue or material adjacent to the nervous system that can move independently to the system" (Butler, 1991). Mechanical interfaces are central to an understanding of neurodynamic dysfunction because they represent the most likely sites for the development of movement or force transmission problems. Mechanical interfaces can be hard or bony (e.g., ulnar nerve at the elbow or the vertebral foramen), ligamentous (e.g., carpal tunnel), articular (e.g., zygapophysial joints), or muscular (e.g., supinator muscle in the forearm). Mechanical interfaces can be normal, where movement and function are normal and symptom free, or they can be pathologic, where something happens to compress or restrict movement of the nervous system at the interface. Examples of pathologic interfaces include osteophytes, extensive bruising, or ligamentous swelling that could occupy space at the mechanical interface to restrict

normal range of motion and inhibit independent function of the nervous system and the interface. In this scenario, range of motion of the nervous system can be compromised, which would presumably lead to the abnormal mechanical response in our definition of neurodynamic dysfunction.

As the nervous system winds its way through its anatomic course, it will be required to stretch, slide (longitudinal or transverse), and become compressed. Stretch is defined as the elongation of the nerve relative to a starting length (Topp & Boyd, 2006). However, nerves are not solid structures, and stretch causes internal compression due to displacement of nerve tissue/fluid (Topp & Boyd, 2006). The physiologic effects of stretch and compression include changes in intraneural blood flow, conduction, and axoplasmic transport. Research has shown that an 8% stretch of a peripheral nerve for 30 minutes results in a 50%

decrease in blood flow, and an 8.8% stretch for 1 hour results in a 70% decrease in blood flow. Further, a 15% stretch for 30 minutes will cause 80% to 100% blockage in blood flow (Ogata & Naito, 1986; Driscoll et al., 2002). Wall et al. (1992) were able to demonstrate that 6% stretch or strain of a peripheral nerve for 1 hour resulted in a 70% decrease in action potentials, and 12% stretch or strain for 1 hour caused complete conduction block. Interestingly, other studies have demonstrated that from end-range wrist and elbow flexion to end-range wrist and elbow extension, the median nerve has to adapt to a nerve bed that is 20% longer (Millesi, 1986; Zoech et al., 1991). Similar data have been provided by Beith et al. (1995) with respect to the sciatic/tibial nerve. Obviously, there must be some mechanical and physiologic adaptations within peripheral nerves to accommodate such significant changes in length and to cope with prolonged stretching or strain. The effects of compression have also been studied, with as little as 20 to 30 mm Hg causing decreased venous blood flow and 80 mm Hg causing complete blockage of intraneural blood flow (Rydevik et al., 1981; Ogata & Naito, 1986). Compression has also been shown to alter axonal transport (Dahlin et al., 1993) and action potential conduction (Fern & Harrison, 1994).

Nerves can be seen to move relative to their adjacent tissues; this motion has been described as sliding or excursion (McLellan & Swash, 1976; Wilgis & Murphy, 1986). Excursion occurs both longitudinally and transversely. This sliding or excursion is considered an essential aspect of neural function because it serves to dissipate tension and distribute forces within the nervous system. Instead of stretching (and thereby developing tension), the nervous system can move longitudinally and/or transversely and distribute itself along the shortest course between fixed points; hence, it can equalize tension throughout the neural tract. An excellent example of transverse sliding or excursion can be seen at the wrist. Using real-time ultrasound at the carpal tunnel, one can appreciate transverse sliding of the median nerve relative to the flexor tendons during performance of the upper limb neurodynamic test and other arm movements (Erel et al., 2003; Greening et al., 2005; Shacklock, 2005).

The proposed mechanisms contributing to the generation of headache symptoms have been well covered elsewhere in this text. If there is a neurodynamic component to a patient's headache, as has been shown to be present in 7.4% to 18% of patients with cervicogenic headaches (Jull et al., 2002; Zito et al., 2006; von Piekartz et al., 2007), we must consider the neurobio-

mechanics of the structures involved. There must be some change in the neurobiomechanics, either proximal or distal, that affects the space, movement, and/or blood flow of the neural structures that contribute to the development of a headache. Direct compression on the upper cervical spine nerve roots, dorsal root ganglion, and greater occipital nerves has been documented in patients with headache (Hildebrandt & Jansen, 1984; Jansen et al., 1989a, 1989b; Pikus & Phillips, 1995, 1996); however, it has not correlated well with symptom production. It appears that pressure alone may not be enough to generate symptoms and that other factors are likely involved in the development of mechanosensitivity of a nerve (Howe et al., 1977; Calvin et al., 1982). It might well be that compression, in combination with reduced sliding movement and/or blood flow to a nerve, may lead to the increased sensitivity of neural tissue and symptom generation.

In two studies on cervicogenic headache, neurodynamics were assessed using passive upper cervical flexion along with either the straight leg raise or placement of the upper limb in an upper limb neurodynamic position (Jull et al., 2002; Zito et al., 2006). In these studies, only 8% to 10% of the subjects experienced any increase in their headache symptoms with the added neural tissue load. Von Piekartz et al. (2007) investigated the difference in cervical flexion and sensory responses (intensity and location) during the long sitting slump (LSS) test in 123 children aged 6 to 12 years. The test was performed on children with migraine or cervicogenic headache and a control group; it was found that 18% of the headache subjects felt the responses in their head. The results indicated that the intensities of the sensory response rate were highest in the migraine and cervicogenic headache groups as compared with the control group. The children with cervicogenic headaches had cervical flexion ranges that differed significantly (P <0.0001) from both the control group and the migraine headache group. Although these preliminary studies suggest that only a small percentage of headache patients may have a neurogenic component, additional research related to neurodynamic tests and treatment strategies is certainly warranted.

NEURODYNAMICS IN THE MANAGEMENT OF PATIENTS WITH HEADACHE

Clinical neurodynamics is best described as the clinical application of the systematic assessment of the mechanics and physiology of a relevant part of the nervous system. Butler (1991) proposed a base test system for neurodynamic evaluation. It is a clinically intuitive system that evolved for ease of handling and to fulfill a perceived clinical demand. It is based on existing tests and the basic principles of neurodynamics already discussed, and, in most clinical situations, the tests are refined or adapted based on reasoned hypotheses and the clinical presentation of the patient. The base tests for the axial skeleton include passive neck flexion and slump (Butler, 1991, 2000). Neurodynamic base tests for the lower extremity include the straight leg raise and prone knee bend, and the base tests for the upper extremity include four variations of the upper limb neurodynamic test (ULNT) (Butler, 1991, 2000), which evolved from Elvey's initial test (Elvey, 1979).

All neurodynamic tests are focused on a major neural pathway and the major sensitizing movements of those pathways. *Sensitizing movements* are movements that increase movement or force in the neural structures in addition to those movements employed in the standard neurodynamic test (Butler, 1991; Shacklock, 2005). An example of a sensitizing movement is the addition of cervical contralateral lateral flexion to the upper limb neurodynamic test, which might increase the symptom response around the axilla, upper arm, and forearm. Sensitizing movements should not be confused with differentiating movements. Sensitizing movements can be useful in loading or moving the nervous system beyond the effects of the standard neurodynamic test (i.e., strengthening the test). However, they also load and move musculoskeletal structures and are therefore not as helpful as differentiating movements in determining the existence of neurodynamic impairment. *Differentiating movements* are movements that emphasize the nervous system by producing movement in the neural structures in the area in question rather than moving the musculoskeletal structures in the same area (Butler, 1991; Shacklock, 2005). Differentiating movements place emphasis on the nervous system without affecting the other structures and are therefore used to help establish the existence of a neurodynamic problem. An example of a differentiating movement for a patient with a hypothesized neurodynamic headache might be the addition of ankle dorsiflexion to passive neck flexion while maintaining a slump position with a straight leg raise. It would be the observed effect of movement of a distal segment (ankle dorsiflexion) that would add neurodynamic load upon the proximal symptom (in this case, headache) that would imply structural differentiation.

Studies have shown that the starting position and the sequencing of limb movement during neurodynamic tests affect the degree of excursion along the nerve. Dilley et al. (2003) examined the median nerve at the distal part of the upper arm and midforearm using two different starting positions—elbow in full extension and shoulder at 45° or at 90° abduction. They then performed wrist extension from neutral to 45° and found that greater excursion of the median nerve occurred when the shoulder was in a more slackened position (45° abduction). When the shoulder was abducted 45°, the excursion was 2.4 mm distally at the distal arm and 4.7 mm distally at the midforearm. When the shoulder was abducted 90°, the excursion was 1.8 mm distally at the distal arm and 4.2 mm distally at the midforearm. The sequence of movements has also been shown to affect the distribution of symptoms in response to neurodynamic testing (Shacklock, 1989; Zorn et al., 1995). These authors reported a greater likelihood of producing a response that is localized to the region that is moved first or more strongly. Tsai (1995) conducted a cadaveric study in which strain in the ulnar nerve at the elbow was measured during ulnar neurodynamic testing in three different sequences: proximal-to-distal, distal-to-proximal, and elbow-first sequence. The elbow-first sequence consistently produced 20% greater strain in the ulnar nerve at the elbow than the other two sequences. Coppieters and Butler (2008), in a cadaveric biomechanical study, investigated the longitudinal strain and excursion in the ulnar and median nerve at the wrist and proximal to the elbow during different types of neurodynamic movements. They found that sliding techniques resulted in more than twice as much excursion of the nerves than tensioning techniques, and that the increased excursion was associated with significantly lower strain. Their findings illustrate how different neurodynamic movements have different mechanical effects on the nervous system. Therefore, it can be argued that greater strain in the nerves occurs at the site that is moved first—that is, the first component of a neurodynamic test or treatment technique—and that sliding techniques actually generate more movement with less strain than tensioning techniques.

THE BASE TESTS FOR PATIENTS WITH HEADACHE

It is recommended that all neurodynamic tests be performed actively before passively. This allows the therapist to gauge the patient's willingness to move and provides an approximate measure of the range of motion likely to be encountered during any subsequent passive test. It also may decrease the patient's fears and anxieties about the test and symptoms likely to be elicited during the test. Finally, if the active examination is found to be sensitive, a reasoned decision may be made not to perform the tests passively in order to avoid symptom exacerbation.

Some important handling issues with respect to performance of neurodynamic tests include the following.

- Have a clinically sound reason for doing the test in the first place. Establish hypotheses based on the clinical reasoning and suspected pathobiological mechanisms prior to the test, likely specific dysfunctions to be found on examination, precautions, and sources of symptoms.
- It is important to explain to patients exactly what you are going to do and what you want them to do. It is vital that patients be comfortable with reporting any responses to testing, anywhere in their body.
- Starting positions should be consistent each time, and any variations from normal practice should be noted and recorded.
- Note symptom responses, including areas and nature (type of response) with the addition of each component of the test.
- Watch for antalgic postures and other motor responses during the test (e.g., cervical movements or trapezius muscle activity).
- Test for symmetry between sides.
- Explain your findings to your patient.
- Repeat the test gently a number of times before recording an actual measurement.

Passive Neck Flexion Test

Passive neck flexion can be used to apply tension to the spinal cord and its surrounding innervated tissues (dura). As the neck is flexed, the cervical canal elongates, the canal and intervertebral foramina open, and the neural tissues in the neck are tensioned and slide relative to their interfacing tissues (Shacklock, 2005). The pattern of sliding that occurs involves caudad movement in the upper cervical spine and cephalad movement in the lower cervical spine (Breig, 1978). This movement pattern has been described as a "tissue-

borrowing phenomenon" whereby the neural tissues encased within the vertebral canal must adapt to the increased length by sliding toward the center (Breig, 1978; Johnson & Chiarello, 1997). Along with the caudad movement of the neural tissues in the upper cervical spine, the brain is pulled downward toward the foramen magnum (Shacklock, 2005).

A detailed description of the passive neck flexion test is available in previously published texts (Butler, 1991, 2000; Shacklock, 1995b). The key points involved are that the patient lies supine, arms by the side, with no pillow if possible, and with the body straight. The therapist stands to one side of the patient's head and places his or her cephalad hand under the patient's occiput and the other hand overlying the chin (**Figure 30.3**). The movement performed is passive cervical flexion, and, as with all neurodynamic tests, the symptom responses, range of movement, and resistance encountered should be noted and analyzed. For the patient

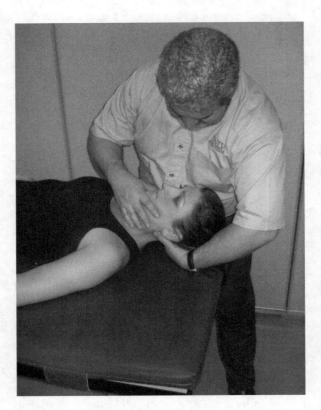

Figure 30.3 Passive Neck Flexion Test. Therapist stands to one side of the patient's head and places the cephalad hand (left) under the patient's occiput and the other hand (right) overlying the chin.

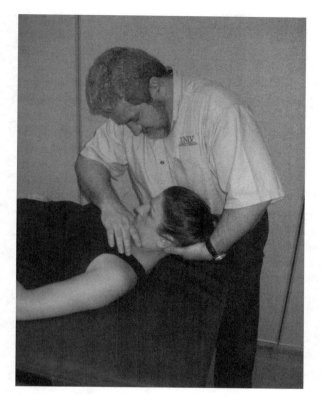

Figure 30.4 Passive Neck Flexion Test. The therapist can localize the passive flexion to the upper cervical spine at first by use of the hand overlying the chin, and then take the head and neck into further flexion as needed and depending on symptom response.

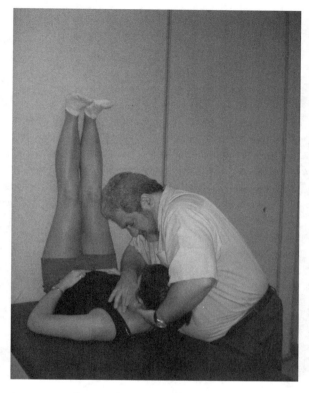

Figure 30.5 Passive Neck Flexion Test. The test can be structurally differentiated by adding or subtracting bilateral straight leg raise while maintaining neck position, or adding or subtracting passive neck flexion while maintaining bilateral straight leg raise position.

with headache, the therapist may want to localize the technique to the upper cervical spine, in which case the hand overlying the chin can introduce localized upper cervical flexion first, and then the head and neck can be moved into flexion (**Figure 30.4**).

The normal response to the passive neck flexion test is a pulling sensation at the cervicothoracic junction at the end of range (Butler, 1991, 2000). The symptoms evoked during this test are most likely related to joint or muscle tissues rather than the neural tissues; however, structural differentiation can be achieved by maintaining the end-range passive neck flexion position and adding straight leg raise (**Figure 30.5**) or, perhaps, an active upper limb neurodynamic test (**Figure 30.6**). If symptoms reported by the patient (such as suboccipital aching or upper cervical pain) are altered (made worse or better) with the addition of these differentiating movements, then an argument could be made for a neural tissue source of the symptoms.

Indications for the Passive Neck Flexion Test in Patients with Headache

A therapist would consider using the passive neck flexion test where, after detailed subjective evaluation, objective examination, and clinical reasoning, there is a hypothesis of a neurogenic source for symptoms (pain, aching, tightness) in the upper cervical or suboccipital region or there is a hypothesis that the source of the disorder lies in the upper three cervical nerve pathways and receptive fields. Alternatively, the patient may have indicated a pain-provoking movement or position that is similar to the test (e.g., nodding the head forward or looking at the feet).

Slump Test

The slump test is simply an extension of the performance of the straight leg raise test in a seated position

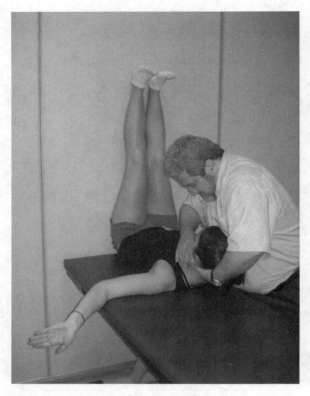

Figure 30.6 Passive Neck Flexion Test. Structural differentiation through use of active upper limb neurodynamic test while maintaining bilateral straight leg raise position.

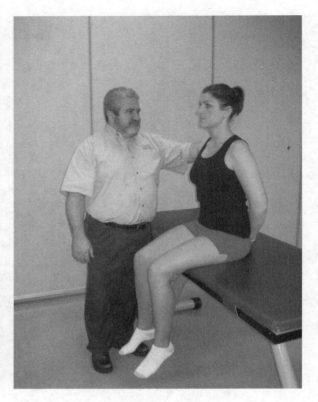

Figure 30.7 Slump Test. Starting position.

(Butler, 1991) and is reported to have been performed as a diagnostic procedure as early as 1909 (Woodhall & Hayes, 1950). Geoffrey Maitland (1979, 1985) is credited with being responsible for introducing the test into manual therapy and medicine.

A detailed description of the slump test is available in previously published texts (Butler, 1991, 2000; Shacklock, 1995b). The key points involved are that the patient sits with thighs fully supported and knees together. The therapist stands beside and close to the patient, perhaps with one leg up on the treatment table. (**Figure 30.7**). Resting symptoms are noted and any new symptoms or alterations in the resting symptoms are checked at each step of the slump test.

1. The patient is asked to slump or sag; gentle hand pressure from the therapist can guide the movement in order to obtain a bowing of the spine rather than hip flexion (**Figure 30.8**).
2. With the slumped trunk position maintained, the patient is asked to flex his or her head and neck forward in a chin-to-chest motion, and the

therapist places a hand behind the patient's head to maintain the position without adding overpressure (**Figure 30.9**).
3. The patient is then asked to extend the knee actively as much as he or she is able to within symptom tolerance (**Figure 30.10**).
4. The cervical flexion is then slowly released and the response assessed (**Figure 30.11**). Usually, patients will report relief of their evoked symptoms and be able to fully extend their knee to tolerance (**Figure 30.12**).

Butler (1991, 2000) reported that studies on the normal responses to the slump test in large groups of South Australian University students included the following:

- 50% of subjects (mean age 20) experienced a central T8-9 area pain when neck flexion was added to the slump position.
- Most subjects were unable to fully extend their leg in the knee extension position due to symptoms usually experienced in the posterior thigh and knee area.

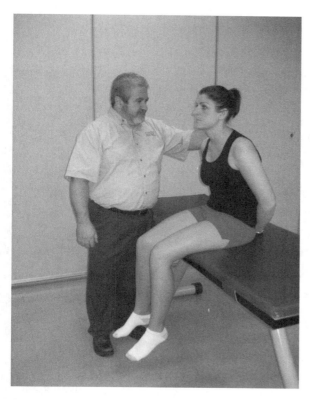

Figure 30.8 Slump Test. Addition of trunk slump or sagging while maintaining head and neck posture.

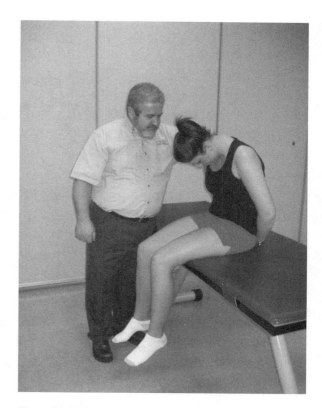

Figure 30.9 Slump Test. Addition of head and neck flexion.

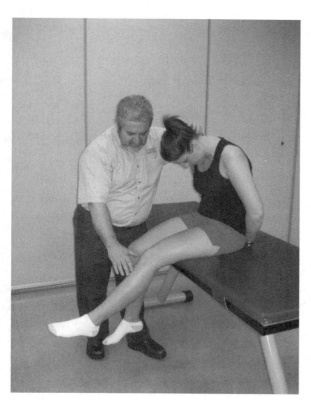

Figure 30.10 Slump Test. Patient is asked to actively extend the left knee as much as he or she is able within symptom tolerance.

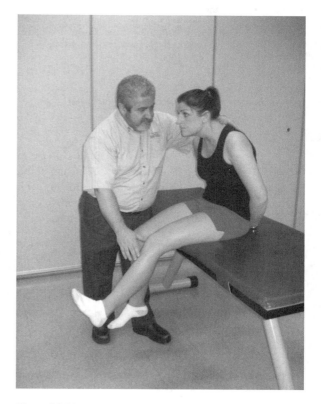

Figure 30.11 Slump Test. Head and neck flexion is then slowly released and the response assessed.

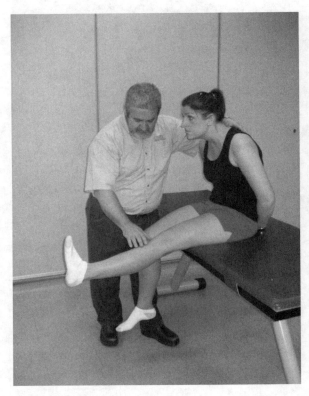

Figure 30.12 Slump Test. With the release of head and neck flexion, patients may report relief of their evoked symptoms and be able to fully extend their knee to tolerance.

- The knee symptoms usually eased when the cervical spine was extended and the knee could extend farther into range.

It is important to note that in the studies of these "normal responses" to the slump test, each stage of the test was firmly held and overpressure was applied. The authors note that this stronger performance of the slump test is not a part of current clinical practice.

Indications for the Slump Test in Patients with Headache

A therapist would consider using the slump test where, after detailed subjective evaluation, objective examination, and clinical reasoning, there is a hypothesis of a neurogenic source for symptoms (pain, aching, tightness) in the upper cervical or suboccipital region and the passive neck flexion test has not provided sufficient data to satisfy the therapist's inquiry. The therapist may clinically reason that a stronger movement or tension

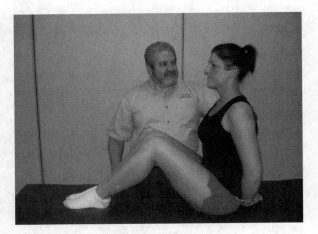

Figure 30.13 Long Sitting Slump Test. Starting position with patient sitting with both knees and hips flexed comfortably. Note: Patients should start with the back upright and not slumped.

on the neural tissues may provide useful findings, and opt to progress the passive neck flexion test into the slump test. Alternatively, the patient may have indicated a pain-provoking movement or position that is similar to the slump test (e.g., bending the head and neck while extending one leg, as in getting into a car).

Long Sitting Slump Test

From the authors' clinical experience, the LSS test can be a particularly useful examination and treatment technique in the management of patients with headache. Butler (2000) describes the technique as "a comfortable way to examine neural tissues in the head, neck and thorax as well as the lumbar spine" (p. 298).

A detailed description of the LSS test is available in Butler (2000). The key points involved are that the patient sits on the treatment table with both knees and hips flexed comfortably. The therapist stands beside and close to the patient (**Figure 30.13**). It is important that the starting position be with the patient sitting up straight and looking forward (neck in neutral). As with the slump test, resting symptoms are noted and any new symptoms or alterations in the resting symptoms are checked at each step of the test.

1. The patient is asked to slump the body, while maintaining the neck neutral posture. The therapist can ask the patient to keep looking forward and provide gentle hand pressure

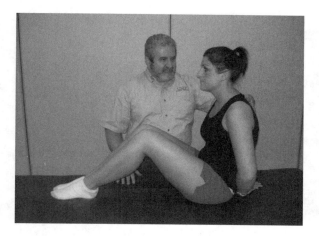

Figure 30.14 Long Sitting Slump Test. Patient is asked to slump the body while maintaining the neck neutral posture.

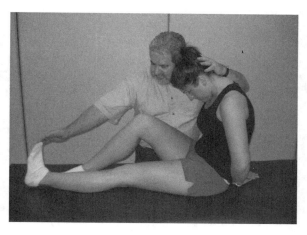

Figure 30.16 Long Sitting Slump Test. The patient is asked to extend his or her knees, one at a time, and compare symptoms evoked.

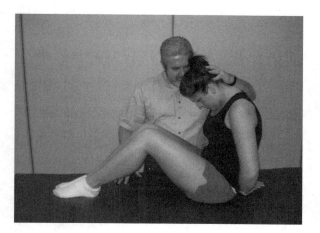

Figure 30.15 Long Sitting Slump Test. The patient is asked to flex the neck and take the chin down to the chest, and the therapist should take note of how easy or difficult the action is.

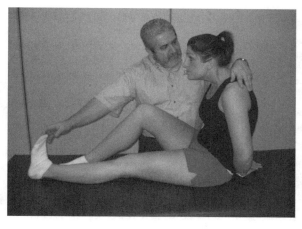

Figure 30.17 Long Sitting Slump Test. With the trunk and lower extremity positions held, the patient is asked to extend the cervical spine (release of cervical flexion), and any changes in symptoms are noted.

to guide the movement in order to obtain the required bowing of the spine (**Figure 30.14**).

2. The patient is asked to flex the neck and take the chin down to the chest. The therapist should take note of how easy or difficult the action is, and if deemed necessary, place a hand on the back of the head and forearm at the cervicothoracic junction to hold the position for the introduction of the next step (**Figure 30.15**).

3. The patient is asked to extend the knees, one at a time, and compare the symptoms evoked (**Figure 30.16**).

4. If necessary, the therapist can ask the patient to add ankle dorsiflexion or plantar flexion for further caudad influence.

5. As the trunk and lower extremity positions are held, the patient is asked to extend the cervical spine (release of cervical flexion), and any changes in symptoms are noted (**Figure 30.17**).

Structural differentiation can be achieved by adding and subtracting elements of the test. For example, if symptoms are evoked in the neck, head, or thorax with the end-range position (**Figure 30.18**), the head and

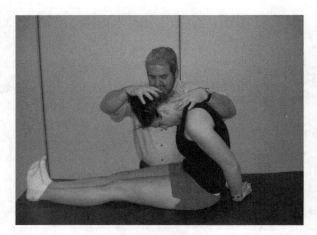

Figure 30.18 Long Sitting Slump Test. Starting position for structural differentiation through release of distal tension (release of knee extension).

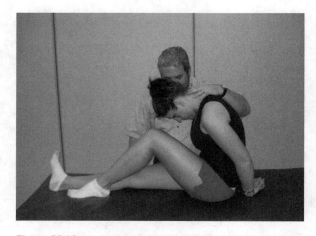

Figure 30.19 Long Sitting Slump Test. Completing structural differentiation through release of distal tension (release of knee extension) while maintaining head and neck flexion. Any changes in symptoms in the neck, head, or thorax should be duly noted.

neck position can be maintained while the patient slowly flexes the knees, one at a time (**Figure 30.19**), and any changes in symptoms in the neck, head, or thorax can be noted. If the symptoms are eased by the knee flexion, there would be a strong argument for a neurodynamic influence to such neck, head, or thorax symptoms. The therapist could then decide to apply treatment in a manner that would address the space, movement, and blood flow demands of the nervous system. Some examples of treatment techniques are presented later in this chapter.

Upper Limb Neurodynamic Tests

The four tests of upper limb neurodynamics are as follows:

ULNT1 (median nerve bias)
ULNT2 (median nerve bias)
ULNT2 (radial nerve bias)
ULNT3 (ulnar nerve bias)

The numbers refer to the powerful sensitizing movements, where 1 is shoulder abduction, 2 represents shoulder girdle depression, and 3 is elbow flexion (Butler, 1991, 2000). There are two tests for the median nerve because this nerve is more commonly injured than the other nerves in the upper limb and it was felt that a test was required to evaluate shoulder girdle depression and glenohumeral elevation independently (Butler, 2000). **Table 30.1** summarizes the movements at each of the joints of the upper limb for each of the four tests.

ULNT1: Median Active Test

If the patient has described a symptom-provoking position or movement, have the patient demonstrate it for you and observe the mechanics involved. If possible, perform a quick structural differentiation. For example, the patient may demonstrate a symptomatic position for his or her elbow pain, and you could have the patient maintain that elbow position and then ask him or her to move the neck to see if that alters the elbow symptoms.

A simple protocol for the active evaluation of the median neurodynamic test (ULNT1) has been described (Butler, 2000). Have patients look at the palm of their hand and extend their elbow, and then get them to extend their arm out sideways with the hand held forward until it comes to just above their head. Then ask them to extend their wrist and tip their head away from the test side. Compare with the opposite side, and note symptom responses as well as what happens to the shoulder girdle. Where the nervous system is sensitive, the shoulder girdle will often elevate (Butler, 2000).

ULNT1: Median Passive Test

A detailed description of the ULNT1 test is available in earlier texts (Butler, 1991, 2000; Shacklock, 1995b). The key points involved are that the patient lies supine, arms by the side, shoulder close to the edge of the

Table 30.1 The Major Components, Movements, Sensitizing Motions, and Differentiating Motions for the Four Distinct Upper Limb Neurodynamic Tests

	ULNT1	UNLT2a	ULNT2b	ULNT3
Nerves tested	Median, anterior interosseous (C5, C6, C7)	Median, anterior interosseous (C5, C6, C7)	Radial	Ulnar, C8, and T1 nerve roots
Shoulder	Stabilized from elevating, and abducted (110°)	Depressed and abducted (10°)	Depressed and abducted (10°)	Depressed and abducted (10° to 90°), hand to ear
Elbow	Extended	Extended	Extended	Flexed
Forearm	Supinated	Supinated	Pronated	Pronated
Wrist	Extended	Extended	Flexed and ulnarly deviated	Extended and radially deviated
Fingers and thumb	Extended	Extended	Flexed	Extended
Rotation of shoulder	Lateral	Lateral	Medial	Lateral
Cervical spine (sensitizing)	Contralateral side flexed	Contralateral side flexed	Contralateral side flexed	Contralateral side flexed
Cervical spine (differentiating)	Ipsilateral side flexed	Ipsilateral side flexed	Ipsilateral side flexed	Ipsilateral side flexed

examination table, with no pillow if possible, and with the body straight. The therapist stands with the near foot placed forward, near hip approximating the table, and faces the patient's head. The therapist's near hand presses on the table above the patient's shoulder in either a knuckles or fist position, but there should not be any downward or caudad pressure on the superior aspect of the patient's shoulder (**Figure 30.20**). The focus of this procedure is to maintain the shoulder position during the performance of the test and prevent any shoulder elevation rather than to passively depress the shoulder girdle. With the other hand, the therapist holds the patient's hand with the thumb extended to apply tension to the motor branch of the median nerve. The therapist's fingers wrap around the patient's fingers distal to the metacarpophalangeal joints. The patient's elbow is flexed at 90° and supported on the therapist's near (front) thigh.

The movements performed, in sequence, are glenohumeral abduction up to 90° to 110°, if available, in the frontal plane (**Figure 30.21**), followed by wrist and finger extension and forearm supination (**Figure 30.22**). Then, glenohumeral external rotation is added to the available range, although it is generally stopped at 90° if the patient is very mobile (**Figure 30.23**). The next component of the test is elbow extension; this should be done gently and with care not to cause any shoulder motion, especially adduction, which would thereby ease off the developing neurodynamic test (**Figure 30.24**). After the

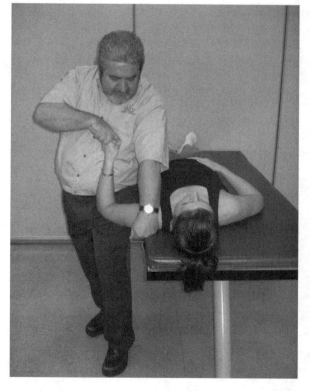

Figure 30.20 Upper Limb Neurodynamic Test 1: Median Passive Test. Starting position with the therapist's left hand providing a block to prevent shoulder girdle elevation.

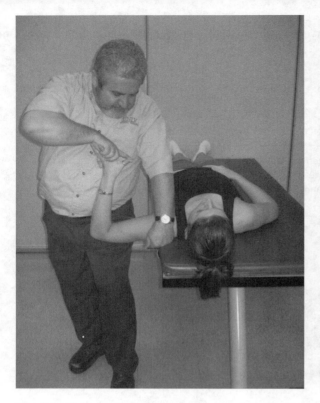

Figure 30.21 Upper Limb Neurodynamic Test 1: Median Passive Test. Addition of shoulder abduction to 90° to 110° as per patient tolerance. Note: The movement should occur in the frontal plane.

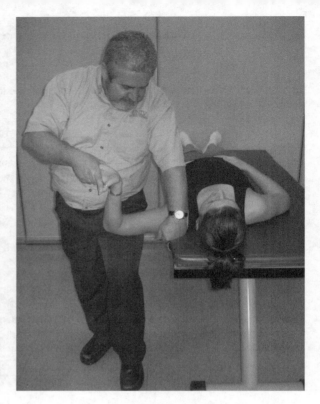

Figure 30.22 Upper Limb Neurodynamic Test 1: Median Passive Test. Addition of wrist and finger extension and forearm supination.

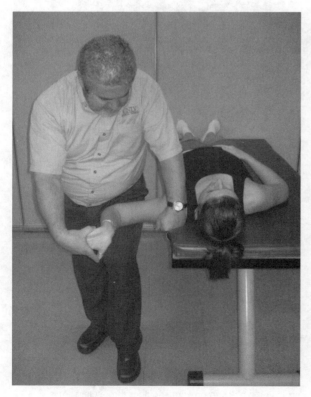

Figure 30.23 Upper Limb Neurodynamic Test 1: Median Passive Test. Addition of glenohumeral external rotation to available range (generally stopped at 90° if patient is very mobile).

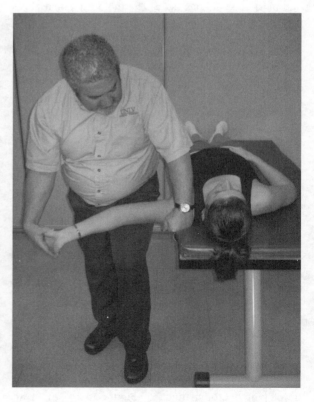

Figure 30.24 Upper Limb Neurodynamic Test 1: Median Passive Test. Addition of elbow extension. This should be done gently and with care not to cause any shoulder motion, especially adduction.

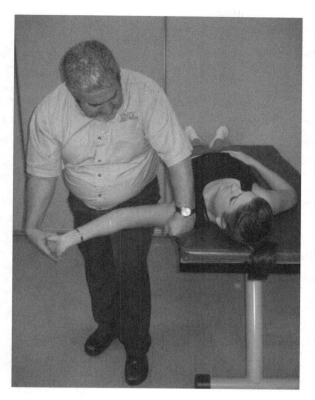

Figure 30.25 Upper Limb Neurodynamic Test 1: Median Passive Test. Structural differentiation through addition of cervical contralateral lateral flexion.

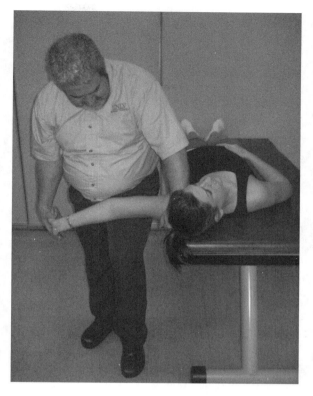

Figure 30.26 Upper Limb Neurodynamic Test 1: Median Passive Test. Structural differentiation through addition of cervical ipsilateral lateral flexion.

addition of each component, the patient is asked to relate any and all symptoms that may be evoked. The final component of the test involves structural differentiation with cervical spine movements; the selection of the correct movement for structural differentiation is based on where the symptoms (if any) are located. If distal symptoms have developed (e.g., forearm and wrist pain) and are to be differentiated, the neck is moved into contralateral lateral flexion, and any change in the distal symptoms would constitute a positive structural differentiation (**Figure 30.25**). If cervical contralateral flexion increases these symptoms and cervical ipsilateral flexion decreases these symptoms (**Figure 30.26**), this would constitute a positive structural differentiation and perhaps lead to a positive neurodynamic test. If proximal symptoms have been developed (e.g., head, neck, and shoulder pain) and are to be differentiated, the wrist is released from its extended position; again, any change in the proximal symptoms would constitute a positive structural differentiation.

A pattern of frequently reported and observed responses has been noted in young asymptomatic subjects (Kenneally, 1985; Kenneally et al., 1988). Stretching, pulling, pain, tingling, and numbing are quite commonly reported sensations even in individuals who are asymptomatic prior to the test. Kenneally et al. (1988) summarized the responses to the ULNT of 400 asymptomatic individuals as follows:

- A deep stretch or ache was felt in the cubital fossa (99% of volunteers) extending down the anterior and radial aspect of the forearm and into the radial side of the hand.
- A definite tingling sensation was felt in the thumb and first three fingers.
- A small percentage felt stretch in the anterior shoulder.
- Cervical lateral flexion away from the side tested increased evoked responses in 90% of subjects.
- Cervical lateral flexion toward the side tested decreased the test response in 70% of subjects.

Indications for the ULNT1 Test

A therapist would consider using the ULNT1 test in the clinic where, after detailed subjective evaluation, objective examination, and clinical reasoning, there is a hypothesis of neurogenic pain in the upper limb or there is a hypothesis that the source of the disorder lies in the median nerve pathways and receptive fields. Alternatively, the patient may have indicated a pain-provoking movement or position that is similar to the test (e.g., hanging washing on the line) or to a part of the test (e.g., forearm pronation and supination activities).

ULNT2: Median Active Test

In some cases, it may not be possible or appropriate to abduct the shoulder. This is where the ULNT2 test can be quite useful, because it uses shoulder girdle depression as the sensitizing movement. For the active test, patients can hang their arms naturally by their side and look at their thumb. Have patients point their thumb away, extend the wrist, and then reach their hand down toward the floor. They can use their other hand to depress their shoulder girdle. If necessary, they can then laterally flex their cervical spine away from the test side and compare responses with the other side.

ULNT2: Median Passive Test

For detailed description of the ULNT2 test see earlier texts (Butler, 1991, 2000; Shacklock, 1995b). Once again, the key points involved are that the patient lies supine on a slight diagonal with the shoulder just over the edge of the treatment table to allow for contact with the therapist's thigh. The therapist stands near the patient's shoulder and uses his or her thigh to carefully depress the shoulder girdle (**Figure 30.27**). The therapist's left hand cradles the patient's right elbow, and the right hand controls the patient's wrist and hand. The patient's arm is in approximately 10° of abduction. The second component of the test is elbow extension (**Figure 30.28**) and then whole arm external rotation. Next, add wrist and finger extension (**Figure 30.29**); some specific hand-holds are suggested by authors (Butler, 2000; Shacklock, 2005). Throughout this test, as each component is added, the patient is asked to relate any and all symptoms that may be evoked. Glenohumeral abduction is then added if necessary. In most cases, there will be sufficient symptoms evoked without adding abduction, and structural differentiation can be achieved through

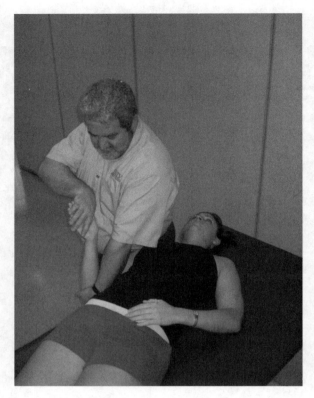

Figure 30.27 Upper Limb Neurodynamic Test 2: Median Passive Test. Starting position with the therapist's left hip providing depression of the shoulder girdle, and the left hand cradling the elbow while the right hand controls the patient's wrist and hand. The patient's shoulder should be in approximately 10° of abduction.

cervical contralateral lateral flexion (**Figure 30.30**). Once again, for positive structural differentiation, the therapist is looking for alteration of evoked symptoms by the addition or subtraction of test components distant to the symptoms. If symptoms are reported distally (e.g., forearm and wrist), then change in the symptoms with cervical movements (increase with contralateral lateral flexion and decrease with ipsilateral lateral flexion) would represent positive structural differentiation.

ULNT2: Radial Active Test

There are many ways to have the patient perform an active ULNT2 radial test. The most common method is to have the patient hold the arm to the side, flex the wrist, look at the palm, and then internally rotate the arm so that he or she can look at the palm over his or her shoulder. The patient can then depress the shoulder and look away to laterally flex the cervical spine if needed.

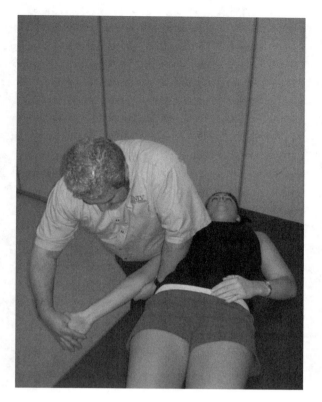

Figure 30.28 Upper Limb Neurodynamic Test 2: Median Passive Test. Addition of elbow extension and whole arm external rotation.

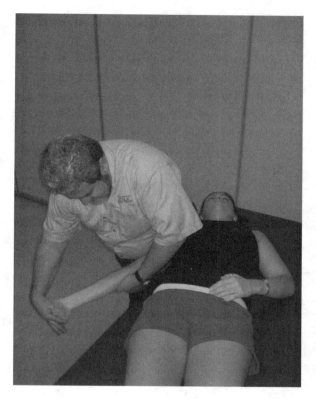

Figure 30.29 Upper Limb Neurodynamic Test 2: Median Passive Test. Addition of wrist and finger extension. Note specific hand hold to add tension to the thumb and thenar eminence.

Symptoms evoked during the performance of the test actively may obviate the need for performing the test passively.

ULNT2: Radial Passive Test

Further detailed descriptions of this test can be found in previously published texts (Butler, 1991, 2000; Shacklock, 1995b). The key points involved in this test, much like the ULNT2 median test, are that the patient lies supine on a slight diagonal with the shoulder just over the edge of the treatment table to allow for contact with the therapist's thigh. The therapist stands near the patient's shoulder and uses his or her thigh to carefully depress the shoulder girdle (**Figure 30.31**). The therapist's left hand cradles the patient's right elbow, and the right hand controls the patient's wrist and hand. The patient's arm is in approximately 10° of abduction. The second component of the test is elbow extension and then whole arm internal rotation. Next, add wrist and finger flexion; it

may also be appropriate to add wrist ulnar deviation and thumb flexion (**Figure 30.32**). As with all the neurodynamic tests, as each component is added, the patient is asked to relate any and all symptoms that may be evoked. Glenohumeral abduction can be added if necessary (**Figure 30.33**), but as with the ULNT2 median test, in most cases there will be sufficient symptoms evoked without adding abduction, and structural differentiation can be achieved through cervical contralateral lateral flexion (**Figure 30.34**).

Yaxley and Jull (1991) investigated the most common responses to the ULNT2 radial test on 50 asymptomatic 18- to 30-year-old subjects. Their findings were a strong painful stretch over the radial aspect of the proximal forearm (84% of all responses), often accompanied by a stretch pain in the lateral aspect of the upper arm (32%) or biceps brachii (14%) or the dorsal aspect of the hand (12%). A response in this area would make the radial nerve at the elbow a candidate for a source of pain (Butler, 2000).

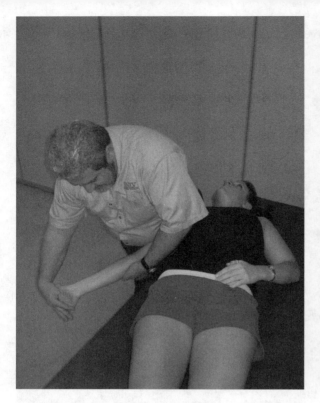

Figure 30.30 Upper Limb Neurodynamic Test 2: Median Passive Test. Structural differentiation can be achieved through cervical contralateral lateral flexion.

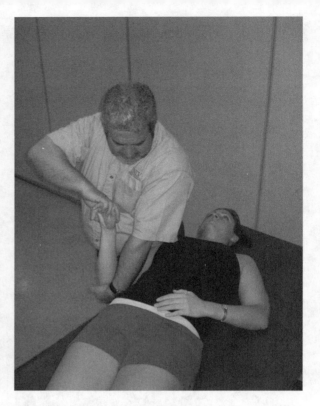

Figure 30.31 Upper Limb Neurodynamic Test 2: Radial Passive Test. Starting position with the therapist's left hip providing depression of the shoulder girdle, and the left hand cradling the elbow while the right hand controls the patient's wrist and hand.

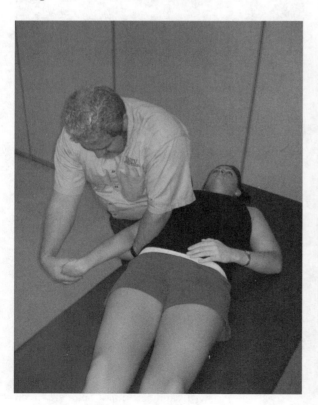

Figure 30.32 Upper Limb Neurodynamic Test 2: Radial Passive Test. Addition of elbow extension and whole arm internal rotation. Also adding forearm pronation, wrist flexion, wrist ulnar deviation, and thumb flexion.

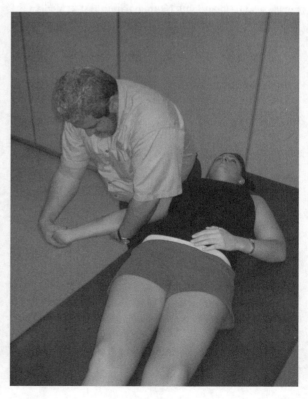

Figure 30.33 Upper Limb Neurodynamic Test 2: Radial Passive Test. Addition of glenohumeral abduction (in cases where no symptoms or insufficient symptoms have been evoked).

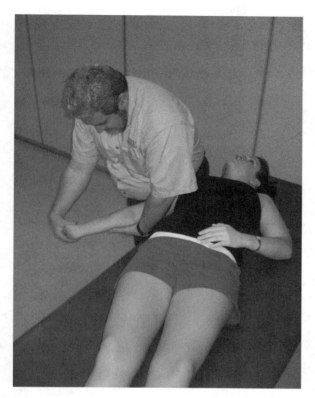

Figure 30.34 Upper Limb Neurodynamic Test 2: Radial Passive Test. Structural differentiation can be achieved through cervical contralateral lateral flexion.

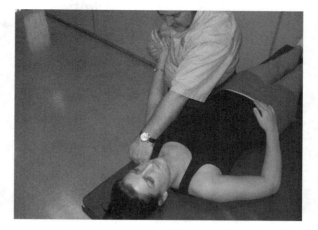

Figure 30.35 Upper Limb Neurodynamic Test 3: Ulnar Passive Test. Starting position with the therapist's left hand applying a downward or caudad pressure on the superior aspect of the patient's shoulder to achieve shoulder girdle depression.

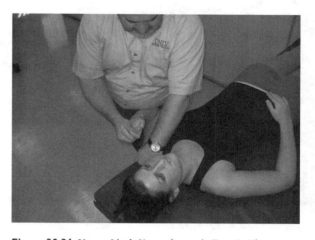

Figure 30.36 Upper Limb Neurodynamic Test 3: Ulnar Passive Test. The wrist and fingers are extended (with perhaps some radial deviation) as the elbow is flexed.

ULNT3: Ulnar Active Test

The active ULNT3 ulnar test can be performed by asking patients to look at their hand and hold it up as though they were holding a tray of drinks. Further loading can then be added by having patients look away, adding more elbow flexion, depressing the shoulder girdle, and adding forearm pronation. Cervical spine retraction is also thought to be another worthwhile sensitizing movement (Butler, 2000). In patients with good range of movement, and especially in younger, flexible patients, an end-range active test may be achieved with the "mask" position, with the index finger and thumbs making circles over the eyes while fingers 3 to 5 are placed on the cheeks, pointing downward.

ULNT3: Ulnar Passive Test

As with the ULNT1 median test, this test has the patient lying supine, arms by the side, shoulder close to the edge of the examination table, with no pillow if possible,

and with the body straight. The therapist stands with the near foot placed forward, near hip approximating the table, and faces the patient's head. The therapist's near hand presses on the table above the patient's shoulder in either a knuckles or fist position, and this time applies a downward or caudad pressure on the superior aspect of the patient's shoulder to achieve shoulder girdle depression (**Figure 30.35**). With the other hand, the therapist holds the patient's hand (palm against palm), and the elbow starts in extension. The wrist and fingers are extended (and perhaps some radial deviation) as the elbow is flexed (**Figure 30.36**).

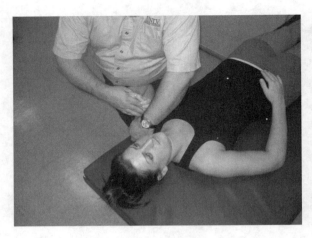

Figure 30.37 Upper Limb Neurodynamic Test 3: Ulnar Passive Test. The forearm is then pronated and the shoulder taken into lateral rotation and abduction.

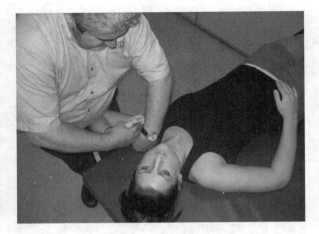

Figure 30.39 Upper Limb Neurodynamic Test 3: Ulnar Passive Test. Addition of cervical contralateral lateral flexion for structural differentiation.

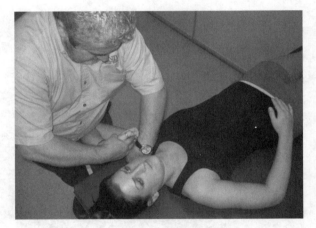

Figure 30.38 Upper Limb Neurodynamic Test 3: Ulnar Passive Test. Shoulder abduction achieved as the therapist "walks" around the point of the patient's elbow within his or her groin.

The forearm is then pronated and the shoulder taken into lateral rotation and abduction (**Figure 30.37**). This is achieved by the therapist "walking" around the point of the patient's elbow within the groin (**Figure 30.38**). The final components added can be cervical contralateral lateral flexion or shoulder girdle depression, depending on symptoms evoked and structural differentiation (**Figure 30.39**). Flanagan (1993) reported normal values for this distal-to-proximal sequencing of the test and found that 82% of subjects reported responses in the hypothenar eminence and medial two fingers, and 64% reported pins and needles in the same area.

The ULNT3 ulnar test is often performed from proximal to distal, with shoulder girdle depression and shoulder abduction followed by shoulder external rotation, then elbow flexion, and finally wrist and finger extension with forearm pronation (Butler, 2000). Butler (2000) has suggested that to standardize the base test system, clinicians should make all the tests start from the shoulder girdle.

CLINICAL APPLICATION OF NEURODYNAMICS IN HEADACHE AND NECK PAIN

It is important to keep in mind that healthy mechanics of the nervous system within the neck and upper quadrant facilitates pain-free posture, movement, and function. In the presence of neural tissue pathomechanics (e.g., adaptive shortening or neural tissue entrapment), symptoms may be provoked during activities of daily living such as nodding one's head to say "yes," combing one's hair, or tucking in one's shirt. The aim of using neurodynamic tests in assessment is to mechanically stimulate and move neural tissues in order to gain an impression of their mobility and sensitivity to mechanical stresses. It follows that the purpose of treating patients with these techniques is to improve the mechanical and physiologic function of the neural tissues (Shacklock, 1995a).

Mechanosensitivity, as described in Chapter 20, is the chief mechanism by which neural tissue causes pain with movement. If a nerve is not mechanically sensitive, then it will not respond (cause pain) to mechanical forces applied to it. Mechanosensitivity can be defined as the ease with which impulses can be activated from a site in the nervous system when a mechanical force is applied (Butler, 2000; Shacklock, 2005). Normal nerves can be mechanosensitive (given sufficient force) and, therefore, respond to applied forces (Lindquist et al., 1973; Rosenbleuth et al., 1953). This is an important point to consider when making judgments about the contribution of the neural tissues within the upper cervical spine and upper quadrant to a patient's symptoms. Responses to neurodynamic testing can be normal or abnormal, relevant or irrelevant (Butler, 2000; Shacklock, 2005). Normal neurodynamic test responses are typically symmetric, in a normal location (relative to normative data), generate a normal quality of symptoms, and display a normal range of movement for the segment being evaluated. A neurodynamic test response might be considered abnormal if it occurs in a different location than normal, has a different quality of symptoms, and/or the range of movement of the limb or trunk segment is different from normal (or the uninvolved side, if extremity movements are used). In most cases, there is reproduction of the patient's symptoms. The next clinical question would consider whether the test response is relevant or irrelevant. Relevance, in this case, would mean that the test response is causally related to the patient's current problem (meaning that the response is directly related to the patient's condition), and an irrelevant finding would be a test response that is not causally related to the patient's current problem.

The symptoms evoked on a neurodynamic test can be inferred to be neurogenic (a positive test in a clinical sense) if:

- Structural differentiation supports a neurogenic source
- There are differences left to right and to known normal responses
- The test reproduces the patient's symptoms or associated symptoms
- There is support from other data such as history, area of symptoms, imaging tests, and so on

The greater the number of these factors present, the stronger the case for a clinically relevant test.

The information required from a neurodynamic test is the symptom response, the resistance encountered, and the effect it has on the symptom response as each component of the test is added or subtracted. The infor-

mation gleaned from the neurodynamic test, along with the patient history, subjective and objective examination, and so forth, should give the clinician the ability to provisionally diagnose the site of neuropathodynamics and then reassess after a potential treatment has been administered. It is important to realize that the treatment need not be a mobilizing technique for the nervous system, since the clinician may decide to mobilize or treat the mechanical interface. In any event, treatment should focus on addressing issues of space, movement, and blood flow to the nervous system. It is also important to consider that sensitivity to a neurodynamic test could be from a combination of primary (tissue-based) or secondary (central nervous system–based) processes (Butler, 2002).

When designing the treatment program, it is important to note that current best evidence indicates that a multimodal approach consisting of manual therapy and specific exercise improves outcomes in patients with cervicogenic headaches (Gross et al., 2004, 2006; Jull et al., 2002). As stated in Chapter 20, this is important because neural tissue mobilization involves both hands-on treatment and active exercises (Butler, 1991, 2000; Shacklock, 2005). Although the focus of this chapter has been on outlining the hands-on passive evaluation techniques, it should be clear to the clinician that they may be easily modified to form active exercises that will complement the required multimodal approach. Some general guidelines would include using sliders early in the program before advancing to the more neurodynamically challenging tensioners (Coppieters & Butler, 2008).

Sliders are neurodynamic maneuvers performed in order to produce a sliding movement of neural structures relative to their adjacent tissues (Butler, 2000; Shacklock, 2005; Coppieters & Butler, 2008). Sliders involve application of movement/stress to the nervous system proximally while releasing movement/stress distally, and then the sequence may be reversed. An example in patients with headache symptoms would be to have them sit in the slumped position and perform knee extension and ankle dorsiflexion at the same time as they extend their head and neck; then, alternate so that they perform knee flexion and ankle plantar flexion at the same time as they flex their head and neck. Sliders allow for larger ranges of motion, provide a means of distraction from the painful area, and should provide multitissue, nonpainful, and, it would be hoped, fear-reducing novel inputs into the central nervous system (Butler, 2002). Sliders are generally better tolerated by patients with irritable conditions.

Tensioners are neurodynamic maneuvers performed in order to produce an increase in tension (not stretch) in neural structures, which may improve neural viscoelastic and physiologic functions (help neural tissue accommodate to increased tension) (Butler, 2000; Shacklock, 2005; Coppieters & Butler, 2008). Tensioners are the opposite of sliders in that movement/stress is applied proximally and distally to the nervous system at the same time, and then released. As an example once more in our patients with headache symptoms, they would sit in the slumped position and perform knee extension and ankle dorsiflexion at the same time as they flex their head and neck (tensioner); then, they would release the tension by performing knee flexion and ankle plantar flexion at the same time as they extend their head and neck. Tensioners may better challenge stiffness and more long-lasting physical dysfunction (Butler, 2002) and are generally better tolerated by patients with nonirritable conditions.

Clinicians should keep in mind the underlying principles of addressing the issues of space, movement, and blood for the nervous system. Accordingly, performance of any neurodynamic techniques (either passively or actively) should involve smooth, controlled, gentle, large-amplitude movements. Sustained or vigorous stretching of the nervous system tissues is not at all indicated, given that prolonged stretching has been shown to reduce intraneural blood flow (Ogata & Naito, 1986; Driscoll et al., 2002). It is also important to consider the most probable sites (mechanical interface) for compression of the nervous system in each presenting case and to develop treatment approaches that might address opening the mechanical interface and help create needed space for the neural tissues.

CASE STUDY

The purpose of the following case study is to illustrate the practical application of neurodynamics in the management of a patient with headache consulting an outpatient orthopaedic physical therapy clinic. The patient was a 34-year-old woman referred for evaluation and treatment of tension-type headache. She reported a 3-month history of headaches. She stated she had been involved in a rear-end motor vehicle accident approximately 1 month prior to the onset of headaches but did not recall any neck pain or appreciable injuries at the time. To her, it had been a minor event—"a slight jolt"—and she had thought nothing of it at the time. About a month after the onset of her headaches, she went to see her primary care physician. She had plain films taken of the head and neck, which were reported to be normal. She reported that her physician did not know what was causing the headaches and simply recommended she take Excedrin as needed. When her headaches persisted, she spoke to her physician about referring her for physical therapy.

Subjective Complaints

The patient's primary complaint was intermittent suboccipital headache with radiation into both frontal areas. A secondary complaint was "aching" in her neck, which she described as central, with one side not greater than the other. Finally, she felt an unusual stiffness between her shoulder blades, like she had "an annoying strap on her bra" (**Figure 30.40**). She had no symptoms radiating into the shoulders, arms, forearms, or hands. She had no symptoms in her lower back or

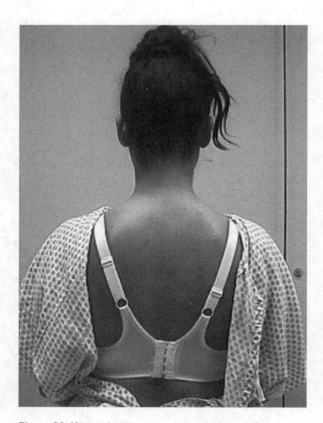

Figure 30.40 Headache Case Study Patient Seen from Behind. The patient reported an unusual stiffness between her shoulder blades at this location that felt like she had "an annoying strap on her bra."

lower extremities. The headache was brought on, and made worse, if she had a hectic day or was stressed in any way. She worked as a receptionist at a dental practice. Using the phone or working too long at the front office computer gave her the headache, and the neck ache and midthoracic stiffness were mostly present at the end of her day and only noticeable if she had a headache. She rated her headache as usually 6/10, neck aching as 2/10, and the stiffness between the shoulder blades as a 1/10 level. The Headache Disability Index (HDI) (Jacobson et al., 1994) was administered, and she scored 38, indicating mild disability.

Functional Level

The patient reported she was independent with all of her activities of daily living and was generally without pain most times. Her sitting tolerance was 45 to 60 minutes without significant pain, and she could only tolerate driving for 45 to 60 minutes without significant pain. She could walk 1 hour or more without significant pain. Her ability to tolerate computer work was limited to 15 to 30 minutes without significant pain, and talking on the phone was also limited to 15 to 30 minutes without significant pain. She reported that she had a regular handset that she habitually cradled between her right ear and right shoulder.

Medical History

She reported that her current medications included Excedrin as needed, but she felt it was not helping. She reported her general health as excellent and denied any preexisting conditions, prior injuries, or other health concerns.

Objective Testing

Seated cervical spine active range of motion testing revealed a range within normal limits and no pain for flexion, left rotation, and left lateral flexion. Extension was full range, but overpressure of the upper cervical component of extension reproduced her neck ache symptom. Right rotation was approximately 75% of normal range, but she had no pain at end range, and there was a firm end-feel. Right lateral flexion was approximately 75% normal range, but with no pain at end range, and also exhibited a firm end-feel. The right upper cervical quadrant (Maitland, 1986) strongly reproduced the suboccipital headache, whereas the left upper cervical quadrant was negative for symptom reproduction or discomfort. Thoracic spine range of motion was normal, and no pain was elicited with end-range overpressure. Bilateral shoulder range of motion was normal, with no pain. Vertebral artery testing and subjective questioning were negative for signs of vertebrobasilar insufficiency (Magarey et al., 2000).

Manual palpation revealed tenderness and hypomobility at C2-C3 with passive accessory intervertebral motion testing, and passive physiological intervertebral motion testing revealed stiffness and pain with right rotation and right lateral flexion at C1-C2 and C2-C3 levels. Palpation of the thoracic spine revealed generalized hypomobility (no significant level) but no tenderness. Firm and sustained bilateral pressure into the suboccipital musculature and tissues reproduced her headache, and relief of the pressure reduced or relieved her headache completely.

Assessment

The initial hypothesis was that of a motion restriction problem at C1-C2 and C2-C3 leading to headaches, and perhaps that the neck aching and stiffness were associated with muscular fatigue or upper trapezius tension when her headache was present.

Initial Treatment

A Maitland approach was taken and unilateral posterior-anterior (PA) mobilizations were performed on the right C1-C2 and C2-C3, grade IV minus (Maitland, 1986). This was performed for 45 seconds, with oscillations at each level to try to improve rotation and lateral flexion to the right. However, reassessment immediately after treatment revealed no change in the range or comfort of right rotation or lateral flexion. An alternative mobilization technique was chosen. A unilateral PA mobilization with the neck in full left rotation was performed directly over the left C1-C2 and C2-C3 articular pillar, grade IV minus (45 seconds of oscillations at each level); afterward, reassessment revealed improved right rotation (to 90%) but no change in right lateral flexion. The initial treatment was completed with topical application of pulsed ultrasound to the right suboccipital region, and then the patient was educated in a home program consisting of seated chin retraction as per McKenzie (1998), shoulder shrugs, and active range of motion for upper cervical flexion with elbows together and hands behind the neck.

Second and Third Visits
Subjective

The patient reported that her headaches were the same, and her neck aching and midthoracic stiffness were no better. She felt she could move her neck a lot better, but the symptoms were essentially the same. The HDI score improved only minimally—to 32 from the original score of 38—indicating no significant change (Jacobson et al., 1994).

Objective

The upper cervical spine rotation and lateral flexion to the right had improved to about 95% range and remained pain free and had the same firm end-feel. Treatments were advanced to include high-velocity, low-amplitude thrust techniques into left rotation (upslope glide) and left lateral flexion (downslope glide) in order to gap the right C1-C2 and C2-C3 levels.

Assessment

The patient's physical signs (motion restriction and end-feel) were improving, but her subjective complaints remained the same. Something was being missed.

Fourth Visit
Subjective

No change since the last two visits.

Objective

Upper cervical spine rotation and lateral flexion to the right were unchanged. A decision was made to look for a possible neurodynamic problem as a source of her headaches. The seated slump test was performed, with cervical flexion causing onset of midthoracic stiffness ("that's the feeling I get like there's an annoying strap on my bra"); addition of either-side knee extension with same-side ankle dorsiflexion intensified the sensation, but she was unable to fully extend either knee. Release of the cervical flexion immediately relieved the midthoracic stiffness and she was able to extend her knees into full locking. There did not appear to be any significant difference in symptoms or resistance to movement with either right or left knee extension/ankle dorsiflexion. Bilateral knee extension/ankle dorsiflexion did not produce a greater symptom response.

Assessment

The patient appeared to have a neurodynamic restriction with slump and straight leg raise; therefore, a slump slider was performed. The seated trunk slumped posture was sustained while the patient alternated between flexing her neck, flexing her knees, and relaxing her ankle, and then extending her neck while extending her knee and maximally dorsiflexing her ankles. This active exercise has been affectionately termed "kicking your head off your shoulders" (Butler, 2000). This was performed for three to four sets of 45 seconds each, and then the complete slump was reassessed. Knee extension range and patient symptoms during slump were improved.

Final Three Visits
Subjective

During the last three treatment sessions, the patient reported gradual clearing of her headaches. She had been headache free for 2 weeks by the last visit. She reported feeling 100% better in that she felt she was not restricted in her work and had no neck aching or midthoracic stiffness after working. She had managed to arrange for a hands-free headset to be supplied by her employer, and she felt she was back to her usual state of being, "perhaps a little better." The HDI was readministered at the last visit, and she scored 2, which was a greater than 29-point decrease from her original 38 and subsequent 32. According to Jacobson et al. (1994), a 29-point change (95% CI) or greater in the total HDI score must occur before the changes can be attributed to treatment effects. She had not scored a perfect 0 because she had answered "sometimes" to question F4, "I restrict my recreational activities (e.g., sports, hobbies) because of my headaches."

Objective

During the last three treatment sessions, the slump test was rechecked each time, and with each testing, it was only possible to reproduce the familiar midthoracic stiffness with the fully wound-out tension sequence (i.e., full cervical flexion and full knee extension/ankle dorsiflexion). Structural differentiation was achieved each time with change or relief of symptoms with the release of cervical flexion. The patient's treatment sessions progressed from seated slump sliders to tensioners, and then long sitting slump sliders to tensioners. Manual therapy techniques were also continued for the upper cervical spine, including unilateral and central PA as well as supine upper cervical longitudinal distraction mobilizations. Therapeutic exercises and postural education regarding optimal upper and lower cervical positions and movements were provided.

Discussion

The addition of the slump neurodynamic technique with progression from sliders to tensioners appeared to clear the patient's headache symptoms. She still had some movement restriction into right rotation and right lateral flexion at C1-C2 and C2-C3, but this had not changed significantly with mobilization or specific manipulation techniques.

On the second to last visit, a manipulative technique was added to the midthoracic spine region (supine posterior-to-anterior thrust), and this appeared to help her slump range considerably.

The patient was discharged with a home program that included monitoring her slump range for nervous system mobility and capacity for stress or tension, as well as a comprehensive gymnasium program to further her upper body strength and promote improved upright posture.

REFERENCES

Beith I, Robins E, Richards P. An assessment of the adaptive mechanisms within and surrounding the peripheral nervous system, during changes in nerve bed length resulting from underlying joint movement. In: Shacklock MO, ed. *Moving In on Pain*. Australia: Butterworth-Heinemann; 1995.

Breig A. *Biomechanics of the Central Nervous System*. Stockholm: Almqvist and Wiksell; 1960.

Breig A. *Adverse Mechanical Tension in the Central Nervous System*. Stockholm: Almqvist and Wiksell; 1978.

Breig A, El-Nadi FA. Biomechanics of the cervical spinal cord. *Acta Radiol* 1966;4:602–624.

Breig A, Marions O. Biomechanics of the lumbo-sacral nerve roots. *Acta Radiol* 1963;1:1141–1160.

Breig A, Troup J. Biomechanical considerations in the straight leg raising test. *Spine* 1979;4:242–250.

Butler DS. *Mobilization of the Nervous System*. London: Churchill Livingstone; 1991.

Butler DS. *The Sensitive Nervous System*. Adelaide: Noigroup Publications; 2000.

Butler DS. Upper limb neurodynamic test: clinical use in a "big picture" framework. In: Grant R, ed. *Physical Therapy of the Cervical and Thoracic Spine*. London: Churchill Livingstone; 2002.

Calvin WH, Devor M, Howe JF. Can neuralgias arise from minor demyelination? Spontaneous firing, mechanosensitivity, and after-discharge from conducting axons. *Exp Neurol* 1982;75:755–763.

Coppieters MW, Butler DS. Do 'sliders' slide and 'tensioners' tension? An analysis of neurodynamic techniques and considerations regarding their application. *Man Ther* 2008 13(3):213–221.

Dahlin LB, Archer DR, McLean WG. Axonal transport and morphological changes following nerve compression: an experimental study in the rabbit vagus nerve. *J Hand Surgery (Br)* 1993;18:106–110.

Dilley A, Lynn B, Greening J, DeLeon N. Quantitative in vivo studies of median nerve sliding in response to wrist, elbow, shoulder and neck movements. *Clin Biomech* 2003;18: 899–907.

Driscoll PJ, Glasby MA, Lawson GM. An in vivo study of peripheral nerves in continuity: biomechanical and physiological responses to elongation. *J Orthopaedic Res* 2002;20:370–375.

Elvey RL. Brachial plexus tension tests and the patho-anatomical origin of arm pain. In: Idczak R, ed. *Aspects of Manipulative Therapy*. Melbourne: Manipulative Physiotherapists Association of Australia; 1979:105–110.

Erel E, Dilley A, Greening J, Morris V, Cohen B, Lynn B. Longitudinal sliding of the median nerve in patients with carpal tunnel syndrome. *J Hand Surgery (Br)* 2003;28: 439–443.

Fern R, Harrison PJ. The contribution of ischaemia and deformation to the conduction block generated by compression of the cat sciatic nerve. *Exp Physiol* 1994;79:583–592.

Flanagan M. *The Normal Response to the Ulnar Nerve Bias Upper Limb Tension Test* [Master's thesis]. University of South Australia; 1993.

Ginn S, Cartwright M, Chloros G, et al. Ultrasound in the diagnosis of a median neuropathy in the forearm: case report. *J Brachial Plex Peripher Nerve Inj* 2007;2:23.

Greening J, Dilley A, Lynn B. In vivo study of nerve movement and mechano-sensitivity of the median nerve in whiplash and non-specific arm pain patients. *Pain* 2005;115: 248–253.

Gross AR, Hoving JL, Haines TA, et al. A Cochrane review of manipulation and mobilization for mechanical neck disorders. *Spine* 2004;29:1541–1548.

Gross AR, Hoving JL, Haines TA, et al. Manipulation and mobilization for mechanical neck disorders. *Cochrane Library* 2006;1:CD004249.

Hall T. Manually detected impediments in the straight leg raise test. In: Jull G, ed. *Clinical Solutions. Proceeding of the Ninth Biennial Conference of the Manipulative Physiotherapists' Association of Australia*. Gold Coast: Manipulative Physiotherapists' Association of Australia; 1995:48–53.

Hildebrandt J, Jansen J. Vascular compression of the C2 and C3 roots—yet another cause of chronic intermittent hemi-crania? *Cephalalgia* 1984;4:167–170.

Howe JF, Loeser JD, Calvin WH. Mechanosensitivity of dorsal root ganglia and chronically injured axons: a physiological basis for the radicular pain of nerve root compression. *Pain* 1977;3:25–41.

Jacobson GP, Ramadan NM, Aggarwal SK, Newman C. The Henry Ford Hospital Headache Disability Inventory (HDI). *Neurology* 1994;44:837–842.

Jansen J, Bardosi A, Hildebrandt J, Lucke A. Cervicogenic, hemi-cranial attacks associated with vascular irritation or compression of the cervical nerve root C2: clinical manifestations and morphological findings. *Pain* 1989a;39:203–212.

Jansen J, Markakis E, Rama B, Hildebrandt J. Hemi-cranial attacks or permanent hemi-crania: a sequel of upper cervical root compression. *Cephalalgia* 1989b;9:123–130.

Johnson EK, Chiarello CM. The slump test: the effects of head and lower extremity position on knee extension. *J Orthop Sports Phys Ther* 1997;26:310–317.

Jull G, Trott P, Potter H, et al. A randomized controlled trial of exercise and manipulative therapy for cervicogenic headache. *Spine* 2002;27:1835–1843.

Kenneally M. The upper limb tension test. In: *Proceedings of the Fourth Biennial Conference, Manipulative Therapists Association of Australia*. Brisbane: Manipulative Therapists Association of Australia; 1985.

Kenneally M, Rubenach H, Elvey RL. The upper limb tension test: the SLR test of the arm. In: Grant R, ed. *Physical Therapy of the Cervical Spine: Clinics in Physical Therapy*. Edinburgh: Churchill Livingstone; 1988.

Kleinrensink G, Stoeckart R, Vleeming A. Mechanical tension in the median nerve: the effects of joint positions. *Clin Biomech* 1995;10:240–244.

Kleinrensink GJ, Stoeckart R, Mulder PG, et al. Upper limb tension tests as tools in the diagnosis of nerve and plexus lesions: anatomical and biomechanical aspects. *Clin Biomech* 2000;15:9–14.

Lindquist C, Nilsson BY, Skoglund CR. Observations on the mechanical sensitivity of sympathetic and other types of small-diameter nerve fibers. *Brain Res* 1973;49:432–435.

Magarey M, Coughlan B, Rebbeck T. *Clinical Guidelines for Pre-manipulative Procedures for the Cervical Spine*. Melbourne: Australian Physiotherapy Association; 2000.

Maitland GD. Negative disc exploration: positive canal signs. *Aust J Physiother* 1979;25:129–134.

Maitland GD. The slump test: examination and treatment. *Aust J Physiother* 1985;31:215–219.

Maitland G. *Vertebral Manipulation*. 5th ed. Sydney: Butterworth; 1986.

McKenzie R. *Treat Your Own Neck*. 3rd ed. Waikanae, New Zealand: Spinal Publications; 1998.

McLellan DL, Swash M. Longitudinal sliding of the median nerve during movements of the upper limb. *J Neurol Neurosurg Psychiatry* 1976;39:566–570.

Millesi H. The nerve gap: theory and clinical practice. *Hand Clinics* 1986;2:651–663.

Nordin M, Nystrom B, Wallin U, Hagbarth KE. Ectopic sensory discharges, and paresthesiae in patients with disorders of peripheral nerves, dorsal roots and dorsal columns. *Pain* 1984;20:231–245.

Ogata K, Naito M. Blood flow of peripheral nerve: effects of dissection, stretching and compression. *J Hand Surgery (Am)* 1986;11:10–14.

Omar N, Alvi F, Srinivasan M. An unusual presentation of whiplash injury: long thoracic and spinal accessory nerve injury. *Eur Spine J* 2007;16(suppl 3):275–277.

Pikus HJ, Phillips J. Characteristics of patients successfully treated for cervicogenic headache by surgical decompression of the second cervical root. *Headache* 1995;35:621–629.

Pikus HJ, Phillips JM. Outcome of surgical decompression of the second cervical root for cervicogenic headache. *Neurosurgery* 1996;39:63–70.

Richardson C. The de-load model of injury. In: Richardson C, Hodges P, Hides J, eds. *Therapeutic Exercise for Lumbo-Pelvic Stabilization: A Motor Control Approach for the Treatment and Prevention of Low Back Pain*. Edinburgh: Churchill Livingstone; 2004:105–117.

Rosenbleuth A, Buylla A, Ramos G. The responses of axons to mechanical stimuli. *Acta Physiol Latinoamericana* 1953;3:204–215.

Rydevik B, Lundborg G, Bagge U. Effects of graded compression on intra-neural blood blow: an in vivo study on rabbit tibial nerve. *J Hand Surgery (Am)* 1981;6:3–12.

Selvaratnam P, Glasgow E, Matyas T. Strain effects on the nerve roots of brachial plexus. *J Anatomy* 1988;161:260–264.

Shacklock M. *The Plantar-Flexion Inversion Straight Leg Raise* [MS thesis]. Adelaide: University of South Australia; 1989.

Shacklock M. Neurodynamics. *Physiotherapy* 1995a;81:9–16.

Shacklock M. Clinical application of neurodynamics. In: Shacklock MO, ed. *Moving In on Pain*. Australia: Butterworth-Heinemann; 1995b:123–131.

Shacklock M. *Clinical Neurodynamics: A New System of Neuro-musculoskeletal Treatment*. Sydney: Butterworth-Heinemann; 2005.

Shacklock M, ed. *Biomechanics of the Nervous System: Breig Revisited*. Adelaide: Neurodynamic Solutions; 2008.

Topp K, Boyd B. Structure and biomechanics of peripheral nerves: nerve responses to physical stresses and implications for physical therapist practice. *Phys Ther* 2006;86:92–109.

Tsai Y. *Tension Change in the Ulnar Nerve by Different Order of Upper Limb Tension Test* [MS thesis]. Chicago: Northwestern University; 1995.

Van der Heide B, Allison GT, Zusman M. Pain and muscular responses to a neural tissue provocation test in the upper limb. *Man Ther* 2001;6:154–162.

Von Piekartz HJM, Schouten S, Aufdemkampe G. Neurodynamic responses in children with migraine or cervicogenic headache versus a control group: a comparative study. *Man Ther* 2007;12:153–160.

Wall EJ, Massie JB, Kwan MK, et al. Experimental stretch neuropathy: changes in nerve conduction under tension. *J Bone Joint Surgery (Br)* 1992;74:126–129.

Wilgis EF, Murphy R. The significance of longitudinal excursion in peripheral nerves. *Hand Clinics* 1986;2:761–766.

Woodhall B, Hayes B. The well leg raising test of Fajerztajn in the diagnosis of ruptured inter-vertebral disc. *J Bone Joint Surgery* 1950;32:786–792.

Wright TW, Glowczewskie F Jr, Cowin D, Wheeler DL. Ulnar nerve excursion and strain at the elbow and wrist associated with upper extremity motion. *J Hand Surgery (Am)* 2001;26:655–662.

Yaxley GA, Jull GA. A modified upper limb tension test: an investigation of responses in normal subjects. *Aust J Physiother* 1991;37:143–152.

Zito G, Jull G, Story I. Clinical tests of musculoskeletal dysfunction in the diagnosis of cervicogenic headache. *Man Ther* 2006;11:118–129.

Zochodne DW, Ho LT. Stimulation-induced peripheral nerve hyperemia: mediation by fibers innervating vasa nervorum? *Brain Res* 1991;546:113–118.

Zoech G, Reihsner R, Beer R, et al. Stress and strain in the peripheral nerves. *Neuro-Orthopedics* 1991;10:73.

Zorn P, Shacklock M, Trott P, Hall R. The effect of sequencing the movements of the upper limb tension test on the area of symptom production. In: *Proceedings of the 9th Biennial Conference of the Manipulative Physiotherapists' Association of Australia*. Gold Coast: Manipulative Physiotherapists' Association of Australia; 1995:166–167.

Needling of Head, Neck, and Shoulder Muscle Trigger Points Relevant to Headache

Jan Dommerholt, PT, MPS, and Robert D. Gerwin, MD

Muscle trigger points (TrPs) can be treated manually by needling the TrP without injection of substances (dry needling) or by trigger point injection (TrPI) of substances, most often local anesthetics. The clinician who performs either dry needling or TrPI must be familiar with the functional anatomy of the muscle (the origin and insertion and function of the muscle) and of the surrounding structures to avoid needling the wrong structures, causing unwanted complications. This chapter provides basic guidance to needling or injection of muscle TrPs. The reader must not be misled into thinking that this presentation will qualify clinicians to perform TrP needling or injection. Skill in needling or injecting TrPs can only come from hands-on experience, usually gained in courses or from mentors.

The best results in needling or injecting TrPs come from placing the needle in the most responsive part of the TrP. That point usually corresponds with the region of greatest hardness and greatest tenderness, two characteristics most often found at the same region in a taut band of the muscle. Finding the region of the muscle taut band that is most hard requires training and practice in order to develop the sensitivity to appreciate subtle changes in tissue compliance. The trigger zone is easy to find in some muscles but more difficult in others. Identification of TrPs by palpation is not a difficult skill to learn, but is nevertheless a learned skill (see Chapter 16).

Needling or injecting muscle requires an awareness of the structures in the vicinity of the trigger zone. Vessels can be punctured, nerves can be injured, and organs can be penetrated. These kinds of complications can be avoided by knowing the local anatomy and by being careful to identify the landmarks relevant to the muscle that is to be injected. Needling or injecting muscles also requires a well-developed kinesthetic awareness. At all times, the clinician must be able to visualize the pathway the needle takes within the body. Finally, postneedling or postinjection care will prevent or minimize local bleeding, help restore and maintain range of motion, and facilitate a return to normal function. Hemostasis must be accomplished. In general, the use of Coumadin (warfarin) is a contraindication to needling, except for the very experienced clinician. The use of platelet inhibitors is generally not a contraindication to needling, but requires care to achieve hemostasis.

APPROACH TO NEEDLING TRIGGER POINTS IN ALL MUSCLES

The following general steps apply to needling or injecting a trigger point in a muscle:

1. Palpate the muscle(s) to identify the TrP(s) responsible for a given referred pain pattern.
2. Palpate along the trigger point taut band to identify the region of greatest hardness (greatest resistance) and tenderness.
3. Identify the landmarks associated with the muscle to be treated (e.g., the borders of the muscle or of underlying bone, such as the infraspinatus muscle and the borders of the scapulae).
4. Prepare to use the needle for dry needling, or the solution for injection.
5. Recheck the landmarks, making certain to identify or note the structures that are to be avoided when placing the needle.
6. Disinfect the skin at the needle site with an alcohol wipe or spray.
7. Determine the angle of needle entry into the skin and muscle before penetrating the skin.
8. Injection of an anesthetic such as lidocaine 0.25% can be done using a hypodermic needle (30 gauge for facial muscles, 25 gauge for neck and shoulder muscles) with the same technique for muscle entry as with a solid filament needle.

9. The needle is moved in and out (or up and down) and is directed through a circumference of muscle by drawing the needle back to the skin and reinserting it into the muscle until there are no more twitch responses at that location.
10. In all muscles, the needle is directed to various parts of the muscle within reach of the needle by withdrawing the needle from the muscle and its fascia, but staying under the skin. The needle direction can be changed, and the needle reinserted into the muscle. If the needle remains within the muscle (i.e., not withdrawn sufficiently), it will follow the same original path through even if the direction of the needle above the skin is changed. In that case, the needle will curve as it is inserted back into the muscle.
11. Postneedling muscle stretching is always done in a direction opposite the action of the muscle. Stretching is done to restore normal muscle length. Overstretching is not necessary. Stretching may not be indicated in patients who are systemically hypermobile.
12. The patient should always be lying down when being needled, because of the possibility of vasodepressive syncope.
13. If the clinician is not absolutely certain where the needle is going, needling should not be done. When in doubt, stay out!

HEAD MUSCLES

Corrugator Muscle

- *Anatomy:* The corrugator muscle is located in the medial aspect of the eyebrow, lying deep to the orbicularis oris and the frontalis muscles. At the medial insertion it may arch downward over the eyebrow.
- *Function:* The corrugator muscle draws the eyebrow medially, furrowing the forehead.
- *Innervation:* Facial nerve (temporal branches).
- *Needling technique:* The patient is supine, and the clinician is seated at the head of the table. The muscle is palpated with the free hand. The approach is either from the medial or the lateral aspect of the muscle, directed toward its midportion. The needle is inserted through the skin at a shallow angle, and advanced into the

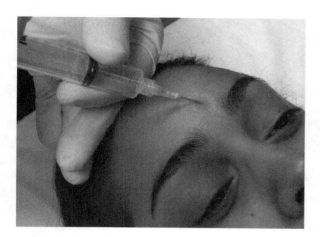

Figure 31.1 Needling of the Corrugator Muscle

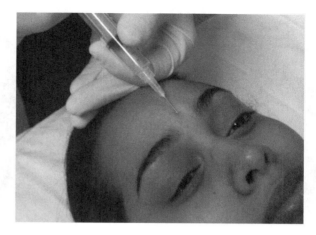

Figure 31.2 Needling of the Procerus Muscle

muscle. The entire muscle may be approached with one penetration (**Figure 31.1**).
- *Precautions:* None.

Procerus Muscle

- *Anatomy:* The procerus muscle covers the bridge of the nose, with fibers arising from the nasal fascia.
- *Function:* Wrinkles the skin of the bridge of the nose.
- *Innervation:* Facial nerve (buccal branches).
- *Needling technique:* The patient is supine, and the therapist sits at the head of the table. The needle is directed from superior to inferior, coming from the forehead toward the nose. The needle is inserted through the skin at a shallow angle. The needle is directed to various parts of the muscle, keeping a shallow angle (**Figure 31.2**).
- *Precautions:* None.

Masseter Muscle

- *Anatomy:* Three layers arising from the zygomatic process. The superficial layer inserts into the angle and lateral surface of the mandible. The middle layer inserts into the mid-portion of the mandibular ramus. The deep layer inserts into the upper mandibular ramus and the coronoid process.
- *Function:* Closes the mouth by elevating the mandible.

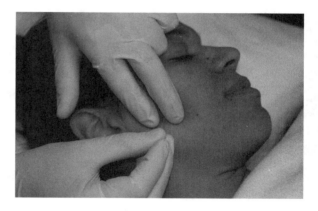

Figure 31.3 Dry Needling of the Masseter Muscle

- *Innervation:* Mandibular branch of trigeminal nerve.
- *Needling technique:* The patient is in supine or lateral decubitus position, whereas the clinician is seated at the head of the table. The needle is inserted perpendicularly to the skin, directly into the TrP taut band identified by palpation (**Figure 31.3**).
- *Precautions:* None.

Temporalis Muscle

- *Anatomy:* The muscle arises in the temporal fossa; the insertion is the mandibular coronoid process and the posterior mandibular ramus.
- *Function:* Closes the mouth by elevating the mandible.

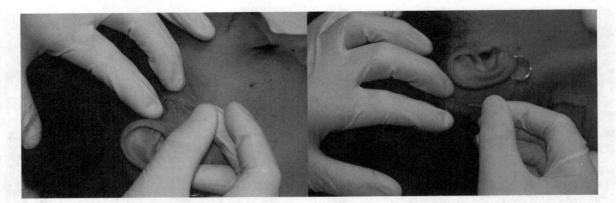

Figure 31.4 Dry Needling of the Temporalis Muscle

- *Innervation:* Trigeminal nerve, mandibular branch.
- *Needling technique:* The patient is supine or in lateral decubitus position, and the therapist sits at the head of the table or at the side. TrP taut bands are identified by palpation and fixed in place by the index and long fingers of the nonneedling hand. The needle is inserted perpendicularly to the skin directly into the taut band (**Figure 31.4**).
- *Precautions:* Identify the superficial temporal artery to avoid penetrating it with the needle.

Zygomatic Muscle

- *Anatomy:* The zygomatic major and minor muscles arise from the zygomatic bone and insert into the muscles of the mouth (the orbicularis oris, levator, and depressor anguli oris).
- *Function:* Elevates the angle of the mouth, as in smiling.
- *Innervation:* Facial nerve.
- *Needling technique:* The patient is supine and the clinician is standing or sitting at the patient's head. The muscle is identified by pincer or flat palpation. With the pincer palpation, one palpating digit is inside the cheek against the buccal mucosa and one digit is on the external surface of the skin. With the flat palpation, the taut band is held in between the fingers. The muscle may be thin and difficult to feel. The needle is inserted at the most tender spot and angled toward the zygomatic bone. The needle is moved in and out of the muscle, keeping the palpating fingers in place while needling the TrP (**Figure 31.5**).
- *Precautions:* None.

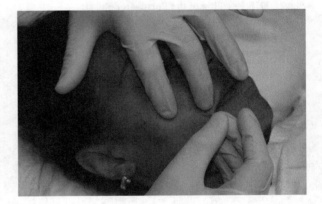

Figure 31.5 Dry Needling of the Zygomatic Muscle

NECK MUSCLES

Splenius Capitis Muscle

- *Anatomy:* The muscle arises from the occipital ligamentum nuchae of the mastoid process, and inserts on the posterior spinous processes of C7 to T3/4.
- *Function:* Extension, lateral bending, and rotation of the neck.
- *Innervation:* Cervical spinal nerves.
- *Needling technique:* The patient is in lateral decubitus or prone position, whereas the clinician is standing or sitting at the patient's head. TrPs are identified manually. One finger is placed on the distal part of the taut band. The needle is inserted into the taut band in a rostral (superior) to caudal (inferior) direction (**Figure 31.6**).
- *Precautions:* Avoid needling in a rostral direction to be absolutely certain that the needle will not pass through the foramen magnum.

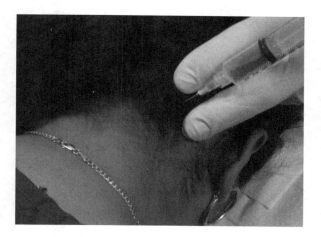

Figure 31.6 Needling of the Splenius Capitis Muscle

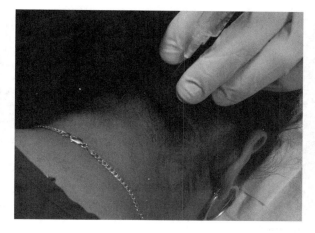

Figure 31.7 Needling of the Semispinalis Capitis Muscle

Semispinalis Capitis Muscle

- *Anatomy:* The muscle arises from the occipital ligamentum nuchae and inserts on the articular processes of C4 to C6 and the transverse processes of T1 to T6.
- *Function:* Extension, lateral bending, and rotation of the neck.
- *Innervation:* Cervical spinal nerves.
- *Needling technique:* The patient is in lateral decubitus or prone position, and the therapist is sitting or standing at the patient's head. If the patient is in lateral decubitus position, the clinician is positioned behind the patient. The needle is directed downward from the most rostral part of the TrP in upper neck TrPs. In more caudal TrPs, the needle can be directed more perpendicularly into the muscle (**Figure 31.7**).
- *Precautions:* The downward or caudal direction of the needle ensures that the vertebral artery will not be penetrated and that the needle will not penetrate the cervical spine. The caudal direction of the needle also ensures that the foramen magnum will not be penetrated.

Splenius Cervicis Muscle

- *Anatomy:* The superior attachment is to the anterior aspect of the transverse processes of C1 to C3. The inferior or caudal attachment is to the posterior spinous processes of T2 to T6.
- *Function:* Extension of the neck and rotation of the head.

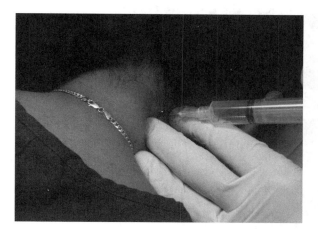

Figure 31.8 Needling of the Splenius Cervicis Muscle

- *Innervation:* Cervical spinal nerves.
- *Needling technique:* The patient is in prone or lateral decubitus position, whereas the therapist is standing or sitting at the patient's head. If the patient is in the lateral decubitus position, the clinician is positioned behind the patient. The TrP is fixed between two fingers. The needle is inserted perpendicularly to the skin over the muscle into the taut band at the area of maximum tenderness. The needle may be directed medially because the muscle is situated laterally away from the cervical spine foramina. The insertion may be through the upper fibers of the trapezius muscle (**Figure 31.8**).
- *Precautions:* None.

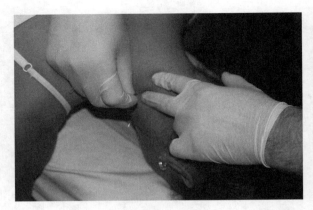

Figure 31.9 Dry Needling of the Semispinalis Cervicis Muscle

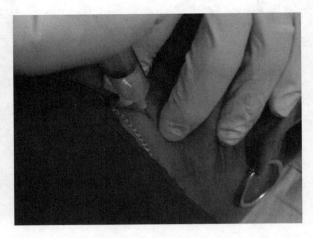

Figure 31.10 Needling of the Multifidi Muscles

Semispinalis Cervicis Muscle

- *Anatomy:* The rostral (superior) attachment is to the posterior spinous processes of C2 to C5. The inferior attachment is to the transverse processes of T1 to T5/6.
- *Function:* Neck extension and contralateral cervical rotation.
- *Innervation:* Cervical nerves.
- *Needling technique:* The patient is in prone or lateral decubitus position. The therapist is standing or sitting at the patient's head. If the patient is in lateral decubitus position, the clinician is positioned behind the patient. The taut band of the TrP is fixed by the index and long fingers of the nonneedling hand. The needle is inserted perpendicularly to the skin at the most tender part of the taut band. The needle may be directed parallel to the posterior processes or slightly laterally (**Figure 31.9**).
- *Precautions:* The vertical or slightly lateral direction of the needle minimizes the danger of inserting the needle through the spine into the epidural space, the subarachnoid space, or the spinal cord.

Multifidi Muscles

- *Anatomy:* The rostral (superior) attachment is the posterior processes of C2 to C5. The caudal (inferior) attachment is the articular processes of C2 to C7. The muscle crosses two to four vertebral levels.

- *Function:* Stabilization of the cervical spine. They may assist in extension and rotation of the spine.
- *Innervation:* Cervical nerves.
- *Needling technique:* The patient is in prone or lateral decubitus position, and the clinician is sitting or standing by the head of the patient. If the patient is in the lateral decubitus position, the clinician is behind the patient. TrPs are not palpable directly. The level to be treated is identified by determining the level of neurotrophic changes in the skin (changes in skin moisture, edema, or segmental sensitivity to noxious stimuli, such as pinpoint drag across the skin). The level can also be determined by identifying the innervation of neck and shoulder muscles affected by muscle TrPs. For example, the multifidi at C5 are treated if the C5 innervated infraspinatus muscle has active TrPs. Once the level is identified, the needle is inserted perpendicular to the skin and parallel to the posterior spinous processes, about 1 cm lateral to the spinous process. The level above and the level below can be reached from one needle insertion (**Figure 31.10**).
- *Precautions:* Avoid directing the needle medially to minimize the risk of penetrating the structures within the spinal canal (epidural or subarachnoid space, spinal cord).

Suboccipital Muscles

- *Anatomy:* The rectus capitis posterior major muscle and oblique capitis inferior attach

medially to the posterior spinous process of the
axis (C2). The rectus capitis posterior minor
muscle attaches medially to the posterior
spinous process of the atlas (C1). The oblique
capitis superior attaches inferiorly and laterally
to the transverse process of the atlas. The rectus
capitis posterior major and minor and the
oblique capitis superior muscles all attach to
the occiput. The oblique capitis inferior muscle is
the only one that does not attach to the skull. It
attaches to the transverse process of the atlas
(C1).

- *Function:* The rectus capitis posterior major and
  minor and the oblique capitis superior muscles
  extend the neck. The oblique capitis superior
  assists in ipsilateral side bending. These three
  muscles are more postural control muscles than
  primary movers of the head. The oblique capitis
  inferior is a powerful ipsilateral rotator of the
  head.

- *Innervation:* C1 nerve.

- *Needling technique:* Only the oblique capitis
  inferior muscle is easily and safely needled
  because of the proximity of the vertebral artery
  above the arch of the atlas. The patient is in
  prone or lateral decubitus position, whereas the
  clinician is sitting or standing at the patient's
  head. The clinician is behind the patient when
  the patient lies in lateral decubitus position. The
  muscle is located by placing one finger on the
  transverse process of C1 and the other finger on
  the posterior process of C2. The point to be
  needled is midway between these two markers.
  The needle is inserted perpendicular to the skin
  directly into the muscle. A small radius of muscle
  can be needled from one skin penetration
  (**Figure 31.11**).

- *Precautions:* Avoid directing the needle upward
  or needling too laterally in order to prevent
  inadvertent penetration of the vertebral artery.

Sternocleidomastoid Muscle

- *Anatomy:* The two heads of the
  sternocleidomastoid muscle attach superiorly to
  the mastoid process by a single tendon. The
  sternal or medial head attaches inferiorly to the
  manubrium. The clavicular or lateral head
  attaches inferiorly to the medial third of the
  clavicle.

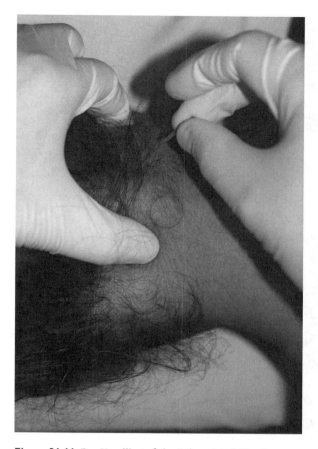

Figure 31.11 Dry Needling of the Suboccipital Muscles

- *Function:* Acting together, the two
  sternocleidomastoid muscles flex the neck
  against resistance or against gravity. Acting
  unilaterally, the muscle side-bends the head to
  the same side, and rotates the head to the
  opposite side. It also tilts the chin upward and to
  the opposite side.

- *Innervation:* The muscle is innervated by the
  accessory nerve (XI pars) and by the C2 and C3
  spinal nerves.

- *Needling technique:* The patient is in supine or
  lateral decubitus position, and the therapist is
  sitting or standing at the head of the patient.
  When the patient is in the lateral decubitus
  position, the muscle is easily reached by coming
  over the top of the patient's head. The muscle is
  grasped by pincer palpation after identifying the
  carotid artery. The two heads, clavicular and
  sternal, must both be grasped within the fingers.
  The needle is inserted either perpendicular to the

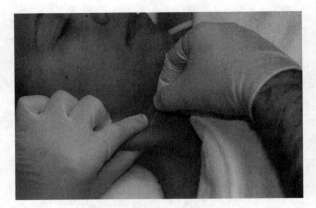

Figure 31.12 Dry Needling of the Sternocleidomastoid Muscle

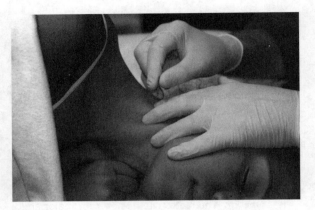

Figure 31.13 Dry Needling of the Levator Scapulae Muscle (Superior Portion)

skin in a posterior direction or in a posterior-lateral direction. The needle should penetrate both heads of the muscle. Two insertions of the needle may be needed to clear the TrPs (**Figure 31.12**).

- *Precautions:* The carotid artery lies medial to the sternocleidomastoid muscle, next to the trachea. Lift the sternocleidomastoid away from the carotid artery and only needle between the fingers holding the muscle in a pincer grasp, directing the needle as described above, to avoid needling the carotid artery.

Levator Scapulae Muscle: Superior Portion

- *Anatomy:* The cervical portion of the levator scapulae muscle is palpated on its lateral border that is identified as the first muscle belly ventral to the upper part of the trapezius muscle. It is generally felt as a ropy muscle of about 5 mm diameter in lateral extent, between the anterior (ventral) border of the upper trapezius and the transverse process of C1. The inferior attachment is to the lateral border of the scapula between the scapular spine and the superior medial border of the scapula.
- *Function:* The levator scapulae muscle extends and side-bends the neck. When the head is turned to the opposite side and forward flexed, the levator scapulae rotates the head toward the midline. The muscle rotates the scapula glenoid fossa downward when the neck is fixed. Acting with the trapezius, the two muscles elevate the shoulder.

- *Innervation:* Cervical spinal nerves 3 and 4, and C5 through the dorsal scapular nerve.
- *Needling technique:* The patient is in lateral decubitus position, whereas the clinician is sitting or standing behind the patient. The muscle is identified and fixed along its length between the index and long fingers. The needle is inserted perpendicular to the skin at the most tender point (**Figure 31.13**).
- *Precautions:* Do not needle the lowest 2 centimeters of the muscle above the anterior border of the upper trapezius because of the danger of penetrating a high-positioned apex of the lung.

Scalene Muscles

- *Anatomy:* The anterior scalene lies deeply beneath the sternocleidomastoid muscle, originating on the anterior aspect of the transverse processes of C3 to C6. It inserts on the first rib anterior to the neurovascular bundle. The medium scalene arises from the transverse processes of C3 to C7. It attaches inferiorly to the first rib posterior to the neurovascular bundle.
- *Function:* Side bending to the same side. The anterior scalene also assists in rotating the head to the opposite side. Both anterior and medial scalene muscles are accessory respiratory muscles through elevation of the first rib.
- *Innervation:* The anterior scalene is innervated by spinal nerves C4 to C6. The medium scalene is innervated by C3 to C8.

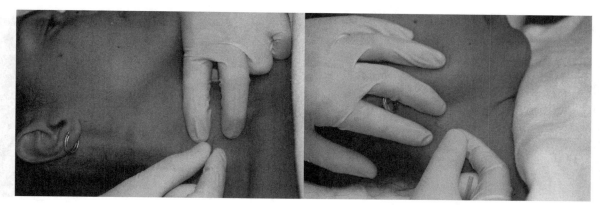

Figure 31.14 Dry Needling of the Scalene Muscles

- *Needling technique:* The patient is in supine or lateral decubitus position, and the therapist is sitting or standing behind the patient. The muscles can be identified by having the patient sniff sharply (activation of the respiratory component of the muscle function). The anterior scalene is reached in the triangle formed by the jugular vein laterally, the lateral edge of the clavicular head of the sternocleidomastoid muscle, and the clavicle as the base (**Figure 31.14**).
- *Precautions:* The medial head of the scalene muscle must not be needled at the base of the neck. Needle it only one fingerbreadth or more above the base of the neck to avoid a high-positioned apex of the lung.

SHOULDER MUSCLES

Trapezius Muscle: Upper Portion

- *Anatomy:* The superior attachment is to the medial third of the occipital nuchal ridge. The midfibers attach to C7 posterior spinous processes. The horizontal fibers attach to the lateral third of the clavicle, to the acromion process, and to the scapular spine.
- *Function:* Unilaterally—ipsilateral side bending of the head, contralateral rotation of the head, and elevation of the shoulder; bilaterally—extension of the neck.
- *Innervation:* Accessory nerve (C11) and cervical spinal nerves C3 and C4.
- *Needling technique:* The patient is in lateral decubitus position, whereas the clinician is

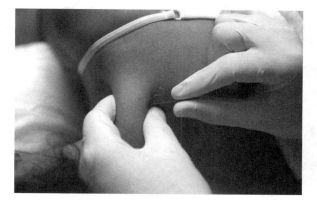

Figure 31.15 Dry Needling of the Trapezius Muscle (Upper Portion)

sitting or standing behind the patient. The TrP taut bands are identified and fixed either with flat palpation (as in the neck) or by pincer palpation at the shoulder. The needle is inserted perpendicular to the skin, and the needle is advanced into the muscle. The needle is kept between the fingers in the shoulder. The needle can be inserted downward from the top of the muscle, always staying between the fingers, or it can be inserted from anterior to posterior or posterior to anterior, always needling toward the opposing finger. Several passes may be required to clear the upper trapezius of TrPs (**Figure 31.15**).

- *Precautions:* The most common serious adverse event arising from needling the upper trapezius is penetrating the lung and producing a pneumothorax. The danger of this occurring can be minimized by needling strictly between the fingers holding the muscle in a pincer grasp, or needling to the opposing finger.

Levator Scapulae: Inferior Portion

- See the section "Levator Scapulae: Superior Portion" for anatomy, function, and innervation.
- *Needling technique:* The patient is in lateral decubitus position and the therapist is sitting or standing behind the patient. The insertion of muscle on the scapula is located at the medial border of the scapula between the scapular spine and the upper medial border of the scapula. The needle is inserted through the skin at a shallow angle, directed toward the upper, medial border of the scapula. Movement of the needle is directed toward the scapula (**Figure 31.16**).
- *Precautions:* The danger with needling the levator scapula in the thorax is penetration of the lung

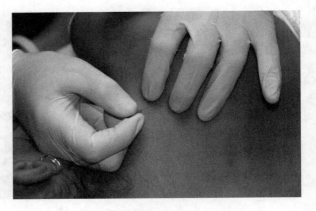

Figure 31.16 Dry Needling of the Levator Scapulae (Inferior Portion)

with consequent pneumothorax. This danger is minimized by keeping the angle of the needle shallow and directing the needle toward the medial border of the scapula.

Botulinum Toxin A in the Treatment of Headaches

Robert D. Gerwin, MD

Headache management remains difficult, despite significant gains made in the treatment of headache in recent years. Headache is treated as an acute illness with medications that abort headache, such as nonprescription analgesics or triptans, and as a chronic condition with prophylactic medications, such as the anticonvulsant topiramate or the calcium channel blocker verapamil. Triptans have been highly successful in the acute treatment of migraine, although the acute treatment of tension-type headache is more problematic. Although the anticonvulsant drugs, calcium channel blockers, and dual reuptake antidepressant drugs (SNRIs) are effective in the prevention of migraine headaches, the plethora of manual and alternative medicine treatments testifies to the inadequacy of any one treatment to effectively prevent headache, particularly chronic daily headache, whether transformed migraine or tension type.

Binder, an otolaryngologist, treated patients with botulinum toxin A (BTxA) for cosmetic purposes. He found that the migraineurs among his patients had fewer headaches. A retrospective assessment of headache response following treatment with BTxA for other purposes was then published with Brin, Blitzer, and Schoenrock (Binder et al., 2000). Among the patients treated were 77 who fulfilled the International Headache Society (IHS) criteria for migraine. Of these, 51% reported complete alleviation of migraine headaches for an average of a little over 4 months. A partial response was reported by 38% of patients. Some patients with acute migraine reported improvement within 2 hours of injection, an observation that continues to be made in patients treated with botulinum toxin (BTx) for migraine. Their report triggered a series of studies of the effect of botulinum toxin injections in a variety of headaches: migraine headache (MH), chronic tension-type headache (CTTH), and episodic tension-type headache (ETTH). Initially, many of these were open-label or retrospective studies that were promising, but lacked the credibility of randomized, controlled studies.

431

Botulinum toxin has been used in the treatment of headache syndromes since the report by Binder et al. (2000). Its use remains controversial, however. The majority (but not all) of randomized, controlled, double-blinded studies to date have failed to show a consistent benefit of BTx over placebo. However, improvement with BTx has been shown in some subpopulations and in some secondary outcome measures, so that the studies have not been uniformly negative. Published studies used different injection site and dosing protocols, so there has been no uniform approach to the question. The placebo response in many of the studies has been robust and has confounded their interpretation. The end result has been that there is no clear-cut body of evidence that supports the use of BTx in the management of headaches, particularly in migraine. Nevertheless, a general consensus has developed among clinicians that BTx is effective, resulting in the widespread use of BTx in headache management. A backlash among some headache specialists has occurred in response to the present use of BTx, strongly stating that it should not be used until it can be proven to be effective in the treatment of various headache types by randomized, controlled studies.

In addition to questioning the role of BTx in headache management, the controversy has reactivated an old question about the role of muscle trigger points (TrPs) in headache, including MH without aura, that is commonly associated with CTTH or chronic daily headache. Tfelt-Hansen et al. (1981) used the term *myogenic headache* to indicate the contribution of muscle TrPs to headache. Disagreement still occurs about whether muscle TrPs initiate headache or result from headache-induced central sensitization, as illustrated by a recent exchange of letters to the editor between Gerwin and Dodick (2006). Gerwin proposed that muscle TrPs could initiate the trigeminovascular cascade that results in migraine, or cause the pain of tension-type headache through referred pain mechanisms, whereas Dodick opined that myofascial TrPs resulted from the central sensitization caused by the headache itself.

The general acceptance of the use of BTx in headache management in the face of inconsistent medical evidence in the studies to date has also led to a suggestion that there are two kinds of migraine. One kind of migraine is associated with extracranial innervation that leads to an "imploding," crushing headache that responds to BTx treatment, and the other kind of migraine is associated with a buildup of pressure inside the head ("exploding" headache), not responsive to

BTx, mediated by intracranial innervation (Jakubowski et al., 2006). In an exchange of letters to the editor (Fernández-de-las-Peñas et al., 2007), it was argued that botulinum toxin–responsive headaches were possibly related to the presence of myofascial TrPs in head, neck, and shoulder muscles, a view that was refuted by the authors of the original paper, who noted that muscle tenderness was not prominent in their patients before the migraine attack, and no different between imploding and exploding headaches. Moreover, argued the authors, cutaneous sensitivity, a manifestation of allodynia seen in acute migraine, was not prevented by BTx, even in the responders. Thus, the question of the role of BTx in headache management is very much alive today and relates not only to efficacy of treatment but also to issues of the pathogenesis of headache.

Finally, the response of those patients whose migraine or tension-type headache improves after treatment with BTx is often very fast, as mentioned earlier, sometimes within hours, often within 1 to 2 days, far faster than would be expected if the effect were only mediated through the known action of BTx at the neuromuscular junction, where BTx prevents the release of acetylcholine from the presynaptic nerve terminal. Studies have now shown that BTx has an antinociceptive effect, as well as a paralytic effect, at the neuromuscular junction.

MECHANISM OF ACTION OF BOTULINUM TOXIN
Effects at the Neuromuscular Junction

Botulinum toxin acts to inhibit muscle contraction by preventing the vesicles in the presynaptic nerve terminal from docking or attaching to the cell membrane, thereby preventing the release of acetylcholine (ACh), the neurotransmitter that initiates depolarization of the muscle fiber membrane at the motor endplate. This subject has been well reviewed by Royal (2001). Each myelinated motor axon terminates in unmyelinated branches at the muscle fiber. The unmyelinated nerve terminals each contain about 300 active sites opposite a motor endplate. Acetylcholine is stored in vesicles in the motor nerve terminal. There are about 500,000 such vesicles per neuromuscular junction. These vesicles store more than ACh. They also store glutamate (an excitatory amino acid), nitric acid, calcitonin gene-related peptide (CGRP, a neurotransmitter), and substance P. These substances, capable of modulating activity at the neuromuscular junction, are co-released with ACh. Acetylcholine is released both in response to evoked stimulation of the nerve by efferent nerve impulses and spontaneously without axonal nerve activation (Bukharaeva et al., 2002; Augustine, 2001; Samigullin et al., 2005; Wessler, 1996). Exocytosis in response to evoked stimulation is dependent on calcium influx, which in turn is modulated by a large number of factors, including facilitory and inhibitory adenosine receptor activation, α- and β-adrenergic receptor activation, CGRP-induced increase in ACh release, muscle fiber length, frequency of endplate potential discharge, and feedback from muscle fiber cytosolic calcium concen-

tration (Gerwin, 2008). Whether ACh release is evoked or spontaneous, nerve terminal vesicles must first dock at the nerve terminal cell membrane before their contents are released by exocytosis through a fusion pore in the synaptic space. Botulinum toxin acts by blocking the docking of ACh-containing vesicles to the nerve terminal cell membrane.

Botulinum toxin undergoes four steps in its process of blocking ACh release (**Figure 32.1**). It first binds to the cell membrane surface of the nerve terminal; it does this through the heavy chain portion of the molecule. It is then incorporated or internalized intracellularly in the nerve terminal. Step 3 is the cleavage of the heavy chain

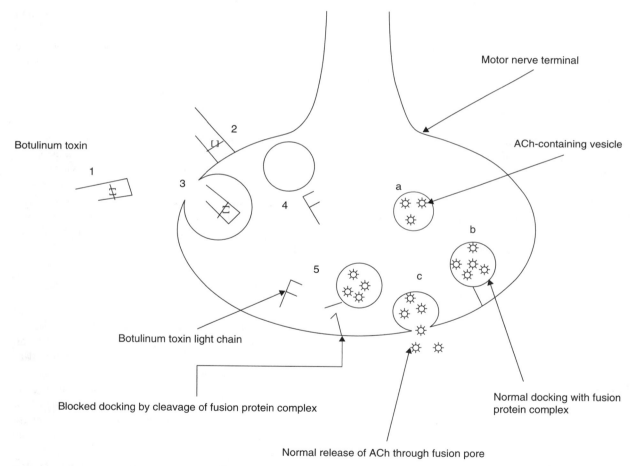

Figure 32.1 **The Mechanism of Action of Botulinum Toxin in the Prevention of the Release of Acetylcholine (ACh) from the Motor Nerve Terminal.** Step 1: Botulinum toxin is in the interstitial fluid as a heavy and a light chain bound by a disulfide bond. Step 2: Botulinum toxin binds to the motor nerve terminal by the heavy chain. Step 3: Botulinum toxin is incorporated into the motor nerve terminal in acidic vesicles. Step 4: The light chain is cleaved from the heavy chain. Step 5: The action of the botulinum toxin light chain cleaves the fusion protein complex, thereby preventing the docking of the ACh-containing vesicle and the release of ACh. a, An ACh-containing vesicle; b, the vesicle docking in a normal manner to the cell membrane via a fusion protein complex; c, the normal release of ACh through the fusion pore.

from the light chain. Botulinum toxin is composed of a heavy and a light chain connected by a disulfide bond that is cleaved when the toxin is internalized in the cell. Step 4 is the cleavage of either synaptosomal-associated protein, a 25-kDa protein (SNAP25), or synaptobrevin (also known as vesicle-associated membrane protein, or VAMP) by the light chain, thereby preventing the binding of ACh-containing vesicles to the cell membrane. The entire process, from binding to cleavage of the docking proteins, can take from 3 to 5 days.

There are seven serotypes of BTx, two of which have found clinical applications. These two are types A and B. Type A is marketed in the United States as Botox and in Europe as Dysport. Dysport may soon be marketed in the United States as well. Botulinum toxin type B is marketed in the United States as Myobloc. The different serotypes have different sites of action. All serotypes of BTx act by interfering with the protein binding of the ACh-containing vesicle to the cell membrane. They do this by cleaving one or another of the docking-complex proteins. Botulinum toxin type A cleave SNAP25 between glycine and arginine. Botulinum toxin type B cleaves synatobrevin between glycine and phenylalanine. When either docking protein is cleaved, the vesicle cannot bind to the cell membrane and exocytosis cannot occur.

The serotypes are not interchangeable on a dose-to-dose basis. Botulinum toxin type A is the most potent serotype. Potency is measured in mouse units. One mouse unit corresponds to the median lethal dose for a reference mouse. The usual doses for Botox are in the range of 1 to 400 units, whereas the usual doses for Myobloc are in the range of 500 to 20,000 units total. Botulinum toxin A and BTxB also differ in the postinjection pain induced by injection. A double-blind, controlled comparison of pain induced by the different types of BTx given intradermally showed that BTxB caused significantly more pain than either a commercial preparation of BTxA or saline (Kranz et al., 2006). Finally, the two commercially available preparations of BTxA are not interchangeable. The dose efficacy to safety ratio for Botox is calculated as 8.6, whereas that for Dysport is 3.3 (Royal, 2001). One has to become familiar with the dosing for particular conditions and for individual muscles for each available preparation of BTx. Thus, higher doses per muscle are used in treating spasticity and dystonia, where weakening muscle is a predominant consideration. Lower doses per muscle are used when the intention is to treat pain while preserving function.

Botulinum toxin has few significant side effects, and they are mostly transient, limited to the duration of action of BTx and to the recovery of muscle. The most serious one is muscle atrophy and weakness, a direct consequence of its action at the neuromuscular junction. This is of considerable importance when BTx is injected in the anterior cervical muscles, because there can be weakness of the pharyngeal muscles that interferes with swallowing. This adverse reaction can be minimized or avoided by reducing the dosage administered to such muscles as the sternocleidomastoid, and by injecting only one side of the anterior cervical muscles. Another adverse consequence of anterior cervical muscle injections is dry mouth, the result of interference with the cholinergic nerve-mediated action of the salivary glands. Muscle atrophy occurs with continued use of BTx.

Recovery of neuromuscular junction function is a two-step process. Botulinum toxin causes the motor nerve terminal to be nonfunctional. New nerve terminals sprout from the original terminal nerve axon to form new neuromuscular junctions in the neighborhood of the original neuromuscular junction. The motor endplate zone under the original nerve terminal elongates, and acetylcholine receptors are upregulated to extend to the endplate zone under the newly created terminal nerve sprouts (dePaiva et al., 1999). This usually begins within 45 to 60 days of injection, and varies with the species injected. As the original motor nerve terminal recovers in the course of 1 year, the secondary sprouts retract and disappear.

Effect of Botulinum Toxin on Nociception

When dystonia is treated with BTx, dystonia-associated pain is reported to be reduced or eliminated well before the effect of BTx on the neuromuscular junction can occur. This effect has also been noted in patients with acute migraine headache who are treated for headache prophylaxis, who report that their headache is gone within hours to 1 or 2 days. The mechanism of action of BTx in these situations cannot be explained by its effect at the neuromuscular junction. Instead, there must be another action that affects nociception. Therefore, the effect of botulinum toxin on peripheral and central aspects of nociception has been investigated.

The effect of BTxA on cutaneous nociception in humans was studied in a randomized, controlled trial (RCT) of thermal pain thresholds (Blersch et al., 2002). Heat and cold pain thresholds and electrically induced pain thresholds did not increase significantly from baseline in the BTxA-treated forearms compared with placebo. The study failed to show a direct peripheral antinociceptive effect on BTxA in humans. However, in another RCT of BTx effect on neuropeptide release from peripheral nociceptive fibers, the sweating response was inhibited as early as day 2 (P <0.001). Electrically induced flare was likewise inhibited by BTxA (P <0.005). Electrically induced pain was reduced by 10% (P <0.001) (Krämer et al., 2003). Hyperalgesia to pinprick and allodynia after electrical stimulation were unchanged. Thus, peripheral neuropeptide release involved in sweat gland activation and in the flare response was inhibited by BTxA, but peripheral activation of nociceptors was little affected. Nociceptive sensitization that could be peripheral or central was not affected by BTxA.

Botulinum toxin failed to affect thermal pain threshold and neuroselective current sensory testing, and also failed to attenuate the effect of capsaicin (Voller et al., 2003). Thus, BTxA could not be demonstrated to affect peripheral and central pain processing or axon flare in this study. Sycha et al. (2006) found no effect of BTxA on pain or inflammation, or on primary or secondary hyperalgesia. Another study of human cutaneous pain and inflammation induced by capsaicin failed to show either a direct peripheral antinociceptive effect of BTxA (Dysport) or a significant effect on neurogenic inflammation (Schulte-Mattler et al., 2007). However, BTxA was found to reduce capsaicin-induced pain and neurogenic vasodilation without affecting thermal and thermal-pain modalities in a study of capsaicin-induced cutaneous pain in a double-blind human forearm model (Tugnoli et al., 2007). Reduction in capsaicin-induced pain occurred only when capsaicin was injected into the BTxA-pretreated area. Reduction in neurogenic vasodilation did not contribute to the analgesic effect of BTxA. Thus, although studies of the effect of BTx on pain perception and axon reflex have been mixed, there is evidence that neuropeptide release from peripheral sensory neurons is inhibited by BTx.

In support of the concept that BTxA affects sensory neuropeptide release, Aoki (2005) reported that BTxA inhibited the release of substance P in in vitro cell culture systems, inhibited the release of glutamate, and prevented the usual release of the immediate early gene c-fos following exposure of BTxA. These results suggested that BTxA blocks both peripheral and central sensitization. Aoki (2005) also showed that BTxA inhibited formalin-induced glutamate release and inhibited excitation of dorsal horn neurons in the rat hind paw model, demonstrating a direct inhibitory effect of BTxA on peripheral sensitization and an indirect effect on central sensitization. A study of carageenan- and capsaicin-evoked pain and carageenan-induced paw edema in rats showed that pretreatment with BTxA 6 days before injection with either carageenan or capsaicin reduced or abolished pain response, but not associated edema (Bach-Rojecky & Lacković, 2005). Pretreatment with BTxA 24 hours before injection of these irritants did not affect pain or inflammation. This study demonstrated that BTxA was effective in blocking the pain component of the inflammatory response in rats, and that the effect is time dependent, consistent with the hypothesized requirement that BTxA be incorporated into nerve endings before it can be effective.

Botulinum toxins type A and type B were injected subcutaneously in the hind paw and intraventricularly in the brain to evaluate peripheral and central antinociceptive effects of BTx (Luvisetto et al., 2006). Licking response and behavioral responses were recorded for 40 minutes after injection. Botulinum toxin A partially attenuated the licking response in the second phase of the formalin test, whether peripherally or centrally administered. It did not affect the first phase of the formalin test. Botulinum toxin B attenuated the licking response in the first phase, but not the second phase of the response. Intraventricular injection of BTxB had a hyperalgesic effect on the interphase of the formalin test. Botulinum toxin therefore has a central effect that selectively modulates inflammatory pain depending on serotype and on route of administration. Mechanical allodynia was strongly attenuated by BTxA, with a single injection of BTxA inducing antiallodynic effects for at least 3 weeks, in a mouse model of neuropathic pain using chronic sciatic nerve constriction (Luvisetto et al., 2007).

The interest in the antinociceptive effect of BTxA in migraine has prompted a great number of studies of the effect of BTxA on the release of neurotransmitters from trigeminal nerve afferents. The effect of BTx on the release of CGRP is of particular interest because CGRP can induce vasodilation and neurogenic edema, essential elements of the neurogenic inflammatory response that occurs in migraine. Cultures of rat trigeminal ganglia were exposed to a control solution or to capsaicin, or to an inflammatory cocktail of bradykinin, prostaglandin, serotonin, and histamine. Trigeminal ganglion cell cultures were pretreated before exposure to these substances with either control medium or with therapeutic concentrations of BTxA, and the amount of CGRP secreted by these cells into the culture media was determined. Pretreatment with BTxA of the cell cultures exposed to the inflammatory cocktail alone did not alter the amount of CGRP secreted by the trigeminal ganglia cells. However, when the trigeminal nerve ganglia were exposed to a depolarizing amount of potassium chloride (KCl), there was significant suppression of CGRP release in the cell cultures exposed to the inflammatory cocktail and BTxA. This was the first study that demonstrated that BTxA directly decreases the release of CGRP from trigeminal ganglia neurons (Durham et al., 2004).

CGRP was found in rat trigeminal neurons, as were the three exocytotic soluble N-ethylmaleimid-sensitive factor attachment protein receptors (SNAREs): SNAP25, synaptobrevin (SBr), and synaptotagmin (Meng et al., 2007). CGRP release is stimulated by cell membrane depolarization with KCl, less so by capsaicin, and still less by bradykinin. Using different serotypes of BTx, Meng et al. (2007) demonstrated that stimulated release of CGRP was inhibited by BTxA, with the greatest inhibition from the KCl-stimulated cells. Botulinum toxin B did not affect exocytosis in the rat model, unlike BTxA, but did in the mouse model. SBr isoforms I and II each form separate SNARE complexes that bind vesicles to the cell membrane. SBr I and SNAP25 were implicated in exocytosis of large dense-core vesicles, and SBr I in exocytosis of small synaptic vesicles. Thus, different isoforms of SNARE complex molecules have different roles in exocytosis, and there is a species-specific action of BTx serotypes on the release of CGRP.

Human studies of the modulation of trigeminal nerve sensitization by BTxA have used intramuscular injections of BTxA in pericranial, neck, and shoulder muscles prior to intradermal forehead injection of capsaicin (Gazerani et al., 2006). There was a significant reduction in pain, flare, and secondary hyperalgesia at 1, 4, and 8 weeks after BTxA injections. The pain intensity area was smaller in the BTxA group compared with saline ($P = 0.01$). The flare area was significantly reduced ($P < 0.001$). Likewise, the mean area of secondary hyperalgesia was significantly smaller ($P = 0.04$). Capsaicin-induced sensory and vasomotor reactions were remarkably suppressed as early as week 1. These effects are most likely caused by a local peripheral effect of BTxA on cutaneous nociceptors.

In summary, CGRP release from trigeminal nerve neurons appears to be central to the mechanism that may result in an activation of the trigeminovascular cascade. Botulinum toxin has been shown to suppress the release of CGRP from trigeminal neurons in vitro, and to suppress pain and hyperalgesia when injected intramuscularly in the forehead, a trigeminal nerve–innervated area. The rapid action of botulinum toxin reported to occur in migraine headache states may be related to inhibition of the release of CGRP. However, as will be seen in the following section, it is not so clear that botulinum toxin is effective in the treatment of migraine, as might be expected from these studies.

BOTULINUM TOXIN IN HEADACHE TREATMENT

Great interest in the use of botulinum toxin was generated by Binder's report (Binder et al., 2000). The potential use of a drug that was effective in the treatment of various types of headache and that showed little in the way of serious side effects was very attractive. Early reports suggested that BTxA met both of these criteria (Freund & Schwartz, 2000; Mathew, 2006; Freitag, 2007). However, early reviews of the effect of BTx on headache disorders could not find a sufficient number of studies that met current standards of evidence-based medicine to make a recommendation for the general use of BTx in the treatment of headache (Evers et al., 2002).

Preliminary studies of the use of botulinum toxin were open-label studies or retrospective case series. They often showed promise that BTx could be useful in the management of various headaches. For example, Blumenfeld (2003) retrospectively studied botulinum treatment in migraine ($n = 29$), ETTH ($n = 17$), mixed headache ($n = 71$), and chronic daily headache ($n = 154$). All headache patient results were considered together. Headache days dropped 56%, and headache intensity decreased significantly. He concluded that botulinum toxin may be an effective treatment. This and similar uncontrolled studies were encouraging and helped stimulate interest in conducting a number of randomized, placebo-controlled, double-blind studies of the use of BTx in specific headache types. Porta (2000) reported a single-blind, randomized comparative trial of BTxA with methylprednisone. Patients with either ETTH or CTTH were included in the study. Tender sites were injected either with 5 to 15 units of BTxA or 40 mg of methylprednisone. At 60 days post-treatment, but not at 30 days post-treatment, those subjects treated with BTxA had a significantly greater reduction in pain severity than those treated with methylprednisone. One can question the use of methylprednisone as a control, and the selection of tender points from a predetermined set of 13 sites, but nevertheless there was a beneficial effect of BTxA on headache.

Another small, prospective, open-label study of 19 Japanese subjects reported results on 14 patients who completed the 3-month study (Suzuki et al., 2007). Thirteen of the 14 reported subjective improvement. Overall headache frequency and analgesic consumption did not decline, but the frequency of severe headaches was reduced. However, randomized, controlled, double-blind studies must show clearly the benefit of BTx on various headache types before BTx will be accepted throughout the medical community as therapy for headache.

Chronic Daily Headache

Chronic daily headache in the studies reported here is defined as headache occurring for more than 15 days per month. The two subtypes, CTTH and chronic migraine, and the overlap syndrome in which patients suffer both types of headache (now commonly diagnosed as migraine), are considered together in the studies reported here. This distinction has not been made in many of the studies, even though the mechanism of headache may be different.

Ondo et al. (2004) conducted a randomized, double-blind, controlled study in which subjects were followed for 12 weeks, after which all subjects were offered BTxA in an open-label manner. High-dose, concentrated BTxA was used (200 units total, 100 units/mL). Injections were given in a follow-the-pain protocol that included, in some patients, the masseter muscles. The primary efficacy point of headache-free days on headache diaries has been faulted unless patients report in daily, because studies have shown that headache diaries are completed retrospectively. Nevertheless, headache-free days improved from weeks 8 to 12 compared with baseline ($P < 0.05$), but tended to improve strongly only over the entire period of weeks 0 to 12 ($P = 0.07$). The subject and the investigator "global" assessments both improved in the treated group. The group that received two BTxA injections had fewer headache days than the group that was injected only once in the second, open-label 12-week period ($P < 0.05$). Of interest, though not commented on by the authors, the original placebo group that was treated in the open-label BTxA injection second phase of the study did not have a significant increase in headache-free days during the second 12 weeks of the study. The findings were interpreted as

suggesting, but not confirming, the efficacy of BTxA in the treatment of chronic daily headache.

A large RCT that identified placebo responders and placebo nonresponders prior to randomization, conducted for 11 months, showed that the placebo nonresponders treated with BTxA had a greater reduction in headache-free days (almost 7 days less per 30 days at day 180) than those not treated with BTxA (a little over 5 days less), but the difference of 1.5 days between the groups was not statistically significant (Mathew et al., 2005). However, as a secondary outcome measure, a higher percentage of BTxA-treated subjects had a decrease of 50% or greater in headache frequency per 30-day period at day 180 (32.7% vs. 15.0%, $P = 0.027$). The mean change from baseline in headache frequency per 30-day period at day 180 was −6.1 for the BTxA patients versus 3.1 for the placebo patients ($P = 0.013$). Four of the 173 BTxA-treated subjects (2.3%) dropped out of the study because of adverse events. The authors concluded that BTxA showed significant reductions in headache frequency and that treatment was well tolerated.

A subgroup analysis of the above study patients (Mathew et al., 2005) looked at data obtained from those patients who were not receiving any concurrent prophylactic medications (Dodick et al., 2005). There were 228 patients who met this criteria of the 355 patients randomized in the study. Of these, 117 received BTxA and 111 received placebo. Mean frequency of headaches per 30-day period was −7.8 in the BTxA group compared with −4.5 days in the placebo group ($P = 0.032$). The difference continued through a third injection session ($P = 0.023$). In addition, BTxA treatment at least halved the headache frequency in over 50% of the BTxA-treated patients after three injection sessions compared to baseline. The authors concluded that in this subgroup of patients not taking other prophylactic medications, BTxA was effective and well tolerated in the prophylaxis of chronic daily headache.

A double-blind, placebo-controlled, RCT dose-response study was conducted to determine the safety and efficacy of three different doses of BTxA in the treatment of chronic daily headache (Silberstein et al., 2005). Placebo nonresponders were injected with either 75, 150, or 225 total units, and retreated at 90 and 180 days. They were followed for 240 days. The primary efficacy endpoint of mean change from baseline in headache frequency at day 180 was not met, because all groups improved, including the placebo group. However, decrease in headache frequency at day 240 was significantly greater for patients treated with 150 units and 225 units compared with placebo (-8.6, -8.4, and -6.4 respectively; $P = 0.03$ analysis of covariance). Only 3.8% of subjects withdrew from the study because of adverse events.

A large study of the use of BTxA in chronic daily headache reported the results of treating 1,347 patients with a fixed-site, fixed-dose protocol of 100 units (Farinelli et al., 2006). After 12 months of treatment, patients were free of attacks 23 days per month. Adverse effects were noted in only 1.6% of patients, and all were mild and transient.

Undifferentiated Tension-Type Headache

A small RCT of 21 subjects meeting the IHS criteria for tension-type headache treated with pericranial BTxA injection of 10 pericranial sites of 20 units each, evaluated at 4, 8, and 12 weeks, showed no significant difference in headache severity (rated using the Visual Analogue Scale), frequency, or duration (Rollnik et al., 2000).

Chronic Tension-Type Headache

The effectiveness of BTxA in CTTH was evaluated in an RCT in which 20 units of BTxA was injected into frontal and temporal muscles (Schmitt et al., 2001). Patients were followed for 4 weeks pretreatment and for 8 weeks post-treatment. Some improvement was noted in affective variables in the BTxA group, but there was no statistically significant difference between both treatment and placebo groups in the important outcome measures of pain intensity, the number of pain-free days, and the consumption of analgesics.

Another RCT came to the same conclusion, using a fixed-dose, fixed-site injection scheme (Schulte-Mattler et al., 2004). There was no difference between the BTxA group and the placebo group in any measured variable. Transient weakness of eyelids, neck, or both occurred in some patients treated with BTxA.

A study of different dosing schemes (0, 50, 100, and 150 units injected in five sites, or 86 and 100 units injected subcutaneously in three sites) showed no difference in the number of TTH-free days in CTTH subjects (Silberstein et al., 2006). However, even though efficacy was not demonstrated for the primary endpoint, more subjects in three BTxA groups had 50% or greater reduction in TTH days than did those given placebo ($P \leq 0.024$). Adverse effects of BTxA were mild to moderate, and BTxA was considered to be well tolerated.

Migraine

A pilot study was conducted in 10 migraine patients to investigate the mechanism of action of BTxA in migraine headache (Smuts et al., 2004). Botulinum toxin type A (20 units) was injected into the procerus and corrugator muscles. The compound muscle action potential (CMAP) was obtained before and at intervals up to 90 days after injection. A 50% decrease in headache was demonstrated in all subjects by day 7, was maximal at day 30, and was sustained to day 60. Migraine frequency declined by 50% or more in 7 of 10 subjects by day 60. Migraine response did not correlate with the resulting denervation pattern, leading the authors to conclude that relaxation of the corrugator muscles was not the sole factor in producing migraine relief.

A randomized, double-blind, vehicle-controlled study in episodic migraine (frequency of two to eight moderate to severe migraines per month) of BTxA in two total dose levels of 25 units and 75 units injected into predetermined, fixed sites (frontalis, temporalis, and glabellar [procerus and corrugator] muscles) showed that the lower, but not the higher, dose of BTxA was more effective than placebo in treating migraine (Silberstein et al., 2000). At 3 months the subjects treated with a total dose of 25 units of BTxA showed significant improvement in the number of migraine attacks and in the use of medication compared with vehicle. There was no such improvement in subjects treated with a total dose of 75 units of BTxA. However, the subjects treated with 75 units had significantly greater side effects. Improvement was mainly noted at 2 to 3 months. The failure of subjects treated with a total dose of 75 units was thought perhaps to be due to the lower frequency of migraine attacks at baseline.

Another RCT divided subjects into three groups: one group that received 100 units injected into frontal, temporal, and shoulder and neck muscles; one group that received 16 units injected only in the frontalis and temporalis muscles; and a placebo group (Evers et al., 2004). Thirty percent of patients in the two treatment groups had a 50% decrease in headache days, the primary outcome measure. However, 25% of the placebo group also reached that mark. The difference was not significant. This study used a low dose of BTxA in the temporalis muscle compared with doses often used today, and did not include the glabellar muscles.

Botulinum toxin type A in three different dose schedules was evaluated in a study of episodic migraine

(Elkind et al., 2006). Botulinum toxin type A at a total dose of 25 units or 50 units was divided between the frontalis muscles (four sites), the temporalis muscles (two sites), and the glabellar muscles (corrugator and procerus muscles) and given at intervals of 4 months. A group receiving a total of 7.5 units was included as an active control, to evaluate those nontherapeutic doses that might still give a botulinum effect that could unblind the studies. Headache frequency was equally reduced in all groups (high-dose BTxA, low-dose BTxA, and placebo). There was no advantage of any group over placebo. Injection of low doses of BTxA into fixed muscle sites was effective in reducing headache frequency, but no more so than placebo injections.

A small study of 32 migraineurs with headaches occurring more than five times per month compared BTxA with saline placebo (Vo et al., 2007). There was improvement in both groups, but there was no significant difference for headache frequency or severity. Headache index scores, however, worsened for the control group over 3 months, but not for the treated group ($P = 0.02$), suggesting a protective effect of BTxA against headache severity.

A multidose RCT of BTxA for prophylaxis of episodic migraine that employed 75, 150, or 225 units, injected into the frontalis, corrugator, temporalis, splenius capitis, trapezius, semispinalis, and suboccipital muscles failed to show a benefit (decrease in headache) (Relja et al., 2007). This was a fixed-dose, fixed-site study that evaluated the response of placebo nonresponders. All groups, the variable-dose BTxA and the placebo group, showed a decrease in headache frequency, but there was no significant improvement between the BTxA and the placebo groups.

A series of RCTs is being conducted to compare different injection sites and doses of BTxA in the treatment of episodic migraine (Saper et al., 2007). The study of low-dose BTxA (total dose of 25 units) injected in predetermined, fixed sites in the head (corrugator/procerus muscles, frontalis and temporalis muscles) was performed in subjects whose headaches included frontotemporal migraine (Saper et al., 2007). Each subject was injected in one of these areas (glabellar, frontalis, or temporalis) or all three areas. Thus, there were four treatment groups and a placebo group. The primary outcome measure was headache frequency through day 60. There was no statistical difference among the groups at day 60 for headache frequency. A secondary outcome measure was safety. Adverse side effects were recorded in 47% of all patients in the study, with no dif-

ferences between groups, including placebo. Muscle weakness was the most frequently reported adverse side effect in the treatment group, and flu syndrome the most frequently reported adverse event across groups. The adverse side effects were mild to moderate in severity and transient. Lack of efficacy in this trial may reflect one of any number of possibilities. Botulinum toxin type A might not be effective in episodic migraine. The dose used may have been too small. Concomitant medications were taken that may have masked the effect of BTxA. Dosage requirements of BTxA in treatment of migraine have not been established, so that optimal doses may not have been used. Injections were only made in fronto-glabellar-temporal sites, and omitted the occiput and any other trigger sites that might be included in a follow-the-pain protocol.

An RCT of BTxA in episodic migraine using higher doses (mean BTxA dose 190.5 units, range 110–260) used a modified follow-the-pain protocol (Aurora et al., 2007). Subjects were injected in muscles deemed to be relevant to their headache, except that the occipital muscles were always included. Any given muscle treated was injected according to a predetermined schedule of fixed dosages. Botulinum toxin type A was administered every 90 days. Patients were followed to 270 days. Placebo nonresponders (PNR) in the run-in initial 30 days were followed separately to eliminate the effect of a robust placebo response. At day 180, headache frequency in the previous 30-day period decreased 2.4 in the PNR group compared with 2.2 in the placebo control group ($P > 0.9$). There was no statistical difference in the frequency of migraine episodes in any 30-day period between treatment and placebo groups, in the placebo responders (PR) and placebo nonresponders alike. Pooled data of both PNR and PR showed that both groups had a sustained decrease in mean headache frequency from baseline, per 30-day period. A secondary outcome measure of a decrease of 50% or greater in migraine events per 30-day period showed that at least 60% of patients in all treatment groups had a decrease of at least two headaches per month, including the placebo group. A post hoc analysis attempted to identify a subgroup that might have shown a greater response to BTxA. Those with more than 12 headache days per month but less than 15 headache days at baseline constituted a subgroup that was analyzed separately. This subgroup analysis of 88 patients showed that these subjects had greater reduction in migraine frequency at day 180 when treated with BTxA than with placebo (4.0 vs. 1.9, $P = 0.048$). Adverse events were more common among BTxA-treated patients (81%) than placebo (60%). The majorities of adverse events were mild to moderate in severity and were transient. In summary, both placebo and treatment groups improved compared with baseline, but only those patients with the most frequent headaches (>12/month) improved more with BTxA than with placebo.

The use of botulinum toxin in migraine headache was reviewed in 2006 (Schulte-Mattler & Martinez-Castrillo, 2006). The authors noted that despite early indications that botulinum toxin was effective in tension-type and migraine headaches, well-designed RCTs in migraine failed to provide evidence of benefit at doses of up to 200 units of Botox and up to 500 units of Dysport, except that trends favored botulinum toxin. The problem of robust placebo effect, even in studies that were conducted on placebo nonresponders, continued to confound the studies. Ongoing studies attempting to deal more effectively with the issue of placebo responders have yet to be reported.

Anand et al. (2006) reported a randomized, double-blind, vehicle-controlled, parallel-group study of the effect of BTxA injected into pericranial muscles of 32 migraineurs, with and without aura, monitored over 3 months. Fifty units of BTxA or vehicle alone (placebo) was injected into pericranial muscles. About 75% of the patients reported complete relief to mild headache with BTxA, and none reported relief with placebo. No adverse effects were reported.

Finally, three recent articles have appeared addressing the treatment of chronic daily headache with BTxA. All three randomized, controlled studies showed a favorable response to the use of BTxA in the treatment of chronic daily migraine headache. One study identified unilateral migraine as opposed to bilateral migraine and pericranial tenderness as predictors of responsiveness to BTxA in chronic migraine, and pericranial tenderness as a predictor of responsiveness in CTTH (Mathew et al., 2008). Botulinum toxin type A was superior to placebo for the primary endpoint of reduction of headache episodes and for the secondary endpoints of total headache days, headache index, and quality of life measures (Freitag et al., 2008). A third study comparing BTxA with divalproex sodium showed that both were effective prophylactic treatments of chronic daily migraine headache, and showed a trend of decreased headache severity with BTxA (Blumenfeld et al., 2008). In addition, there were less adverse events with BTxA than with divalproex sodium. These studies add further support for the use of BTxA in the treatment of chronic daily headache of the migraine and tension-type headache varieties.

COMMENTARY ON THE STATUS OF BOTULINUM TOXIN IN HEADACHE MANAGEMENT

The results of all the above-mentioned studies taken together are mixed, making interpretation difficult. There are many possible reasons for the variation in study results. The criteria for subject selection among the different studies were not uniform. The application of botulinum toxin was also not uniform in dose or in site of injection. Nevertheless, that the outcome for the primary outcome measures of many of the studies was negative is sobering. However, there is a need to exercise caution when interpreting the negative results of these studies taken as a group. A study that had sufficiently large numbers of subjects (Dodick et al., 2005), for example, did meet the primary outcome of reduced headache frequency. Furthermore, secondary outcome measures were met in many of the studies, with reduced headache severity or intensity, or decreased headache frequency over specific time periods, such as after 180 days (Mathew et al., 2005).

A further complexity was that some studies of chronic daily headache (CDH) combined subjects with MH or subjects having CTTH. Nevertheless, the outcome of studies of BTx in CDH was generally favorable in either subgroup analysis or in secondary outcomes, if not in the primary outcome measures. CTTH was studied as a separate category in many studies, but would qualify as a CDH study, because of the frequency of headache. Most of the study of the use of BTx in migraine included only subjects with four to eight migraines per month, occurring less than 15 days per month, but the inclusion criteria varied, such as one specifying only that subjects must have at least five migraines per month (Vo et al., 2007). The use of botulinum toxin in the doses and sites used to treat chronic daily headache failed to meet the primary study endpoint of reduction in headache days in four of five studies. Only the study of Dodick et al. (2005) evaluating a subset of subjects in a larger trial of chronic daily migraine (Mathew et al., 2005) reported that the primary outcome measure of decrease in mean frequency of headaches per 30 days was met. In addition, in all five studies there was improvement in headache frequency (**Table 32.1**), and at least some secondary objectives were met in each study. This is of great interest, because the study

Table 32.1 Studies of Botulinum Toxin in the Treatment of Headache

Author	Headache Type	Study Type	Primary Endpoint Met	Secondary Endpoint(s) Met
Mathew et al., 2005	CDH	RCT, DB $N = 571$	No. PNR decreased h/a days more than P, but NS.	Yes at 180 days: decrease in h/a intensity and frequency ($P < 0.03$).
Ondo et al., 2004	CDH	RCT, DB $N = 60$	No, but h/a-free days improved in weeks 8 to 12, BTx compared to Pl ($P < 0.07$).	Yes. Improved over Pl: IGI (<0.005), SGI (<0.05), SHI ($P < 0.001$).
Silberstein et al., 2005	CDH	RCT, DB $N = 702$	No. All groups improved, including Pl.	Yes. The 225 U & 150 U groups had > decrease in h/a frequency than Pl at day 240.
Farinella et al., 2006	CDH	5-yr review of treatment with 100 U, FDFS $N = 1,347$	After 12 months Rx, h/a free 23 days/month.	—
Freund & Schwartz, 2000	Cervicogenic h/a	RCT, DB $N = 26$	Yes. Pain and ROM improved ($P < 0.01$).	—
Schmitt et al., 2001	CTTHH	RCT 20 U BTxA in frontal & temporal musc	No.	—
Schulte-Mattler et al., 2004	CTTH	RCT, DB $N = 112$ 500 U BTxAD FDFS	No.	No.
Dodick et al., 2005	CDH:M	RCT, DB $N = 228$ Subgroup analysis	Yes. H/a frequency decreased ($P = 0.032$).	Yes. H/a frequency and severity significantly lower days 180–270.
Silberstein et al., 2006	CTTH	RCT, DB $N = 300$ 5 different doses (50, 100, 150 units, and 86 or 100 units subcut); FDFS	No. NS difference except that Pl was significantly better than 150 units.	Yes. At day 90, more BTx subjects had ≥50% fewer h/a days than Pl ($P < 0.024$).
Siberstein et al., 2000	EM	RCT, DB $N = 123$ 25 or 75 U injected pericranially	Yes. 25 U reduced h/a frequency ($P = 0.011$).	Yes. Reduced h/a severity at 25 U ($P < 0.029$).
Evers et al., 2004	M	RCT, DB $N = 60$ 16 U in neck, or 100 U in neck and frontal muscles	No.	Yes. Post hoc analysis: reduction in accompanying symptoms with 16 U in neck.
Anand et al., 2006	M	RCT, DB $N = 32$ 50 U in pericranial muscles	Yes. 75% of BTxA reported complete relief; Pl no relief.	Yes. QOL improvement in energy/vitality, but work functions and social interaction worsened.
Elkind et al., 2006	M	RCT, DB $N = 418$ 7.5 U, 25 U, or 50 U FDFS	No.	No.
Aurora et al., 2007	EM	RCT, DB 110–260 U to PNR, PR in modified follow-the-pain paradigm $N = 369$	No.	Yes. In group with ≥12 but ≤15 h/a days/month, migraine decreased more than Pl ($P = 0.048$).

Table 32.1 *Continued*

Author	Headache Type	Study Type	Primary Endpoint Met	Secondary Endpoint(s) Met
Vo et al., 2007	M	RCT, DB $N = 32$	No.	Yes. The pattern headache index in BTx group suggested a protective effect.
Relja et al., 2007	EM	RCT, DB $N = 495$ Injection sites included pericranial muscles	No.	No.
Menezes et al., 2007	CM	Open label BTxA in refractory migraine; BTxAD FDFS $N = 15$	Yes. Improvement within 30 days ($P = 0.03$).	Yes. Decreased pain frequency and analgesic use.
Saper et al., 2007	EM	RCT, DB Comparison of different doses and injection sites; low-dose trial of F, T, Gl, or all three, max BTxA 25 U $N = 232$	No.	No.
Suzuki et al., 2007	M	Open label 50 units FDFS $N = 14$	Yes. 13/14 reported improvement; h/a frequency decreased significantly.	Yes. Headache impact on life lessened (improvement in QOL).
Mathew et al., 2007	CM, CTTH	Open-label study to identify predictors of response CM: $N = 71$ CTTH: $N = 11$	Unilateral h/a, scalp allodynia, and pericranial muscle tenderness predicted response in CM.	—

Abbreviations: CDH, chronic daily headache, CDH:M, chronic daily headache (migraine); RCT, randomized, controlled trial; DB, double blind; h/a, headache; Pl, placebo; PNR, placebo nonresponders; NS, nonsignificant; SGI, subject global impressions; IGI, investigator global impressions; SHI, subject change in headache impressions, >dec, greater decrease; FDFS, fixed dose, fixed site; ROM, range of motion; CTTH, chronic tension-type headache; BTxA, botulinum toxin type A (Allergan); musc, muscles; BTxAD, botulinum toxin type A (Dysport); EM, episodic migraine; M, migraine; QOL, quality of life; CM, chronic migraine; F, frontal muscles; T, temporalis muscles; Gl, glabellar muscles.

populations in the five studies of CDH included persons with migraine headache as well as those with tension-type headache and those with both. Thus, there is some support for the use of botulinum toxin in chronic daily headache, whether migraine or tension-type headache.

The studies of episodic migraine (EM) showed contradictory results. Most of the studies included subjects with both migraine with aura and migraine without aura. These two types of MH probably have different etiologies, and perhaps should be studied separately. Migraine without aura may have a specific peripheral trigger that might respond to BTx, whereas migraine with aura might not. For example, a myofascial TrP can act as a muscle trigger point for migraine without aura such that inactivation of the trigger points with BTx may reduce MH frequency and intensity. Inactivation of myofascial TrPs has, in fact, been performed in subjects with MH, using bupivacaine as a local anesthetic, with beneficial results (Giamberardino et al., 2007). In this study, the group treated with trigger point inactivation by local anesthetic had significant reduction in migraine symptoms (intensity and frequency of migraine) compared with the nontreated control group. In addition, an objective parameter measuring reduction in tissue hyperalgesia to electrical stimulation was noted in the treated group, but not in the untreated group. Furthermore, Giamberardino et al. (2007) specifically treated those muscles in which TrP stimulation reproduced headache symptoms. In none of the BTx studies of EM were both the sternocleidomastoid or upper trapezius muscles injected with botulinum toxin, even though TrPs in those muscles are known to refer pain to the forehead or to the occiput in pain patterns typical of migraine headache. The follow-the-pain paradigm used in some studies was restricted only to pericranial muscles such as the splenius capitis and cervicis and the semispinalis capitis and cervicis, omitting other muscles in the neck and shoulder where TrPs are known to refer pain to the head. Relja et al. (2007) injected the splenius capitis and semispinalis capitis, but not the sternocleidomastoid, the oblique capitis inferior, or the splenius cervicis or semispinalis cervicis muscles, all of which may refer trigger-point-induced pain to the head.

Some of the studies of EM were clearly exploring different doses and different injection sites in order to identify effective doses and effective injection sites. One might expect that there would be failure to affect the frequency or intensity of headache at some doses and with some fixed-site protocols. There remain studies in progress looking at different dosing paradigms and different injection protocols, so that the final answers as to effective doses and effective injection sites are yet to come. If BTx continues not to be injected in some muscles where TrPs refer pain to the head, then the trials may continue to fail. A lesson to be learned from the insights of Jakubowsky et al. (2006) about the difference between imploding and exploding migraine headache, and the beneficial effect of inactivation of myofascial TrPs on migraine headache frequency and intensity shown by Giamberardino et al. (2007), is that future trials looking at the effect of BTx on migraine and tension-type headache should both identify the muscle TrPs in the head, neck, and shoulders that reproduce the patient's headache and direct injection of BTx to those TrPs.

As clinicians, we must be honest with ourselves and with our patients at this point and inform them that BTx treatment of headache is an off-label use of BTx in the United States, but that it still looks promising, that there are contradictory results in the studies to date, and that BTx use in headache is still being evaluated. If I were to recommend the off-label use of BTx in the treatment of migraine, I would select patients for whom conventional therapy has failed, and I would identify those muscles where TrP activation reproduces part or the patient's entire headache. I recommend referring patients to enroll in randomized controlled trials of the use of BTx where possible, but only in those studies that identify the muscle trigger points of headache and include them in the muscles injected with botulinum toxin. The relevance of these sites selected by physical examination may be confirmed by a trial of TrP inactivation with local anesthetic, although there is no study published that shows that the outcome is improved if one directs treatment to only those patients in whom there was reduction of headache with trigger point inactivation.

REFERENCES

Anand KS, Prasad A, Singh MM, Sharma S, Bala K. Botulinum toxin type A in prophylactic treatment of migraine. *Am J Ther* 2006;13:183–187.

Aoki KR. Review of a proposed mechanism for the antinociceptive action of botulinum toxin type A. *Neurotoxicology* 2005;26:785–793.

Augustine GJ. How does calcium trigger neurotransmitter release? *Curr Opin Neurobiol* 2001;11:320–326.

Aurora SK, Gawel M, Brandes JL, Pokta S, VanDenbrugh AM, for the BOTOX North American Episodic Migraine Study Group. Botulinum toxin type A treatment of episodic migraine: a randomized, double-blind, placebo-controlled exploratory study. *Headache* 2007;47:486–499.

Bach-Rojecky L, Lacković Z. Antinociceptive effect of botulinum toxin type A in rat model of carageenan and capsaicin induced pain. *Croat Med J* 2005;46:201–208.

Binder W, Brin MF, Blitzer A, et al. Botulinum toxin type A (BOTOX) for migraine: an open-label assessment. *Otolaryngol Head Neck Surg* 2000;123:669–676.

Blersch W, Schulte-Mattler WJ, Przywara S, May A, Bigalke H, Wohlfarth K. Botulinum toxin A and the cutaneous nociception in humans: a prospective, double-blind, placebo-controlled, randomized study. *J Neurol Sci* 2002;205:59–63.

Blumenfeld A. Botulinum toxin type A as an effective prophylactic treatment in primary headache disorders. *Headache* 2003;43:853–860.

Blumenfeld AM, Schim JD, Chippendale TJ. Botulinum toxin type A and divalproex sodium for prophylactic treatment of episodic or chronic migraine. *Headache* 2008;48: 2210–2220.

Bukharaeva E, Samigullin D, Nikolskey E, Vyskocil F. Protein kinase A cascade regulates quantal release dispersion at frog muscle endplate. *J Physiol Lond* 2002;202:837–848.

Cui M, Khanijou S, Rubino J, Aoki KR. Subcutaneous administration of botulinum toxin A reduces formalin-induced pain. *Pain* 2004;107:125–133.

dePaiva A, Meunier FA, Molgo J, Aoki KR, Dolly JO. Functional repair of motor endplates after botulinum neurotoxin type A poisoning biphasic switch of synaptic activity between nerve sprouts and their parent terminals. *Proc Natl Acad Sci* 1999;96:3200–3205.

Dodick DW, Mauskop A, Elkind AH, DeGryse R, Brin MF, Silberstein SD, BOTOX CDH Study Group. Botulinum toxin type A for the prophylaxis of chronic daily headache: subgroup analysis of patients not receiving other prophylactic medications—a randomized double-blind, placebo-controlled study. *Headache* 2005;45:315–324.

Durham PL, Cady R, Cady R. Regulation of calcitonin gene-related peptide secretion from trigeminal nerve cells by botulinum toxin type A: implications for migraine therapy. *Headache* 2004;44:35–43.

Elkind AH, O'Carroll, Blumenfeld A, DeGryse R, Dimitrova R, for the BoNTA-024-026-036 Study Group. A series of three sequential, randomized, controlled studies of repeated treatments with botulinum toxin type A for migraine prophylaxis. *J Pain* 2006;7:688–696.

Evers S, Rahmann A, Vollmer-Haase J, Husstedt IW. Treatment of headache with botulinum toxin A: a review according to evidence-based medicine criteria. *Cephalalgia* 2002;22:699–710.

Evers S, Vollmer-Haase J, Schwaag S, Rahman A, Husstedt I-W, Frese A. Botulinum toxin A in the prophylactic treatment of migraine: a randomized, double-blind, placebo-controlled study. *Cephalalgia* 2004;24:838–843.

Farinelli I, Coloprisco G, De Filippis S, Martelletti P. Long-term benefits of botulinum toxin type A (BOTOX) in chronic daily headache. *J Headache Pain* 2006;7:407–412.

Fernández-de-las-Peñas C, Arendt-Nielsen L, Simons DG. Exploding vs. impoding headache in migraine prophylaxis with botulinum toxin A [letter] and reply by Burstein R, Jakubowski M, McAllister PJ, Bajwa ZH, Ward TN, Smith P. *Pain* 2007;129:363–365.

Freitag FG. Botulinum toxin type A in chronic migraine. *Expert Rev Neurother* 2007;7:463–470.

Freitag FG, Diamond S, Diamond M, Urban G. Botulinum toxin type A in the treatment of chronic migraine without medication overuse. *Headache* 2008;48:201–209.

Freund BJ, Schwartz M. Treatment of chronic cervical-associated headache with botulinum toxin A: a pilot study. *Headache* 2000;40:231–236.

Gazerani P, Staahl C, Drewes AM, Arendt-Nielsen L. The effects of botulinum toxin type A on capsaicin-evoked pain, flare, and secondary hyperalgesia in an experimental human model of trigeminal sensitization. *Pain* 2006;122: 315–325.

Gerwin R, Dodick DW. Chronic daily headache [letters]. *N Engl J Med* 2006;354:1958.

Gerwin R. The taut band and other mysteries of the myofascial trigger point: an examination of the mechanisms relevant to the development and maintenance of the trigger point. *J Musculoskeletal Pain* 2008 (in press).

Giamberadino MA, Tafuri E, Savini A, Fabrizio A, Affaitati G, Lerza R, Ianni LD, Lappena D, Mezzetti A. Contribution of myofascial trigger points to migraine symptoms. *J Pain* 2007;8:869–878.

Jakubowski M, McAllister PJ, Bajwa ZH, Ward TN, Smith P, Burstein R. Exploding vs. imploding headache in migraine prophylaxis with botulinum toxin A. *Pain* 2006;125: 286–295.

Krämer HH, Angerer C, Erbguth F, Schmelz M, Birklein F. Botulinum toxin A reduces neurogenic flare but has almost no effect on pain and hyperalgesia in human skin. *J Neurol* 2003;250:188–193.

Kranz G, Sycha T, Voller B, Gleiss A, Schnider P, Auff E. Pain sensation during intradermal injections of three different botulinum toxin preparations in different doses and dilutions. *Dermatol Surg* 2006;32:886–890.

Luvisetto S, Marinelli S, Lucchetti F, Marchi F, Cobianchi S, Rossetto O, Montecucco C, Pavone F. Botulinum neurotoxins and formalin-induced pain: central vs. peripheral effects in mice. *Brain Res* 2006;1082:124–131.

Luvisetto S, Marinelli S, Cobianchi S, Pavone F. Anti-allodynic efficacy of botulinum neurotoxin A in a model of neuropathic pain. *Neuroscience* 2007;145:1–4.

Mathew NT. The prophylactic treatment of chronic daily headache. *Headache* 2006;46:1552–1564.

Mathew NT, Frishberg BM, Gawel M, Dimitrova R, Gibson J, Turkel C, BOTOX CDH Study Group. Botulinum toxin type A (BOTOX) for the prophylactic treatment of chronic daily headache: a randomized, double-blind, placebo-controlled trial. *Headache* 2005;45:293–307.

Mathew NT, Kailasam J, Meadors L. Predictors of response to botulinum toxin type A (BoNTA) in chronic daily headache. *Headache* 2008;48:194–200.

Meng J, Wang J, Lawrence G, Dolly JO. Synaptobrevin I mediates exocytosis of CGRP from sensory neurons and inhibition by botulinum toxins reflects their antinociceptive potential. *J Cell Sci* 2007;120:2864–2874.

Ondo WG, Vuong KD, Derman HS. Botulinum toxin A for chronic daily headache: a randomized, placebo-controlled, parallel design study. *Cephalalgia* 2004;24:60–65.

Porta M. A comparative trial of botulinum toxin type A and methylprednisone for the treatment of tension-type headache. *Curr Rev Pain* 2000;4:31–35.

Relja M, Poole AC, Schoenen J, Pascual J, Lei X, Thompson C. A multicentre, double-blind, randomized, placebo-controlled, parallel group study of multiple treatments of botulinum toxin type A (BoNTA) for the prophylaxis of episodic migraine headaches. *Cephalalgia* 2007;27: 492–503.

Rollnik JD, Tanneberger O, Schubert M, Schneider U, Dengler R. Treatment of tension-type headache with botulinum toxin type A: a double-blind, placebo controlled study. *Headache* 2000;40:300–305.

Royal M. The use of botulinum toxins in the management of pain and headache. *Pain Practice* 2001;1:215–235.

Samigullin D, Bukharaeva EA, Vyskocil F, Nilolsky EE. Calcium dependence of uni-quantal release latencies and quantal content of mouse neuromuscular junction. *Physiol Res* 2005;54:129–132.

Saper J, Mathew NT, Loder EW, DeGryse R, VanDenburgh AM, for the NoNTA-009 Study Group. A double-blind, randomized, placebo-controlled comparison of botulinum toxin type A injection sites and doses in the prevention of episodic migraine. *Pain Med* 2007;8:478–485.

Schmitt WJ, Slowey E, Fravi N, Weber S, Burgunder JM. Effect of botulinum toxin A injections in the treatment of chronic tension-type headache: a double-blind, placebo-controlled trial. *Headache* 2001;41:658–664.

Schulte-Mattler WJ, Martinez-Castrillo JC. Botulinum toxin therapy of migraine and tension-type headache: comparing different botulinum toxin preparations. *Eur J Neurol* 2006; 13(suppl 1):51–54.

Schulte-Mattler WJ, Krack P, BoNTTH Study Group. Treatment of chronic tension-type headache with botulinum toxin A: a randomized, double-blind, placebo-controlled multicenter study. *Pain* 2004;109:110–114.

Schulte-Mattler WJ, Opatz O, Blersch W, May A, Bigalke H, Wohlfarth K. Botulinum toxin A does not alter capsaicin-induced pain perception in human skin. *J Neurol Sci* 2007;260:38–42.

Silberstein S, Mathew N, Saper J, Jenkins S, for the BOTOX Migraine Clinical Research Group. Botulinum toxin type A as a migraine preventative treatment. *Headache* 2000;40: 445–450.

Silberstein SD, Stark SD, Lucas SM, Christies SN, Degryse RE, Turkel CC, BoNTA-039 Study Group. Botulinum toxin type A for prophylactic treatment of chronic daily headache: a randomized, double-blind, placebo-controlled trial. *Mayo Clin Proc* 2005;80:1126–1137.

Silberstein SD, Göbel H, Jensen R, Elkind AH, Degryse R, Walcott JM, Turkel C. Botulinum toxin type A in the prophylactic treatment of chronic tension type headache: a multicentre, double-blind, randomized, placebo-controlled, parallel group study. *Cephalalgia* 2006;26:790–800.

Smuts JA, Schultz D, Barrnard A. Mechanism of action of botulinum toxin type A in migraine prevention: a pilot study. *Headache* 2004;44:801–805.

Suzuki K, Iizuka T, Sakai F. Botulinum toxin type A for migraine prophylaxis in the Japanese population: an open-label prospective trial. *Intern Med* 2007;46:959–963.

Sycha T, Samal D, Chizh B, Lehr S, Gustorff B, Schider P, Auff E. A lack of antinociceptive or anti-inflammatory effect of botulinum toxin A in an inflammatory human pain model. *Anesth Analg* 2006;102:509–516.

Tfelt-Hansen P, Lous I, Olesen J. Prevalence and significance of muscle tenderness during common migraine attacks. *Headache* 1981;21:49–54.

Tugnoli V, Capone JG, Eleopra R, Quatrale R, Sensi M, Gastaldo E, Tola MR, Geppetti P. Botulinum toxin type A reduces capsaicin-evoked pain and neurogenic vasodilation in human skin. *Pain* 2007;130:76–83.

Vo AH, Satori R, Jabbari B, Green J, Killgore WD, Labutta R, Campbell WW. Botulinum toxin type-a in the prevention of migraine: a double-blind controlled study. *Aviat Space Environ Med* 2007;78(suppl 5):B113–B118.

Voller B, Sycha T, Gustorff B, Schmetter L, Lehr S, Eichler HG, Auff E, Schnider P. A randomized, double-blind, placebo controlled study on analgesic effects of botulinum toxin A. *Neurology* 2003;61:940–944.

Wessler I. Acetylcholine release at motor endplates and autonomic effector junctions: a comparison. *Pharmacol Res* 1996;33:81–94.

Psychological Aspects of Chronic Headache Treatment

Christopher Gilbert, PhD

THE PSYCHOLOGICAL APPROACH

Headaches with similar, if not identical, descriptions may have quite different origins, and the farther back in time and away from the brain one looks, the more varied the potential sources become. For instance, the most proximal (toward consciousness) headache pain source may be in the thalamus, or a certain layer of the sensory cortex, or the insula or cingulate cortex. But those areas relay problems from farther downstream from the brain. One possible source for the headache may be a spastic suboccipital muscle, which stimulates local nociceptive fibers to carry their designated message to the brain, activating synapses that terminate in the sites just mentioned and releasing specific molecules such as substance P (Fernández-de-las-Peñas et al., 2006).

But what activates the suboccipital muscle, in this example? Perhaps the person having the headache overuses the neck muscle to the point of strain or spasm due to forward head posture and lack of mobility (Fernández-de-las-Peñas et al., 2006). Contributing to that problem might be the person's physical setting: a poorly placed computer monitor that skews the head position, perhaps amplifying a bad habit. Beyond that, it could be an urgent work assignment that day which discourages taking a break all morning. Beyond that, it might be a personality trait in this person, who overvalues doing a good job above comfort or rest, coupled with fear of the supervisor's evaluation. Beyond that, it might be the person's general self-concept, level of assertiveness, and habits of self-care, and beyond that is how the person's parents raised him or her.

Of course a headache may stem from many other possible physical mechanisms and emotional factors other than the above examples. This description of the multiple levels of causation leading to a headache at least raises the question of where treatment might begin.

Physicians focus mostly on biochemical interventions, injuries, and structural problems that may interact with behavior and cause headaches. Physical therapists, massage therapists, and body workers in general work with soft structure, habits of body use, and the effects of structural defects on physiology. The psychological approach deals mostly with the areas of how the patient sets priorities for attention and activity, manages emotions, acts on beliefs, chooses headache-provoking social and physical settings, and uses the body. Attention, perception, and behavior are the relevant properties with which psychological specialists deal.

Each therapeutic discipline can obtain good results by intervening somewhere along the etiologic chain. Even with muscle trigger points (TrPs), disciplines have distinct approaches: physicians inject and may prescribe stretching and deactivating; psychologists facilitate multisystem relaxation, which raises pain thresholds and diminishes sympathetic input to the TrPs. Physical therapists address TrPs with manual release methods, stretching, and improved body use.

Physical therapists and physicians have direct approaches to chronic headache treatment when etiology seems to fall within their domain, and often enough the treatment goes well and the headaches subside. But sometimes all does not go so well for various reasons, such as continued poor body use in defiance of advice, mismanaged emotions, unusual sensitivity to pain, or other issues related to a psychological or behavioral aspect. This is not to say headaches are either "organic" or "psychosomatic"—such a clear distinction is too simple to be more than preliminary. It is more realistic to think in terms of a continuum from "strong organic component" to "strong psychological component." When a headache case seems psychologically influenced to a certain degree, this should stimulate investigation into factors arising not only from the person's body but from the person whose body it is.

The patient with chronic headache often has the disadvantage of a genetic and constitutional susceptibility to headaches. The following statement is a good summary regarding migraines: "Multiple genetic factors seem to set the individual trigger threshold for migraine attacks, endogenous and exogenous factors may modulate this set point and attacks involving physiological mechanisms are provoked by patient-specific trigger factors" (Hunt & Koltzenburg, 2005). This latent susceptibility must be activated for headaches to occur, in the same way that fair skin is at risk for sunburn, but only when exposed to sunlight.

Therefore, in the current chapter, the psychological factors and contexts depicted as headache triggers are relevant only for people susceptible to headaches. It does not seem true that the same psychological factors cause headaches in everybody. From 50 years of headache-treatment experience, John Graham summarized his impression of headache susceptibility as a constitutional weakness coupled with excessive demands: "[T]he biological meaning of the migraine attack is that the congenitally poorly equipped neurovascular system has been pushed beyond its limits of adaptation and needs a chance to recuperate" (Graham, 1968).

PSYCHOLOGICAL-MINDEDNESS

This section is offered to help estimate a patient's readiness for considering behavioral and psychological factors. In thinking about the possibility of psychological and behavioral factors contributing to headaches and other pain, it is useful first to consider the term *psycho-logical-mindedness*. This refers to seeing connections among feelings, events, and behavior (e.g., wondering whether a person who is acting unusually generous might feel guilty about something). The capacity to reflect on one's own behavior (such as introspection) and to consider the emotions and attitudes underlying behavior are traits of a more psychologically minded person. Such a person usually has a good vocabulary for feelings and some skill in discriminating small differences in emotional states (e.g., having a range of words for degrees of anger, such as *annoyance, irritation, aggravation, rage,* and *resentment*). Also included would be an ability to tolerate one's emotional distress with some detachment and self-knowledge, rather than with impulsive acting-out behavior, strong somatic reactions, or denial. Finally, psychological-mindedness includes having some interest in the psychological meanings behind behaviors—of both self and others.

One good way to gauge a person's psychological-mindedness is to ask about family interactions and tensions and how the tensions might be explained. If a person is at a loss to explain the backstage action in the minds of family members, shows no interest in the topic, or gives simple, glib answers, this might indicate real limits on processing and expressing emotional information.

Patients on the low end of the psychological-mindedness continuum are less likely to admit that they are experiencing stress, may think very simplistically about it, or may simply dismiss the concept ("I'm not working now, but I'm on disability, so I have no stress"). This trait will lead often to poor insight and poor communication with others about their feelings, and increased social stress. People suffering from low psychological-mindedness may assume they have more control over their feelings than they really do: for example, the belief that they should not or do not want to feel something (such as anger or hurt) is the same as not having the feeling. They make statements such as "What good is it to feel that?" or "I can't afford to feel that." A decision to not have a feeling is equated with actual fact; inconvenient emotions are legislated out of existence.

The downside to this situation is that troubling feelings are not acknowledged and so cannot be understood, shared, or ameliorated. The physiologic aspects of the disowned feelings then persist, reverberating throughout the body and causing symptoms that are mistaken for medical problems. This is one hypothesized route to what is called *somatization*.

ALEXITHYMIA

Alexithymia refers to a poverty of words for feelings: for instance, when asked about some recent traumatic event, being unable to say much more than "It was bad" or "I didn't like it." It also includes relative lack of imagery ability, less introspection, more concrete thinking, and difficulty connecting emotions with bodily feelings. This trait tends to correlate with higher frequency of somatizing and increased likelihood of psychosomatic symptoms, including headache. "In alexithymia, awareness of feelings is short-circuited; the patient is aware only of the physiological concomitants of the affect" (Adler et al., 1987, p. 51).

Conceptually, alexithymia is the opposite of psychological-mindedness. To the extent the trait may be neurologically based, research has suggested a left-right hemispheric and a neocortical-subcortical disconnection, both of which would interfere with full conscious processing of emotions. Therapy for this limitation focuses on learning to label and express feelings through words, which allows understanding and sharing of strong feelings at a different level.

One study of female chronic pain patients found that the alexithymia factor was higher in these women than in a comparable control group (Celike & Saatcioglu, 2006). Okasha et al. (1999) showed that patients with chronic headache displayed significantly more alexithymia than control groups, and also more evidence of personality disorders. Another study conducted with patients with tension-type headache showed significantly higher depression, lower assertiveness, higher alexithymia, and more negative automatic thoughts compared with a control group (Yücel et al., 2002). Brosschot and Aarsse (2001) studied women with chronic pain from fibromyalgia and found higher alexithymic traits and poorer emotional processing. The therapist or clinician who is not very psychologically minded may not even be reading this chapter, and some of the suggestions and explanations will be more useful for those having some psychological insight, or at least interest. Applying psychological techniques awkwardly may go badly or seem insincere; they work better coming from personal conviction and experience.

If a person is reluctant to inquire about another's emotional life for fear of "opening up something" or feels unable to cope with the possible responses (crying, recalled trauma, neediness, or rejection of the inquiry), then that reluctance could hinder the process. Feeling that such questioning would take too much time is another block, and in fact it is difficult to limit a patient's answer to an exploratory question. Yet the answer may reveal a fruitful new dimension to explore.

MATCH AND MISMATCH OF PSYCHOLOGICAL-MINDEDNESS

Following are four examples in which either the therapist or patient is psychologically minded (YES) or not (NO), with sample dialogue that might take place between them when the question of psychological influence is brought up.

Therapist: NO/Patient: NO

Th: You don't think your headaches are psychosomatic or anything like that, do you?
Pt: Psychosomatic? Nah. The doctor said these are hereditary, or a chemical imbalance or something. Probably, just muscle spasms.

Therapist: YES/Patient: NO

Th: You know, medication and physical therapy may not be enough. Since you're still having headaches, I'm thinking we might need to look deeper for the cause. There are many ways that body habits, lifestyle, or emotions can produce and prolong headaches. Are you willing to widen our focus a little?
Pt: You're saying you can't help me? I thought these were simple muscle spasms! Are you implying I'm crazy?

Therapist: NO/Patient: YES

Th: Do I think your headaches come from stress? I doubt it. I can feel the knots in your shoulders—they're real.
Pt: But it seems like my headaches get worse when my boss is around. I think that he makes my muscles tense. I may not seem like it, but I worry a lot, and I hold grudges longer than I should.

Therapist: YES/Patient: YES

Th: Headaches can happen when you're struggling to meet the demands of life, and maybe feeling overwhelmed sometimes. You have heard people say "He gives me a headache" or "This project is going to be a real headache." I'm not sure

whether this applies to you, but have you ever thought about it?
Pt: Yeah, I'm glad you brought it up. I struggle all the time! Anyone would have a headache with a life like mine. I know you're not a shrink, but can we just talk for a minute?

WHAT THE PSYCHOLOGICALLY MINDED NONPSYCHOLOGIST CAN DO

Interviewers in a hurry tend to ask for yes/no responses, and they may even have a form with such boxes to check off. It is easier to process yes/no responses than to extract useful information from a stream of words, but the stream of words is usually easier for the patient to produce, and in the end provides much more information. Phrasing questions in dichotomous terms ("Are you depressed? Yes or no?") can terminate an inquiry prematurely and result in inaccurate polarization. On the other hand, some patients might not want to elaborate and may prefer yes/no responses. To get maximum information yield, use broad, open-ended questions, but make sure you have the time to listen to the answer. For example, instead of "Is stress a factor in your headaches?" say "Is there anything about your headache pattern that makes you wonder whether stress is involved?" Or instead of "Do you think muscle tension is causing your headaches?" try "Muscles don't get tense for no reason. Do you have an idea what might be behind all your muscle tension?"

Quick Psychological Screening

If the patient displays signs that worry you, consider the extent of depression, especially the risk of suicide. A simple question in a suitable context, such as "Are you losing your will to live?" or "Do you ever think about suicide?" will either bring a reassuring answer or something else that prods you to inquire further. Depression interferes with everything therapeutic: it will sap the motivation to follow directions, work against good health habits, interfere with natural relaxation and sleep, generally magnify pain and the emotional impact of it, and discourage adequate exercise.

Bipolar disorder occurs with migraine far higher than chance would predict (Low et al., 2003). A cyclic pattern of periodic excess energy with little need for sleep, over-ambitious plans, overcommitment, and an unusual lack of fatigue is the manic or hypomanic part; alternating with periods of lethargy, excess sleep, and depression, the whole picture could indicate bipolar disorder, which complicates headache management enormously by working against the steadiness and stability that seems to protect against migraine.

Be curious about physical or psychological trauma history and significant events around when the headache started, and correlations between recurring situations and headache (school finals, holidays, visits to family relatives, family disruptions, marital arguments, or job conflicts). Major changes in employment or residence disrupt routines and increase stress.

Signs That a Headache Pattern May Be Psychologically Influenced

Describing the headache process in physiologic terms does not exclude some psychological factors, just as describing headaches as products of perception, behavior, and emotion does not exclude the biological factors. Headaches with clear psychological input, however, might be labeled *psychologically influenced*. Any of the following signs would be suggestive:

- The patient does not respond to treatment. This item may be used as a way to blame the patient, but if an emotional or behavioral factor is maintaining a headache pattern and that factor is not addressed, then cure is being sought in the wrong place. A strong emotion may be affecting an intermediary system such as muscles, blood vessels, or biochemistry in a way that makes it resistant to medication.
- Symptoms respond a little, and then return or transform to another symptom. This may illustrate a transient placebo effect or it may show some aspect of the mind insisting on being heard.
- Half-hearted participation by the patient may indicate that the headache is being reinforced, serving a purpose, and the patient is ambivalent about eliminating it.
- Avoidance of psychological discussions could mean avoidance of an uncomfortable but important issue, or low interest or belief in psychological approaches, indicating a lack of psychological-mindedness—which probably makes the patient more susceptible to walled-off emotional effects. Much psychosomatic research supports the claim that lower psychological-mindedness increases the chance that strong feelings will be expressed somatically.
- Pain distribution is not anatomically accurate, but is symbolically meaningful—for example, the whole hand is numb rather than a particular dermatome. This happens with conversion disorder, for example.
- Headache is reliably aggravated or amplified by anxiety, especially anxiety about the headache. Asking about what the headache means to the patient might reveal fear of a brain tumor, for example, or evidence of personal weakness.

To check for certain kinds of headache etiology, ask about anniversary reactions and the circumstances surrounding when the headaches first began. Are there family members or friends with similar headaches? Just as husbands of pregnant wives can sometimes develop abdominal symptoms (sympathetic pregnancy, or *couvade*), developing headaches may provide symbolic or sympathetic identification with a loved one who has a cranial aneurysm or other secondary headache.

Listening to the Patient

Simple reassurance offered by a clinician who works with headaches should not be underestimated. Pain is a complex phenomenon that mixes together somatic sensations and emotions of anticipation, anxiety, suffering, and anger, along with fantasies of what is happening in the head to create the pain. The anterior cingulate cortex, a limbic brain structure, has been characterized as integrating distress signals from bodily and nonsomatic (social or psychological) sources, yielding a final amplification factor of suffering and distress. Reducing the psychological part of the equation by explanation and meaningful reassurance can create the equivalent of a placebo effect, which in matters of pain is not negligible.

It is natural for clinicians to listen to a patient with a problem-solving mind-set, staying alert for clues that might lead to solutions, eager to start helping, but this is not the only useful way to listen. Empathic listening, attending to a person's words without the helping agenda in mind, may feel risky, but sometimes it is a relief for both parties. Before agreeing to follow directions, patients want to feel understood; they need explanations about the cause of their headaches, and they need to have their fears addressed. Their bodies are not automobiles presented to a mechanic for repair. In the words of Dr. Charles Adler (1987): "The symptoms may not be helped by listening, but the patient is."

Non–mental health specialists can be very helpful, but it is important to realize one's limits—for instance, do not ask too much about a case of unresolved trauma. It can quickly get complicated, with surges of emotion, dissociation, and florid anxiety symptoms. Psychotherapists acquire a reluctance to open the box if they are not prepared to deal with the results.

Ways to Suggest Referral to Mental Health Care

Referral to a mental health practitioner or a headache management group can be for consultation, for parallel, adjunctive work while body-oriented therapy continues, or to take over the case because further physical therapy does not seem indicated. To make such referrals more effective, here are some sample phrasings:

- "I'd be in over my head, going into this, but I think you'd benefit from talking things over with someone. Just try one session and see if it interests you."
- "In your situation, it doesn't make sense to leave any possibility untried, because your headaches are really interfering with your life."
- "See what the psychologist (or other mental health professional) has to say. If you don't like how things are going, you can walk out. You're in control of what you do and say, so it can't hurt to get more information."
- "This referral doesn't mean I think you're mentally ill, or that you are making up your symptoms. But I know that strong emotions create physical changes that can underlie headaches."
- "You strike me as pretty smart and flexible; you could probably learn to manage better any emotions that have gotten stuck in your body."
- "Sometimes headaches happen for reasons that medicine and exercises just can't touch. For instance, there are 'anniversary headaches' that happen once a year on the date when someone died. Events can cause thoughts and feelings that affect the body and increase the chance of headaches."
- "The stressful situations you've named might not be the ones responsible for headaches; it's the

barely noticed underground reactions and feelings that can persist in the body."

However it is phrased, conveying that a psychological referral is simply a consultation with another specialist lessens the impression that the clinician is giving up or is desperate. It need not be a one-way referral, either, if the patient is reassured that his or her care is not being transferred to an unknown person in an unfamiliar discipline, and especially if a follow-up appointment is offered.

WHAT HAPPENS UPON REFERRAL TO A PSYCHOTHERAPIST?

In trying to change a chronic headache pattern from the psychological/behavioral angle, there are three broad categories of factors to consider: predisposing, situational, and triggering. The predisposing factors include genetic susceptibility and biological liabilities such as prior injury, as well as long-term emotional biases and distortions of attitudes and behavior. Situational factors might include issues in the realms of family, job setting, physical environment, favored activities, and emotional management. Trigger factors are thought to interact with the first two factors to provoke specific headaches. An excellent source for more detail on this kind of analysis can be found in *Psychological Management of Chronic Headaches* (Martin, 1993).

Psychotherapists vary in theoretical orientation, assumptions, and style, but when working with headaches, most would assume that since headaches are episodic, they might be related to episodic life events. This could mean physical triggers such as alcohol, glare, or loud noise, or subtler issues such as lack of sleep, prolonged fixed posture, or muscle overuse. More subtle yet are factors such as frustration, suppressed anger, perpetual time urgency, or a harsh, self-critical attitude. In each of these domains can be found an element of choice—whether conscious or not, intentional or not. A psychodynamic therapist might look for the deeper patterns; a behaviorist might emphasize current events in light of punishments and reinforcements; a cognitive-behavioral therapist would examine how thoughts affect behavior. Experienced psychotherapists usually are able to incorporate elements from a wide range of approaches, as appropriate to the individual case.

Even a simple, straightforward headache trigger may be complicated by the patient. For instance, suppose that fishing in mid-day on open water without sunglasses is identified as a headache trigger. The patient is advised to wear sunglasses when fishing, but several obstacles might appear: first, he keeps forgetting the sunglasses or he neglects to use them because he doubts they can prevent headaches, or he feels that sunglasses impair his visual acuity, or he resents being told to wear sunglasses when his father didn't have to wear them, or he may covertly be looking forward to his wife's care and concern that night upon returning home with a crippling headache. As soon as the occurrence of a trigger is subject to personal choice, psychology is involved, with factors such as motivation, self-awareness, self-discipline, memory, acceptance of limits, foresight, and intelligence hovering in the background to complicate a simple and reasonable proposal: wear sunglasses when you go fishing.

For another trigger example, consider lack of sleep: many factors can perpetuate the habit of skimping on sleep, and avoiding a headache may not be the patient's top priority. Reluctance to leave a party early, feeling unfairly restricted, fondness for late-night privacy, simple habit, a favorite late-night TV show, or some other factor can sabotage a plan for getting enough sleep. A therapist will most likely approach this as a behavior problem first, then consider emotional factors, and finally look at the possibility of self-sabotage.

Case Example: Victory over Parents

A 49-year-old man living alone had chronic, near-daily migraines clearly linked with how much sleep he got the night before. He usually chose to stay up as late as he possibly could. He was participating in a headache group, and his late-bedtime behavior, even though it guaranteed a headache the next day, piqued the attention of the group. Their questioning prompted him to look more deeply inside, and he finally identified the reason for his obstinacy regarding staying up late: in his childhood, his parents had demanded that he go to bed at a certain time. That activated a perpetual power struggle such that if he stayed up later than they authorized, he felt more grown up.

His parents were no longer in the picture, but he had internalized them, as if they were always mentally present. He felt victorious when he refused to give in to sleepiness, even though the grown-up part of him could acknowledge that it was foolish to deprive himself of rest and then suffer a headache the next day. The good feeling he derived from staying awake as long as he wanted was more powerful than logic. It felt good to him in the way a drink or a chocolate donut did.

Only after extended discussion in the group was he able to begin to devalue the "victory" he kept having. When he went to bed at a reasonable time, he felt better the next day. He could not do this every night, but he slowly increased his sleep time and reduced his headaches. Thus, a simple trigger turned out to have a tangle of other motives maintaining it.

Overcommitment to a job or family role is a familiar context for chronic headaches. The lack of breaks, the disdain for judicious pacing of tasks, the unquestioned rule to keep working until near-collapse—the entire pattern should become the focus of treatment rather than only the headaches. Presenting the concept of "preventive rest" may be effective only when framed as a way to prolong work time and ultimately get more work done. If the person feels that personal happiness can come only from more and better productivity, then a therapist's attempts to activate self-nurturing behavior may be futile. But if resting before the breakdown point can either postpone or prevent the next headache, this leads in the end to actually getting more work done. Everyone who drives has learned the advantage of refilling the gas tank before running out of gas, and this can be offered as a parallel to what might work with headache management.

Self-defeating patterns appear frequently when working with headache, chronic pain, or other health problems, and they confound the commonsense expectations of clinicians of every discipline. If a patient requests help with a particular symptom yet continues to defy or complies poorly with a therapeutic plan, it is easy to blame the patient for not cooperating. But this lack of cooperation should be included as an integral part of the problem, rather than considered only as an obstacle to the cure. The proper target of treatment is the headaches plus the behavior or emotions leading to the headaches, plus the resistance to change.

One way out of this impasse is to discern what, for the individual, seems more important than avoiding pain. Also to be considered is the self-regulating function of headaches: without the periodic headaches and the enforced interruption of the work pace, how else would this person obtain any rest?

Case Example: Art Versus Corporation

A 45-year-old aspiring artist was disabled by chronic migraines two to three times per week, and also had a fairly continuous tension-type headache focused in her neck and shoulders. Medication use was minimal, well below recommended limits. Her promising art career had been interrupted by the headache pattern, aggravated by shoulder tension from prolonged work with a paintbrush, so that she had to drop out of a painting class. She had sold some work at art shows and hoped to continue on this path. She enrolled in a group chronic headache program.

Some improvement occurred during the group as she learned to warm her hands and relax her shoulders. She learned many strategies and techniques, but no major advance happened until she spoke in the group about what would happen if her headaches went away. "I would have to go back to work," she said. She was asked to repeat it, because the group had assumed that she wanted to return to her art. She explained that before pursuing her art activities she had been working full time in a corporation. Lately her husband had said that she would have to return to that job because of the steady income, and she did not want to. The woman was generally unassertive, with a cheery, noncomplaining manner no matter what happened. She acknowledged that she was not good at expressing anger or resentment, and she denied any anger toward her husband for his rule. But during discussion, she saw that many other people would be resentful toward her husband in the situation she was in, and with sudden revelation she became aware of her own anger also.

The headaches were helping her to postpone returning to the job, but they were blocking her art work also. Her art was being sacrificed to keep her independent, and so she was unable to do anything productive. Once this situation was clarified, she understood that anger suppression was probably maintaining her headaches, and that they were also being reinforced by helping her to avoid returning to a job she did not want.

She tentatively discussed with her husband her wish to try returning to art before returning to a corporate job, and he was more flexible than she expected. They compromised with a plan for her to finish college classes that would qualify her to teach art; meanwhile, she could pursue her art career. The next week and thereafter, the headaches were down to about 20% of their former level.

STRESS

Definitions of human stress generally describe it as the response to a demand to cope with something. But there is great variability in designating what is stressful.

A job that is very demanding for one person is easy for another, depending on a person's attitude and experience. For instance, being hospitalized may reduce stress if a burden of responsibility is suspended; that is, being hospitalized offers a respectable opportunity for a rest. On the other hand, if the person cannot accept a break in responsibilities, then the hospitalization will be very stressful.

Any requirement to adapt is going to create at least temporary stress. This does not guarantee a headache, of course, but the activation of stress responses involving the hypothalamic-pituitary-adrenal axis, including more secretion of catecholamines and other stress hormones and neurotransmitters, destabilizes the nervous system and in some way puts a burden on the mechanism out of which headaches emerge—particularly the muscles of the head, neck, and shoulders, the intracranial and extracranial circulation, muscle TrPs, and the cortical neurons that are put under demand for continuous or enhanced performance. These biochemical and physiologic adjustments maximize physical readiness for some kind of threat or challenge, and headache prevention, or any kind of maintenance function, is given low priority biologically.

Stress, however, no matter how objectively measurable, is a subjective matter to the person who has it, and through habituation can be ignored, minimized, or denied. When asking a patient whether stress is likely to be a factor in headaches, the answer can be accepted without being automatically believed. The information given reveals something about what the person believes, but the interviewer should reserve judgment about whether stress is a factor until more information is gathered.

Emotional Stress and Psychological Factors in Headaches

Many surveys have concluded that stress, with various names, is a major contributor to chronic headaches. For instance, Henryk-Gutt and Rees (1973), in a large study of migraines in which patients kept records over a 2-month period, found that more than half of the 120 recorded migraines were due to emotionally stressful events. Also, more than half of these subjects reported that their first migraine occurred during a stressful period.

Lanzi et al. (1983), studying children suffering from migraine, found that 85% demonstrated repressed anger before an attack, and Maratos and Wilkinson (1982) found that "emotional upset" was the most frequently reported precipitating factor (86%) in the headaches of 47 migrainous children.

In the workplace and at home, psychological and social conflict can enhance noradrenaline release and stimulation of sympathetic dominance and tensing of muscles via intrafusal fibers of the muscle spindles. Opportunities for rest and recovery are bypassed, and quiet inner signals signaling head and neck imbalance are easily ignored. Emotional flare-ups and conflicts emerge as headache risk factors from many psychological studies of headache proneness.

The following are some common situations that have special potential for triggering, in susceptible people, not just single headaches but a pattern of recurrent headaches, whether migraine or tension-type, that can eventually turn chronic: (a) leaving home, (b) submitting to a domineering spouse, (c) marital tension (marriage ending or beginning), (d) work and career problems, (e) sexual and relationship problems, (f) disruption of home life (new additions or subtractions to the family unit that disrupt the social balance), (g) increased or decreased dependence, (h) transitions such as beginning a job, college, or new job, and (i) events leading to guilty feelings.

Case Example of a Psychological Trigger

The following example, though true, could be a prototype script for how to get a headache. A man in his 40s with migraines once or twice a week, participating in a weekly headache management program, had often discussed in the group his high sense of loyalty and duty toward his wife. He suspected that it could be a factor in his headache pattern in two ways: guilt over being unable to function during a headache attack, and compulsion to do what he thought was his duty as a husband.

One afternoon he was driving his wife across town to an early movie, with a grim determination to arrive on time. Commuter traffic was heavy, and he was frustrated, angry, and guilty over not planning well enough to get there on time. His wife, anticipating that he was developing a headache that would disable him most of the weekend, assured him that it was fine if they missed the movie or entered late, and that he should not push so hard just for her. He would not hear of it, but continued to plow his way through the traffic toward the theater. They arrived in time for the start of the movie, but by that time the warning signs of migraine were apparent, and he was disabled for most of the weekend.

This behavior was a common pattern for him, with only the specific task varying. Discussion in the group brought out that his wife felt that having his pain-free company for the weekend was more important to her than getting to a movie on time. Yet he had become so single-minded about keeping his promise to her that he could not turn off his headache-eliciting behavior. This stubbornness became the focus for self-change in the ensuing weeks as he kept his diary about his progress.

RELAXATION TRAINING

Many procedures and practices are designed to reduce overall arousal and facilitate relaxation in order to counteract tension that may be contributing to headaches. Research seems to support the efficacy of most of them if practiced sufficiently and applied on either a regular basis or as needed to prevent headache occurrence. Theories of how relaxation helps include reducing muscle ischemia, raising pain thresholds, soothing anxiety, rebalancing the autonomic nervous system, lowering sympathetic input to TrPs, reducing adrenaline output, and increasing feelings of control.

Autogenic training consists of a series of phrases to be repeated to oneself while imagining the desired change, always in the direction of homeostasis and improved functioning. These formulas constitute a structured form of self-hypnosis, on which the technique was originally modeled in the 19th century. "My hands are warm and heavy" (facilitating peripheral vasodilation and muscle relaxation), "my forehead is cool" (promoting cephalic vasoconstriction), and other phrases intended to normalize breathing, heart rate, and abdominal circulation can be powerful agents for normalizing bodily functioning. Results are not immediate; learning this type of self-regulation can take weeks to months. But extensive research on autogenic training shows good results with headaches (Linden, 1994).

Progressive muscle relaxation consists of sequential focusing on major muscle groups: slight tensing followed by thorough release while studying the waning sensation. This too can take many weeks to become effective: Although its domain is exclusively muscular, it still has autonomic effects and has been found effective in headache treatment (Blanchard et al., 1990). It is often used as a control condition against which other self-regulation methods are compared. Recommending that a patient learn either progressive relaxation or autogenics can be a nonthreatening way of introducing a patient to the possibility that his or her headaches can be provoked by stress. This can stimulate more thinking about psychological factors without suggesting mental disorder.

There is also good research evidence for meditation, controlled breathing, hypnosis, the relaxation response, guided imagery, and several other techniques for alleviating headaches. They all have in common taking time out to perform a structured exercise directed toward interrupting ongoing activities (perhaps simply a disguised rest period) in which a patient intends, in a noneffortful way, to self-regulate. The targets are a combination of thought content, emotionality, and physiologic state. The somatic factors that may seem to underlie chronic headaches may be only mediators between headache phenomena and psychological strain. Penzien et al. (2002) review and summarize the evidence for behavioral management of recurrent headaches. The U.S. Headache Consortium (Campbell et al., 2000) studied many such strategies and routines and concluded that there was "Grade A" evidence (multiple well-designed clinical trials) for thermal and electromyographic (EMG) biofeedback, cognitive therapy, and relaxation training; they all could be recommended for headache treatment.

BIOFEEDBACK

Biofeedback has been prominent in headache intervention for many years, despite vaguely specified mechanisms involving extracerebral circulation, neck and head muscle tension, central nervous system calming, and generalized arousal. When aberrant physiologic states are found to correlate with either specific headache events ("state") or with individuals who are subject to headaches ("trait"), it is tempting to assume causation and then attempt to change the physiologic state via biofeedback training. In principle this resembles teaching a dog to wag its tail to make it happy. Success would indicate a bidirectional relationship between a central and a peripheral state. A similar concept underlies biofeedback training, and often enough, it works, suggesting that with chronic headaches, the symptom complex can be interdicted at many different levels. Although biofeedback is based on altering some aspect of physiology underlying a given symptom, the nonspecific effect, in common with the relaxation techniques detailed earlier, may be the more important factor.

Biofeedback usually involves displaying to a patient the moment-to-moment status of the relevant body variable, usually muscle tension, hand temperature, peripheral or temporal pulse pressure (pulse volume amplitude), or other somatic variables measurable from the body surface. Learning to control such things takes practice, close self-observation, and faith in the process, because improvement is rarely immediate.

It is not a "treatment" in the usual sense, but more like tutoring and learning a specific kind of self-regulation, similar to assigning stretching as homework. Success with biofeedback often depends on the patient learning the skill to specific criteria with the aid of an instrument to reflect the process, and then applying the skill in real life without the biofeedback available. It can be applied either for routine preventive maintenance or as a response to warning signs of impending headache. The biofeedback apparatus provides a temporary learning aid, with objective indicators of progress. Although a nonspecific relaxation effect is hard to rule out, some studies have shown a specific advantage of biofeedback for headaches over other relaxation techniques (Arena et al., 1995; Silberstein, 2000; Nestoriuc & Martin, 2007).

Work with headaches using biofeedback typically utilizes surface electromyography and/or hand temperature, with instruments able to detect and display tiny moment-to-moment physiologic changes. Several model approaches are commonly used, as described in the following subsection.

Sample Biofeedback Approaches

- Scan resting muscle tension in cervical, facial, and scalp muscles and compare with norms. If too high, train down to criteria with and then without the feedback. Train the patient to accurately detect and control excess muscle tension.
- Provide EMG biofeedback from certain muscles thought to contribute to the headache; display to the patient fluctuations in tension correlated with postures and movements (such as fixed computer-related positions) and find an optimal combination of body use or position and minimal muscle tension.
- Using generalized relaxation as a goal, give feedback of overall muscle tension, peripheral skin temperature, skin conductance, variables of breathing, heart rate variability, and perhaps electroencephalography. Train for maximum relaxation and the ability to reach the state without feedback.

- Set voluntary peripheral vasodilation as the goal, and give hand temperature biofeedback to reinforce tiny rises in skin temperature (this correlates with autonomic nervous system shift toward parasympathetic dominance). Train the ability to do this without biofeedback. Monitor somatic variables while the patient talks about stressful incidents suspected to contribute to the headaches. Point out the body effects of the descriptions or recollections.
- Monitoring the relevant physiology, demonstrate the bodily effects of activities thought to be related to the headaches (e.g., operating equipment, occupational actions, computer work). Show the effect of rest breaks and prolonged activity without a break.

Reaching and holding a physiologic criterion, and being able to do it without the aid of biofeedback, is the essence of the biofeedback approach. The assumption is that extending the individual's influence into normally automatic domains confers power to self-regulate away from a headache. The learning process normally takes weeks to months, but can provide hope and goal-directed engagement long before that. Monitoring various muscle groups, temporal pulse volume, and variables of breathing, skin conductance, hand temperature, and direct current (DC) scalp potential can help patients interact and gain influence over their biological self. Further procedural details can be found in Schwartz and Andrasik (2003).

More esoteric methods not easily available clinically have supported the general potential of biofeedback of the components of headaches. For instance, McGrady et al. (1994) and Vasudeva et al. (2003) both used feedback blood flow velocity in the middle cerebral artery using transcranial Doppler. Migraineurs showed significant improvement compared with self-directed relaxation.

Functional magnetic resonance imaging (real-time monitoring of subcortical brain activity) has been used to provide a feedback loop to subjects from the anterior cingulate cortex (ACC), a brain structure involved in both negative affect and pain perception (deCharms et al., 2005). Subjects observed a visual display that reflected in near real time the activity of the ACC, and they tried to affect its activity by various kinds of concentration. Reducing this signal—watching one's brain in the act of hurting—resulted in temporary pain reduction. This technique has not been specifically applied to

headaches, but it does offer promise for chronic pain control in general.

Contingent Negative Variation: Slow Cortical Potential

The variable of cortical potential, measured from the scalp, is now being studied in relation to migraines. The resting DC potential of the cerebral cortex becomes more negative when primed to respond to a stimulus or making a choice based on stimulus discrimination. Compared with control groups without migraine, migraineurs seem to be closer to this primed state much of the time, especially before the onset of a migraine. This may indicate that the brain is in a greater state of readiness to respond, and is supported by increased noradrenaline release. Furthermore, habituation to a repeated stimulus (getting used to something) is delayed in migraineurs compared with controls, which fits with greater readiness to respond. Some studies show that this difference is maintained between headaches, but the cortical negativity is most likely to appear 1 to 3 days before a migraine, and goes away when the headache subsides (Siniatchkin et al., 1999). Presenting a challenging achievement task also changed the brains of migraineurs toward negativity, compared with non-migrainous controls (Siniatchkin et al., 2006).

Research so far has been mostly on the basic mechanism rather than using contingent negative variation (CNV) as a biofeedback training procedure, but one controlled study did show clinical improvement. Migrainous children learned to reduce their CNV in response to a vigilance-discrimination task during a series of 10 training sessions. As their CNV normalized, their headaches significantly improved (Siniatchkin et al., 2000). In another study, treatment of migraineurs with metoprolol (a beta-blocker) reduced headache frequency and also made the CNV pattern closer to normal (Siniatchkin et al., 2007). Future research may determine whether noradrenaline- and/or adrenaline-reducing relaxation procedures can approximate the effects of beta-blockers on headaches, using CNV as an indicator.

This research extends earlier conclusions about the role of prolonged attention and mental tension in creating a fertile climate for migraines. Early observers such as Friedman (1982) and Graham (1968), did not know the specifics of modern brain electrophysiology, but they generally agreed on the attention style, behavior, and attitude that made headaches more likely.

Becoming less primed for choice or action, and adapting more quickly to things that are routine and predictable, may be an effective self-generated antimigraine remedy.

Jaw clenching and grinding are often cited as headache triggers, yet it has not been conclusively shown that chronic headache patients actually have tighter jaw muscles. Hypersensitivity of muscles with normal tension is an alternate possibility rarely explored. One interesting study of jaw tension and headaches (Jensen & Olesen, 1996) asked two groups of subjects (headache-prone and non–headache-prone) to maintain mild tooth clenching for 30 minutes. Both groups experienced jaw tenderness afterward, but in the subjects prone to tension-type headaches, 69% developed head pain within 24 hours. Of the nonheadache subjects, only 17% did. The authors speculated about a deficiency in pain modulation in chronic headache patients, perhaps from central sensitization or increased sensitivity to incoming stimuli. This study illustrates the point made earlier, that identical bodily stresses will create headaches in some people and not others, depending on prior susceptibility to headaches.

SELF-REGULATION: FROM PASSIVE TO ACTIVE

Many patients with chronic headaches enter treatment with the idea that their headaches are similar to weather changes: occurring out of the blue, independent of anything the patient does, and responsive only to medication, manipulation or massage, or perhaps a vacation. They may believe that they are simply deficient in their preferred medication, and if they only take enough then everything will be fine.

The concept of avoidable headache triggers challenges the headache victim's view that the headaches are independent events, and introduces instead the idea of self-care and taking some responsibility for headache occurrence. If avoiding triggers was considered at all, it was typically in a superficial way, for instance, "I tried not drinking red wine and not eating blue cheese, and I still had headaches." But triggers can be more subtle than that, and more psychological.

A simple starting approach would be to begin giving greater priority to headache prevention than to other considerations, such as getting more work done, continuing service to others (at the extreme, semivoluntary servitude), or honoring commitments no matter what. Deciding to take preventive breaks, not just stopping

activity because a headache makes it impossible anyway, means adopting some responsibility for the headaches rather than seeing them as an inconvenience to be banished with medication.

John Graham (1968) wrote, "Migraine is the ticket given by Nature's policeman for speeding." This statement can be expanded to describe the path taken by many chronic headache patients. The speeding ticket or headache is the undesirable endpoint of a process that can usually be prevented. Watching one's speed is comparable to monitoring one's emotions, body state, exposure to known triggers, and so on. If the speed stays within normal limits, then police attention is not attracted and there is no ticket or headache.

But suppose the habitually speeding driver becomes frustrated with the tickets and takes his car to a mechanic: "This car keeps going too fast, and I keep getting tickets. Can you fix it?" The mechanic could install a speed governor to limit the speed (beta-blocker, tricyclic antidepressant, or other medication). Or he could give the driver a special "No ticket, please, my brother is on the force" card to show to the officer (abortive medication). But chances are the mechanic will mention something like "You're driving your car too fast!" The driver, feeling blamed for the problem, might then ask a surgeon to weaken his calf muscle, thinking the problem is that his leg is pressing down too hard on the accelerator pedal. The surgeon explains that the problem starts higher up, with his decision to drive fast and ignore the speed limit. The driver might then go to a psychiatrist for a medication that removes the speeding urge, or he might at last come to terms with the need to take responsibility for the speeding tickets.

COGNITIVE-BEHAVIORAL THERAPY

Cognitive-behavioral therapy is a widely used and well-researched style of psychotherapy that focuses on "automatic thoughts," the near-reflexive default reactions and interpretations that may pop into consciousness or stay underground but either way can trigger particular feelings and behavior. Many automatic thoughts are desirable and useful; for instance, as a response to persuasion ("Resist sales pressure!"), sensing physical danger ("That car's going to hit me!"), and noting social disapproval ("I just said the wrong thing"). Automatic thoughts (Beck, 1976) serve the function of initial orientation to ongoing reality.

But trouble arises when these rapid responses are inaccurate and misleading. Nobody is correct all the time, but perceiving reality accurately is generally a good thing. The concept of cognitive distortions deals with how an individual reacts to something with an interpretation that does not fit with the reality of the moment. This error often reflects a fixed bias in responding based on childhood learning, traumatic experience, or excessive anxiety.

Related to headaches, there are two areas of distortion to consider: reactions to the headache already under way and reactions to preheadache events that could increase the chance of a headache.

Reaction to Onset of Headache: Example

A person may tend to feel overwhelmed and panicky at the first migraine warning sign. The feeling does not emerge from nowhere, but is triggered by a quick "flash" thought interposed between noticing the warning sign and reacting in some dysfunctional way such as bracing the neck muscles in expectation of pain, taking premature medication beyond the recommended dosage, or canceling work that day because of certainty that the headache will be disabling.

This automatic thought would be something such as "Oh my God, here we go again!" or "This is going to be bad. I can't do anything about this." But if the headache warning sign has not always led to a major headache, the catastrophic interpretation of the warning sensation could be in error. Note that the interpretation of the sensation precedes and triggers the emotional response, if only by a few seconds. Changing that interpretation, and therefore the emotion and the behavior, is the goal of cognitive-behavioral therapy.

If this person were asked to consider alternate interpretations of the warning sensation, he or she may initially resist but could probably, with prompting, agree that yes, this warning sign has not always led to a bad headache, and yes, there may be some constructive action he or she could take, and yes, sometimes the headache is only moderate and not disabling. There will usually be emotional resistance to these alternatives, and so a therapist would proceed slowly, leading a review of the evidence for the cognitive distortion and helping the patient to see the discrepancy between the distorted version and the more accurate version.

After this, the therapist and patient would explore how a more constructive emotional response to the warning sign would lead to different behavior: for example, using a relaxation technique, taking a stretch break, applying ice preventively, postponing medication or using it as prescribed, and perhaps not calling in sick for the day (or week). These alternate behaviors increase the chance of avoiding a major headache, but become options only when the cognitive distortion is challenged. This therapeutic process can take several sessions to engage the patient's active participation, but eventually a pattern is established that can be applied to many other situations.

Preheadache Stage: Example

The previous example applies to the headache itself. The other arena for change is in the preheadache stage, upstream, where an individual has much more potential influence. Habitual behaviors and emotional biases are the target here: posture, body use, overwork and fatigue, choices about rest and sleep, attitudes toward work and family, and managing hostility, anxiety, and anger are all subject to change.

A chronic headache patient is told that forward head posture is a risk factor for his chronic headaches. He is advised to correct and limit this head position, and in the therapist's office, he can do this. The daily habit, however, is the appropriate target. Just as a person can drive under the speed limit when a policeman is nearby but at other times routinely drives too fast, changing body use with full attention in a therapeutic context may not generalize to everyday behavior because of competing priorities.

Suppose prolonged computer work is the problem. In competition with good head and neck positioning is the desire to meet a work deadline, or grinding persistence until the project is finished, or resenting that coworkers do not worry about their head position or need to take breaks. Perhaps the person looks at the clock and sees work time diminishing. The automatic thought here would be "I have to finish this on time," which leads to anxiety about not finishing on time, which leads to continuing to work through a break time, with the end result being yet another headache. Or, close to the end of the task, the thought flashes: "Don't give up until it's finished. Keep going until you're done." Either of these thoughts gives rise to an emotion (time urgency, anxiety, resolve to keep pushing) and also to an associated behavior: continuing to work at the computer with head forward and shoulders tensed.

The automatic thought happens so quickly that it cannot be blocked, only noted and resisted. But reflection will reveal other possibilities about what to think. Challenging the "I have to finish on time" commandment can diminish the urge to rush. The "Keep going until you're done" imperative may come from a belief that the project is so complicated that interrupting it will cause it to crash down, or that the creative magic will disappear. That belief too can be subjected to rational scrutiny. In this case, a 5-minute break, resting and changing the head position, may make a difference between headache and no headache. This self-care moment becomes suddenly available only because an automatic thought was questioned.

Thinking "My coworkers don't have to worry about their head position, and they don't get headaches!" may lead to resentment and self-denial, but could be inaccurate, or, even if accurate, irrelevant to the desire of the patient to prevent personal headaches. A more adaptive thought might be "I do seem to have to worry about headaches more than other people, but so what if I do? My coworkers probably have other problems that I don't."

Learning to identify an automatic thought as only a tentative guide for feelings and behavior, rather than the only possible interpretation, helps the patient to consider alternatives and promotes greater behavioral flexibility, including better body use, better emotional management, and wiser use of time.

Cognitive Distortions

Here are some other common cognitive distortions often relevant to headache management. These all contain automatic thoughts that usually occur quickly, without reflection, in response to provoking situations. They all express a reflexive bias that encourages premature closure and limits further consideration. These distortions all have in common the potential to activate physiologic stress responses and hypervigilance, which can initiate and prolong chronic headaches.

Catastrophic Thinking

Catastrophic thinking is the tendency to anticipate the worst possible outcome and leap to dire conclusions. It distorts reality in the direction of disaster, activates physiologic alarms, and works against rational thought. When used to excess, it creates a perpetual alarm state, bracing for what seems like certain disaster. It is a frequent component of depressive and anxiety disorders.

Example: A warning sign of approaching headache is noticed.

Response: "Here we go again. I'm in for it this time. Why bother going to work? I'll probably just have to come home."

This response bypasses self-help moves and ignores evidence that the warning sign does not always lead to a disabling headache. This style can be hard to give up, even though the catastrophic prediction is usually wrong. There may in fact develop a superstitious linkage between the negative prediction and the usually positive outcome, so that if this sequence recurs often enough, it seems as if the negative thinking causes the positive outcome. A person with this bias may actually fear optimistic thinking because it could put him or her at risk of being caught unprepared. This distortion works like a tinder-dry forest flaring up from one spark. "I must have a brain tumor that they're not telling me about" is one example, or "I'll never get better," or "I'll lose my job, family, or sanity."

Denial

Denial is a protective strategy. By postponing conscious recognition of an undesirable possibility, peace is prolonged and negative facts are ignored. Facing an unpleasant fact may mean changing one's activities and adjusting to something, so this is delayed by denying a warning sign. The mind scrambles for facts that support the denial against the onslaught of evidence to the contrary.

Example: A person rushing to complete a project begins to feel cold hands, and sounds seem louder.

Response: Keep rushing and ignore the warning signs of approaching migraine.

By denying the evidence that a headache is trying to happen and giving the project priority, the work can continue. Taking a break, doing some stretches, taking an abortive medication, or even postponing the project may prevent the headache, and the project could still be finished.

"Should" and "Should Not" Statements

"Should" and "should not" statements refer to rigid thinking and concern with "right" and "wrong" thoughts, feelings, and behaviors. They lead to being critical, either of the self ("I should be doing better") or of other people

("I shouldn't be treated this way"). The stricter the standards, the more impossible they are to meet. These types of automatic thoughts are filled with negative judgments and evaluations, and either condemnations or demands for improvement. The headache itself can be a trigger: "I should be able to prevent these things" or "This shouldn't be happening to me."

Black-or-White Thinking

Black-or-white thinking refers to artificially clear-cut dichotomous categories: something is either good or bad, successful or not successful, with no in-between. Partial failure with a headache treatment feels the same as a complete failure. With this distortion, headaches are seen as organically caused or psychologically caused, but not both. This strict categorical thinking may be efficient in emergencies when quick decisions are essential ("friend or enemy?"), but in headache management it impairs progress because improvements usually start small and build with practice. The slow, steady progress required to break a headache pattern, either by persisting with treatment or applying self-care techniques, is incompatible with black-or-white thinking.

Overgeneralization

Akin to black-or-white thinking, overgeneralization involves making premature conclusions without enough data. It discourages thoughtful consideration of evidence. Such a person is likely to use the terms *always* and *never*. If aged cheese seems to trigger a headache just once, the individual prone to rapid closure will see the cheese as a headache trigger forever. If a bit of negative feedback occurs at work, it means a pattern of criticism that will go on and on. When such dire conclusions are reached too soon, emotional flares are triggered inappropriately.

Magnification and Minimization

The twin distortions of magnification and minimization usually serve a negative bias, so that evidence of personal shortcomings, errors, and negative feedback loom large, whereas successes and compliments are discounted or do not seem to count much. Minimizing a 10% improvement in headache intensity, for example, will lessen the patient's interest in further treatment or more self-care. Setbacks are magnified out of proportion, so that objective learning from setbacks is made difficult.

Mind Reading

The essence of mind reading is skipping past the usual rules of evidence to a dire conclusion without requiring more proof. Thus, a person may be convinced of being snubbed socially because of not being greeted on the street. The person may be certain that the physiotherapist is frustrated about progress, that the doctor does not believe the pain report, or that friends are not calling because they are scornful of the continuing headaches. Evidence to the contrary (the therapist is merely being patient, the doctor accepts the pain report as valid, and friends feel awkward about bothering the patient in case she has a headache) is not sought or considered.

Emotional Reasoning

Saddled with the distortion pattern of emotional reasoning, people give little credence to actual evidence other than their feelings. Whatever they feel is, they are certain, objectively true. Respecting one's intuition has a place if it has usually been successful in predicting the future or helping to make good choices, but feelings can be based on many things other than reality: a traumatic past, powerful wishing, phobias, associating present events with past ones, and so on.

This pattern leads to inappropriate emotional reactions, which flare up the physiology and exacerbate or create headaches. It also may cause resistance to headache-prevention advice ("I feel better when I take long drives. So how could it be bad for my headaches?").

Pain Catastrophizing

The cognitive variable of pain catastrophizing is defined as a tendency to focus excessively on pain sensations. The Pain Catastrophizing Scale (PCS, first developed by Sullivan [1995]) consists of 13 items such as "I can't stop thinking about how much it hurts," "I worry that something serious might happen," and "There is nothing I can do to stop the intensity of the pain." Its three subscales are Helplessness, Rumination, and Magnification (*rumination* refers to repetitive worrying). The PCS has successfully predicted responses of both pain patients and normal control subjects to various experimental pain measures such as the cold pressor test (Michael & Burns, 2004). The authors concluded: "Catastrophizing about pain may affect pain severity and distress of chronic pain patients through a bias toward processing the most disturbing elements of a painful stimulus."

Pain catastrophizing is a relatively stable and enduring trait (Sullivan et al., 2001). In a study of the PCS's ability to predict severity of symptoms in patients with upper respiratory tract illness (Devoulyte & Sullivan, 2003), the subscale of Rumination seemed to best predict intensity of reported symptoms. A study of 169 chronic pain patients using analysis of pain diaries showed that the Helplessness subscale was the best predictor of pain level, and that passive pain coping and helplessness combined were the best predictors of disability (Samwel, 2006).

Thorn et al. (2007) demonstrated that chronic headache patients engaged in intensive cognitive therapy to alter pain catastrophizing achieve significant improvements. Headache frequency and peak intensity, as well as depression, catastrophizing, and anxiety, were all affected positively. These results from brief therapy indicated a broad positive effect not only on headache itself, but also on several associated psychological variables that improve the life of patients and may help alleviate the conditions that create the headache pattern.

OTHER PSYCHOLOGICAL INPUTS TO HEADACHE

Headaches can be triggered or worsened by some ongoing psychophysiologic effect in which events arouse emotions that act as a bridge between mental and physical domains. For instance, habitual neck and head muscle bracing may be tied to continuing anger, fear, or conflict. Biochemical effects, vasoconstriction, and general sympathetic arousal may be chronically activated from anger, resentment, or anxiety. Choices about how to use one's body include issues such as prolonged static tension without a break, postural abnormalities, and simple habit. Choosing to stay in noxious, trigger-laden environments can boost headache risk in a direct way. Adler et al. (1987) mention that fixed facial expressions, such as the frozen grin of the receptionist or flight attendant, constitute prolonged isometric muscle contraction with limited excursion (this may apply even to the extraocular eye muscles from doing close work). If the person is either stuck in a single emotional expression or is stuck simulating it, there are consequences for muscle circulation, with tissue nutrient replenishment reduced. To the fixed grin might be added a perpetual look of interest via raised eyebrows, or a grim, determined look as

expressed by a tight jaw. Neck muscles may also be subject to the same strain if they are deprived of the usual head turning and nodding, and subjected instead to an unvarying expression or posture.

Anger

From the early observation in 1743 by the physician Junkerius, "*Ira, in primus tacita et suppressa*" ("Initially anger, unspoken and suppressed"), headache researchers and clinicians have often pinpointed suppressed anger as a prime emotional factor in triggering headaches. Frieda Fromm-Reichmann (1937) describes the fear of being cast out of a group or family for expressing hostility, and how commonly her migraine patients maintained ambivalence about their anger toward a loved one, ever fearful of rebuke for disloyalty. Other writers mention the frequent discovery, in the families of migraine patients, of "house rules" discouraging expression of anger.

Charles Adler, a psychiatrist, headache specialist, and first author of *Psychiatric Aspects of Headache*, had a descriptive phrase for this condition: "Anger that cannot be acted upon yet cannot be forgotten" (Adler et al., 1987, p. 117).

Much research on the psychological concomitants to chronic migraines has concluded that anger is involved somehow, but it was often confounded in the research with anxiety, depression, and other emotions, and the distinction between anger expression and suppression was not fully examined. Arena et al. (1997) used a specific measure of anger suppression, the "anger-in" scale of the State-Trait Anger Expression Inventory, to conclude that tension headache patients scored significantly higher on this dimension than a control group. Kerns (1994) also found that a style of inhibiting angry feelings was the strongest predictor of chronic pain intensity, interference with daily life, and pain behavior. Kerns's subjects were chronic pain patients rather than headache patients only. Nicholson et al. (2003) examined differences in dimensions of anger between headache and nonheadache subjects, and again found that although trait anger, depression, and anxiety were all important to headache intensity, anger suppression ("anger-in") was the strongest predictor of headache status.

Other Psychological Factors

Apart from suppressed anger, other psychological factors often mentioned are depression, unreasonable

Chapter 33 | Psychological Aspects of Chronic Headache Treatment | 463

persistence without a break, rigid standards for self and others, and reluctance to rest, or in Harold Wolff's words, "unwillingness to bow to low points in their energy cycle." There is often a combination of self-imposed extra responsibilities and high standards, perpetual time pressure, and self-criticism. Wolff mentions "Fear of failure to *excel*" (not just fear of failure). Wolff also mentions that migraineurs are unusually preoccupied with moral and ethical problems and do not understand why their peers are not. W. C. Alvarez (1965), after studying 500 patients with migraine, observed a prevalence of excessive commitments, a tendency to overwork, and that "they always kept their engines at the strain." A general conflict between expectation and reality seems to aggravate headache tendencies. In Australia, migraines are often referred to as "trap headaches," referring to the insoluble conflicts and unresolvable vicious circles, such as being forbidden to say or do something for which one has a strong need or urge.

Seymour Diamond, director of the Headache Clinic in Chicago for many years, stated: "Depression is probably the single most prevalent cause of headache" (1987). The route from emotional states to physiologic dysregulation and eventual headache has not been fully elucidated, but probably involves behavioral, self-care, emotional, biochemical, and neurologic factors.

Arnold Friedman, after years of running a headache clinic at Montefiore Hospital in New York, concluded from over 5,000 chronic headache cases that psychological factors were relevant to over 90% of them. He named as prime factors difficulty handling aggression (either the patient's or that of others) and early training to value the approval of others more than the patient's own (Friedman, 1982).

Accidental Reinforcement

If a naturally occurring headache accidentally results in some advantage or favorable outcome, it may become reinforced and be more likely to recur. Headaches can serve a function that to the patient is more important than avoiding pain. For instance, a headache can postpone or terminate an argument, help avoid sex, serve as a cry for help from an otherwise unhelpful spouse, buy time, or postpone an obligation. A recurring headache pattern can prevent divorce, avoid job promotion or the start of school, or provide an excuse to take pills that sedate or reduce anxiety.

Headaches may allow a person to take a break from duties otherwise not easily escaped. A headache pattern can disrupt a marriage or can keep it together by activating caretaking and better treatment by the spouse. Headaches can serve as a cry for help or provide an excuse for taking narcotics or tranquilizers. Headaches can both express guilt and provide expiation from self-condemnation. All this can go on unconsciously in the service of the patient's needs.

"Marital migraine" is often mentioned anecdotally, often with sardonic humor. But one study of 40 married couples, compared with an unmarried control group, observed the response of chronic headache patients to prophylactic medication. Seventy-one percent of the unmarried patients responded, but only 17% of the married patients (Featherstone & Beitman, 1984).

MYOFASCIAL TRIGGER POINTS AND SYMPATHETIC INPUT

Though still unknown to many physicians, myofascial TrPs are quite capable of generating and referring pain plus autonomic symptoms. When located in the neck, shoulder, or facial muscles, they can be contributory or causative for both tension-type and migraine headaches (Fernández-de-las-Peñas et al., 2006). Trigger points are not completely static structures, but are somewhat variable in activity and may switch from active to latent status. They are susceptible to emotional influence through the sympathetic nervous system, which can be modulated by relaxation techniques and aggravated by strong negative emotions. McNulty et al. (1994) showed that trigger point activity, measured by EMG, increased under greater sympathetic load brought on by mentally stressful tasks such as mental calculations. Chung et al. (2004) demonstrated that increasing sympathetic outflow to a myofascial painful area (TrP) increased its electromyographic activity, and Ge et al. (2006) found that increasing sympathetic activity lowered pain-pressure thresholds in TrPs. Injecting phentolamine, a sympathetic blocker, into the arterial system reduced spontaneous electrical activity from muscle TrPs in rabbits (Chen et al., 1998). Thus, by several experimental tests, it seems that sympathetic nervous system activity, whether activated physiologically or by emotional stress, will increase myofascial pain and also the electrical activity of the TrP itself. Not only short-term stress but more chronic states of anxiety and depression—also associated with sympathetic excess (Hughes et al.,

2004)—could be considered potentiators of trigger points and thus chronic headaches.

PLACEBO AND NOCEBO EFFECTS

The placebo effect would be better named "expectation" because it does not depend on the well-known inert pill but on the anticipation of relief from the pill. People vary in how readily they believe that help is on the way, but the power of that belief is considerable. For instance, a study of 1,420 headache patients seen in several British neurologic clinics (Fitzpatrick & Hopkins, 1981) examined which factor most strongly predicted improvement over the year following the consultation. Those who felt that the consultation was valuable in relation to their concerns (assessed during the visit) experienced the best results in the following year. Drug treatment initiation or changes were less important than satisfaction with the consultation, including matters such as explanations, reassurance, and rapport.

Modern headache research usually includes a placebo condition because a 30% to 50% response to any medication can be expected, and positive response to the active agent must be substantially higher than the placebo response rate. To the researcher, this self-generated improvement is probably annoying and complicates the research process. But to the patient and the clinician, the placebo response offers nonpharmaceutical promise that does not require deception. The placebo phenomenon implies that specific techniques used for headaches by practitioners of every discipline will yield good results at least a third of the time. This success is not due to the technique itself, but to the patient's psychological response to it—that is, the anticipation of relief, which not only feels good but has biochemical consequences. The magnitude of this response may depend on personality variables, but attempts to define a "placebo personality" have not been successful. Although sometimes assumed by physicians and patients alike, gullibility and low intelligence do not seem to be responsible, and neither does the variable of hypnotizability. (Hypnosis works its effects in a way that does not involve endorphins.)

Placebo response cannot be reduced to self-deception, distraction, ability to ignore pain, or any strictly psychological explanation. In an early study (Levin et al., 1978), endorphin release was seen to be enhanced during apparent placebo responses, and was diminished by naltrexone, an opiate antagonist. More recently, endorphin secretion has been extensively studied in the context of placebo responses (Zubieta et al., 2005). Using positron emission tomography (PET) monitoring of several brain regions involved in pain modulation, including the anterior cingulate and nucleus accumbens, researchers found that activity in the brain's mu-opioid receptor system corresponded with how much pain relief subjects felt from (unknown to them) inert substances. The neurotransmitter dopamine was also found to correlate with both degree of pain relief and degree to which the subject expected pain relief (dopamine rises in response to amphetamine, nicotine, and cocaine). In other words, the amount of benefit anticipated by a person from a given painkiller, genuine or spurious, modulates the increase in both dopamine and endorphins, which then reduce pain intensity. Subjects varied in their capacity to block their own pain by belief; some subjects were labeled "high placebo responders" and others had less response. Whether this is a stable personality trait or can be altered through manipulating belief factors awaits research.

Wager et al. (2007) have shown via PET scans that the biological facet of the placebo response correlates with activity in the frontal and limbic structures that are part of the descending inhibitory pain-modulation system: the periaqueductal gray matter and anterior cingulate in particular. These structures participate in evaluating the probable danger of noxious stimuli, and they facilitate pain reduction via both neurologic (synaptic inhibition) and biochemical (endogenous opiate) mechanisms. This is also consonant with the pain gate concept of Melzack and Wall (1965).

These recent findings may seem to place placebo responding more in the physiologic realm than the psychological, but the psychological factor still comes first, activating the expectation and belief needed to activate pain suppression by biochemical means.

Nocebo: The Negative Effect of Pain Anxiety

Relaxation procedures have in common the reduction of anxiety, apprehension, and emotional agitation, and success seems to carry the bonus of somatic consequences, such as reducing noradrenaline and TrP sensitivity. Because of this nonspecific factor, matching a specific technique with the particular pain pathophysiology may not matter so much. But this mental input to pain control has been found to work both ways: research with "nocebo" responses has shown that the peptide hormone cholecystokinin (CCK) seems to oppose endorphins, amplifying pain. A nocebo is the opposite of a placebo, meaning harm resulting from expectation alone, and Benedetti et al. (2007) found that negative expectations about pain increased pain through the mediation of CCK, which facilitates pain transmission. Biochemical antagonists to CCK were found to block the rise in pain. If CCK is a biochemical expression of pain catastrophizing, then it seems important to attend to the inner expectations of people in pain in order to prevent what amounts to anxiety-based hyperalgesia.

CONCLUSIONS

Headache management and treatment usually proceeds with some tool or outside aid, such as medication or injections from the physician or hands-on techniques from the physical therapist. Psychologists must depend for their effectiveness mainly on words, reaching and influencing aspects of a person in a way that alters their biochemistry, neural activity, and physiology. Words, by triggering thoughts and feelings, can manipulate physiology as surely as hands and chemicals can, though the effects are more subtle and interact with the mind of the patient. Rudyard Kipling wrote, "Words are, of course, the most powerful drug used by mankind. Not only do words infect, egotize, narcotize, and paralyze but they enter into and color the minutest cells of the brain" (Kipling, 1923).

That the ultimate causes of pain and headaches seem to be chemical and physiologic does not mean that only physiologic factors are relevant; positive expectations, apprehension, anxiety, and calmness all create physiologic changes that are like bodily shadows of the mind.

REFERENCES

Adler CS, Adler SM. Psychodynamics of head pain: an introduction. In: Adler CS, Adler SM, Packard RC, eds. *Psychiatric Aspects of Headache*. Baltimore: Williams & Wilkins; 1987.

Alvarez WC. A life-time study of migraine. *Headache* 1965;5: 35–37.

Arena JG, Bruno GM, Hannah SL, Meader KJ. Comparison of frontal electromyographic biofeedback training, trapezius electromyographic biofeedback training, and progressive muscle relaxation therapy in the treatment of tension headache. *Headache* 1995;35:411–419.

Arena JG, Bruno GM, Rozantine GS, Meador KJ. A comparison of tension headache sufferers and nonpain controls on the State-Trait Anger Expression Inventory: an exploratory study with implications for applied psycho-physiologists. *Appl Psychophysiol Biofeedback* 1997;22:209–214.

Beck AT. *Cognitive Therapy and the Emotional Disorders*. New York: International Universities Press; 1976.

Benedetti F, Lanotte M, Lopiano L, Colloca L. When words are painful: unravelling the mechanisms of the nocebo effect. *Neuroscience* 2007;147:260–271.

Blanchard EB, Appelbaum KA, Radnitz CL, Michultka D, et al. Placebo-controlled evaluation of abbreviated progressive muscle relaxation and of relaxation combined with cognitive therapy in the treatment of tension headache. *J Consult Clin Psychol* 1990;58:210–215.

Brosschot JF, Aarsse HR. Restricted emotional processing and somatic attribution in fibromyalgia. *Int J Psychiatry Med* 2001;31:127–146.

Campbell JK, Penzien D, Wall EM. Evidence-based guidelines for migraine headache: behavioural and physical treatments. *Neurology* [serial online]. Available at: http://www.aan.com/professionals/practice/pdfs/g10089.pdf. Accessed July 20, 2008.

Celike FC, Saatcioglu O. Alexithymia and anxiety in female chronic pain patients. *Ann Gen Psychiatry* 2006;5:13.

Chen JT, Chen SM, Kuan TS, Chung KC, et al. Phentolamine effect on the spontaneous electrical activity of active loci in a myofascial trigger spot of rabbit skeletal muscle. *Arch Phys Med Rehabil* 1998;79:790–794.

Chung JW, Ohrbach R, McCall WD. Effect of increased sympathetic activity on electrical activity from myofascial painful areas. *Am J Phys Med Rehab* 2004;83:842–850.

deCharms RC, Fumiko M, Glover GH, Ludlow D, et al. Control over brain activation and pain learned by using real-time functional MRI. *Proc Natl Acad Sci USA* 2005;102: 18626–18631.

Devoulyte K, Sullivan MJ. Pain catastrophizing and symptom severity during upper respiratory tract illness. *Clin J Pain* 2003;19:125–133.

Diamond S. Depression and headache: a pharmacological perspective. In: Adler CS, Adler SM, Packard RC, eds. *Psychiatric Aspects of Headache*. Baltimore: Williams & Wilkins; 1987:272.

Featherstone HJ, Beitman BD. Marital migraine: a refractory daily headache. *Psychosomatics* 1984;25:30–38.

Fernández-de-las-Peñas C, Arendt-Nielsen L, Simons, D. Contributions of myofascial trigger points to chronic tension type headache. *J Manual Manip Ther* 2006;14:222–231.

Fitzpatrick RM, Hopkins A. Patients' satisfaction with communication in neurological outpatient clinics. *Psychosom Res* 1981;25:329–334.

Friedman AP. Psycho-physiological aspects of headache. In: *Phenomenology and Treatments of Psychophysical Disorders*. New York: Spectrum; 1982.

Fromm-Reichmann F. Contribution to the genesis of migraine. *Psychoanalytic Rev* 1937;24:26–33.

Ge HY, Fernández-de-las-Peñas C, Arendt-Nielsen L. Sympathetic facilitation of hyperalgesia evoked from myofascial tender and trigger points in patients with unilateral shoulder pain. *Clin Neurophysiol* 2006;117: 1545–1550.

Graham JR. Migraine: Clinical aspects. In: Vinken PJ, Bruyn GW, eds. *Handbook of Clinical Neurology*. Amsterdam: North Holland; 1968:45–58.

Henryk-Gutt R, Rees WL. Psychological assessment of migraine. *J Psychosom Res* 1973;17:141–153.

Hughes JW, Watkins L, Blumenthal JA, Kuhn C, et al. Depression and anxiety symptoms are related to increased 24-hour urinary nor-epinephrine excretion among healthy middle-aged women. *J Psychosom Res* 2004;57:353–358.

Hunt SP, Koltzenburg M. *The Neurobiology of Pain*. New York: Oxford University Press; 2005:343.

Jensen R, Olesen J. Initiating mechanisms of experimentally induced tension-type headache. *Cephalalgia* 1996;16:175–182.

Kerns RD, Rosenberg R, Jacob MC. Anger expression and chronic pain. *J Behav Med* 1994;17:57–67.

Lanzi G, Balottin U, Gamba N, Fazzi E. Psychological aspects of migraine in childhood. *Cephalagia* 1983;3(suppl 1):218–220.

Levin JD, Gordon NC, Fields HL. The mechanism of placebo analgesia. *Lancet* 1978;2:654–657.

Linden W. Autogenic training: narrative and quantitative review of clinical outcome. *Biofeedback Self Reg* 1994;19:227–264.

Low NC, du Fort G, Cervantes P. Prevalence, clinical correlates, and treatment of migraine in bipolar disorder. *Headache* 2003;43:940–949.

Maratos J, Wilkinson M. Migraine in children: a medical and psychiatric study. *Cephalalgia* 1982;2:179–187.

Martin PR. (1993). *Psychological Management of Chronic Headaches*. New York: Guilford Press.

McGrady A, Wauquier A, McNeil A, Gerard C. Effect of biofeedback-assisted relaxation on migraine headache and changes in cerebral blood flow velocity in the middle cerebral artery. *Headache* 1994;34:424–428.

McNulty WH, Gevirtz R, Hubbard DR, Berkoff GM. Needle electromyographic evaluation of TrP response to a psychological stressor. *Psychophysiology* 1994;31:313–316.

Melzack R, Wall PD. Pain mechanisms: a new theory. *Science* 1965;150:971–979.

Michael ES, Burns JW. Catastrophizing and pain sensitivity among chronic pain patients: moderating effects of sensory and affect focus. *Ann Behav Med* 2004;27:185–194.

Nestoriuc Y, Martin A. Efficacy of biofeedback for migraine: a meta-analysis. *Pain* 2007;128:111–117.

Nicholson RA, Gramling SE, Ong JC, Buenevar L. Differences in anger expression between individuals with and without headache after controlling for depression and anxiety. *Headache* 2003;43:651–663.

Okasha A, Ismail MK, Khalil AH, el Fiki R, Soliman A, Okasha T. A psychiatric study of nonorganic chronic headache patients. *Psychosomatics* 1999;40:233–238.

Penzien DB, Rains JC, Andrasik F. Behavioral management of recurrent headache: three decades of experience and empiricism. *Appl Psychophysiol Biofeedback* 2002;27:163–181.

Samwel HJ. The role of helplessness, fear of pain, and passive pain-coping in chronic pain patients. *Clin J Pain* 2006;22:245–251.

Schwartz M, Andrasik F. *Biofeedback: A Practitioner's Guide*. New York: Guilford Press; 2005.

Silberstein SD. Practice parameter: evidence-based guidelines for migraine headache (an evidence-based review): report of the quality standards subcommittee of the American Academy of Neurology. *Neurology* 2000;55:754–762.

Siniatchkin M, Gerber WD, Kropp P, Vein A. How the brain anticipates an attack: a study of neuro-physiological periodicity in migraine. *Funct Neurol* 1999;14:69–77.

Siniatchkin M, Hierundar A, Kropp P, Kuhnert R, et al. Self-regulation of slow cortical potentials in children with migraine: an exploratory study. *Psychophysiol Biofeedback* 2000;1:13–32.

Siniatchkin M, Averkina N, Andrasik F, Stephani U, et al. Neuro-physiological reactivity before a migraine attack. *Neurosci Lett* 2006;400:121–124.

Siniatchkin M, Andrasik F, Kropp P, Niederberger U, et al. Central mechanisms of controlled-release metoprolol in migraine: a double-blind, placebo-controlled study. *Cephalalgia* 2007;27:1024–1032.

Sullivan MJ, Bishop SR, Pivik J. The Pain Catastrophizing Scale: development and validation. *Psychol Assess* 1995;7:524–532.

Sullivan M, Thorn B, Haythornthwaite J, Keefe F, et al. Theoretical perspectives on the relation between catastrophizing and pain. *Clin J Pain* 2001;17:52–64.

Thorn B, Pence L, Ward C, Kilgo G, et al. Cognitive-behavioral therapy reduces chronic headache frequency. *J Pain* 2007;8:938–949.

Vasudeva S, Claggett AL, Tietjen GE, McGrady AV. Biofeedback-assisted relaxation in migraine headache: relationship to cerebral blood flow velocity in the middle cerebral artery. *Headache* 2003;3:245–250.

Wager TD, Scott DJ, Zubieta JK. Placebo effects on human μ-opioid activity during pain. *Proc Natl Acad Sci USA* 2007;104:11056–11061.

Yücel B, Kora K, Ozyalçin S, Alçalar N, et al. Automatic thoughts, alexithymia, and assertiveness in patients with tension-type headache. *Headache* 2002;42:194–199.

Zubieta JK, Bueller JA, Jackson LR, Scott DJ, et al. Placebo effects mediated by endogenous opioid activity on opioid receptors. *J Neurosci* 2005;25:7754–7762.

Physical Therapy Diagnosis and Management of a Patient with Chronic Daily Headache: Translating Knowledge to Clinical Practice

Tamer S. Issa, PT, BSc, DPT, OCS, and
Peter A. Huijbregts, PT, MSc, MHSc, DPT, OCS, MTC, FAAOMPT, FCAMT

The preceding chapters of this textbook have provided an in-depth discussion of the epidemiology, pathophysiology, diagnosis, and management of patients presenting with headache. The emphasis has been focused on tension-type headache, cervicogenic headache, or headache associated with temporomandibular pain disorders. However comprehensive these preceding chapters, the most important goal of this textbook is to help therapists and physicians improve diagnosis and management of real-life patients with headache presenting to their clinic. This final chapter is a case report describing an actual patient seen in a physical therapy (PT) clinic for a complaint of chronic daily headache using the five components of patient management (examina-

tion, evaluation, diagnosis, prognosis, plan of care, and intervention) introduced in Chapter 13. The intent of this last chapter is to allow for a translation of the comprehensive information from the preceding chapters to real-life diagnosis and management of this often complex and challenging group of patients.

CASE DESCRIPTION

History

The patient was a married 48-year-old woman with four teenage children, two dogs, one cat, and a horse, which made for a busy home life. She was referred to PT

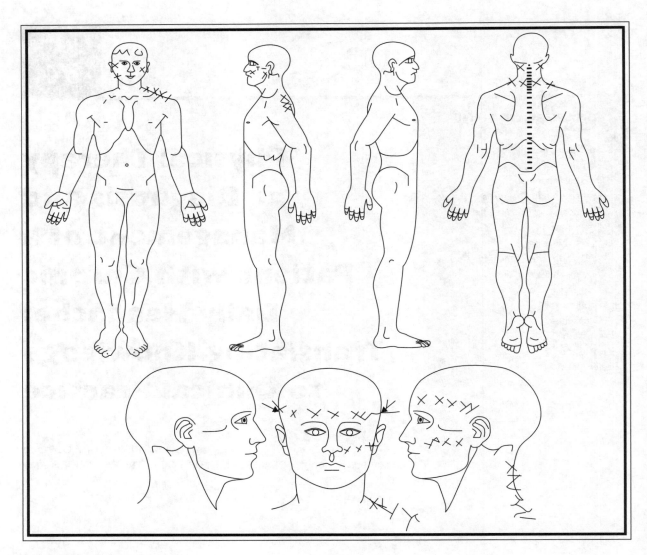

Figure 34.1 Pain Diagram

within a multidisciplinary pain management practice with a medical diagnosis of common migraine headache, chronic tension-type headache, and temporomandibular disorder. The patient worked as a full-time general counsel attorney and had been at her current job for 6 months. The work environment was sedentary, with physical demands related to sitting deskwork with some time spent using the computer and telephone. She had not lost any work time because of her headaches. The patient was a nonsmoker and drank two glasses of wine per week and one cup of caffeinated coffee per day. The wine and coffee were not reported as triggers for her headaches. Recreational

activities included yoga once a week, aerobic and resistance training three times a week, and reading.

Prior to the initial evaluation, the patient was asked to complete a pain drawing (**Figure 34.1**) and two outcome assessment tools: the Henry Ford Hospital Headache Disability Inventory, or HDI (**Figure 34.2**), and the Neck Disability Index, or NDI (**Figure 34.3**). The HDI and NDI were chosen as outcome measures to assess the response to treatment on the patient's headache and related self-perceived disability. Psychometric and content information on the HDI and NDI outcomes is provided in Chapter 13, where the history-taking process for patients with headache disorders is

HEADACHE DISABILITY INDEX

Patient Name _____   Date 10/18/04 _____

INSTRUCTIONS: Please CIRCLE the correct response:
 1. I have headache: (1) 1 per month (2) more than 1 but less than 4 per month **(3)** <u>more than one per week</u>
 2. My headache is: (1) mild   (2) moderate   **(3)** <u>severe</u>

Please read carefully: The purpose of the scale is to identify difficulties that you may be experiencing because of your headache. Please check off "YES", "SOMETIMES", or "NO" to each item. Answer each question as it pertains to your headache only.

YES	SOMETIMES	NO		
____	X	____	E1.	Because of my headaches I feel handicapped.
____	X	____	F2.	Because of my headaches I feel restricted in performing my routine daily activities.
____	X	____	E3.	No one understands the effect my headaches have on my life.
X	____	____	F4.	I restrict my recreational activities (eg, sports, hobbies) because of my headaches.
X	____	____	E5.	My headaches make me angry.
X	____	____	E6.	Sometimes I feel that I am going to lose control because of my headaches.
X	____	____	F7.	Because of my headaches I am less likely to socialize.
____	X	____	E8.	My spouse (significant other), or family and friends have no idea what I am going through because of my headaches.
____	X	____	E9.	My headaches are so bad that I feel that I am going to go insane.
____	X	____	E10.	My outlook on the world is affected by my headaches.
____	____	X	E11.	I am afraid to go outside when I feel that a headaches is starting.
____	X	____	E12.	I feel desperate because of my headaches.
X	____	____	F13.	I am concerned that I am paying penalties at work or at home because of my headaches.
____	X	____	E14.	My headaches place stress on my relationships with family or friends.
____	X	____	F15.	I avoid being around people when I have a headache.
X	____	____	F16.	I believe my headaches are making it difficult for me to achieve my goals in life.
____	____	X	F17.	I am unable to think clearly because of my headaches.
X	____	____	F18.	I get tense (eg, muscle tension) because of my headaches.
____	____	X	F19.	I do not enjoy social gatherings because of my headaches.
X	____	____	E20.	I feel irritable because of my headaches.
____	____	X	F21.	I avoid traveling because of my headaches.
____	____	X	E22.	My headaches make me feel confused.
X	____	____	E23.	My headaches make me feel frustrated.
____	X	____	F24.	I find it difficult to read because of my headaches.
____	____	X	F25.	I find it difficult to focus my attention away from my headaches and on other things.

OTHER COMMENTS: 36 yes + 20 sometimes = 56/100 _____

_____
                                                          Examiner

With permission from: Jacobson GP, Ramadan NM, et al. *The Henry Ford Hospital headache disability inventory (HDI).* *Neurology* 1994;44:837–842.

Figure 34.2 Initial Headache Disability Index

The Neck Disability Index

Patient name: _____ File# _____ Date: 10/18/04 _____

Please read instructions:
This questionnaire has been designed to give the doctor information as to how your neck pain has affected your ability to manage everyday life. Please answer every section and mark in each section only the ONE box that applies to you. We realize that you may consider that two of the statements in any one section relate to you, but please just mark the box that most closely describes your problem.

SECTION 1-PAIN INTENSITY

I have no pain at the moment.
The pain is very mild at the moment.
The pain is moderate at the moment.
The pain is fairly severe at the moment.
The pain is very severe at the moment.
The pain is the worst imaginable at the moment.

SECTION 2-PERSONAL CARE (Washing, Dressing, etc.)

I can look after myself normally, without causing extra pain.
I can look after myself normally, but it causes extra pain.
It is painful to look after myself and I am slow and careful.
I need some help, but manage most of my personal care.
I need help every day in most aspects of self care.
I do not get dressed; I wash with difficulty and stay in bed.

SECTION 3-LIFTING

I can lift heavy weights without extra pain.
I can lift heavy weights, but it gives extra pain.
Pain prevents me from lifting heavy weights off the floor, but I can manage if they are conveniently positioned, for example, on a table.
Pain prevents me from lifting heavy weights off the floor, but I can manage light to medium weights if they are conveniently positioned.
I can lift very light weights.
I cannot lift or carry anything at all.

SECTION 4-READING

I can read as much as I want to, with no pain in my neck.
I can read as much as I want to, with slight pain in my neck.
I can read as much as I want to, with moderate pain in my neck.
I can't read as much as I want, because of moderate pain in my neck.
I can hardly read at all, because of severe pain in my neck.
I cannot read at all.

SECTION 5-HEADACHES

I have no headaches at all.
I have slight headaches that come infrequently.
I have moderate headaches that come infrequently.
I have moderate headaches that come frequently.
I have severe headaches that come frequently.
I have headaches almost all the time.

SECTION 6-CONCENTRATION

I can concentrate fully when I want to, with no difficulty.
I can concentrate fully when I want to, with slight difficulty.
I have a fair degree of difficulty in concentrating when I want to.
I have a lot of difficulty in concentrating when I want to.
I have a great deal of difficulty in concentrating when I want to.
I cannot concentrate at all.

SECTION 7-WORK

I can do as much work as I want to.
I can do my usual work, but no more.
I can do most of my usual work, but no more.
I cannot do my usual work.
I can hardly do any work at all.
I can't do any work at all.

SECTION 8-DRIVING

I can drive my car without any neck pain.
I can drive my car as long as I want, with slight pain in my neck.
I can drive my car as long as I want, with moderate pain in my neck.
I can't drive my car as long as I want, because of moderate pain in my neck.
I can hardly drive at all, because of severe pain in my neck.
I can't drive my car at all.

SECTION 9-SLEEPING

I have no trouble sleeping.
My sleep is slightly disturbed (less than 1 hr sleepless).
My sleep is mildly disturbed (1–2 hrs sleepless).
My sleep is moderately disturbed (2–3 hrs sleepless).
My sleep is greatly disturbed (3–5 hrs sleepless).
My sleep is completely disturbed (5–7 hrs sleepless).

SECTION 10-RECREATION

I am able to engage in all my recreation activities, with no neck pain at all.
I am able to engage in all my recreation activities, with some neck pain at all.
I am able to engage in most, but not all, of my usual recreation activities, because of pain in my neck.
I am able to engage in few of my recreation activities, because of pain in my neck.
I can hardly do any recreation activities, because of pain in my neck.
I can't do any recreation activities at all.

Instructions:

1. The NDI is scored in the same way as the Oswestry Disability Index.

2. Using this system, a score of 10–28% (i.e., 5–14 points) is considered by the authors to constitute mild disability; 30–48% is moderate; 50–68% is severe; 72% or more is complete. **Score: 38/100**

Figure 34.3 Initial Neck Disability Index

discussed. The results of the HDI for this patient (Figure 34.2) indicated severe headache intensity, a headache frequency greater than one per week, and a total score of 56/100 (emotional 26/52, functional 30/48). The NDI questionnaire results for this patient (Figure 34.3) indicated a 38% score (i.e., moderate disability).

On the pain drawing (Figure 34.1), the patient indicated headache, facial pain, and neck pain. The headaches were located in the bilateral frontal head region, the facial pain was in the left cheek and jaw region, and the neck pain was in the bilateral suboccipital, lower neck, and left back of neck. The headache was described as severe, daily, and bandlike across the front of the head with tenderness of the head and occasional ringing in the left ear. The neck pain was described as tenderness.

The patient denied complaints of dizziness, loss of consciousness or balance, sensation disturbances, weakness, nausea, vomiting, or visual disturbances. These symptoms were asked about in order to screen for central nervous system dysfunction—including cord compression, cranial nerve dysfunction due to undiagnosed central processes, vertebral or carotid artery compromise, postconcussive syndrome, and other intracranial pathology—that might be causing the current complaints of headache (Roy, 2002). The diagnostic accuracy of these symptoms for implicating the mentioned pathologies has not been validated.

The patient reported that symptoms were improved by local application of heat, stretching, sometimes doing nothing, and Imitrex (a triptan-class migraine drug), if in fact the headache was a migraine-type headache. The patient identified this migraine-type headache as the headache that caused pain behind her left eye; this identification was confirmed by the positive response to medication specific for a migraine headache (i.e., Imitrex). However, the patient noted that the use of Imitrex did not always relieve the present headache, which would seem to indicate the presence of more than one type of headache. Symptoms were aggravated by bright light, certain smells, hunger, hot weather, exercise, and change in barometric pressure. No diurnal pattern of symptoms was noted. Sleep was undisturbed in a habitual left and/or right side-lying position with use of a cervical pillow.

A review of the available physician medical records and radiologic reports indicated a history of migraine since age 17. The onset time and cause of her neck pain was unknown. Onset of the newly described headache was 3 years before, and a neurologist who specialized in

headache management supervised its diagnosis and management. Follow-up with the physician had occurred approximately a year prior because of the onset of left tinnitus. The patient was then referred to a dentist due to suspicion of temporomandibular disorder (TMD). The dentist prescribed a night splint, which the patient wore on and off. She continued to see her dentist regularly until her mother died in February of 2004. Headaches had become more intense in March of 2004 and continued to become progressively worse over the next 6 months. The patient was unable to relate possible reasons contributing to the onset or worsening of the complaints.

Her neurologist referred the patient to a pain management outpatient practice in August 2004, where she was seen by a physician who was both a neurologist and pain management specialist. This physician reported increased and abnormal tone of the left arm and pronounced slowness of finger tapping of the left hand. He was concerned with the facts of increasing severity of headaches, worsening of symptoms when lying down compared with being upright, and motor dysfunction with the left arm when raised. The physician ordered a magnetic resonance imaging (MRI) study; findings showed no focal signal abnormality or mass lesions in the brain. MRI and magnetic resonance angiography (MRA) studies of the brain done approximately 2 years earlier were again evaluated and found normal. The patient had a follow-up visit with the same physician 1 month later with continued complaints of headache more than 50% of the time. At the time of the initial PT evaluation, the headache was daily during some weeks, but at other times the patient could go several days without a headache. At times she took the Imitrex daily or even twice daily, but the effect varied from none to satisfactory headache relief. The temporomandibular joint (TMJ) remained uncomfortable, but the dentist told the patient that improvement as a result of wearing the splint would take time. The neurologist had recommended botulinum toxin injections for selected neck, shoulder, and facial muscles in combination with PT, but the patient elected against these injections.

The medical history for this patient included migraine, asthma, depression, and a fractured pelvis and nose as a result of a motor vehicle accident (MVA) 5 years before. Her surgical history included tubal ligation, laser surgery for cervical dysplasia, and tonsillectomy. Current medications included Celexa 20 mg once a day (QD) (antidepressant), Imitrex 50 mg as needed (PRN), Zanaflex PRN (short-acting muscle relaxant),

Advair Diskus QD (asthma treatment), and Yasmin (birth control).

A screening examination using a systems approach revealed that the patient was receiving psychological counseling once a week. The patient's family history included the father alive at 69 with high blood pressure and diabetes and the mother deceased at age 69 from an overdose. The patient provided no further details on her mother's death. There was no indication in the family history of headaches, including migraine. First-degree relatives of persons who never had migraine are at no increased risk of migraine without aura (relative risk = 1.11; 95% confidence interval [CI]: 0.83–1.39) or with aura (relative risk = 0.65; 95% CI: 0.36–0.94) (Gardner, 2006).

Physical Examination

The patient stood 5 feet, 7 inches at 155 pounds, with a mesomorphic body type. Postural observation of this patient from the side using a three-point grading system (increased, normal, decreased) revealed decreased lumbar lordosis, increased thoracic kyphosis, and increased craniocervical extension resulting in a forward head posture (FHP). Observation from the back revealed symmetric iliac crest and shoulder heights; the head was side-bent to the right. Fedorak et al. (2003) noted fair intrarater ($\kappa = 0.50$) and poor interrater reliability ($\kappa = 0.16$) for visual assessment of cervical and lumbar lordosis using a similar three-point rating system.

Craniocervical, cervical, and upper thoracic spine active range of motion (AROM) testing in a sitting position assessed quality of motion, range, and pain provocation; limitations were estimated visually, with the following findings:

- Craniocervical flexion limited by 50%; extension not limited
- Craniocervical rotation right limited by 50%
- Cervical flexion limited by 25% with tightness reported in the upper back; extension hypermobility with an apex of the curve observed at C5-C6
- Cervical side-bending right limited by 75% with tightness in the contralateral neck; side-bending left limited by 25% with restriction noted ipsilateral
- Cervical rotation right limited by 25% with contralateral tightness; rotation left limited by 75% with no symptoms

- Upper thoracic (T1-T4) and midthoracic (T4-T8) extension limited without pain; all other directions were within normal limits

Bilateral shoulder functional AROM assessed by way of visual estimation was within normal limits. Interrater reliability for visual estimation of cervical ROM is poor overall compared with goniometric techniques (Youdas et al., 1991). Interrater agreement for visual estimation of shoulder AROM tests is poor to good (ICC = 0.15–0.88) but decreases when pain and disability are present. However, with the exception of horizontal adduction, it is suitable for distinguishing between the affected and normal side, indicating that its use here as a screening tool was appropriate (Terwee et al., 2005).

A neuroconductive examination yielded bilateral normal (5/5) results for C2-T1 myotomal muscle strength tests. Reflex testing yielded a 2+ bilateral for the brachioradialis, biceps, and triceps deep tendon reflexes. Sensation testing for bilateral C1-C5 distribution was normal for light touch and pinprick. Spine compression through the head in sitting position was negative for pain reproduction. Spine distraction in sitting position was negative for pain reproduction or pain relief. Extension quadrant AROM to the right revealed slight limitation with complaints of left anterior neck tightness, but to the left produced no limitations or symptoms.

Jepsen et al. (2004) noted fair to good ($\kappa = 0.25$–0.72) interrater reliability for upper limb manual muscle testing; Bertilson et al. (2003) reported poor to moderate ($\kappa = 0.20$–0.57) reliability for myotomal (C2-C8) strength tests and poor interrater reliability ($\kappa = -0.09$) for reflex testing. Sensitivity to pain with use of a pinwheel has shown moderate to substantial ($\kappa = 0.46$–0.79) interrater reliability (Bertilson et al., 2003). Using a three-point rating scale, Jepsen et al. (2006) reported median interrater κ values of 0.69 for sensitivity to light touch and 0.48 for sensitivity to pinprick. Neck compression and traction tests for reproduction or traction tests for relief have shown moderate ($\kappa = 0.44$, $\kappa = 0.41$, and $\kappa = 0.63$, respectively) interrater reliability (Bertilson et al., 2003).

Palpation for condition of the cervical spine in sitting position revealed no aberrant findings for skin temperature, skin moisture, paravertebral muscle tone, or swelling. Palpation for soft-tissue condition of the spine, neck, and head was also performed in supine and prone positions. This revealed myofascial hypertonicity characterized by palpable taut bands and active muscle trigger points (TrPs) using clinical diagnostic criteria (**Table 34.1**) (Simons et al., 1999) in bilateral upper trapezius (UT) (left worse than the right), sternocleidomastoid (SCM), splenius capitis (SpCap), and suboccipital (SO) muscles, and left masseter and temporalis muscles. Trigger point palpation of the UT produced referred pain into the upper neck, and palpation of the SCM caused referred pain into the forehead.

Reliability studies looking at the various clinical aspects of TrPs have been varied, and clinically relevant agreement in identifying the presence or absence of TrPs has proven to be difficult to achieve (Cummings & White, 2001). Gerwin et al. (1997) found good interrater reliability among four expert clinicians for the identification of tenderness, presence of a taut band, referred pain, local twitch response (LTR), and reproduction of the patient's pain, and when a global assessment was made regarding the presence of a trigger point. Lew et al. (1997) showed poor interrater reliability for locating latent TrPs in the UT; in contrast, Sciotti et al. (2001) found acceptable (G-coef ≥0.8) interrater reliability for the same procedure. Schöps et al. (2000) reported κ values of 0.46 to 0.63 and 0.31 to 0.37 for the interrater agreement on pain on palpation for the SCM and UT, respectively. Interrater agreement on muscle tone for these muscles yielded κ values of 0.22 to 0.37 and 0.20 to 0.30, respectively. Lending validity to the diagnosis of TrPs, the treating clinician later confirmed the above manual identification of TrPs with the elicitation of LTRs during treatment. Hong et al. (1997) concluded

that an LTR was more frequently elicited by needling than by palpation. They also noted that there was a significant ($P < 0.01$) correlation between the incidence of referred pain and the pain intensity of an active TrP and the occurrence of an LTR.

Palpation for position in sitting position revealed a decreased functional space between the occiput and spinous process of C2. Without reference to research, Rocabado (2001) noted that this functional space is adequate if a minimum of two fingers can be placed between the base of the occiput and the C2 spinous process. Palpation for position of the C1 vertebrae in sitting position revealed that the right transverse process of the C1 was anterior and superior compared with the left and was tender to palpation compared with the left. Positional palpation of C1 has moderate interrater reliability (κ = 0.63) (Metcalfe & Reese, 2007). Palpation for position in supine position revealed no aberrant findings for palpation of the articular pillars of the cervical spine, bony landmarks of the scapula, or for the first and second ribs. Lewis et al. (2002) noted surface palpation as a valid tool for determining scapular position.

Palpation for passive mobility of the cervical spine was performed in supine position and of the thoracic spine in prone position. Passive intervertebral motion (PIVM) was tested using the Paris (1999) grading system (**Table 34.2**). This yielded the following findings:

C0-C1: Pain-free grade 1 restriction for flexion and left side-bending
C1-C2: Painful grade 1 restriction for right rotation
T1-T4: Pain-free grade 1 restriction for extension
T4-T8: Pain-free grade 2 restriction for extension

Palpation for mobility is used by manual medicine clinicians to identify mobility dysfunctions that may

Table 34.1 Recommended Criteria for Identifying Latent and Active Trigger Points

---

Essential Criteria

1. Palpable taut band (if muscle accessible)
2. Exquisite spot tenderness of a nodule within the taut band
3. Pressure of tender nodule elicits patient's current pain complaint (identifies an active trigger point)
4. Painful limitation to full range of motion stretch

Confirmatory Findings

1. Visual or tactile identification of a local twitch response
2. Referred pain or altered sensation with pressure of tender nodule
3. Electromyographic demonstration of spontaneous electrical activity in the tender nodule of a taut band
4. Imaging of a local twitch response induced by needle penetration of tender nodule

---

Modified from Simons et al., 1989.

Table 34.2 Grading System for Passive Intervertebral Mobility Tests

Grade	Description
0	Ankylosis or no detectable movement
1	Considerable limitation in movement
2	Slight limitation in movement
3	Normal (for the individual)
4	Slight increase in motion
5	Considerable increase in motion
6	Unstable

Modified from Paris, 1999.

contribute to spinal disorders (Jull et al., 1997; Fjellner et al., 1999; McGregor et al., 2001; Huijbregts, 2002; Humphreys et al., 2004; Pool et al., 2004). Palpation for mobility in the cervical and thoracic spine has demonstrated both intra- and interrater agreement varying from no better than chance to perfect (Huijbregts, 2002). Most relevant to this case report, however, Jull et al. (1997) reported near excellent to perfect interrater agreement (κ = 0.78–1.00) for identifying a C0-C3 joint restriction considered relevant to cervicogenic headache (CeH). Jull et al. (1988) also examined the construct validity of cervical palpation for mobility tests and found 100% sensitivity and specificity when comparing palpation tests with single facet blocks. Zito et al. (2006) reported 80% sensitivity for a finding of painful upper cervical joint dysfunction with manual examination in the differential diagnosis of patients with CeH from those with migraine headache (MH) and controls. Aprill et al. (2002) found a 60% positive predictive value for occipital headaches originating in the C1-C2 joint with a combination of findings including pain in the (sub)occipital region, tenderness on palpation of the lateral C1-C2 joint, and restricted C1-C2 rotation.

All tests described above were performed during the initial visit. A TMJ evaluation on the 14th visit revealed decreased AROM of mouth opening to 30 mm measured with a ruler. During mouth opening, lateral anterior translation of the left condyle was noted. There was also maximal limitation with right lateral excursion (LE), moderate limitation with left LE, and moderate limitation for protrusion. The latter three movements were evaluated using visual estimation on a four-point scale (none, minimal, moderate, and maximal). Bilateral TMJ traction and compression tests were negative. Tenderness was evident with palpation of the left TMJ. At this time—and different from the first visit—myofascial hypertonicity and TrPs were noted in bilateral masseter and temporalis muscles.

Walker et al. (2000) noted near-perfect interrater agreement for measuring mouth opening with a ruler (ICC = 0.99). Manfredini et al. (2003) noted moderate agreement (κ = 0.48–0.53) for palpation for pain of the TMJ. Lobbezoo-Scholte et al. (1994) reported moderate interrater agreement (κ = 0.40) for pain on compression, and near-absent agreement for restriction (κ = 0.08) and end-feel (κ = 0.07) with traction and translation tests. Pain on palpation of the lateral and posterior aspects of the TMJ carried a positive likelihood ratio of 1.16 to 1.38 for the presence of TMJ synovitis (Holmlund & Axelsson, 1996; Israel et al., 1998); ab-

sence of joint crepitus carried a negative likelihood ratio of 0.70 with regard to TMJ osteoarthritis (Israel et al., 1998).

Evaluation and Diagnosis

The evaluation and diagnosis of this patient with a complex presentation involved answering two questions:

1. Was this patient appropriate for physical therapy management, or was a referral for medical diagnosis and (co)management warranted?
2. If appropriate for physical therapy management, which were the relevant neuromusculoskeletal impairments and resultant limitations in activity and restrictions in participation amenable to interventions within the physical therapy scope of practice?

Determining whether this patient was appropriate for physical therapy management required the therapist both to exclude with a sufficient degree of diagnostic confidence potential serious pathology responsible for the current presentation and to ascertain that the provided medical headache diagnoses fit with the signs and symptoms noted during the history and physical examination.

In the authors' clinical opinion, serious pathology was ruled out sufficiently by the comprehensive examination of the referring neurologist and the findings from the history and examination noted earlier. However, it should be noted that data on the diagnostic accuracy of history items and physical examination, as discussed earlier, is either absent or insufficient to confidently exclude central nervous system pathology potentially capable of producing similar signs and symptoms. Therefore, this decision was made mainly on clinician experience and interpretation of the tests based on a pathophysiologic rather than research-based rationale.

The International Headache Society (IHS) has long aimed to improve upon the understanding, diagnosis, and management of headache disorders. The IHS published the first internationally accepted and clinically useful headache classification system in 1988 with the first edition of the *International Classification of Headache Disorders* (ICHD); a second edition (ICHD-II) was published in 2004 (Olesen, 2005). The ICHD-II classified over 300 different types of headaches within two categories: primary headaches and secondary headaches. Primary headaches are the most common headache types and have no other underlying cause.

They include MH, tension-type headache (TTH), cluster headache and additional trigeminal autonomic cephalalgias, and other primary headaches. Secondary headaches are classified according to their causes and are classified in 10 separate categories. Diagnostic criteria for the various headache types are contained in other chapters in this book; most notably, diagnostic criteria for tension-type, migraine, cervicogenic headache, and headache due to temporomandibular disorders (TMD) can be found in Chapter 13.

This patient came with medical diagnoses of chronic tension-type headache, migraine, and temporomandibular disorder. As discussed previously, these, but also many other headache types within the ICHD-II, could potentially present with the same signs and symptoms as collected during the history and physical examination. Although it is not the role of the physical therapist to make a medical diagnosis, it is his or her responsibility to ascertain that the provided medical diagnosis fits with the history and physical examination findings. Discrepancies between the diagnosis provided and the signs and symptoms observed should lead to medical referral. Only when the signs and symptoms observed fit with the diagnosis provided will a PT examination and diagnosis indicate whether the patient might benefit from PT intervention. A clinical decision-making process consisting of an evaluation of history and examination findings was performed to confirm or cast doubt on the provided medical diagnosis. In this case, key differential diagnostic data were derived from the headache onset, nature, severity, chronicity, characteristics, associated symptoms, and physical examination findings.

Of the primary headache groups noted in the ICDH-II, only migraine and tension-type headache required further diagnostic consideration. With this patient presentation, the diagnostic criteria for migraine without aura (1.1) (see Chapter 13) were not entirely met. The patient had at least five attacks (criterion A), the headaches lasted 4 to 72 hours (criterion B), and the headaches were of severe intensity (criterion 4C). However, the patient did not fulfill a second characteristic out of the four in criterion C. She did describe a unilateral location (behind the left eye), but this was not part of her primary headache. The patient described aggravation by exercise, but not aggravation by or avoidance of routine physical activity (e.g., walking or climbing stairs). She also did not describe a pulsating quality to her headaches. With regard to criterion D, the patient described aggravation by bright light (photopho-

Table 34.3 Diagnostic Criteria for New Daily Persistent Headache

A. Headache >3 months fulfilling criteria B–D
B. Headache is daily and unremitting from onset or from <3 days from onset
C. At least two of the following pain characteristics
  1. Bilateral location
  2. Pressing/tightening (nonpulsating) quality
  3. Mild or moderate intensity
  4. Not aggravated by routine physical activity such as walking or climbing stairs
D. Both of the following:
  1. No more than one of photophobia, phonophobia, or mild nausea
  2. Neither moderate or severe nausea nor vomiting
E. Not attributed to another disorder

Modified from Olesen et al., 2004.

bia), but she did not mention phonophobia, nausea, or vomiting. Typical migraine with aura (1.2.1) (see Chapter 13) was not a consideration mainly because her symptoms were not accompanied by any aura. She did not meet the frequency and chronic nature of chronic migraine (1.5.1), as outlined in criterion A. However, with a report of symptomatic relief of her unilateral headache with a triptan-class medication, a diagnosis of migraine without aura was considered probable despite the patient not meeting all diagnostic criteria.

Episodic TTH (2.1) and frequent episodic TTH (2.2) (see Chapter 13) could be eliminated because the frequency per month of her headaches exceeded criteria for both, leaving chronic TTH (2.3) (see Chapter 13) and new daily persistent headache (4.8) (**Table 34.3**). Their criteria are very similar, and the patient's headache fulfilled criteria for both types; however, new daily persistent headache (4.8) is daily and unremitting since or very close to a time of onset that is clearly recalled and unambiguous (Olesen, 2004). This was not evident in this case, with the onset of daily headache for this patient being described as insidious and vague. Chronic TTH (2.3) exists in two forms: associated (2.3.1) and not associated with pericranial tenderness (2.3.2), described as local tenderness to manual palpation by the second and third finger on muscles of the head and neck (i.e., frontalis, temporalis, masseter, pterygoid, SCM, splenius, and trapezius muscles) (Olesen, 2004). Palpation of the neck and head musculature in this patient revealed tenderness, characterized by palpable taut bands and active TrPs, making a diagnosis of chronic

Table 34.4 Competing Secondary Headache Diagnoses Related to Whiplash and Head or Neck Trauma

Type	Diagnostic Criteria
Chronic headache attributed to whiplash injury (5.4)	A. Headache, no typical characteristics known, fulfilling criteria C and D B. History of whiplash (sudden and significant acceleration/deceleration movement of the neck) associated at the time with neck pain C. Headache develops within 7 days after whiplash injury D. Headache persists for >3 months after whiplash injury
Chronic headache attributed to other head and/or neck trauma (5.6.2)	A. Headache, no typical characteristics known, fulfilling criteria C and D B. Evidence of head and/or neck trauma of a type not described above C. Headache develops in close temporal relation to, and/or other evidence exists to establish a causal relationship with, the head and/or neck trauma D. Headache persist for >3 months after the head and/or neck trauma

Modified from Olesen et al., 2004.

tension-type headache associated with pericranial tenderness (2.3.1) very plausible.

A medical history of suspected TMD, an MVA 5 years prior during which the patient sustained a fractured nose, and neuromusculoskeletal impairments found during the examination warranted further inquiry regarding the secondary headache groups. Whether to classify a headache as secondary depends on a few factors. If a headache is a new headache that presents with another disorder known to be capable of causing it, then it is described as a secondary headache (Olesen, 2004). If a primary headache already exists, factors that support adding a secondary headache diagnosis include a close temporal relation to a causative disorder, a discernible worsening of the primary headache, good evidence that the causative disorder can exacerbate the primary headache, and improvement or resolution of the headache after relief of the presumed causative disorder (Olesen, 2004). In respect to the improvement or resolution of the headache, in many cases there is insufficient follow-up time, or a diagnosis needs to be made prior to the end of expected time for remission. In these cases, it is recommended to describe the headache as a headache probably attributed to the disorder; a definitive diagnosis can only be made once the time-sensitive outcome criterion D is fulfilled (Olesen, 2004).

Of the secondary headache groups, headache attributed to head and/or neck trauma and headache or facial pain attributed to a disorder of cranium, neck, eyes, ears, nose, sinuses, teeth, mouth, or other facial or cranial structures required further investigation as competing secondary headache diagnoses for this patient (Olesen, 2004). The presentation did not fulfill the criteria for chronic headache attributed to whiplash injury (5.4)

(**Table 34.4**), because the patient did not describe a discernable whiplash injury after her MVA and the headache did not develop within 7 days after a possible or suspected whiplash injury. A fractured nose might constitute possible head trauma, but there was no evidence that the headache developed in close temporal relation to the trauma, thereby making chronic headache attributed to other head and/or neck trauma (5.6.2) (Table 34.4) also unlikely. Although the clinician suspected headache due to TMD, and this suspicion was to some degree substantiated later based on the examination findings for the TMJ noted above, this case did not meet the established criteria for headache or facial pain attributed to temporomandibular joint disorder (11.7) (see Chapter 13); evidence of TMD established by way of X-ray, MRI, and/or bone scintigraphy was not available (criterion B). Also, the time-dependent outcome criterion D could not be met. Cervicogenic headache (11.2.1) (see Chapter 13) was a possible secondary headache diagnosis because the examination findings met criteria A, B, and C1. Again, the time-sensitive outcome criterion D could not be confirmed. Clinical findings that supported the diagnosis of CeH included forward head posture, suboccipital tenderness, and upper cervical positional abnormalities and mobility restrictions.

In summary, after the initial evaluation, the relevant signs and symptoms associated with the patient's headaches seemed to be consistent with and fulfill ICDH-II diagnostic criteria (Olesen, 2004) for:

1. Chronic tension-type headache associated with pericranial tenderness
2. Probable migraine without aura
3. Probable cervicogenic headache

As noted earlier, the ICHD-II is an update of the original 1988 classification and includes expanded definitions and clarifications (Olesen, 2004, 2005). Few studies have examined the reliability and validity of this new edition. Relevant to this patient is the fact that there is considerable symptom overlap between the diagnostic criteria for TTH and CeH (Haldeman & Dagenais, 2001), yet some evidence shows that they are distinct disorders (Fernández-de-las-Peñas et al., 2006b; Nilsson & Bove, 2000). It should be noted that the absence of data on diagnostic accuracy of the ICHD-II does and should affect the level of diagnostic confidence with regard to the established headache diagnoses.

After excluding serious underlying undiagnosed pathology and establishing the seeming appropriateness of the headache diagnoses provided by the referring physician, the next step in the diagnostic process was to ascertain whether neuromusculoskeletal impairments caused or contributed to the patient's headaches and neck pain. The patient presented with several physical examination findings of the musculoskeletal system of the head and neck that have been shown to contribute to various headache types. Myofascial trigger points have been noted to cause referred pain to the head, neck, and face contributing to TTH, MH, and CeH (Graff-Radford et al., 1986; Han & Harrison, 1997; Davidoff, 1998; Simons et al., 1999; Graff-Radford, 2001; Alvarez & Rockwell, 2002; Borg-Stein, 2002; Freund & Schwartz, 2002; Fernández-de-las-Peñas et al., 2005, 2006a). Cervical spine joint dysfunction has been noted to contribute to CeH due to referred pain from the facet joints and influence of neural and vascular structures of the head and neck (Niere & Robinson, 1997; Pollmann et al., 1997; Alix & Bates, 1999; Biondi, 2000; Haldeman & Dagenais, 2001; Jull et al., 2002; Petersen, 2003; Martelletti & van Suijlekom, 2004; Moore, 2004; Jensen, 2005). Forward head posture with posterior rotation of the cranium may lead to adverse effects on the structure and function of the cervical spine and TMJ, increasing the incidence of neck, interscapular, and headache pain (Mannheimer & Rosenthal, 1991; Griegel-Morris et al., 1992; Marcus et al., 1999; Alvarez & Rockwell, 2002; Agustsson, 2004; Moore, 2004).

In light of this complex patient presentation, the clinician decided to assess for a suspected TMD at a later date due to a lack of time and a lower assigned priority. TMD constitutes a variety of conditions involving the TMJ, muscles of mastication, and other associated structures. The diagnosis of TMD is varied, and a con-

sensus is lacking on the pathophysiologic mechanisms involved (Freund & Schwartz, 2002). At some point during the course of treatment, the patient mentioned the onset of jaw pain. It was at that time that a TMJ evaluation was performed. The diagnostic criteria of the American Academy of Orofacial Pain (AAOP) for TMD classify two major subgroups (Okeson, 1996):

1. Temporomandibular joint articular disorders including congenital and developmental disorders, disc derangement disorders, dislocation, inflammatory conditions, arthritides, ankylosis, and fracture
2. Masticatory muscle disorders divided into myofascial pain, myositis, myospasm, myofibrotic contracture, local myalgia (unclassified), myofibrotic contracture, and neoplasia

The TMJ evaluation indicated diagnoses of myofascial pain and left condylar hypermobility based on the history and on active and passive movement and palpation findings. The patient reported being under high stress and complained of jaw pain, stiffness, and pain with chewing. Limitations were present during mouth opening with anterior-lateral translation of the left condyle, bilateral lateral excursion (right worse than left), and protrusion. Palpation revealed myofascial hypertonicity and pain in the muscles of mastication and over the left TMJ. No joint sounds were noted. Therefore, the patient clearly met the diagnostic inclusion criteria for TMJ myofascial pain (**Table 34.5**) (Okeson, 1996). But the myofascial pain diagnosis did not explain the anterior-lateral translation of the left condyle, the discrepancy between left and right lateral excursion, and the pain with palpation of the left TMJ. Further investigation of the TMJ articular disorders did not show any plausible diagnosis for which all inclusion criteria were met. With the absence of joint sounds and without radiographic imaging, disc displacement disorders, inflammatory, and osteoarthritic disorders could not be excluded nor included (Okeson, 1996). The diagnosis of left condylar hypermobility is not a classified disorder named by the AAOP, but it has been used to describe an articular condition that is likely to precede disc derangement disorders of the TMJ (Rocabado, 2001). It is characterized by excessive condylar rotation (anterior translation) with mouth opening and could explain the lateral excursion restrictions as well as the pain on palpation of the TMJ (Rocabado, 2001).

Table 34.5 Temporomandibular Disorders: Diagnostic Criteria for Myofascial Pain

1. Regional dull, aching pain; pain aggravated by mandibular function when the muscles of mastication are involved
2. Hyperirritable sites (trigger points) frequently palpated within a taut band of muscle tissue or fascia; provocation of these trigger points altering the pain complaint and often revealing a pattern of pain referral
3. Greater than 50% reduction of pain with vapocoolant spray or local anesthetic injection of the trigger point followed by stretch

The following may accompany the above:

1. Sensation of muscle stiffness
2. Sensation of acute malocclusion not verified clinically
3. Ear symptoms, tinnitus, vertigo, toothache, tension-type headache
4. With masticatory muscle involvement, decreased mouth opening; passive stretching of the elevator muscles increasing mouth opening by more than 4 mm (soft end-feel)
5. Hyperalgesia in the region of the referred pain

Modified from Okeson et al., 1996.

It should be noted that data on diagnostic accuracy for most tests used in the examination are limited to reliability data; frequently, interrater reliability is insufficient for clinical decision making, thereby encouraging us to question our test results. The patient met all three criteria (pain in suboccipital region, pain on palpation of right C1, and restricted C1-C2 rotation) for CeH originating in C1-C2 (Aprill et al., 2002), and the painful C1-C2 restriction also indicated CeH rather than migraine as the cause of at least some of the headache complaints (Zito et al., 2006). However, it should be again noted that a positive predictive value of 60% and a positive finding in light of data only on sensitivity might be considered insufficient for confident diagnostic decision making. The AAOP's TMD classification system has not been studied for reliability or validity. The assumption made here that the patient presented with a muscular and not as much an articular TMD was neither supported nor contradicted by the likelihood ratios noted previously for pain on TMJ palpation and the absence of joint crepitus; values close to 1.0, as discussed earlier, do little to affect post-test probability either way. However, in the authors' opinion, for this patient the psychometric data on TrP palpation and especially on palpation for mobility permitted a physical therapy

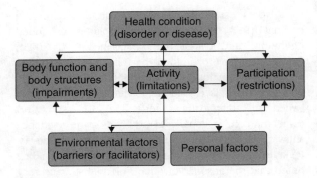

Figure 34.4 ICF Biopsychosocial Framework
Source: Modified from Stucki, 2005.

Table 34.6 ICF: Definition of Terms

Health condition Diseases, disorders, injuries.
Body functions The physiological functions of body systems, including psychological functions. *Impairments* are problems in body function as a significant deviation or loss.
Body structures Anatomic parts of the body, such as organs, limbs, and their components. *Impairments* are problems in structure as a significant deviation or loss.
Activity The execution of a task or action by an individual. Activities may be *limited* in nature, duration, or quality.
Participation The involvement in a life situation. Participation may be *restricted* in nature, duration, or quality.
Environmental factors The makeup of the physical, social, and attitudinal environment in which people live and conduct their lives; includes *barriers* or *facilitators*.
Personal factors Factors that impact on functioning (e.g., lifestyle, habits, social background, education, life events, race/ethnicity, sexual orientation, and assets of the individual).

Modified from World Health Organization, 2006.

diagnosis with regard to TrPs and segmental mobility dysfunction that had sufficient diagnostic confidence to identify impairments potentially amenable to PT intervention.

The International Classification of Functioning, Disability, and Health (ICF) (World Health Organization, 2007) disablement model was used to describe the patient's diagnosis, current functioning, and level of disability (**Figure 34.4**), because the full personal impact of headache disorders can be illustrated well using the ICF classification (Leonardi et al., 2005). ICF terms and definitions are described in **Table 34.6**. Stucki (2005)

Table 34.7 Physical Therapy Diagnosis in Accordance with the ICF Format

Health condition

1. Headaches	• Chronic tension-type headache associated with pericranial tenderness
	• Cervicogenic headache
	• Probable migraine headache
2. Neck pain	• Impaired joint mobility, motor function, muscle performance, and range of motion associated with connective tissue dysfunction
	• Impaired posture

Body function & structure (impairments)

1. Active TrPs contributing to myofascial hypertonicity and tenderness	• Bilateral: Upper trapezius, sternocleidomastoid, splenius capitis, and suboccipital muscles
	• Left: Masseter and temporalis
2. Spinal mobility restrictions	• Left C0/C1 for FB and SBL
	• Left C1/C2 for RR
	• U/T and M/T for BB and axial extension
3. Decreased muscle flexibility	• Bilateral: Upper trapezius, sternocleidomastoid, cervical/thoracic paraspinals, and suboccipital muscles
4. Postural dysfunction	• Forward head posture with craniocervical extension
5. Stress/Tension	• Related to busy home and work life, and possible grieving over death of her mother earlier in the year
6. Craniomandibular disorder	• Assessed at a later date

Activity (limitations)

1. Functional limitations with:	• Routine daily activities, personal care, lifting, work activities, concentration, reading, recreational activities, driving
2. Emotional feelings of being:	• Handicapped, isolated, angry, tense, irritable, frustrated, insane, desperate, unable to maintain control

Participation (restrictions)

Restrictions with life situations	• Less likely to socialize
	• Concerned about consequences on work, home, and relationships with others
	• Perceived difficulty achieving life goals

TrPs, trigger points; FB, forward bending; SBL, side-bending to left; RR, right rotation; U/T, upper thoracic; M/T, midthoracic; BB, backward bending.

suggested that the ICF is moving toward becoming the generally accepted framework and classification system in medicine, specifically rehabilitation medicine. **Table 34.7** summarizes the involved health conditions, impairments, activity limitations, and participation restrictions in accordance with the ICF.

Another diagnostic framework used increasingly within PT in the United States is the preferred practice patterns contained in the *Guide to Physical Therapist Practice* (American Physical Therapy Association [APTA] 2001). For this patient, diagnosis using this model with regard to the cervical and thoracic spine included the following:

1. Pattern B: Impaired posture
2. Pattern D: Impaired joint mobility, motor function, muscle performance, and range of motion associated with connective tissue dysfunction

The PT diagnosis with regard to the TMD, again following the second edition of the *Guide to Physical Therapist Practice* (APTA, 2001), was pattern D (impaired joint mobility, motor function, muscle performance, and range of motion associated with connective tissue dysfunction). Although promoted for use in PT diagnosis, prognosis, and treatment planning, this diagnostic framework has not been studied for reliability and validity.

Prognosis

The patient described in this case report presented with a number of poor prognostic indicators. It was not clear whether this patient had suffered a whiplash injury during the MVA 5 years ago or if her chronic neck pain should be attributed to previous neck injury or chronic tension-type headache. Patients with chronic neck pain and chronic pain and disability related to "late whiplash syndrome" present with central sensitization. It has been proposed that in patients with chronic tension-type headache, prolonged nociceptive stimuli from pericranial muscle tissue contribute to supraspinal facilitation leading to central sensitization, which in turn results in an increased general pain sensitivity (Jensen et al., 1998; Bendtsen, 2000; Schulman, 2001). Signs of central sensitization include hyperalgesia, allodynia, and widespread and stimulus-independent pain (Moog et al., 2002). Central sensitization as might exist in this patient poses an obstacle to therapeutic success because of the negative consequences of maintained pain perception and the increased excitatory state of the central nervous system in response to peripheral inputs.

Emotional stress and depression are relevant psychological impairments that serve as poor prognostic indicators for this patient diagnosed with both tension-type headache and migraine. High levels of depression and anxiety are common in patients with chronic TTH (Choi et al., 1995; Holroyd et al., 2000). Significant functional and well-being impairments have been noted in chronic tension-type headache patients, including adversely affected sleep, energy levels, emotional well-being, and performance in daily responsibilities. In contrast, work and social functioning are generally only severely impaired in a small minority (Holroyd et al., 2000). Leistad et al. (2006) showed the deleterious effect of cognitive stress on electromyographic (EMG) muscle activity and reported pain in patients with migraine and tension-type headache and in healthy controls. Although EMG peak activity revealed no between-group differences, the TTH patients recorded higher pain responses in the temporalis and frontalis muscles, a higher increase of pain during the cognitive test, and delayed pain recovery in all muscle regions when compared with controls. They also had delayed EMG recovery in the trapezius compared with controls and migraine patients. The migraine patients developed more pain in the splenius and temporalis than did the controls; pain responses were higher in the neck and trapezius compared with patients with tension-type headache with delayed pain recovery in the trapezius and temporalis muscles (Leistad et al., 2006).

In this patient, the history revealed both multiple emotional stressors and a history of depression. First, her mother died earlier in the year from a medication overdose: headache symptoms became worse a month after her death. The patient had a 30-year history of migraine as a physical stressor. Also, the patient had a history of depression and was seeing a therapist and used antidepressive medication. She noted work- and home-related stress to her physicians and physical therapist, yet she maintained a successful career as an attorney and managed a household of four teenage children and three pets. The responses to her perceived emotional and functional disability on the HDI and NDI questionnaires were revealing with regard to perceived stress levels (Table 34.7). The patient reported feeling handicapped, isolated, angry, tense, irritable, frustrated, insane, desperate, and unable to maintain control. From a functional standpoint, she reported limitations with routine daily activities, personal care, lifting, work activities, concentration, reading, recreational activities, and driving. All of these findings were significant in that they most likely contributed to pain through a stress-related increase of muscular tension and pain perception.

The prolonged nature of the complaints and the worsening of the condition over time despite the medical management by various health-care providers seemed to also indicate an unfavorable prognosis. The patient had increased her headache medication intake to daily use and sometimes twice daily. One had to surmise that to expect this patient's chronic pain condition to improve with time on its current course and without specific therapeutic intervention would be unrealistic.

On the other hand, this patient presented with a number of musculoskeletal impairments that might indicate the potential for successful treatment of the chronic headache and neck pain by way of an orthopaedic manual physical therapy (OMPT) approach. Manual therapy techniques to address spine joint dysfunction and soft-tissue or myofascial restrictions, combined with exercise therapy to address postural imbalances and poor cervical muscle activation or endurance, have been noted to be effective treatment approaches both individually and collectively in the treatment of headaches (Jull, 1997; Niere & Robinson, 1997; Bronfort et al., 2001; Karakurum et al., 2001; Jull et al., 2002; Mills Roth, 2003; Moore, 2004; Hanten et al., 2005). Studies have shown that trigger point dry needling relieved symptoms related to myofascial pain (Cummings & White, 2001) and that it improved headache indices, tenderness, and neck mobility in TTH patients (Karakurum et al., 2001). In some studies, spinal manipulation has been shown to be efficacious in the treatment of chronic tension-type headache, migraine, and CeH (Bronfort et al., 2001). In this patient, the noted moderate to high headache intensity and chronic nature of headaches were not predictors of a negative outcome in the treatment of CeH using therapeutic exercise and manipulative therapy (Jull & Stanton, 2005).

Another positive prognostic indicator—although not known at the time of the evaluation—was the significant within-session improvements of pain and neck mobility observed early in the intervention period. Tuttle (2005) reported that positive within-session changes in cervical mobility and pain could predict between-session changes for PT treatment of the cervical spine: the odds ratios (ORs) for within-session changes to predict between-session changes using an improved/not improved categorization for cervical mobility ranged from 2.5 (95% CI: 0.6–4.3) to 21.3 (95% CI: 10.1–96.1); for pain intensity, the OR was 4.5 (95% CI: 1.2–14.4). The positive likelihood ratio for cervical mobility improvements ranged from 2.1 (95% CI: 0.7–6.2) to 5.0 (95% CI: 2.6–9.9); for pain intensity improvements, it was 2.5 (95% CI: 1.3–4.6).

Intervention

Following the initial evaluation, the patient was initially seen twice a week for approximately 6 weeks for a total of 11 visits, after which there was a period she was out of town for almost 3 weeks. After this absence from therapy, she was seen 9 times over the next 3 months and finally 1 month later, for a total of 21 visits. As noted previously, specific assessment and treatment of the TMD began on the 14th visit. The patient was reassessed at each visit, and treatment on that visit was dependent on subjective reporting and objective reassessments.

The treatment progression was based on the therapist's clinical experience. After the initial evaluation, the findings, recommended treatment plan, and expected outcome were outlined to the patient using charts and other skeletal aids. In the authors' opinion, educating a patient on her or his problem and how it will be treated may be extremely important for optimal success and patient compliance with exercise and self-management concepts. This also established patient responsibility with regard to self-management.

The initial therapy focus was to decrease pain by addressing the most pertinent myofascial and spinal dysfunctions, to initiate a home exercise program (HEP) for relaxation and flexibility, and to establish whether continuation of the plan of care was indeed warranted indicated by patient progress. The progression of therapy emphasized monitoring self-perceived disability ratings, addressing remaining muscle dysfunctions established upon each new reevaluation, monitoring and maintaining spinal mobility, progressing the HEP for mobility and coordination of movement, and further assessing and treating the TMD. It was the clinician's belief that treating the myofascial and upper cervical spine restrictions first would improve the probability of successfully addressing any possible TMD that might be present or that might be contributing to the patient's headaches.

Once a plateau of improvement was reached, as indicated by a decrease of headache frequency to one or less per month of mild intensity, the last one to two visits were intended to finalize the patient's HEP, aiming at preventing the onset or exacerbation of the patient's complaints. The following paragraphs explain in more detail the therapeutic interventions used during follow-up visits (**Table 34.8**).

Dry Needling

Trigger point dry needling (TrPDN) is a technique used for releasing muscle TrPs; this release is hypothesized to occur as a result of the elicitation of LTRs with subsequent inactivation of the TrP. The TrPDN treatment utilizes fine solid acupuncture needles, but the technique is in all other aspects different from traditional acupuncture (**Table 34.9**) (Gunn, 1996). Other terminology used in the literature describing similar techniques includes *intramuscular stimulation* (IMS), *twitch-obtaining intramuscular stimulation*, and *deep dry needling*. Other variations of dry needling include superficial dry needling, which involves placing an acupuncture needle in the skin overlying a TrP, and electrical twitch-obtaining intramuscular stimulation, which applies electricity through a monopolar EMG needle electrode at motor endplate zones. Sometimes the term IMS is used to refer to a specific system of diagnosis and treatment for myofascial pain of hypothesized radiculopathic origin as developed by Gunn (1996).

Table 34.8 Physical Therapy Visits and Treatment Interventions

Treatment Date	Myofascial OMPT Techniques	Articular OMPT Techniques	Exercise Therapy	Education
10/18/04 (initial eval) NDI: 38/100, HDI: 56/100	(Trial treatment) 1. TrPDN: Lt UT and SCM 2. STM & PIR		1. Self-stretch: UT and SCM for HEP	1. Eval findings & recommended Tx plan 2. Postural instruction in sitting
10/25/04 *Comments:* Significant initial improvement of HA complaints.	1. TrPDN: Rt UT and SCM 2. STM & PIR	1. Reverse NAGS: T1-4 2. LAD: C0-2 3. Rt lateral glide (Gr. IV): C0/1 4. SNAG: C1/2 RR 3×	1. Self-stretch: SOs & SpCap for HEP 2. Review of HEP	1. Education for stress reduction through breathing and relaxation of head, neck, and jaw
10/28/04 *Comments:* MTrPs reproduced HA pain.	1. TrPDN: Bil UT and Lt SCM 2. STM & PIR	1. Reverse NAGS: T1-4 2. PA (prog. osc.): T4-8 3. Rt lateral glide (Gr. IV): C0/1 4. SNAG: C1/2 RR 5×	1. Review of HEP	
11/01/04 *Comments:* Onset of midback pain. Pain in midback with axial EXT. Patient brought in her cervical pillow from home.	1. TrPDN: Lt LT 2. STM & PIR: Bil UT, SCM, SpCap, SOs 3. SID	1. Reverse NAGS: T1-4 2. PA (prog. osc.): T4-8 3. LAD: C0-2 4. Rt lateral glide (Gr. IV): C0/1 5. SNAG: C1/2 RR 5×	1. Self-stretch: Lower trapezius for HEP	1. Education for proper neck and head positioning during sleep with use of towel roll 2. Education for suboccipital release self-treatment
11/04/04	1. TrPDN: Rt SCM 2. STM & PIR: Bil UT, SCM, SpCap, SOs 3. SID	1. PA (prog. osc.): T1-8		1. Review of self-Tx for SO release
11/08/04	1. STM & PIR: Bil UT, SCM, SOs 2. SID	1. PA (prog. osc.): T1-8	1. Neck clocks 2. AROM AR of the head/axial EXT 3. Shoulder clocks	
11/11/04 NDI: 28/100, HDI: 42/100 *Comments:* Notes overall improvement.	1. TrPDN: Bil UT, Lt SCM 2. STM & PIR 3. SID	1. PA (prog. osc.): T1-8	1. Review of exercises issued last visit	
11/18/04	1. TrPDN: Lt UT & LT 2. STM & PIR 3. SID	1. Traction mob Gr. V: T4-8		
11/29/04	1. TrPDN: Lt UT & LT 2. STM & PIR 3. SID	1. Traction mob Gr. V: T4-8		

Table 34.8 *Continued*

Treatment Date	Myofascial OMPT Techniques	Articular OMPT Techniques	Exercise Therapy	Education
12/02/04	1. TrPDN: Bil temporalis, masseter, SCM 2. STM & PIR (mouth opening)			1. Proper tongue position, resting jaw position, and nasal diaphragmatic breathing 2. Self-STM of temporalis and masseter for HEP
12/7/04 *Comments:* Noted excellent improvement.	1. TrPDN: Bil temporalis, masseter 2. STM & PIR (mouth opening) 3. SID	1. LAD: C0-2		
Interruption of physical therapy intervention due to vacation and holiday obligations				
1/03/05 *Comments:* Recent exacerbation of pain complaints.	1. TrPDN: Lt UT 2. STM: UT, SCM, SOs 3. SID	1. Traction mob Gr. V: T1-8 2. LAD: C0-2		
1/13/05 NDI: 12/100, HDI: 24/100	1. TrPDN: Bil UT 2. STM & PIR: SCM, SOs, masseter, temporalis 3. SID	1. Traction mob Gr. V: T1-8 2. LAD: C0-2		
Interruption of physical therapy intervention of headaches and neck pain due to acute onset of left anterior-lateral shoulder pain				
2/8/05 *Interim history:* Series of headaches in past week. Most likely due to stress. Jaw pain in past week. Pain with chewing. TMJ examination performed.	1. TrPDN: Bil masseter, temporalis 2. STM & PIR (mouth opening)	1. LAD, medial glide, lateral glide Gr. 3: Bil TMJ	1. AROM: 10 mm MO, 10 mm Rt LE, 10 mm MO in Rt LE	1. Patient education for TMJ findings and self-care
2/10/05 *Comments:* Reports much less pain and tightness of her jaw. Decrease in HA intensity and frequency.	1. TrPDN: Bil masseter, temporalis 2. STM & PIR (mouth opening)	1. LAD, medial glide, lateral glide Gr. 3: Bil TMJ	1. AROM: 10 mm MO, 10 mm Rt LE, 10 mm MO in Rt LE	
2/16/05 *Comments:* Reports improvement of jaw pain and mouth opening, but still with some soreness and headaches.	1. STM: Bil masseter, temporalis, SCM, SOs 2. PIR: mouth opening	1. LAD, medial glide, lateral glide Gr. 3: Bil TMJ	1. AROM: 10 mm MO, 10 mm Rt LE, 10 mm MO in Rt LE	1. Proper tongue position, resting jaw position, and nasal diaphragmatic breathing 2. Self-STM of masseter and temporalis

Table 34.8 *Continued*

Treatment Date	Myofascial OMPT Techniques	Articular OMPT Techniques	Exercise Therapy	Education
2/18/05 Comments: Reports some return of jaw pain, and headaches.	1. TrPDN: Bil masseter, temporalis 2. STM & PIR (mouth opening)	1. LAD, medial glide, lateral glide Gr. 3: Bil TMJ	1. AROM of TMJ for HEP	1. Review of postural positioning and breathing education
2/23/05 Comments: Reports much improved mouth opening, less jaw pain, and resolution of headaches. Minimal limitation with Lt LE and Pro, and moderate limitation with mouth opening and Rt LE. Good condylar stability with mouth opening. Hypertonicity of Bil masseter and temporalis improved.	1. TrPDN: Bil UT, SCM 2. STM: Bil UT, SCM, masseter, temporalis 3. SID	1. FB, SB, Rot Gr. IV Passive mobs: upper cervical spine		
3/24/05 Comments: Continued improvement of mouth opening, jaw pain, and headaches.	1. TrPDN: Bil UT, SCM 2. STM: Bil UT, SCM, masseter, temporalis 3. SID	1. FB, SB, Rot Gr. IV Passive mobs: upper cervical spine		
3/31/05 NDI: 20/100, HDI: 20/100 Comments: Reports some neck soreness with one HA.	1. STM: Bil UT 2. SID	1. FB, SB, Rot Gr. IV Passive mobs: upper cervical spine		
4/25/05 Comments: Doing very well. No HA in the past month.		1. Traction mob Gr. V: T4-8	1. Issued neck program 2. Reviewed & performed the relaxation and postural aspects of program	1. Next visit will review, perform, and finalize the flexibility and strength aspects of the neck program

OMPT, orthopaedic manual physical therapy; HA, headache; TMJ, temporomandibular joint; eval, evaluation; Tx, treatment; HEP, home exercise program; NDI, Neck Disability Index; HDI, Headache Disability Inventory; Lt, left; Rt, right; Bil, bilateral; UT, upper trapezius; SCM, sternocleidomastoid; LT, lower trapezius; SpCap, splenius capitus; SOs, suboccipital muscles; TrPDN, trigger point dry needling; STM, soft-tissue manipulation; PIR, postisometric relaxation; SID, subcranial inhibitive distraction; NAGS, natural apophyseal glides; LAD, long-axis distraction; SNAG, sustained natural apophyseal glide; PA (prog. osc.), posterior-anterior progressive oscillations; Gr, grade; mob, mobilization; AROM, active range of motion; EXT, extension; FB, forward bending; SB, side bending; Rot, rotation; MO, mouth opening; LE, lateral excursion; Pro, protrusion.

Table 34.9 Differences Between Traditional Acupuncture and Dry Needling or Intramuscular Stimulation

Acupuncture	Dry Needling or Intramuscular Stimulation
Medical diagnosis not relevant	Medical diagnosis is pertinent
Medical examination not pertinent	Medical examination essential
Needle insertions along nonscientific meridians according to Chinese philosophy	Needled insertions in trigger points or motor points according to examination
Knowledge of anatomy not pertinent	Knowledge of anatomy essential
No immediate objective changes anticipated	Immediate subjective and objective effects often expected

Modified from Gunn, 1996.

Travell et al. (1942) first described the use of muscle TrP injections in the treatment of myofascial pain in a 1942 paper. Travell's work subsequently led to the development of the TrPDN technique, which is different from trigger point injections (also used by Travell) in that no substance is injected. In 1979, Lewit described the "needle effect" as the immediate analgesia that was produced by needling the painful spot. Both Travell and Lewit, as well as many others, agreed that it is the mechanical stimulus of the needle that likely results in beneficial therapeutic effects and not necessarily the substance being injected (Lewit, 1979; Hong, 1994; Simons et al., 1999; Chen et al., 2001). Several case reports have described dry needling techniques in the treatment of various musculoskeletal conditions by other medical professionals (Ingber, 1989, 2000; Gozon et al., 2001; Gunn et al., 2001; Kaye, 2001; Chu et al., 2004a; Cummings, 2003a, 2003b), but to date, only one case report in the PT literature exists on the inclusion of the TrPDN technique in PT intervention (Issa & Huijbregts, 2006).

Although there may be no reported cases of complications related to dry needling and despite the differences noted earlier between dry needling and acupuncture (Table 34.9), precautions and complications related to the insertion of acupuncture needles must be considered. Contraindications to dry needling include acute trauma with hematoma, local or generalized circulatory problems (i.e., varicosis, thrombosis,

and ulceration), diminished coagulation, and local or generalized skin lesions or infections (Gerwin & Dommerholt, 2001). Complications related to dry needling may include vasodepressive syncope; hematoma; penetration of visceral organs such as lung, bowel, or kidney; increased spasm and pain of the muscle treated; and muscle edema (Gerwin & Dommerholt, 2001).

Serious complications related to acupuncture are rare but include pneumothorax, cardiac tamponade (compression of the heart caused by blood or fluid accumulation in the space between the myocardium and the pericardium), and spinal cord lesions (Peuker & Gronemeyer, 2001). Serious injuries to abdominal viscera, peripheral nerves, and blood vessels are also rare (Peuker & Gronemeyer, 2001). A prospective survey study of adverse events following acupuncture in 32,000 consultations by 78 acupuncturists reported 2,178 events—that is, an incidence of 684 per 10,000 consultations (White et al., 2001). Most included minor events, with the following mean incidence per 10,000 (95% CI): bleeding or hematoma in 310 cases (160 to 590), needling pain in 110 (48 to 247), aggravation of complaints in 96 (43 to 178), faintness in 29 (22 to 37), drowsiness after treatment in 29 (16 to 49), stuck or bent needle in 13 (0 to 42), headache in 11 (6 to 18), and sweating in 10 cases (6 to 16) (White et al., 2001). Forty-three events were considered significant minor adverse events, a rate of 14 per 10,000 (95% CI: 8–20), and one seizure event was considered serious (White et al., 2001). Another prospective study of 34,000 consultations by 574 practitioners revealed similar findings (MacPherson et al., 2001): transient minor events, 15% (95% CI: 14.6–15.3), included mild bruising, pain, bleeding, and aggravation of symptoms. Forty-three significant minor events were reported—that is a rate of 13 per 10,000 (95% CI: 0.9–1.7) (MacPherson et al., 2001). Significant minor events included severe nausea and fainting; severe, unexpected, and prolonged exacerbation of symptoms; prolonged pain and bruising; and psychological and emotional reactions (MacPherson et al., 2001). No serious major adverse events that required a hospital admission or a prolonged hospital stay or that caused permanent disability or death were reported (95% CI: 0–1.1 per 10,000 treatments) (MacPherson et al., 2001).

The most common side effects of dry needling include soreness, hematoma, and muscle edema (Gerwin & Dommerholt, 2001). General precautions for dry needling include establishing competence through adequate training and competency testing, clinical experience, and—last but not least—using common sense. Although there is limited evidence to suggest a significant risk of spread of infection through acupuncture, universal precautions are still important (Walsh, 2001). Specific precautions that should be taken include proper patient positioning, use of surgical gloves to protect the clinician against needlestick injuries, knowledge of detailed clinical anatomy, and knowledge of muscle-specific precautions (Gerwin & Dommerholt, 2001).

For this patient, the initial trial treatment using dry needling was meant to serve two purposes:

- Confirm the clinical diagnosis of active TrPs through reproducing or relieving the patient's symptoms
- Assess patient tolerance during and after treatment to this sometimes painful procedure

For this reason, the initial trial was performed for a minimal period of time (i.e., approximately 5 minutes). The patient was thoroughly educated on the basic premise of TrPDN treatment, how this technique differs from traditional acupuncture, what to expect during and after the treatment, the type of needle used, precautions used, possible side effects, and expected outcomes. Clinician education, training, and clinical experience with TrPDN were made clear to the patient. The patient provided informed consent for the suggested treatment including TrPDN. In this case, the UT and SCM were chosen for the trial treatment because manual palpation of the muscle TrPs in these muscles causes referred pain into the neck, head, and face that was similar to the patient's complaints. Treating these muscles first could then serve as a diagnostic indicator for the contribution of TrPs to the patient's total presentation.

For this patient, individually packaged stainless steel acupuncture needles in plastic insertion tubes were used. The needle sizes (diameter × length) used were 0.30 × 30 mm, 0.30 × 50 mm, and 0.20 × 13 mm. The taut band and TrP were identified by palpation with the dominant or nondominant hand; the needle in its tube was then fixed against the suspected area by the nondominant hand either by using a pincer grip or flat palpation depending on the muscle orientation, location, and direction of penetration. With the dominant hand, the needle was gently loosened from the tube, and then a flick or tap of the top of the needle was performed to quickly penetrate the layers of the skin. This is done to ensure pain-free penetration of the needle. The needle

was then guided toward the taut band until resistance was felt at a particular direction and depth. Gentle, small-amplitude withdrawals and penetrations of the needle were performed until a trigger point zone had been found that was clinically identified by the elicitation of an LTR. Within the context of TrPDN, the elicitation of an LTR is considered essential in obtaining a desirable therapeutic effect (Hong, 1994; Gunn, 1996; Simons et al., 1999; Chu, 2000, 2002; Chu & Schwartz, 2002; Chu et al., 2004b). The needle was focused in this area or other areas by drawing the needle back toward the skin and then redirecting the needle toward suspected areas. Numerous LTRs can generally be reproduced; sometimes more than 20 LTRs can be elicited from several TrPs in a focused trigger point zone. The needle was removed once few LTRs were attained (none in three to five passes) or until palpable and/or visible release of the taut band had been determined. The needle could be placed back in the tube to be used immediately on the same patient or discarded in a sharps container while pressure was being applied to the treated area with the nondominant hand for approximately 10 to 30 seconds. Generally, if the needle had been used twice or if it had been bent or dulled during the procedure, it was discarded. During the procedure, the patient was closely monitored for tolerance and for reproduction of local or referred pain sensations. If the patient had not tolerated the treatment due to numerous or strong LTRs, the treatment would have been paused for several seconds until the patient indicated the ability to continue. As clearly communicated to the patient, the treatment would be stopped at any time upon her request or if it was clear that she was not tolerating the treatment.

Immediately after TrPDN, manual myofascial therapy was performed to relieve soreness, increase circulation, decrease myofascial hypertonicity, and improve flexibility. The application of a cold pack or moist heat was used at the end of the session dependent on the outcome of that session. A cold pack was used if treatment was intensive and edema was visible or palpable. Moist heat was used if no visible or palpable edema was present. At the end of the TrPDN session, the patient was educated as to the following post-treatment care. The patient should expect soreness in the treated area typically for 1 to 2 days (occasionally more than 2 days). This soreness should be clearly identified as due to treatment and should always resolve. Soreness might make it difficult to judge previous complaints, but the effects would be easy to judge once soreness had

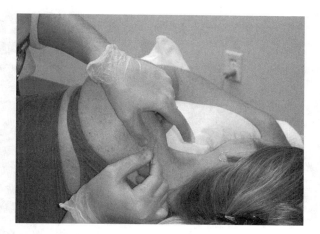

Figure 34.5 Trigger Point Dry Needling of Upper Trapezius Muscle in Side-Lying Position

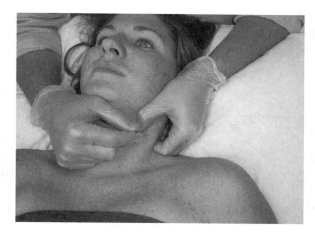

Figure 34.7 Trigger Point Dry Needling of Sternocleidomastoid Muscle

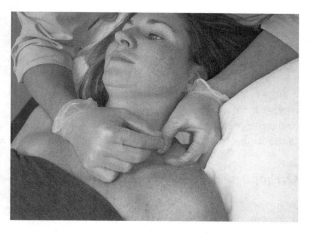

Figure 34.6 Trigger Point Dry Needling of Upper Trapezius Muscle in Supine Position

subsided. Post-treatment soreness could be decreased with moist heat, gentle massage of treated area, self-stretch, and over-the-counter pain medication as necessary.

For the UT muscle, TrPDN was performed with patient in side-lying position (**Figure 34.5**) and/or supine position (the anterior fibers, **Figure 34.6**) and the therapist standing to the side or at the head of the patient. The pincer grip was used in side-lying position, and the taut band and contraction knot were grasped with the nondominant hand while the dominant hand performed the needling procedure in the inferior-lateral, anterior-superior, or anterior-lateral direction. The therapist took care only to needle the muscle fibers accessible between the thumb and index finger. Using flat palpation, the UT taut band and contraction knot were fixed in

between the index and middle finger against the superior portion of the scapula. Using the pincer grip in supine position, the muscle was needled in the posterior direction toward the index finger. For this technique, the 0.30 × 30 mm and 0.30 × 50 mm needle are used depending on patient physical makeup and the location and direction of the treated area. Precautions included that the needle should never be directed in the anterior-medial or inferior direction to avoid puncturing the apex of the lung.

For the SCM muscle, TrPDN was performed in supine or side-lying position with the neck and head adequately supported and with the therapist standing to the side or at the head of the patient (**Figure 34.7**). In supine position, the pincer grip was used to grasp both heads of the muscle while the needle was directed from the medial side to the posterior-lateral and/or anterior-to-posterior direction between the thumb and index finger. For this muscle, the 0.30 × 30 mm needle was used. Precautions for dry needling of the SCM included that the carotid artery should be identified medial to the SCM and that the direction of the needle should not be in the medial direction to avoid puncturing said artery.

For the lower trapezius (LT) muscle, TrPDN was performed in side-lying or prone position with the therapist standing to the treated side (**Figure 34.8**). The diagonally oriented taut band was fixed between the index and middle finger with the contraction knot firmly over a rib. The index finger and middle finger were subsequently located in the intercostal space. The needle was directed anteriorly against the rib or laterally at a shallow angle tangential to the chest wall. For this muscle the 0.30 × 30 mm needle was again used. Precautions for

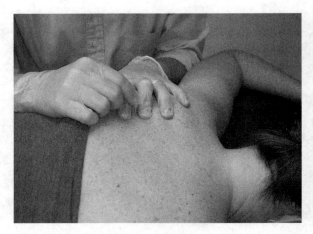

Figure 34.8 Trigger Point Dry Needling of Lower Trapezius Muscle

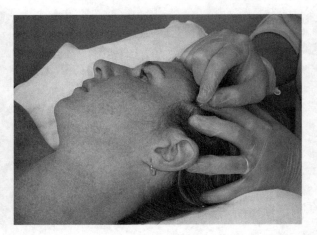

Figure 34.10 Trigger Point Dry Needling of Temporalis Muscle

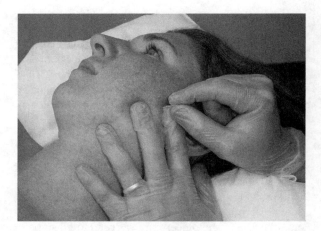

Figure 34.9 Trigger Point Dry Needling of Masseter Muscle

needling this muscle included avoiding penetration of the lung by needling over a rib or tangentially to the chest wall.

For the masseter muscle, TrPDN was performed in side-lying or supine position with the neck and head supported by a pillow and the therapist standing to the side or at the head of the patient (**Figure 34.9**). The taut bands and sensitive knots in the superficial and deep masseter muscle were identified by pincer grip or flat palpation. The treated area was fixed between the index and middle fingers, and the needle was directed between the fingers. For this technique, the 0.20 × 13 mm needle was used because precautions included avoiding needlestick injury to the facial nerve.

For the temporalis muscle, TrPDN was performed in side-lying or supine position with the neck and head

supported by a pillow and with the therapist again standing to the side or at the head of the patient (**Figure 34.10**). The temporal artery was first palpated, and then the taut bands and sensitive knot were identified and fixed against the temporal bone between the index and middle finger. The needle was then directed toward the contraction knot. The 0.20 × 13 mm needle was used, because the precaution for this technique was avoidance of the superficially located temporal artery.

Orthopaedic Manual Physical Therapy

Well integrated into physical therapy, OMPT includes manipulation techniques with purported effects on either soft tissue or joints. Soft-tissue manipulation uses manual techniques aimed at relaxing muscles, increasing circulation, breaking up adhesions or scar tissue, and easing pain in the soft tissues. Soft-tissue manipulation techniques include manual trigger point therapy, strain-counterstrain, muscle energy technique, neuromuscular technique, myofascial release, and other therapeutic massage techniques. Paris (1999) defined joint manipulation as "the skilled passive movement to a joint." Joint manipulation techniques are aimed at restoring motion at a joint and modulating pain. Joint manipulation techniques include nonthrust, thrust, and traction forces applied at various grades and directions (Paris & Loubert, 1999).

Soft-tissue manipulation is used to describe therapeutic massage and manual techniques for mobilizing soft tissue (e.g., muscles, connective tissue, fascia, tendons, ligaments) to improve the function of the muscular, circulatory, lymphatic, and nervous systems

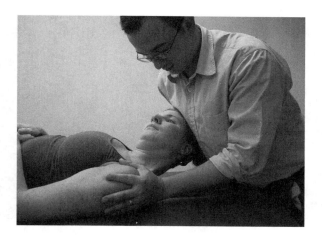

Figure 34.11 Postisometric Relaxation of Upper Trapezius Muscle

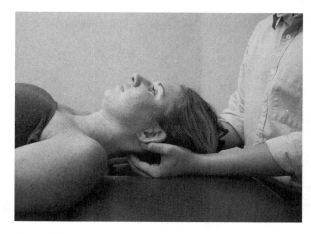

Figure 34.12 Subcranial Inhibitive Distraction

(Johnson & Johnson, 2001). Some techniques are general for treating large areas using the palm of the hand and the forearm, for example, whereas other techniques are specific, such as deep stroking, transverse friction, and trigger point compression release using the thumb and fingertips.

Postisometric relaxation (PIR) was a soft-tissue manipulation technique used for this patient with the goal of achieving muscle relaxation and elongation (Lewit & Simons, 1984; Simons et al., 1999). With the patient relaxed and the body supported, the therapist passively lengthened the muscle to its first barrier. The patient then performed a minimal isometric contraction of the muscle (10–25%) for 5 seconds during an inhalation while the therapist stabilized the muscle to be stretched. Then the patient relaxed completely and exhaled, while the therapist passively stretched the muscle to the new barrier. The technique was then repeated three to five times. This technique is very similar to contract/relax and hold/relax techniques. Specific muscles treated with this technique are indicated in Table 34.8, with the technique illustrated for the UT muscle in **Figure 34.11**.

Subcranial inhibitive distraction (SID) is a myofascial technique described by Paris (1999) that is aimed at releasing tension in suboccipital soft tissue and suboccipital musculature (**Figure 34.12**). The patient was lying supine with head supported. The therapist placed the three middle fingers just caudal to the nuchal line, lifted the fingertips upward, resting the hands on the treatment table, and then applied a gentle cranial pull, causing a long-axis extension. The procedure was performed with this patient for 2 to 5 minutes, as indicated in Table 34.8. A pilot study of the effect of SID

on cervical flexion AROM showed a trend for the largest postintervention changes in AROM among subjects with mechanical neck pain who complained of headaches, indicated lower levels of pain, and had suffered pain for greater than 6 months (Briem et al., 2007).

Mulligan (1999, 2000) described *reverse natural apophyseal glides* as a mid- to end-range oscillatory mobilization indicated from the C7 vertebra down that were intended to aid in treatment of end-range loss of neck mobility, postural dysfunction (FHP with UT pain), and degenerative lower cervical or upper thoracic spine segments. The patient was seated and the therapist stood to the side and cradled the head to the body with the forearm, maintaining some neck flexion. Flexing the index finger interphalangeal joint and extending the metacarpophalangeal joints constituted the mobilizing handgrip. The thumb and index finger formed a V-shape that made contact with the articular pillars; then an anterior-cranial mobilization was applied, gliding the inferior facet up on the superior one (**Figure 34.13**).

Rocabado (2002b) described *long-axis distraction of the upper cervical spine* (C0-C2). The patient was lying supine with head in neutral. The therapist was sitting behind the patient and cradled the occiput with one hand while placing the same shoulder on the frontal bone to prevent head elevation. The opposite hand stabilized C2 with a pincer grip (**Figure 34.14**). Gentle cranial grade III distractions were applied six times with 6-second duration.

Sustained natural apophyseal glides (SNAGS) involve concurrent accessory joint gliding and active physiological movement with overpressure at the end of range

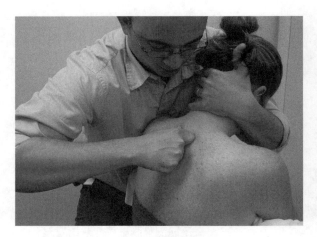

Figure 34.13 Reverse Natural Apophyseal Glides

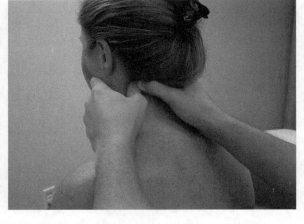

Figure 34.15 Sustained Natural Apophyseal Glide: C1-C2

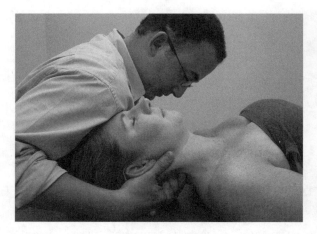

Figure 34.14 Long-Axis Distraction: Upper Cervical Spine

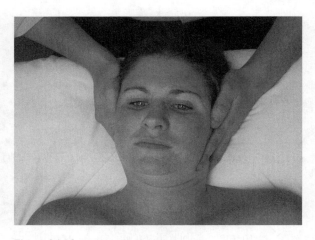

Figure 34.16 Right Lateral Glide: C0-C1

(Mulligan, 1999, 2000). In this case, a C1-C2 SNAG to improve C1-C2 right rotation was performed with the patient sitting or standing and with the therapist behind the patient (**Figure 34.15**). The lateral border of the left thumb was placed on the lateral border of the left C1 transverse process and then reinforced with the right thumb to give an anterior glide. The patient was asked to slowly turn her head to the right while the therapist maintained the anterior glide, also during return to starting position. The horizontal plane of the glide was maintained throughout the movement. If the procedure was pain free, it was repeated five times.

Right lateral glide at C0-C1 was performed to improve C0-C1 left side-bending (Rocabado, 2002b) (**Figure 34.16**). The patient was lying supine with head in neutral.

The therapist was sitting behind the patient, grasping the head by placing the medial side of the index finger on the mastoid process. A right lateral grade III glide was performed with the left hand using the nose as the center of rotation; this was repeated for three sets of 10 repetitions. The right hand simultaneously moved with the head to maintain stability.

Posterior-anterior (PA) glide progressive oscillations were performed to address restrictions of upper and midthoracic extension (Paris, 1999) (**Figure 34.17**). The patient was prone, and the therapist stood facing the patient. The therapist's cranial hand, with elbow slightly bent, was placed on the thoracic spine, with the spinous process fitting in the hollow part of the hand just distal to the pisiform bone. In time with the patient's breathing, at midexhalation, a series of four short progressive

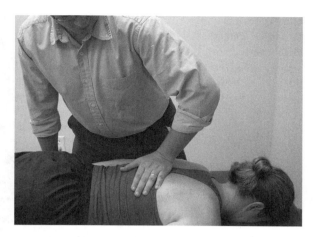

Figure 34.17 Posterior-Anterior Glide with Progressive Oscillation: Midthoracic Spine

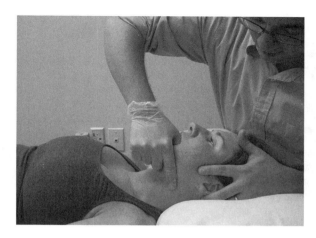

Figure 34.19 Temporomandibular Long-Axis Distraction

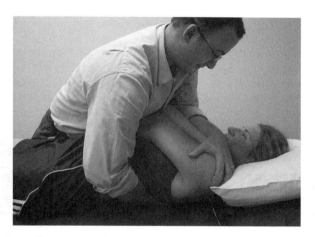

Figure 34.18 Traction Manipulation: Upper and Midthoracic Spine

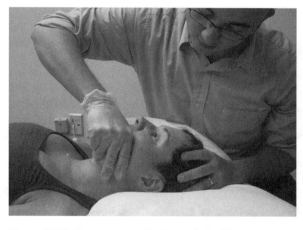

Figure 34.20 Temporomandibular Medial Glide

impulses were given in the PA direction, ending at the patient's end range (grade IV–IV++).

Traction manipulation as described by Kaltenborn et al. (2003) was performed for slight facet restrictions of upper and midthoracic extension (**Figure 34.18**). The patient lay supine with arms folded across the chest and hands on opposite shoulders. The therapist faced the patient and pulled her into a left side-lying position with the right hand. The therapist's left hand fixated the caudal vertebra of the segment with the thenar eminence on the right transverse process and the flexed third finger on the left transverse process. The therapist then rolled the patient back into a supine position with the right hand, maintaining the position of the left hand on the pa-

tient's back. The right hand and forearm were placed over the patient's crossed arms, with the chest over the elbows. During an exhalation, a grade V linear mobilization was applied with the right arm and body moving the upper trunk in a posterior direction at a right angle to the treatment plane through the facet joints.

TMJ long-axis distraction (**Figure 34.19**), *medial glide* (**Figure 34.20**), and *lateral glide* (**Figure 34.21**) were done to improve TMJ position, mobility, and stability as described by Rocabado (2002b). Bilateral TMJ manipulation was performed in this case; described here is an example of the procedure on the left. The patient was supine, with the therapist sitting at the head of the table. The patient was asked to open her mouth minimally

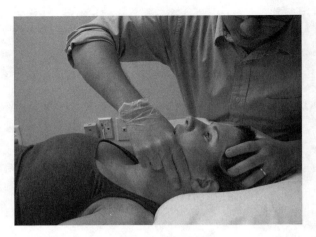

Figure 34.21 Temporomandibular Lateral Glide

(10 mm). Using the right hand and wearing gloves, the therapist placed the palmar side of the thumb on the cranial aspect of the bottom row of teeth on the left hand side toward the molars while the index finger gently grasped the mandible. A gentle long-axis distraction was applied by performing an ulnar deviation of the wrist. To perform a medial glide or lateral distraction of the joint, the therapist changed the position of the hand to place the thumb on the inside aspect of the bottom row of teeth and grasped the lateral aspect of the mandible with the index finger. The therapist then performed an ulnar deviation of the wrist, resulting in a medial glide. To do a lateral glide or medial distraction of the joint, the therapist kept the same hand position as the medial glide, but the left hand was placed on the vertex of the head. The glide was performed by stabilizing the mandible with the right hand and performing a left head side-bend motion using the left hand, resulting in a relative lateral glide of the joint. These TMJ manual interventions were performed as grade III mobilizations and repeated six times each. In between each direction, the hand was removed from the mouth and the patient was encouraged to swallow. Details regarding when these articular OMPT procedures were performed on this patient can be found in Table 34.8.

Exercise Therapy

Self-stretch exercises were provided for each muscle treated and were aimed at reducing muscle tension, decreasing pain, and improving flexibility. The general approach of performing the exercise was based on teaching the patient to stabilize one end of the muscle and then to passively stretch the other end to feel a gentle stretch. Directions were provided to hold the stretch for 20 seconds for three repetitions, two to three times per day. Slow, relaxed breathing was encouraged during the stretch. Neuromuscular reeducation included verbal and manual cues that were used to provide proprioceptive feedback and promote quality of movement.

The *neck clock exercise* was used to induce relaxation, decrease pain, and improve mobility and coordination of the head and neck complex (Johnson & Johnson, 2001). This exercise involved the patient lying on her back with a towel roll to support the neck, knees bent, and feet flat. The patient was instructed to imagine the head against the face of a clock. Using the eyes or nose as a guide and the clock as a reference, she was asked to move the head into the 12:00 and 6:00 positions, then to repeat this for the 3:00 to 9:00 positions, then to move the head in a clockwise direction and finally in a counterclockwise direction. The patient was asked to repeat each direction 10 times.

The *shoulder clock exercise* was aimed at inducing relaxation, reducing pain, and improving mobility and coordination for the neck and shoulder-girdle complex (Johnson & Johnson, 2001). This exercise involved the patient lying on the side that was not targeted and imagining the shoulder against the face of a clock, where 12:00 is toward the head, 6:00 toward the hip, 3:00 toward the front, and 9:00 toward the back. The shoulder blade was moved between the different positions and directions, as it was for the neck clock exercise, and this was repeated 10 times in each direction.

AROM for anterior rotation of the head on the neck (also known as craniocervical flexion or axial extension) emphasized cervical muscular postural training and strengthening, craniocervical flexion mobility, and lengthening of the posterior craniocervical musculature, often shortened in FHP as noted in this patient (Johnson & Johnson, 2001; Rocabado, 2002b). The patient was again lying on her back with a towel roll to support the neck, knees bent, and feet flat. She was then instructed to perform a chin tuck and lift the back of the head upward off the floor, holding this position for 6 seconds for six repetitions. Feedback was given to isolate the deep cervical flexors and to prevent an overcompensatory contraction of the SCM.

TMJ exercises were aimed at relieving joint irritation, promoting muscle relaxation, and reestablishing joint stability (Rocabado, 2001, 2002a). The patient performed AROM for 10-mm mouth opening (MO), 10 mm of right lateral excursion (LE), and 10 mm MO in LE for six repetitions each (Rocabado, 2001, 2002a). AROM for 10-mm MO was performed by applying gentle compression using thumb or fingertips through the bilateral shaft of the mandible, followed by a small excursion of mouth opening (equal to a small separation of the teeth) while keeping the tongue positioned against the palate at the roof of the mouth. AROM for 10-mm LE was performed to the opposite side of dysfunction or hypermobility, in this case to the right; 10 mm of LE is an approximate excursion equal to bringing the upper canine in line with the lower canine. The patient performed AROM of 10-mm MO in opposite LE by gently opening the mouth in the right lateral position. Throughout these exercises, the tongue was positioned at the roof of the mouth to maintain a minimal amount of stress to the TMJ. Manual guiding for these movements may initially be necessary to provide proprioceptive feedback and to encourage quality of motion.

The *Neck Program* is a patient education booklet that includes information on neck pathology and body mechanics, with daily activities and exercises. The exercises can be performed in a short period of time and address four components of musculoskeletal neck care: relaxation, posture, flexibility, and strengthening. During the last visit, the patient was given the booklet, and the relaxation and posture sections were reviewed and performed. One additional visit was recommended to review and perform the flexibility and strengthening aspects, but the patient did not schedule another visit.

Education

Education for this patient included postural education, instruction on relaxation, self-application of a suboccipital release technique, and a TMJ self-care program. The therapist explained to the patient the role that posture played in relation to her complaints and musculoskeletal impairments, and what constituted good and bad postural alignment using the aid of a spine skeleton. Then functional tests were performed with the patient seated in front of a mirror to demonstrate the consequences of poor sitting posture. The patient was asked to assume her habitual posture. A vertical compression test was performed through the shoulders to assess alignment and stability. The patient was encouraged to see and feel any spinal instability as well as to note any pain. The posture was subsequently manually corrected and the test repeated so that the patient might note the positive changes in stability and discomfort. In her habitual posture, the patient was then directed to slowly turn her neck in each direction and then to raise her arms overhead, noting ease of mobility and discomfort. After posture correction, the patient was directed to repeat the movements and note improvement in range and reduction in discomfort.

The patient was taken through a series of postural adjustment steps that she could use to aid in correcting her posture. First, the concepts of base of support through the feet and chair adjustment were reviewed. The patient was then asked to roll her pelvis forward and backward, noting the range of mobility, and then asked to overcorrect the lumbar lordosis, followed by slowly releasing the lordosis until she felt that her pelvis was in a comfortable, neutral position. The patient was encouraged to feel the pressure on the ischial tuberosities, and the therapist explained how this was her neutral position. The patient was then shown the adjustment of the shoulder girdle into neutral while preventing the anterior ribs from elevating. The patient was instructed in the adjustment of the head position into neutral by performing a gentle chin tuck guided passively using the fingertips of the index finger and releasing the chin tuck at the point of a comfortable position. The patient was then shown strategies for maintaining the corrected sitting position using active sitting, a lumbar or sacral roll, or broader lumbar supports. Finally, the patient was educated in body mechanics with proper dynamic posturing for home and work activities. These postural education concepts were based on the treating therapist's personal experience, this therapist's education, and teachings by Paris (1999) and Johnson (2001).

Relaxation was addressed through teaching of relaxed positioning of the head, neck, and jaw incorporated with breathing techniques as described by Rocabado (2001). The positions of the head, jaw, and tongue have been shown to have potential adverse effects on TMJ compression, TMJ mobility, and periarticular muscle activity (Rocabado, 2001). The patient was directed to lie in a supine position with towel support under the neck and pillow support under the head and then to note the resting positions of her head, jaw, and tongue and to recognize her breathing pattern (e.g., through nose or mouth, with chest or abdomen). The patient was then directed to find the neutral position of the head, to position the tongue to the roof of the mouth with the tip behind the top two teeth, and to close the mouth but keep a small separation of the teeth. The patient was then directed to inhale through the nose, allowing the breath to initiate from the abdomen by letting it naturally rise rather than via the chest, and then to exhale slowly through the nose, allowing the abdomen to naturally fall. This relaxation exercise was also instructed in a corrected sitting or standing posture and recommended as needed to relieve stress and tension. Conscious correcting of her posture and performance of these relaxation exercises were encouraged once every hour for any duration.

A suboccipital release self-treatment technique was taught to address tension at the base of the head as well as for relieving headaches. The patient was educated on placing two tennis balls in a thin sock and then tying the sock to maintain stability of the balls. The technique was to be performed in a quiet dark room lying supine with the use of a neck roll to support the neck and a pillow to support the head with knees supported. The tennis balls were to be placed above the neck roll at the base of the head with additional support as needed under the head to prevent craniocervical extension. Lying in this position for 5 minutes while focusing on relaxation and breathing exercises, patients have described good success with the release of tension and pain as well as reducing or warding off headaches.

A TMJ self-care program was instructed for reducing pain, relaxing muscles, relieving intrajoint irritation, and maintaining gains achieved from therapeutic intervention (Rocabado, 2001). Advice for self-care included a soft, nonchewy diet, no wide opening of mouth (maximum of two fingers' width), no biting, no gum chewing, prevention of direct pressure on the mandible or sleeping on the problematic side, yawning with tongue against the palate, tongue against the palate at rest, nasal breathing maintaining free airway space, and maintaining good posture.

Outcomes

On the patient's last visit, she reported doing very well, with no headache in the preceding month. The PT recommended that the patient follow up for one additional visit to perform the flexibility and strengthening portions of the issued *Neck Program* booklet and review the entire program prior to discontinuation of therapy. However, the patient did not schedule another appointment for an unknown reason, so unfortunately objective data and outcome measures could not be reassessed.

Overall, the patient noted a significant decrease in headache frequency, with progressive improvement since the start of therapy from more than once per week (daily) to one to four per month and finally to none in the month preceding her last therapy visit. Headache intensity also progressively improved since therapy onset from a reported severe to a mild intensity. Throughout the duration of PT treatment, the patient also reported cessation of tinnitus, less neck tenderness, and improved jaw and neck mobility and function. The patient reported improvement with the following activities of daily living: she was now able to do as much work as she wanted, able to drive longer distances with only slight neck pain, able to read as much as she wanted with only slight neck pain, and experienced some neck pain related only to a few recreational activities.

The last set of outcome measures completed by the patient was on the second to last visit. The results of the four HDI (**Table 34.10**) and NDI (**Table 34.11**) outcome measures completed throughout the treatment period are illustrated in **Figures 34.22** and **34.23**. The results of the HDI outcome measure showed a 31% improvement for the emotional score, a 42% improvement for the functional score, and a 36% improvement in the total score between the time of the initial evaluation and the second to last visit. During the same time period, the results of the NDI outcome measure showed an 18% improvement and—at one time—a 26% improvement for an earlier assessment date. Although specific subjective and objective signs of improvement were not assessed on the last visit date, which was approximately

Table 34.10 Headache Disability Index: Outcome Measures

	10/18/04	11/11/04	1/13/05	3/31/05
Frequency	>1/wk	>1/wk	1–4/month	1–4/month
Intensity	Severe	Moderate	Mild	Not completed
Emotional score (max. 52)	26	18	12	10
Functional score (max. 48)	30	24	12	10
Total score (max. 100)	56	42	24	20

Table 34.11 Neck Disability Index: Outcome Measures

	10/18/04	11/11/04	1/13/04	3/31/05
Total score (max. 50)	19	14	6	10
Disability score	38%	28%	12%	20%
Disability	Moderate	Moderate	Mild	Mild

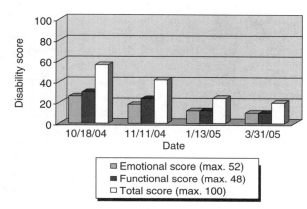

Figure 34.22 Headache Disability Index Outcome Measures Scores

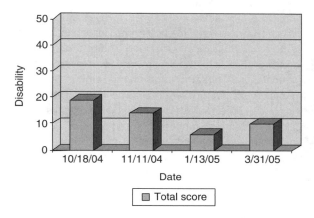

Figure 34.23 Neck Disability Index Outcome Measures Scores

1 month after the previous follow-up, significant improvement was noted through the assessment of self-perceived outcome measures used in this case. A 29% change in the HDI total score constitutes the minimally detectable change score (MDC_{95}) for this measure (Jacobson et al., 1994). A 7-point or 14% change in the NDI score constitutes the minimum clinically important difference (MCID) for the NDI (Cleland et al., 2006). The change in the total score of the HDI outcome measure in this case was a decrease of 36%, which indicates that the MDC was exceeded and that a true change had indeed occurred in pain and disability due to the headache complaints. Similarly, the change in NDI score, which exceeded the established MCID for this measure, indicated that a true and meaningful change in neck-related disability had occurred during the course of treatment.

DISCUSSION

The patient described in this case report had a very complex presentation. Medical diagnoses included chronic tension-type headache associated with pericranial tenderness, probable migraine without aura, proba-

ble CeH, and TMD. Impairments identified during the PT examination included postural deviations (FHP), muscle TrPs and decreased length in the neck and jaw muscles, hypomobility in the C0-C2 and T1-T8 segments, and hypermobility of the left TMJ. Poor prognostic indicators, including the presence of possible central sensitization, emotional stress, depression, and the worsening nature of a chronic condition, further complicated the patient's presentation.

Despite this complexity, the patient clearly improved over the course of treatment. She exceeded the MDC on the HDI, indicating that a true improvement had occurred with regard to headache-related disability, and exceeding the MCID on the NDI implied that a true and clinically meaningful improvement also occurred for disability due to neck pain. In addition, the patient reported on the last visit after 1 month of no treatment that she had not experienced a single headache in the preceding month. This is especially significant considering that the patient initially described daily headaches.

Although a case report does not allow us to infer a cause-and-effect relationship between intervention and outcome, true and meaningful changes in a previously worsening, chronic condition do imply that the PT management described was at least contributory to the positive changes noted.

CONCLUSION

This chapter provides a detailed account of the PT diagnosis and management of a patient with chronic headaches, facial pain, and neck pain. After ascertaining that there were no contraindications to PT examination, the therapist used the ICHD-II and AAOP classification systems to classify the headache and TMJ complaints. Physical examination findings were evaluated based on a pathophysiologic and research-based rationale, and relevant impairments amenable to PT management were identified. The ICF disablement model was used to describe the patient's diagnosis, impairments, current functioning, and level of disability. The preferred practice patterns from the *Guide to Physical Therapist Practice* (APTA, 2001) were used as broad consensus-based guidelines for the development of a plan of care.

Treatment incorporated TrPDN, OMPT, exercise therapy, and education. Over the course of treatment, true and meaningful changes were documented with regard to headache and neck pain–related disability. The patient also reported a noted decrease in headache frequency from daily to none over the month preceding the last visit. True and meaningful changes in a previously worsening, chronic condition do imply that the PT management described was at least contributory to the positive changes noted. As the authors, we hope that this chapter providing a clinical illustration of a real-life patient will help the reader achieve the main objective of this text: to improve diagnosis and management of patients with a primary complaint of headache presenting to therapists and physicians.

This chapter was based largely on the following article: Issa TS, Huijbregts PA. Physical therapy diagnosis and management of a patient with chronic daily headache: A case report. *J Manual Manipulative Ther* 2006;14:E88–123. The authors would like to acknowledge and thank the *Journal* for permission to use this material in this context.

REFERENCES

Agustsson H. *Evaluation and Treatment of the Craniomandibular System*. St. Augustine, FL: University of St. Augustine; 2004.

Alix M, Bates DK. A proposed etiology of cervicogenic headache: the neurophysiologic basis and anatomic relationship between the dura mater and the rectus posterior capitis minor muscle. *J Manipulative Physiol Ther* 1999;22:534–539.

Alvarez DJ, Rockwell PG. Trigger points: diagnosis and management. *Am Fam Physician* 2002;65:653–660.

American Physical Therapy Association. Guide to Physical Therapist Practice (2nd edition). *Phys Ther* 2001;81:9–746.

Aprill C, Axinn MJ, Bogduk N. Occipital headaches stemming from the lateral atlanto-axial (C1-2) joint. *Cephalalgia* 2002;22:15–22.

Bendtsen L. Central sensitization in tension type headache: possible patho-physiological mechanisms. *Cephalalgia* 2000;20:486–508.

Bertilson BC, Grunnesjo M, Strender LE. Reliability of clinical tests in the assessment of patients with neck/shoulder problems: impact of history. *Spine* 2003;28:2222–2231.

Biondi DM. Cervicogenic headache: mechanisms, evaluation, and treatment strategies. *J Am Osteopath Assoc* 2000;100:S7–14.

Borg-Stein J. Cervical myofascial pain and headache. *Curr Pain Headache Rep* 2002;6:324–330.

Briem K, Huijbregts P, Thorsteinsdottir M. Immediate effects of inhibitive distraction on active range of cervical flexion in patients with neck pain: a pilot study. *J Manual Manipulative Ther* 2007;15:82–92.

Bronfort G, Assendelft WJ, Evans R, Haas M, Bouter L. Efficacy of spinal manipulation for chronic headache: a systematic review. *J Manipulative Physiol Ther* 2001;24:457–466.

Chen JT, Chung KC, Hou CR, Kuan TS, Chen SM, Hong CZ. Inhibitory effect of dry needling on the spontaneous electrical activity recorded from myofascial trigger spots of rabbit skeletal muscle. *Am J Phys Med Rehabil* 2001;80:729–735.

Choi YC, Kim WJ, Kim CH, Lee MS. A clinical study of chronic headaches: clinical characteristics and depressive trends in migraine and tension-type headaches. *Yonsei Med J* 1995;36:508–514.

Chu J. Twitch-obtaining intramuscular stimulation (TOIMS): long term observations in the management of chronic partial cervical radiculopathy. *Electromyogr Clin Neurophysiol* 2000;40:503–510.

Chu J. The local mechanism of acupuncture. *Zhonghua Yi Xue Za Zhi (Taipei)* 2002;65:299–302.

Chu J, Schwartz I. The muscle twitch in myofascial pain relief: effects of acupuncture and other needling methods. *Electromyogr Clin Neurophysiol* 2002;42:307–311.

Chu J, Takehara I, Li TC, Schwartz I. Electrical twitch obtaining intramuscular stimulation (ETOIMS) for myofascial pain syndrome in a football player. *Br J Sports Med* 2004a;38:E25.

Chu J, Yuen KF, Wang BH, Chan RC, Schwartz I, Neuhauser D. Electrical twitch-obtaining intramuscular stimulation in lower back pain: a pilot study. *Am J Phys Med Rehabil* 2004b;83:104–111.

Cleland JA, Fritz JM, Whitman JM, Palmer JA. The reliability and construct validity of the Neck Disability Index and patient specific functional scale in patients with cervical radiculopathy. *Spine* 2006;31:598–602.

Cummings M. Referred knee pain treated with electro-acupuncture to iliopsoas. *Acupunct Med* 2003a;21:32–35.

Cummings M. Myofascial pain from pectoralis major following trans-axillary surgery. *Acupunct Med* 2003b;21:105–107.

Cummings TM, White AR. Needling therapies in the management of myofascial trigger point pain: a systematic review. *Arch Phys Med Rehabil* 2001;82:986–992.

Davidoff RA. Trigger points and myofascial pain: toward understanding how they affect headaches. *Cephalalgia* 1998;18:436–448.

Dommerholt J. Dry needling in orthopaedic physical therapy practice. *Orthop Phys Ther Pract* 2004;6:11–16.

Fedorak C, Ashworth N, Marshall J, Paull H. Reliability of the visual assessment of cervical and lumbar lordosis: how good are we? *Spine* 2003;28:1857–1859.

Fernández-de-las-Peñas C, Cuadrado ML, Gerwin RD, Pareja JA. Referred pain from the trochlear region in tension-type headache: a myofascial trigger point from the superior oblique muscle. *Headache* 2005;45:731–737.

Fernández-de-las-Peñas C, Alonso-Blanco C, San-Roman J, Miangolarra-Page JC. Methodological quality of randomized controlled trials of spinal manipulation and mobilization in tension-type headache, migraine and cervicogenic headache. *J Orthop Sports Phys Ther* 2006a;36:160–169.

Fernández-de-las-Peñas C, Alonso-Blanco C, Cuadrado ML, Gerwin RD, Pareja JA. Myofascial trigger points and their relationship to headache clinical parameters in chronic tension-type headache. *Headache* 2006b;46:1264–1272.

Fjellner A, Bexander C, Faleij R, Strender LE. Inter-examiner reliability in physical examination of the cervical spine. *J Manipulative Physiol Ther* 1999;22:511–516.

Freund B, Schwartz M. Post-traumatic myofascial pain of the head and neck. *Curr Pain Headache Rep* 2002;6:361–369.

Gardner KL. Genetics of migraine: an update. *Headache* 2006;46:S19–S24.

Gerwin RD, Dommerholt J. *Trigger Point Needling: Seminar Manual.* Bethesda, MD: Janet G. Travell Seminar Series; 2001.

Gerwin RD, Shannon S, Hong CZ, Hubbard D, Gevirtz R. Interrater reliability in myofascial trigger point examination. *Pain* 1997;69:65–73.

Gozon B, Chu J, Schwartz I. Lumbo-sacral radiculopathic pain presenting as groin and scrotal pain: pain management with twitch-obtaining intramuscular stimulation. A case report and review of literature. *Electromyogr Clin Neurophysiol* 2001;41:315–318.

Graff-Radford SB. Regional myofascial pain syndrome and headache: principles of diagnosis and management. *Curr Pain Headache Rep* 2001;5:376–381.

Graff-Radford SB, Jaeger B, Reeves JL. Myofascial pain may present clinically as occipital neuralgia. *Neurosurgery* 1986;19:610–613.

Griegel-Morris P, Larson K, Mueller-Klaus K, Oatis CA. Incidence of common postural abnormalities in the cervical, shoulder, and thoracic regions and their association with pain in two age groups of healthy subjects. *Phys Ther* 1992;72:425–431.

Gunn CC. *The Gunn Approach to the Treatment of Chronic Pain: Intramuscular Stimulation for Myofascial Pain of Radiculopathic Origin.* 2nd ed. New York: Churchill Livingstone; 1996.

Gunn CC, Byrne D, Goldberger M, et al. Treating whiplash-associated disorders with intramuscular stimulation: a retrospective review of 43 patients with long-term follow-up. *J Musculoskel Pain* 2001;9:69–89.

Haldeman S, Dagenais S. Cervicogenic headaches: a critical review. *Spine J* 2001;1:31–46.

Han SC, Harrison P. Myofascial pain syndrome and trigger-point management. *Reg Anesth* 1997;22:89–101.

Hanten WP, Olson SL, Lindsay WA, Lounsberry KA, Stewart JK. The effect of manual therapy and a home exercise program on cervicogenic headaches: a case report. *J Manual Manipulative Ther* 2005;13:35–43.

Holmlund AB, Axelsson S. Temporomandibular arthropathy: correlation between clinical signs and symptoms and arthroscopic findings. *Int J Oral Maxillofac Surg* 1996;25:178–181.

Holroyd KA, Stensland M, Lipchik GL, Hill KR, O'Donnell FS, Cordingley G. Psychosocial correlates and impact of chronic tension-type headaches. *Headache* 2000;40:3–16.

Hong CZ. Lidocaine injection versus dry needling to myofascial trigger point: the importance of the local twitch response. *Am J Phys Med Rehabil* 1994;73:256–263.

Hong CZ, Kuan TS, Chen JT, Chen SM. Referred pain elicited by palpation and by needling of myofascial trigger points: a comparison. *Arch Phys Med Rehabil* 1997;78:957–960.

Huijbregts PA. Spinal motion palpation: a review of reliability studies. *J Manual Manipulative Ther* 2002;10:24–39.

Humphreys BK, Delahaye M, Peterson CK. An investigation into the validity of cervical spine motion palpation using subjects with congenital block vertebrae as a "gold standard." *BMC Musculoskeletal Disord* 2004;5:19.

Ingber RS. Iliopsoas myofascial dysfunction: a treatable cause of "failed" low back syndrome. *Arch Phys Med Rehabil* 1989;70:382–386.

Ingber RS. Shoulder impingement in tennis/racquetball players treated with sub-scapularis myofascial treatments. *Arch Phys Med Rehabil* 2000;81:679–682.

Israel HA, Diamond B, Saed-Nejad F, Ratcliffe A. Osteoarthritis and synovitis as major pathoses of the temporomandibular joint: comparison of clinical diagnosis with arthroscopic morphology. *J Oral Maxillofac Surg* 1998;56:1023–1027.

Issa TS, Huijbregts PA. Physical therapy diagnosis and management of a patient with chronic daily headache: a case report. *J Manual Manipulative Ther* 2006;14:E88–E123.

Jacobson GP, Ramadan NM, Aggarwal SK, Newman CW. The Henry Ford Hospital Headache Disability Inventory (HDI). *Neurology* 1994;44:837–842.

Jensen S. Neck related causes of headache. *Aust Fam Physician* 2005;34:635–639.

Jensen R, Bendtsen L, Olesen J. Muscular factors are of importance in tension-type headache. *Headache* 1998;38:10–17.

Jepsen J, Laursen L, Larsen A, Hagert CG. Manual strength testing in 14 upper limb muscles: a study of inter-rater reliability. *Acta Orthop Scand* 2004;75:442–448.

Jepsen JR, Laursen LH, Hagert CG, Kreiner S, Larsen AI. Diagnostic accuracy of the neurological upper limb examination I: inter-rater reproducibility of selected findings and patterns. *BMC Neurol* 2006;6:8.

Johnson GS, Johnson VS. *Functional Orthopedics I: Soft Tissue Mobilization, PNF and Joint Mobilization. Course Manual.* Baltimore, MD: Institute of Physical Art; 2001.

Jull G. Management of cervical headache. *Man Ther* 1997;2: 182–190.

Jull GA, Stanton WR. Predictors of responsiveness to physiotherapy management of cervicogenic headache. *Cephalalgia* 2005;25:101–108.

Jull G, Bogduk N, Marsland A. The accuracy of manual diagnosis for cervical zygapophyseal joint pain syndromes. *Med J Aust* 1988;148:233–236.

Jull G, Zito G, Trott P, Potter H, Shirley D. Inter-examiner reliability to detect painful upper cervical joint dysfunction. *Aust J Physiother* 1997;43:125–129.

Jull G, Trott P, Potter H, et al. A randomized controlled trial of exercise and manipulative therapy for cervicogenic headache. *Spine* 2002;27:1835–1843.

Kaltenborn FM, Evjenth O, Kaltenborn TB, Morgan D, Vollowitz E, Kaltenborn F. *Manual Mobilization of the Joints: The Spine*. 4th ed. Minneapolis, MN: OPTP; 2003.

Karakurum B, Karaalin O, Coskun O, Dora B, Ucler S, Inan L. The dry-needle technique: intramuscular stimulation in tension-type headache. *Cephalalgia* 2001;21:813–817.

Kaye MJ. Evaluation and treatment of a patient with upper quarter myofascial pain syndrome. *J Sports Chiropractic Rehabil* 2001;15:26–33.

Leistad RB, Sand T, Westgaard RH, Nilsen KB, Stovner LJ. Stress-induced pain and muscle activity in patients with migraine and tension-type headache. *Cephalalgia* 2006;26:64–73.

Leonardi M, Steiner TJ, Scher AT, Lipton RB. The global burden of migraine: measuring disability in headache disorders with WHO Classification of Functioning, Disability and Health (ICF). *J Headache Pain* 2005;6:429–440.

Lew PC, Lewis J, Story I. Inter-therapist reliability in locating latent myofascial trigger points using palpation. *Man Ther* 1997;2:87–90.

Lewis J, Green A, Reichard Z, Wright C. Scapular position: the validity of skin surface palpation. *Man Ther* 2002;7: 26–30.

Lewit K. The needle effect in the relief of myofascial pain. *Pain* 1979;6:83–90.

Lewit K, Simons DG. Myofascial pain: relief by post-isometric relaxation. *Arch Phys Med Rehabil* 1984;65:452–456.

Lobbezoo-Scholte AM, de Wijer A, Steenks MH, Bosman F. Interexaminer reliability of six orthopaedic tests in diagnostic subgroups of cranio-mandibular disorders. *J Oral Rehabil* 1994;21:273–285.

MacPherson H, Thomas K, Walters S, Fitter M. A prospective survey of adverse events and treatment reactions following 34,000 consultations with professional acupuncturists. *Acupunct Med* 2001;19:93–102.

Manfredini D, Tognini F, Zampa V, Bosco M. Predictive value of clinical findings for temporomandibular joint effusion. *Oral Surg Oral Med Oral Pathol Oral Radiol Endod* 2003;96: 521–526.

Mannheimer JS, Rosenthal RM. Acute and chronic postural abnormalities as related to craniofacial pain and temporomandibular disorders. *Dent Clin North Am* 1991;35:185–208.

Marcus DA, Scharff L, Mercer S, Turk DC. Musculoskeletal abnormalities in chronic headache: a controlled comparison of headache diagnostic groups. *Headache* 1999;39:21–27.

Martelletti P, van Suijlekom H. Cervicogenic headache: practical approaches to therapy. *CNS Drugs* 2004;18: 793–805.

McGregor AH, Wragg P, Gedroyc WM. Can interventional MRI provide an insight into the mechanics of a posterior-anterior mobilisation? *Clin Biomech* 2001;16:926–929.

Metcalfe S, Reese H. The effect of high-velocity low-amplitude manipulation on cervical spine muscle strength: a randomized clinical trial. *J Manual Manipulative Ther* 2007;15:E45–E63.

Mills Roth J. Physical therapy in the treatment of chronic headache. *Curr Pain Headache Rep* 2003;7:482–489.

Moog M, Quintner J, Hall T, Zusman M. The late whiplash syndrome: a psychophysical study. *Eur J Pain* 2002;6: 283–294.

Moore MK. Upper crossed syndrome and its relationship to cervicogenic headache. *J Manipulative Physiol Ther* 2004;27: 414–420.

Mulligan B. *Manual Therapy: "NAGS," "SNAGS," "MWMS" etc*. 4th ed. Wellington, New Zealand: Plane View Services; 1999.

Mulligan B. *The Mulligan Concept: Spinal and Peripheral Manual Therapy Treatment Techniques*. Baltimore, MD: Northeast Seminars; 2000.

Niere K, Robinson P. Determination of manipulative physiotherapy treatment outcome in headache patients. *Man Ther* 1997;2:199–205.

Nilsson N, Bove G. Evidence that tension-type headache and cervicogenic headache are distinct disorders. *J Manipulative Physiol Ther* 2000;23:288–289.

Okeson JP, ed. *Orofacial Pain: Guidelines for Assessment, Classification, and Management*. Chicago: Quintessence Publishing; 1996.

Olesen J. The International Classification of Headache Disorders: 2nd edition. *Cephalalgia* 2004;24(suppl):1–150.

Olesen J. The International Classification of Headache Disorders, 2nd ed: application to practice. *Funct Neurol* 2005;20:61–68.

Paris SV. *Introduction to Spinal Evaluation and Manipulation: Seminar Manual*. 3rd ed. St. Augustine, FL: Institute of Physical Therapy, University of St. Augustine for Health Sciences; 1999.

Paris SV, Loubert PV. *Foundations of Clinical Orthopaedics*. 3rd ed. St. Augustine, FL: Institute Press; 1999.

Petersen SM. Articular and muscular impairments in cervicogenic headache: a case report. *J Orthop Sports Phys Ther* 2003;33:21–30.

Peuker E, Gronemeyer D. Rare but serious complications of acupuncture: traumatic lesions. *Acupunct Med* 2001;19: 103–108.

Pollmann W, Keidel M, Pfaffenrath V. Headache and the cervical spine: a critical review. *Cephalalgia* 1997;17: 801–816.

Pool JJ, Hoving JL, De Vet HC, Van Mameren H, Bouter LM. The inter-examiner reproducibility of physical examination of the cervical spine. *J Manipulative Physiol Ther* 2004;27: 84–90.

Rocabado M. *TMJ: Evaluation and Treatment of the Craniomandibular System. Course Notes.* St. Augustine, FL: University of St. Augustine; 2001.

Rocabado M. *Advanced Cranio-Facial: Course Notes.* St. Augustine, FL: University of St. Augustine for Health Sciences; 2002a.

Rocabado M. *Intermediate Cranio-Facial: Course Notes.* St. Augustine, FL: University of St. Augustine for Health Sciences; 2002b.

Roy M. *Level I Differential Diagnosis Part A: Course Manual.* Fairfax, VA: North American Institute of Orthopaedic Manual Therapy; 2002.

Schöps P, Pfingsten M, Siebert U. Reliability of manual medical examination techniques of the cervical spine: study of quality assurance in manual diagnosis [in German]. *Z Orthop Ihre Grenzgeb* 2000;138:2–7.

Schulman EA. Overview of tension-type headache. *Curr Pain Headache Rep* 2001;5:454–462.

Sciotti VM, Mittak VL, DiMarco L, et al. Clinical precision of myofascial trigger point location in the trapezius muscle. *Pain* 2001;93:259–266.

Simons DG, Travell JG, Simons LS. *Travell and Simons' Myofascial Pain and Dysfunction: The Trigger Point Manual.* Vol. 1. *Upper Half of Body.* 2nd ed. Philadelphia: Lippincott Williams & Wilkins; 1999.

Stucki G. International Classification of Functioning, Disability, and Health (ICF): A promising framework and classification for rehabilitation medicine. *Am J Phys Med Rehabil* 2005;84:733–740.

Terwee CB, de Winter AF, Scholten RJ, et al. Inter-observer reproducibility of the visual estimation of range of motion of the shoulder. *Arch Phys Med Rehabil* 2005;86: 1356–1361.

Travell J, Rinzler S, Herman M. Pain and disability of the shoulder and arm: treatment by intramuscular infiltration with procaine hydrochloride. *J Am Med Assoc* 1942;120: 417–422.

Tuttle N. Do changes within a manual therapy treatment session predict between-session changes for patients with cervical spine pain? *Aust J Physiother* 2005;51:43–48.

Walker N, Bohannon RW, Cameron D. Discriminate validity of temporomandibular joint range of motion measurements obtained with a ruler. *J Orthop Sports Phys Ther* 2000;30: 484–492.

Walsh B. Control of infection in acupuncture. *Acupunct Med* 2001;19:109–111.

White A, Hayhoe S, Hart A, Ernst E. Survey of adverse events following acupuncture (SAFA): a prospective study of 32,000 consultations. *Acupunct Med* 2001;19:84–92.

World Health Organization. 2007. The International Classification of Functioning, Disability, and Health. Available at: http://www.who.int/classifications/icf/en/.

Youdas JW, Carey JR, Garrett TR. Reliability of measurements of cervical spine range of motion: comparison of three methods. *Phys Ther* 1991;71:98–104.

Zito G, Jull G, Story I. Clinical tests of musculoskeletal dysfunction in the diagnosis of cervicogenic headache. *Man Ther* 2006;11:118–129.

Index